T0294432

Pediatric Allergy
Principles and Practice

Pediatric Allergy
Principles and Practice

FOURTH EDITION

Donald Y.M. Leung, MD, PhD, FAAAAI

Professor and Head, Division of Pediatric Allergy and Clinical Immunology
Department of Pediatrics, National Jewish Health, Denver, CO, USA

Cezmi A. Akdis, MD

Director and Professor, Swiss Institute of Allergy and Asthma Research (SIAF)
University of Zurich, Davos, Switzerland

Leonard B. Bacharier, MD

Robert C. Strunk Endowed Chair for Lung and Respiratory Research, Division of Allergy, Immunology and Pulmonary Medicine
Department of Pediatrics, Washington University School of Medicine, St Louis, MO, USA

Charlotte Cunningham-Rundles, MD, PhD

Professor of Medicine and Pediatrics, Division of Clinical Immunology
Department of Medicine, Icahn School of Medicine, Mount Sinai Hospital, New York, NY, USA

Scott H. Sicherer, MD

Professor of Pediatrics, Division of Allergy and Immunology, Jaffe Food Allergy Institute
Department of Pediatrics, Icahn School of Medicine, Mount Sinai Hospital, New York, NY, USA

Hugh A. Sampson, MD

Kurt Hirschhorn Professor of Pediatrics, Division of Allergy and Immunology, Jaffe Food Allergy Institute
Department of Pediatrics, Icahn School of Medicine, Mount Sinai Hospital, New York, NY, USA

For additional online content visit ExpertConsult.com

ELSEVIER

Elsevier

First edition 2003
Second edition 2010
Third edition 2016

Notices

Practitioners and researchers must always rely on their own experience and knowledge in evaluating and
using any information, methods, compounds or experiments described herein. Because of rapid advances
in the medical sciences, in particular, independent verification of diagnoses and drug dosages should be
made. To the fullest extent of the law, no responsibility is assumed by Elsevier, authors, editors, or contributors for any injury and/or damage to persons or property as a matter of products liability, negligence or
otherwise, or from any use or operation of any methods, products, instructions, or ideas contained in the
material herein.

ISBN: 978-0-323-67462-1
e-ISBN: 978-323-67463-8
INK: 978-0-323-67464-5

Content Strategist: Robin Carter
Content Development Specialist: Nani Clansey
Project Manager: Joanna Souch
Design: Bridget Hoette
Illustration Manager: Teresa McBryan
Marketing Manager: Kate Patton

Printed in the USA

Last digit is the print number: 9   8   7   6   5   4   3   2   1

 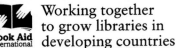

Working together
to grow libraries in
developing countries

www.elsevier.com • www.bookaid.org

Contents

Contributors

Mark J. Abzug, MD
Professor of Pediatrics (Infectious Diseases), Vice Chair for Academic Affairs, Department of Pediatrics, University of Colorado School of Medicine and Children's Hospital Colorado, Aurora, CO, USA
Chapter 18

Cezmi A. Akdis, MD
Director and Professor, Swiss Institute of Allergy and Asthma Research (SIAF), University of Zurich, Christine Kühne-Center for Allergy Research and Education (CK-CARE), Davos, Switzerland
Chapter 20

Cem Akin, MD, PhD
Professor of Medicine, Internal Medicine, University of Michigan, Ann Arbor, MI, USA
Chapter 45

Katrina Allen, MBBS, BMedSc, FRACP, PhD
Professor, Department of Paediatrics, University of Melbourne; Director, Centre for Food and Allergy Research, Murdoch Children's Research Institute, Parkville, VIC, Australia
Chapter 36

Lisa Arzt-Gradwohl, MSc, PhD
Department of Dermatology and Venerology, Medical University of Graz, Graz, Austria
Chapter 43

Leonard B. Bacharier, MD
Robert C. Strunk Endowed Chair for Lung and Respiratory Research; Professor of Pediatrics, Department of Pediatrics, Washington University, St. Louis, MO, USA
Chapter 25

Mark Ballow, MD
Professor of Pediatrics, Children's Research Institute, University of South Florida at Johns Hopkins Children's Hospital, St. Petersburg, FL, USA
Chapter 10

Erin Banta, MD
Clinical Assistant Professor, NYU Long Island School of Medicine, Division of Rheumatology, Allergy, and Immunology, NYU Winthrop Hospital, Mineola, New York, NY, USA
Chapter 40

Alexia Beauregard, MS, RD, CSP
Chief, Clinical Dietetics, Winn Army Community Hospital; Faculty, Ellyn Satter Institute, Fort Stewart, GA, USA
Chapter 32

Bruce G. Bender, PhD
Professor and Head, Pediatric Behavioral Health, National Jewish Health, Denver, CO, USA
Chapter 28

M. Cecilia Berin, PhD
Professor of Pediatrics, Jaffe Food Allergy Institute, Icahn School of Medicine at Mount Sinai, New York, NY, USA
Chapter 30

Brett P. Bielory, MD
Medical Director, Department of Ophthalmology, Riverside Medical Group, Rutherford, NJ, USA; Adjunct Clinical Surgeon, Department of Ophthalmology, New York Eye and Ear Infirmary, Mount Sinai School of Medicine, New York, NY, USA
Chapter 41

Leonard Bielory, MD
Professor of Medicine and Ophthalmology, Hackensack Meridian School of Medicine at Seton Hall University, Nutley, NJ, USA; Professor of Medicine, Thomas Jefferson University Sidney Kimmel School of Medicine, Philadelphia, PA, USA; Professor, Center for Environmental Prediction, Rutgers University, New Brunswick, NJ, USA
Chapter 41

Mark Boguniewicz, MD
Professor, Division of Allergy-Immunology, Department of Pediatrics, National Jewish Health and University of Colorado School of Medicine, Denver, CO, USA
Chapter 38

Andrew Bush, MB BS (Hons), MA, MD, FHEA, FRCP, FRCPCH, FERS, FAPSR, ATSF
Professor of Paediatrics, Imperial College, Professor of Paediatric Respirology, National Heart and Lung Institute; Consultant Paediatric Chest Physician, Royal Brompton Harefield NHS Foundation Trust, London, UK
Chapter 27

Kenny H. Chan, MD
Chief, Department of Pediatric Otolaryngology, Professor of Otolaryngology, University of Colorado School of Medicine, Children's Hospital Colorado, Aurora, CO, USA
Chapter 18

Anne B. Chang, MBBS, FRACP, MPHTM, PhD, FAAHMS
Professor, Menzies School of Health Research, Darwin, NT, Australia; Respiratory and Sleep Medicine, Queensland Children's Hospital; Centre for Children's Health Research, Queensland University of Technology, Brisbane, QLD, Australia
Chapter 19

Mirna Chehade, MD, MPH
Associate Professor of Pediatrics and Medicine, Director, Mount Sinai Center for Eosinophilic Disorders, Icahn School of Medicine at Mount Sinai, New York, NY, USA
Chapter 34

Anca M. Chiriac, MD, PhD
Assistant Professor in Allergology, Pulmonology and Addictology, University Hospital of Montpellier, Montpellier, France
Chapter 42

Lisa Cicutto, RN, ACNP(cert), PhD
Director, Education, Training, and Career Development, Director, Clinical Science Program, Colorado Clinical and Translational Sciences Center Professor, College of Nursing, Director of Clinical Science Program, University of Colorado, Aurora, CO, USA, Director, Clinical Outreach and Research, National Jewish Health, Denver, CO, USA
Chapter 26

Ronina A. Covar, MD
Staff Physician, Department of Pediatrics, National Jewish Health, Denver, CO, USA
Chapter 23

Charlotte Cunningham-Rundles, MD, PhD
Professor of Medicine and Pediatrics, Icahn School of Medicine at Mount Sinai, New York, NY, USA
Chapter 4

Pascal Demoly, MD, PhD
Professor and Head, Département de Pneumologie et Addictologie, Hôpital Arnaud de Villeneuve; Professor, University Hospital of Montpellier, Montpellier, France
Chapter 42

Thomas Eiwegger, PD, Dr. med
Associate Professor, Division of Immunology and Allergy, Food Allergy and Anaphylaxis Program, The Hospital for Sick Children; Departments of Paediatrics and Immunology, University of Toronto; Translational Medicine Program, Peter Gilgan Centre for Research and Learning, Hospital for Sick Children, Toronto, ON, Canada
Chapter 17

Louise Fleming, MD, MRCPCH
Clinical Senior Lecturer, National Heart and Lung Institute, Imperial College; Paediatric Respiratory Consultant, Royal Brompton Hospital, London, UK
Chapter 27

Luz Fonacier, MD
Professor of Medicine, NYU Long Island School of Medicine; Head of Allergy and Immunology, Internal Medicine, NYU Winthrop Hospital, Mineola, NY, USA
Chapter 40

Glenn T. Furuta, MD
Professor of Pediatrics, Department of Pediatrics, University of Colorado School of Medicine; Director, Gastrointestinal Eosinophilic Diseases Program, Digestive Health Institute, Children's Hospital Colorado, Aurora, CO, USA
Chapter 34

Melanie Gleason, MS, PA-C
Senior Instructor, Associate Director, School Based Asthma Programs, Department of Pediatrics, Section of Pediatric Pulmonary and Sleep Medicine, Breathing Institute, Children's Hospital Colorado and University of Colorado, Aurora, CO, USA
Chapter 26

Torie Grant, MD, MHS
Assistant Professor of Pediatrics and Medicine, Johns Hopkins University School of Medicine, Baltimore, MD, USA
Chapter 15

Marion Groetch, MS, RDN
Director of Nutrition Services, Jaffe Food Allergy Institute; Assistant Professor of Pediatrics, Icahn School of Medicine at Mount Sinai, New York, NY, USA
Chapter 32
Chapter 35

Theresa W. Guilbert, MS, MD
Professor of Pediatrics, Director, Asthma Center, Division of Pulmonary Medicine, Cincinnati Children's Hospital Medical Center, University of Cincinnati College of Medicine, Cincinnati, OH, USA
Chapter 21

Malika Gupta, MD
Assistant Professor, Internal Medicine, University of Michigan, Ann Arbor, MI, USA
Chapter 45

Robert G. Hamilton, PhD, D.ABMLI
Professor of Medicine, Johns Hopkins University School of Medicine, Baltimore, MD, USA
Chapter 12

Steven M. Holland, MD
Director, Division of Intramural Research, Chief, Immunopathogenesis Section, Laboratory of Clinical Immunology and Microbiology, National Institute of Allergy and Infectious Diseases, National Institutes of Health, Bethesda, MD, USA
Chapter 8

John W. Holloway, BSc (Hons), PhD
Professor of Allergy and Respiratory Genetics, Human
  Development and Health, University of Southampton,
  Southampton, UK
Chapter 3

Daniel J. Jackson, MD
Associate Professor, Department of Pediatrics and Medicine,
  University of Wisconsin School of Medicine and Public
  Health, Madison, WI, USA
Chapter 22

Shyam R. Joshi, MD
Assistant Professor of Medicine, Section of Allergy and
  Immunology, Oregon Health and Science University,
  Portland, OR, USA
Chapter 39

Meyer Kattan, MD, CM
Professor of Pediatrics, Director Pediatric Pulmonary Division,
  Columbia University Irving Medical Center, New York, NY,
  USA
Chapter 24

David A. Khan, MD
Professor of Medicine and Pediatrics, Internal Medicine, University
  of Texas Southwestern Medical Center, Dallas, TX, USA
Chapter 39

Donald B. Kohn, MD
Professor, Departments of Microbiology, Immunology &
  Molecular Genetics, Pediatrics, and Molecular & Medical
  Pharmacology, University of California Los Angeles, Los
  Angeles, CA, USA
Chapter 11

Jennifer Koplin, PhD
Co-Group Leader, Population Allergy; Director, Centre for Food
  and Allergy Research, Murdoch Children's Research Institute,
  Parkville, VIC, Australia; Senior Research Fellow, School of
  Population and Global Health and Department of Paediatrics,
  University of Melbourne, Carlton, VIC, Australia
Chapter 36

Anna Kovalszki, MD
Assistant Professor of Medicine, Medicine-Allergy and Clinical
  Immunology, University of Michigan, Ann Arbor, MI, USA
Chapter 45

Susanne G. Lau, MD
Professor, Department of Pediatric Pneumology, Immunology
  and Intensive Care, Charité Universitätsmedizin, Berlin,
  Germany
Chapter 19

Donald Y.M. Leung, MD, PhD, FAAAAI
Edelstein Family Chair of Pediatric Allergy-Immunology,
  Department of Pediatrics, National Jewish Health; Professor
  of Pediatrics, Department of Pediatrics, University of
  Colorado Medical School, Denver, CO, USA
Chapter 38

Chris A. Liacouras, MD
Professor of Pediatrics Gastroenterology, Perlman School
  of Medicine at the University of Pennsylvania, School
  of Medicine, Division of Gastroenterology, Hepatology,
  and Nutrition, The Children's Hospital of Philadelphia,
  Philadelphia, PA, USA
Chapter 34

Andrew H. Liu, MD
Director, Airway Inflammation, Resilience & the Environment
  (AIRE) Program, Breathing Institute, Section of Pediatric
  Pulmonary & Sleep Medicine, Children's Hospital Colorado;
  Professor of Pediatrics, University of Colorado School of
  Medicine; Adjunct Professor of Pediatrics, National Jewish
  Health, Aurora, CO, USA
Chapter 2
Chapter 18

Daniel Lozano-Ojalvo, PhD
Postdoctoral Fellow, Jaffe Food Allergy Institute, Icahn School of
  Medicine at Mount Sinai, New York, NY, USA
Chapter 30

Paul J. Maglione, MD, PhD
Assistant Professor, Section of Pulmonary, Allergy, Sleep and
  Critical Care Medicine, Department of Medicine, Boston
  University School of Medicine, Boston, MA, USA
Chapter 5

Julie M. Marchant, MBBS, FRACP, PhD
Associate Professor, Centre for Children's Health Research,
  Queensland University of Technology; Department of
  Respiratory Medicine, Queensland Children's Hospital,
  Brisbane, QLD, Australia
Chapter 19

Jonathan E. Markowitz, MD, MSCE
Medical Director, Pediatric Gastroenterology, Prisma Health
  Children's Hospital-Upstate; Professor and Vice Chair for
  Academic Affairs, Department of Pediatrics, University of
  South Carolina School of Medicine Greenville, Greenville,
  SC, USA
Chapter 34

Fernando D. Martinez, MD
Regents Professor, Asthma and Airway Disease Research Center,
  The University of Arizona, Tucson, AZ, USA
Chapter 2
Chapter 29

Karen M. McDowell, MD
Professor of Pediatrics, Division of Pulmonary Medicine,
  Cincinnati Children's Hospital Medical Center, University of
  Cincinnati College of Medicine, Cincinnati, OH, USA
Chapter 21

Elizabeth C. Matsui, MD, MHS
Professor of Population Health and Pediatrics, Population
  Health, Dell Medical School, University of Texas, Austin, TX,
  USA
Chapter 16

Amanda B. Muir, MD
Assistant Professor of Pediatrics, Perlman School of Medicine at the University of Pennsylvania, School of Medicine, Division of Gastroenterology, Hepatology, and Nutrition, The Children's Hospital of Philadelphia, Philadelphia, PA, USA
Chapter 34

Luigi D. Notarangelo, MD
Chief, Laboratory of Clinical Immunology and Microbiology, National Institute of Allergy and Infectious Disease, National Institutes of Health, Bethesda, MD, USA
Chapter 6

Anna Nowak-Węgrzyn, MD, PhD
Professor of Pediatrics, Allergy and Immunology, Department of Pediatrics, Hassenfeld Children's Hospital New York University School of Medicine, New York, NY, USA
Chapter 33

Joao Bosco Oliveira, MD PhD
Director, Genomics Laboratory, Hospital Albert Einstein, São Paulo, SP, Brazil
Chapter 9

Hanneke (Joanne) N.G. Oude Elberink, MD, PhD
Assistant Professor, Allergology/Internal Medicine, University Medical Center Groningen, Groningen, The Netherlands
Chapter 43

Oscar Palomares, PhD
Professor, Department of Biochemistry and Molecular Biology, School of Chemistry, Complutense University of Madrid, Madrid, Spain
Chapter 20

Elena E. Perez, MD, PhD
Partner, Allergy Associates of the Palm Beaches, North Palm Beach, FL, USA
Chapter 10

Wanda Phipatanakul, MD, MS
Professor of Pediatrics, Harvard Medical School; Director, Asthma Clinical Research Center, Division of Asthma, Allergy, and Immunology, Boston, MA, USA
Chapter 14

Sergio D. Rosenzweig, MD, PhD
Chief, Immunology Service, NIH Clinical Center, National Institutes of Health, Bethesda, MD, USA
Chapter 8

Hugh A. Sampson, MD
Professor of Pediatrics, Pediatrics, Emeritus Director, Jaffe Food Allergy Institute, Division of Pediatric Allergy, Icahn School of Medicine at Mount Sinai, New York, NY, USA
Chapter 31

Amy M. Scurlock, MD
Associate Professor, Department of Pediatrics, University of Arkansas for Medical Sciences; Researcher, Arkansas Children's Research Institute, Little Rock, AR, USA
Chapter 37

William J. Sheehan, MD
Associate Professor of Pediatrics, Allergy and Immunology, Children's National Hospital, George Washington University School of Medicine and Health Sciences, Washington, DC, USA
Chapter 14

Wayne G. Shreffler, MD, PhD
Associate Professor, Department of Pediatrics, Harvard Medical School; Division Chief, Pediatric Allergy Immunology, Massachusetts General Hospital; Principal Investigator, Center for Immunology and Inflammatory Disease, Massachusetts General Hospital, Boston, MA, USA; Associate Member, Food Allergy Science Initiative, Broad Institute, Cambridge, MA, USA
Chapter 37

Scott H. Sicherer, MD
Professor of Pediatrics; Director, Jaffe Food Allergy Institute, Division of Pediatric Allergy, Icahn School of Medicine at Mount Sinai, New York, NY, USA
Chapter 31
Chapter 33

Michael B. Soyka, PD, Dr. med.
Department of Oto-, Rhino-, Laryngology, Head and Neck Surgery, University and University Hospital Zurich, Zurich, Switzerland
Chapter 17

Joseph D. Spahn, MD
Professor of Pediatrics, University of Colorado Medical School and US Medical Affairs, GalxoSmithKline, Denver, CO, USA
Chapter 23

Jeffrey R. Stokes, MD
Professor of Pediatrics, Department of Pediatrics, Washington University School of Medicine, St. Louis, MO, USA
Chapter 25

Gunter J. Sturm, MD, PhD
Associate Professor, Department of Dermatology, Medical University of Graz, Graz, Austria
Chapter 43

Kathleen E. Sullivan, MD, PhD
Professor of Pediatrics, The Children's Hospital of Philadelphia, University of Pennsylvania, Perelman School of Medicine, Philadelphia, PA, USA
Chapter 7

Stanley J. Szefler, MD
Director Pediatric Asthma Research Program and Research Medical Director, The Breathing Institute, Children's Hospital Colorado and Professor of Pediatrics, University of Colorado School of Medicine, Anschutz Medical Campus, Aurora, CO, USA
Chapter 26

Troy R. Torgerson, MD, PhD
Associate Professor, Pediatrics, Immunology and Rheumatology, University of Washington, Seattle Children's Hospital, Seattle, WA, USA
Chapter 9

Pooja Varshney, MD
Pediatric Allergist, Pediatric Allergy, Asthma, and Immunology; Affiliate Faculty in Pediatrics, Dell Medical School, University of Texas, Austin, TX, USA
Chapter 16

Carina Venter, BSc, PhD
Associate Professor, Pediatric Allergy and Immunology, University of Colorado, Denver, CO, USA
Chapter 35

Erika von Mutius, MD, MSc
Professor, Dr. von Hauner Children's Hospital, Department of Pediatrics, Ludwig Maximilian University of Munich, Munich, Germany
Chapter 1

Julie Wang, MD
Professor of Pediatrics, Department of Pediatrics, Icahn School of Medicine at Mount Sinai, New York, NY, USA
Chapter 44

Richard W. Weber, MD
Professor Emeritus, Medicine, National Jewish Health, Denver, CO, USA
Chapter 13

Robert A. Wood, MD
Professor of Pediatrics and International Health, Director, Pediatric Allergy, Immunology, and Rheumatology, Johns Hopkins University School of Medicine, Baltimore, MD, USA
Chapter 15

Preface

These are exciting times for physicians who treat children with allergic and immune-mediated diseases. Recent studies have provided new insights into mechanisms underlying diseases in the areas of pediatric allergy, asthma, and clinical immunology. Many novel research tools such as multiple omics and bioinformatics that enable in-depth and precision research and the development of new treatments are now available. As a result, we are now incorporating into clinical practice novel treatments that have resulted from our improved understanding of the biology and pathophysiology of allergic and immunologic diseases. New management guidelines for various diseases, including food allergy, atopic dermatitis, asthma, and immunodeficiency, have been developed according to evidence-based approaches. The need to document and summarize this remarkable increase in information has necessitated the fourth edition of our textbook in the field of pediatric allergy and clinical immunology for practicing physicians and investigators interested in this clinical and scientific area.

It is often said that children are not simply small adults. In no other subspecialty is this more true than in pediatric allergy and immunology, at the time when the immune system is maturing during the first few years of life. Earlier identification of disease onset offers increased opportunities for prevention and intervention, which are difficult to reverse once disease processes have been established in the older child and adult. Furthermore, many allergic or immunologic diseases encountered in pediatric clinical practice are complex and are thought to result from a multigenic predisposition in combination with exposure to environmental triggers in an evolving immune response. However, the age at which the host is exposed to a particular environmental agent and the resultant immune response are increasingly being recognized as important factors. Furthermore, early intervention is critical to induce tolerance and prevent disease. New disease endotypes and phenotypes are emerging. Increasingly, we are appreciating the complex interaction of genetics, immune response, the microbiome, and various environmental factors, such as diet and stress, in the diseases we see as pediatricians. These concepts have now reached clinical care as we draw attention to population health and prevention.

Pediatric Allergy: Principles and Practice is intended to update the reader on the pathophysiology of allergic responses and allergic diseases, including asthma, food allergy, allergic rhinitis, atopic dermatitis, and immunologic diseases; their socioeconomic impact; and new treatment approaches that take advantage of emerging concepts in the pathobiology of these diseases. An outstanding group of authors who are key opinion leaders in their fields have been assembled because of their personal knowledge, expertise, and involvement with their subject matter in children. Every effort has been made to achieve prompt publication of this book, thus ensuring the content of each chapter is current.

Section A presents general concepts critical to understanding the causes and impact of allergic diseases. These include reviews of the epidemiology and natural history of allergic disease, genetics of allergic disease and asthma, biology of inflammatory effector cells, regulation of immunoglobulin E synthesis, and the developing immune system and allergy. Section B reviews an approach to the child with recurrent infection and specific immunodeficiency and autoimmune diseases frequently encountered by pediatricians. This section discusses emerging important immune-directed therapies, including immunizations, immunoglobulin therapy, stem cell therapy, and gene therapy. Section C examines the diagnosis and treatment of allergic disease. The remainder of the book is devoted to the management and treatment of asthma and specific allergic diseases, such as upper airway disease, food allergy, allergic skin and eye diseases, drug allergy, latex allergy, insect hypersensitivity, and anaphylaxis. In each chapter, the disease is discussed in the context of its differential diagnoses, key concepts, evaluation, environmental triggers, and concepts of established and emerging treatments.

Major advances in this fourth edition include updates on genetics and biomarkers of allergy, inflammatory conditions, and immunodeficiencies; recent guidelines in the treatment of asthma, food allergy, atopic dermatitis, urticaria and angioedema, and immunodeficiencies; prevention strategies; appropriate evaluation of drug allergy; the role of new biologic agents and immunomodulatory therapy in the treatment of inflammatory diseases; and emerging evidence that epithelial barrier dysfunction drives allergic disease.

We would like to thank each of the contributors for their time and invaluable expertise, which are vital to the success of this book. The editors are also grateful to Nani Clansey (Senior Content Development Specialist) and Robin Carter (Executive Content Strategist), who have played a major role in editing and organizing this textbook, and the Elsevier production staff for their expertise in the preparation of this book.

Donald Y.M. Leung, MD, PhD, FAAAAI
Cezmi A. Akdis, MD
Leonard B. Bacharier, MD
Charlotte Cunningham-Rundles, MD, PhD
Scott H. Sicherer, MD
Hugh A. Sampson, MD
2020

1

Epidemiology of Allergic Diseases

ERIKA VON MUTIUS

KEY POINTS

- Large geographic variations in the prevalence of allergic diseases exist worldwide among children and adults.
- Lower prevalences have been reported from developing countries, Eastern European areas, rural areas in Africa and Asia, and farm populations in Europe.

- The prevalence of asthma and allergies has increased over the last few decades. This trend seems to have reached a plateau in affluent countries, but not in low- to middle-income countries.
- Allergic diseases are multifactorial illnesses determined by a complex interplay between genetic and environmental factors.

Introduction

Traditionally, asthma, allergic rhinitis and hay fever, as well as atopic dermatitis and food allergy have been categorized as atopic diseases, yet the relation between clinical manifestations of these diseases and the production of immunoglobulin E (IgE) antibodies to inhalant or food allergens (e.g., atopy) have not been fully clarified. A significant proportion of individuals in the general population will not show any signs of illness despite elevated total and specific IgE levels. In some individuals, various atopic illnesses can be co-expressed, whereas in others, only one manifestation of an atopic illness is present. The prevalence of these four atopic entities therefore only partially overlaps in the general population (Fig. 1.1). Risk factors and determinants of atopy differ from those associated with asthma, atopic dermatitis, and hay fever.

Asthma, atopic dermatitis, and hay fever are complex diseases, and their incidence is determined by an intricate interplay of genetic and environmental factors. Environmental exposures may affect susceptible individuals during certain time windows, before the onset of disease in which particular organ systems are vulnerable to extrinsic influences. Moreover, most allergic illnesses are likely to represent syndromes with many different phenotypes rather than single disease entities. The search for determinants of allergic illnesses must therefore take phenotypes, genes, environmental exposures, and the timing (developmental aspect) of these exposures into account.

Prevalence of Childhood Asthma and Allergies

Asthma is a complex syndrome rather than a single disease entity. Different phenotypes with varying prognosis and determinants have been described, particularly over childhood years, using hypothesis and data-driven approaches.[1] Transient wheezing is characterized by the occurrence of wheezing in infants up to the age of 2 to 3 years, which disappears thereafter and does not progress to childhood asthma. However, there is an increasing body of evidence suggesting that these children may be at risk of developing chronic obstructive pulmonary disease (COPD) in adulthood. The main risk factor for transient wheeze is maternal smoking in pregnancy, which increases the risk of reduced lung function at birth.[1-4] Wheeze among school-aged children can be classified into atopic and nonatopic phenotypes.[5] This differentiation has clinical implications because nonatopic children with wheeze are very likely to outgrow their symptoms and retain normal lung function at school age. In turn, atopic wheezy children are more likely to develop a chronic course of illness, particularly if allergic sensitization to multiple allergens started in the first 3 years of life.[6] A significant proportion of asthmatic children have symptoms that remit over adolescence.[7] Yet those with severe atopy and severe airway hyperresponsiveness are at risk of progression over adolescent years.[8] It is further noteworthy that severe and early-onset atopy, as well as childhood asthma, have been shown to be significant risk factors for later COPD in adulthood.[9,10]

In addition to these investigator-driven classifications, data-driven analyses have been performed in many birth cohorts with latent class analyses over varying length of observations. The transient wheeze phenotype has been confirmed in all of them. There is also consistent evidence that a persistent wheezing phenotype with symptoms starting very early in life and progressing into school age and adulthood exists and affects between 3% and 7% of the population.[11] Intermediate wheeze phenotypes with different ages of onset and remission also have been described, suggesting that a third broad category of wheeze with varying disease manifestation over time exists. This observation suggests that fluctuation of wheeze appearance is a prominent feature of the disease, which may be attributable to developmental clues and the corresponding environmental exposures.

GERMAN 9- TO 11-YEAR-OLD CHILDREN IN MUNICH (*N* = 2612)
VENN DIAGRAM FOR ASTHMA, HAY FEVER, AND ATOPY

☐ Asthma (9.8%) ☐ Hay fever (8.9%) ☐ Atopy (23.1%) None (70.7%)

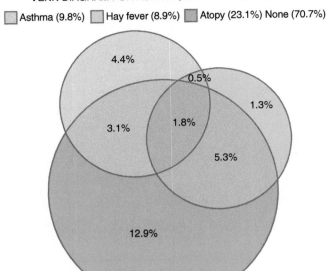

Percentages calculated for all non-missing cases (*N* = 1729)

• **Fig. 1.1** The prevalence of asthma, hay fever, and atopic sensitization only partially overlaps on a population level. Description of findings from the ISAAC Phase II study in Munich, of German children aged 9 to 11 years. (From The International Study of Asthma and Allergies in Childhood [ISAAC]. Lancet 1998;351:1225.)

These phenotypes can be identified only in prospective studies following infants from birth up to school age and through adolescence, enabling the differential analysis of risk factors and determinants for distinct wheezing phenotypes over time. These limitations must be borne in mind when discussing and interpreting findings from cross-sectional surveys. The relative proportion of different wheezing phenotypes is likely to vary among age groups, and therefore the strength of association between different risk factors and wheeze is also likely to vary across age groups.

Similarly, limitations apply with respect to the epidemiology of atopic dermatitis.[12] The definition of atopic eczema varies from study to study, and validations of questionnaire-based estimates have been few. Skin examinations by trained field workers, adding an objective parameter to questionnaire-based data, reflect a point prevalence of skin symptoms at the time of examination, and although they can corroborate questionnaire-based estimates, they will underestimate the true prevalence of disease given its fluctuating appearance.

Finally, identified risk factors in all cross-sectional surveys relate to the prevalence of the condition. The prevalence in turn reflects the incidence and the persistence of a disease. It is therefore often difficult to disentangle aggravating from causal factors in such studies. Only prospective surveys can identify environmental exposures before the onset of an atopic illness and thus infer a potentially causal relationship to the new onset of disease.

Western Versus Developing Countries

In general, reported rates of asthma, hay fever, and atopic dermatitis are higher in affluent, Western countries than in developing countries. The worldwide prevalence of allergic diseases was

assessed in the 1990s by the large-scale International Study of Asthma and Allergy in Childhood (ISAAC).[13] A total of 463,801 children in 155 collaborating centers in 56 countries were studied. Between 20-fold and 60-fold differences were found between centers in the prevalence of symptoms of asthma, allergic rhinoconjunctivitis, and atopic eczema (Fig. 1.2).

The European Community Respiratory Health Survey (ECRHS) studied young adults aged 20 to 44 years.[14] A highly standardized and comprehensive study instrument including questionnaires, lung function, and allergy testing was used by 35 to 48 centers in 22 countries, predominantly in Western Europe, but also in Australia, New Zealand, and the United States. The ECRHS has shown large geographic differences in the prevalence of respiratory symptoms, asthma, bronchial responsiveness, and atopic sensitization, with high prevalence in English-speaking countries and low prevalence rates in the Mediterranean region and Eastern Europe.[15] The geographic pattern emerging from questionnaire findings was consistent with the distribution of atopy and bronchial hyperresponsiveness, supporting the conclusion that the geographic variation in asthma is true and not attributable to methodologic factors such as the questionnaire phrasing, the skin testing technique, or the type of assay for the measurement of specific IgE.

A strong correlation was identified between the findings from children as assessed by ISAAC and the rates in adults as reported by the ECRHS questionnaire.[16] Although differences were found in the absolute prevalences observed in the two surveys, there was good overall agreement, adding support to the validity of both studies.

Dissociations between the prevalence of asthma and atopy, however, have been documented in developing countries.[1,17,18] ISAAC Phase II[19] has demonstrated that the fractions and prevalence rates of wheeze attributable to skin test reactivity correlated strongly with the gross national income of the respective country. These findings suggest that the strength of association between atopy and asthma across the world is determined by affluence and factors relating to affluence.

The East-West Gradient Across Europe

A number of reports have been published demonstrating large differences in the prevalence of asthma, airway hyperresponsiveness, hay fever, and atopy in children and adults between Eastern and Western European areas.[20–24] The prevalence of asthma was significantly lower in all study areas in Eastern Europe compared with that in Western Europe.[21] Among the older age group of 13- to 14-year-old children, the prevalence of wheezing was 11.2% to 19.7% in Finland and Sweden; 7.6% to 8.5% in Estonia, Latvia, and Poland; and 2.6% to 5.9% in Albania, Romania, Russia, Georgia, and Uzbekistan (except Samarkand).

The rates of allergic illnesses have been rising rapidly. After reunification of Germany in 1989 a significantly lower prevalence of allergic diseases was found in East Germany.[20] Only a few years later (1998) differences in the prevalence rates between East and West Germany were no longer observed.[25] The causes underlying the increase in prevalence in East Germany are not fully understood. The drastic decrease in family size after reunification or changes in dietary habits or indoor exposures may have contributed to this trend. Likewise, Poland's accession to the European Union was followed by a rapid and striking increase in the prevalence of atopy in rural areas.[26] This increase may be in part attributable to loss of traditional farming exposures.

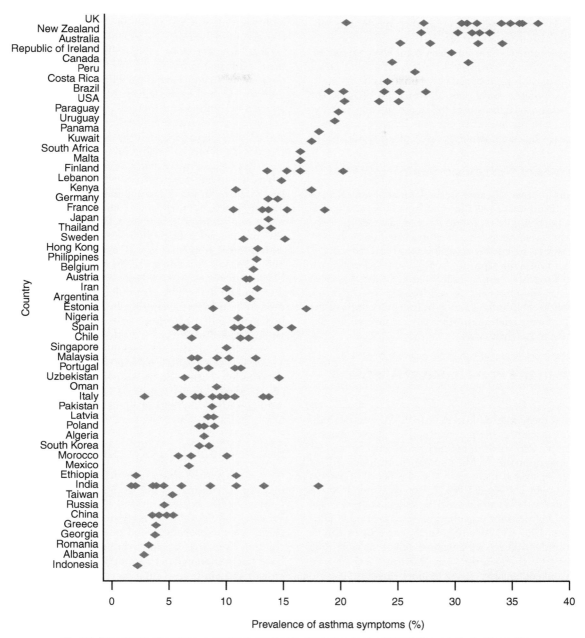

• **Fig. 1.2** Prevalence of asthma symptoms worldwide according to the ISAAC Phase I study. (From The International Study of Asthma and Allergies in Childhood [ISAAC]. Lancet 1998;351:1225.)

Differences Between Rural and Urban Populations

The prevalence of asthma and allergies is increasing not only with westernization and affluence but also with urbanization. The rates of asthma and atopy among children living in Hong Kong are similar to European figures. In some areas of rural China, asthma is almost nonexistent, with a prevalence of less than 1%.[27] In Mongolia, a country in transition from rural, farming lifestyles to an industrial society, marked differences exist in the prevalence of asthma, allergic rhinoconjunctivitis, and atopy.[28] Inhabitants of small rural villages are least affected, whereas residents of the capital city, Ulaanbaatar, have high rates of allergic diseases comparable to those of affluent Western countries.

Across Europe, differences between urban and rural areas are less clear. However, strong contrasts exist on a lower spatial scale, that is, among children raised on a farm compared to their neighbors living in the same rural area but not on a farm.[29] Since 1999, more than 30 studies have corroborated these findings.[30] Children raised on farms retain their protection from allergy at least into adulthood.[31–33] In the United States, children in Amish communities retaining very traditional dairy farming practices are equally protected from asthma and allergies.[34] In contrast, children in Hutterite communities with industrialized farming practices precluding children from early exposures to cow sheds have significantly higher prevalences than Amish children.[34]

The timing and duration of farm exposures seem to play a critical role. The largest reduction in risk of developing respiratory allergies is seen among those who are exposed prenatally and continue to be exposed throughout their life.[35] The protective factors in these farming environments have not been completely unraveled. Contact with farm animals, particularly cattle, confers protection. Also the consumption of unprocessed cow's milk has been shown to be beneficial with respect to childhood asthma and allergies. The structural composition and diversity of the environmental microbiome also contribute to the protective effects in farm homes, which in turn influence the human microbiome of exposed children.[36–39]

Inner City Areas of the United States

Living conditions in inner city areas in the United States are associated with a markedly increased risk of asthma.[40] Several potential risk factors are being investigated, such as race and poverty, adherence to asthma treatment,[41] and factors related to the disproportionate exposures associated with socioeconomic disadvantage, such as indoor and outdoor exposure to pollution and cockroach infestation.[4] Cockroach exposure, at least in early life, has been associated with the development of sensitization to cockroach allergen[42] and wheeze[43] in infants living in inner city areas of the United States. Problems relating to inner city asthma will be discussed in more detail in Chapter 24.

Time Trends in the Prevalence of Allergic Diseases

Data collected over the past 40 years in industrialized countries indicate a significant increase in the prevalence of childhood asthma, hay fever, and atopic dermatitis in repeated cross-sectional surveys using identical questionnaires.[44] Most studies from industrialized countries suggest an overall increase in the prevalence of asthma and wheezing between 1960 and 1990. Twenty-year trends of the prevalence of treated asthma among pediatric and adult members of a large US health maintenance organization were reported.[45] During the period from 1967 to 1987, the treated prevalence of asthma increased significantly in all age-sex categories except males aged 65 and older. In the United States, the greatest increase was detected among children and young adults living in inner cities.[46]

Recent studies suggest that in some areas this trend may have reached a plateau. Studies from Italy showed that among school children surveyed in 1974, 1992, and 1998 the prevalence of asthma had increased significantly during the period 1974 to 1992, whereas it remained stable from 1992 to 1998.[47] Similar findings have been reported from Germany and Switzerland, where prevalence rates have been on a plateau since the 1990s.[48,49] On a global scale, time trends in the prevalence of asthma and allergic rhinoconjunctivitis have been assessed in ISAAC Phase III.[50] The findings indicate that international differences in symptom prevalence have reduced, with decreases in prevalence in English-speaking countries and Western Europe and increases in prevalence in regions where prevalence was previously low, that is, in low- to middle-income countries.

Environmental Risk Factors for Allergic Diseases

Air Pollution

Considerable evidence exists showing that increased exposure to air pollutants is a risk factor for increased morbidity of asthma with worsening of symptoms and lung function.[51] Air pollution is a complex mixture of particulate matter of variable size and various gases. Particulates and polluting gases often co-occur, and their individual contribution to worsening of asthma is hard to disentangle. In panel and time-series studies, air pollutants such as fine particles and ozone reduce lung function in children already affected by asthma and increase symptoms and medication use. Likewise, emergency room visits, general practitioner activities, and hospital admissions for asthma and wheeze are positively associated with ambient air pollution levels.

Mixes of particulate matter, especially those seen with traffic-related exposures, seem to have the most adverse effects. Traffic-related air pollution is a complex mix of particulate matter and primary gaseous emissions, including nitrogen oxides, which lead to the generation of secondary pollutants such as ozone, nitrates, and organic aerosol. Traffic-related pollution decreases quickly with distance from roadways. For adverse effects, distance within 300 to 500 m of roadways seems to be most significant. In large North American cities, 30% to 45% of people live within this distance and so the impact of traffic-related air pollution is significant. The closeness to major roadways may be even greater in cities in Europe and the developing world. Given that disadvantaged families live close to major roadways, other risk factors such as poverty, stress, and cigarette smoking may aggravate the effects.[52]

The role of air pollution in the new onset of asthma and allergic sensitization is less well understood.[51] However, a growing body of prospective studies suggests a causal role for the incidence of asthma among children and adults. In particular, long-term exposure to traffic-related air pollution may again play a significant role.

Environmental Tobacco Smoke

Numerous surveys have consistently reported an association between environmental tobacco smoke (ETS) exposure and respiratory diseases. Strong evidence exists that passive smoking increases the risk of lower respiratory tract illnesses such as bronchitis, wheezy bronchitis, and pneumonia in infants and young children. Maternal smoking during pregnancy and early childhood has been shown to be strongly associated with impaired lung growth and diminished lung function,[2,3] which in turn may predispose infants to develop transient early wheezing. In children with asthma, parental smoking increases symptoms and the frequency of asthma attacks. Banning tobacco smoke in public places has been shown in a number of countries to result in a significant reduction in hospital admissions for asthma.[53]

A series of epidemiologic studies also has been performed to determine the effect of ETS exposure on the new onset of asthma. In most cross-sectional and longitudinal studies, passive and more importantly active smoking appear to be an important risk factor for the development of childhood, adolescent, and adult asthma. In turn, no unequivocal association between ETS exposure, atopic sensitization, and atopic dermatitis was found.

Water Hardness and Dampness

The domestic water supply may be relevant for the inception of atopic dermatitis. An ecologic study of the relation between domestic water hardness and the prevalence of atopic eczema among British school children was performed.[54] Geographic information systems were used to link the geographic distribution of eczema in the study area to four categories of domestic water-hardness data. Among school children aged 4 to 16 years, a significant relation was found between the prevalence of atopic eczema and water hardness, both before and after adjustment for potential confounding factors. The effect on recent eczema symptoms was stronger than on lifetime prevalence, which may indicate that water hardness acts more on existing dermatitis by exacerbating the disorder or prolonging its duration rather than as a cause of new cases. These observations await replication by other studies.

In 2004 a report by the Institutes of Medicine Committee on Damp Indoor Spaces and Health in the United States concluded that there is sufficient evidence of an association between exposure to a damp indoor environment and worsening of asthma symptoms and that there is suggestive evidence of an association between exposure to a damp indoor environment and the development of asthma in children and adults. Dampness can elicit a number of different exposures, for example, fungi, bacteria or their constituents and emissions, or other agents related to damp indoor environments, such as house dust mites and cockroaches. The responsible factors are not known but may vary among individuals or be potentiated in complex mixtures.[55]

Nutrition

Breastfeeding has long been recommended for the prevention of allergic diseases. The epidemiologic evidence is, however, highly controversial.[56] Some studies even suggest that breastfeeding may result in risk of asthma and atopy, but these studies may reflect adherence to recommendations. Likewise, the age at introduction of solid foods has been fiercely debated. Recently the diversity of solid foods introduced in the first year of life has been linked to less atopic dermatitis and asthma later in life.[57] Furthermore, the PEAT Study has elegantly and convincingly shown that the consumption of peanut rather than its avoidance confers protection from peanut allergy in children with atopic eczema (PEAT).[58] Findings from other dietary intervention studies support the notion of early introduction of foods, which may give rise to active tolerance.[59]

Increasing evidence relates body mass index to the prevalence and incidence of asthma in children and adults, males, and, more consistently, adolescent females.[60] It is unlikely that the association is attributable to reverse causation, that is, that asthma precedes obesity because of exercise-induced symptoms. Rather, weight gain can antedate the development of asthma. Weight reduction among patients with asthma can result in improvements in lung function.[60] Obesity has been associated with inflammatory processes, which may contribute to asthma development. Other potential explanations are that mechanical factors promote asthma symptoms in obese individuals or that gastroesophageal reflux as a result of obesity induces asthma. Furthermore, physical inactivity may promote both obesity and asthma.

Fruit, vegetable, cereal, and starch consumption and intake of various fatty acids; vitamins A, C, D, and E; minerals; and antioxidants have all been studied.[44] However, diet is complex and difficult to measure, and standardized tools are still lacking. All methods pertaining to food frequency, individual food items, food patterns, and serum nutrients can introduce substantial misclassification, and the close correlation of many nutrients presents problems when trying to identify independent effects. The evidence from prospective studies and randomized clinical trials for individual food items has been disappointing.[61] Thus, measures such as the Mediterranean diet may better reflect real-world exposures. A Mediterranean diet has in turn been linked to protection from asthma.[62]

Allergen Exposure

Although in some studies a clear, almost linear dose-response relation between allergen exposure and sensitization has been found,[63] others describe a bell-shaped association with higher levels of exposures relating to lower rates of atopic sensitization.[64] Part of the discrepancy may relate to the type of allergen, because mostly cat but not house dust mite allergen exposure has been shown in some studies to exert protective effects at higher levels of exposure. Furthermore, there is some evidence that the presence of a dog or a cat, or both, protects from the development of allergic sensitization, indicating that the presence of an animal is more important than just exposure to its allergens.

The relationship between allergens, particularly house dust mite exposure, and asthma has been studied for many years. Overall, there is little evidence to suggest a positive association between house dust mite exposure and the new onset of childhood asthma.[65] Intervention studies have failed to show convincing evidence of a reduction in asthma risk after the implementation of avoidance strategies.[66] Other co-factors of exposure, such as exposure to microbial compounds, also should be taken into account. For example, levels of endotoxin and other microbial exposures have been shown to modify the effect of allergen exposure.[67–69]

Family Size, Infections, and Hygiene

Strachan[70] first reported that sibship size, the number of children produced by a pair of parents, is inversely related to the prevalence of childhood atopic diseases and thereby proposed the "hygiene hypothesis." This observation has been since confirmed by numerous studies, all showing that atopy, hay fever, and atopic eczema were inversely related to increasing numbers of siblings. In contrast, the relation between family size and childhood asthma and airway hyperresponsiveness is less clear. However, the underlying causes of this consistent protective effect remain unknown.

Viral infections of the respiratory tract are the major precipitants of acute exacerbations of wheezing illness at any age, yet viral respiratory infections are very common during infancy and early childhood and most children do not suffer any aftermath relating to these infections, including infections with respiratory syncytial virus and rhinovirus.[71] Thus, host factors in children susceptible to the development of wheezing illnesses and asthma are likely to play a major role. Deficiencies in innate immune responses have been shown to contribute to a subject's susceptibility to rhinovirus infections, the most prevalent cause of lower respiratory tract viral infections associated with asthma development in infants.[72] Interactions between viral lower respiratory tract infections and early atopic sensitization may play a role; only among children with early onset of atopy may repeated viral infections become a risk factor for developing asthma.[73]

However, an inverse relation between asthma and the overall burden of respiratory infections may also exist. Several studies investigating children in daycare have rather consistently shown that exposure to a daycare environment in the first months of life is associated with a significantly reduced risk of wheezing, hay fever, and atopic sensitization at school age and adolescence.[74,75] It remains unclear, however, whether the burden of infections or other exposures in daycare early in life account for this protective effect. Consistent with the hygiene hypothesis a number of reports have shown that children sero-positive for hepatitis A, *Toxoplasma gondii*, or *Helicobacter pylori* had a significantly lower prevalence of atopic sensitization, allergic rhinitis, and allergic asthma compared with their sero-negative peers.[76]

The use of antibiotics has been proposed as a risk factor for asthma and allergic diseases. In most cross-sectional studies a positive relation between antibiotics and asthma has been found that is most likely to be attributable to reverse causation. Early in life, when it is difficult to diagnose asthma, antibiotics are often prescribed for respiratory symptoms in wheezy children and thus are positively associated with asthma later in life. Most studies using a prospective design, however, have failed to identify antibiotics as a risk factor antedating the new onset of asthma.[77] Recently antibiotics have been newly interpreted as potentially disrupting the intestinal microbiome, but there is still little evidence that the risk between antibiotics and asthma is mediated via intake of antibiotics. Similar problems arise when interpreting the positive relation between paracetamol use and asthma seen in cross-sectional studies.[78] Intervention trials are needed to come to firm conclusions.

Active and chronic helminthic infections were reported to be protective from atopy, but findings are less consistent for wheeze and asthma.[79] Part of the discrepancies in the literature reporting associations between helminths and allergic diseases may be the load of parasitic infestation and the type of helminths in a particular area.

Since the turn of the century an explosion of research studying the role of the microbiome in asthma and allergies has occurred. Much emphasis has been laid on the gut microbiome as part of the Human Microbiome Project. Although descriptions of changes in the gut compositional structure and the maturation of the gut microbiome in the first year of life have been linked to asthma and allergy development,[80] the underlying mechanisms are poorly understood. Experimental studies in mice suggest an important role of microbial metabolites such as short-chain fatty acids and tryptophan for asthma protection,[81,82] but solid evidence in humans is still lacking. Facultative pathogens in the airway and skin microbiome have been linked to the development of asthma and atopic dermatitis, respectively, in particular *Haemophilus influenzae, Moraxella catarrhalis,* and *Streptococcus pneumoniae* in the airways[83] and *Staphylococcus aureus* on the skin.[84] Microbiome structures allowing such outgrow of facultative pathogens such as, for example, decreased diversity, may contribute to the disease process and may in turn be shaped by the environmental microbiome through pet, farm animal, and sibling contacts.[38]

Gene-Environment Interactions

The genetics of asthma will be discussed in Chapter 3 and are touched on here only in the context of environmental exposures. In general, the identification of novel genes for asthma suggests that many genes with small effects, rather than a few genes with strong effects, contribute to the development of asthma and atopy.[85] These genetic effects may, in part, differ with respect to a subject's environmental exposures, although some genes may also exert their effect independently of the environment.

A number of gene-environment interactions have been found, which are discussed in detail by von Mutius[85] and Le Souef.[86] These interactions confer additional biologic plausibility for the identified environmental exposures in the inception of asthma and allergic diseases. For example, the interaction of polymorphisms in the *TLR2* gene with a farming environment or daycare settings is highly suggestive of microbial exposures underlying this observation. Conversely, the more detrimental effects of passive smoking in people with genetically determined insufficient detoxification (e.g., glutathione S-transferase [GST] null genotypes) highlight the importance of taking a host's susceptibility into account when estimating the effect size of harmful exposures.[87] Thus, the analysis of gene-environment interactions may result in the identification of individuals who are particularly vulnerable to certain environmental exposures.

Conclusions

Large variations in the prevalence of childhood and adult asthma and allergies have been reported. In affluent, urbanized centers, prevalences are generally higher than in poorer centers, with the exception of the inner city environments in the United States, where prevalences are particularly high. Lower levels are seen, especially in some rural areas in Africa and Asia and among farmers' children in Europe. Numerous environmental factors have been scrutinized, but no conclusive explanation for the rising trends has been found. Future challenges are to tackle the complex interplay between environmental factors and genetic determinants.

The reference list can be found on the companion Expert Consult website at http://www.expertconsult.inkling.com.

2

Natural History of Allergic Diseases and Asthma

ANDREW H. LIU, FERNANDO D. MARTINEZ

KEY POINTS

- The atopic disorders—atopic dermatitis, food and inhalant allergies, allergic rhinoconjunctivitis and asthma—tend to cluster in individuals, families, and locales.
- A developmental "allergic march" of childhood begins with atopic dermatitis, food allergies, and bronchiolitis episodes in the first few years of life and progresses to inhalant allergic sensitization, allergic rhinoconjunctivitis, and atopic asthma.
- Although persistent asthma commonly begins in the first few years of life, most infants and toddlers who have recurrent bronchiolitis episodes do not go on to have persistent asthma in later childhood and adulthood. Early-life predictive factors for

  disease persistence include allergic march manifestations (i.e., atopic dermatitis, allergic sensitization to inhalant allergens), recurrent bronchiolitis episodes triggered by common rhinoviruses, and parental asthma.
- Epidemiologic evidence suggests that atopic disorders are caused by environmental and lifestyle factors in the susceptible host.
- Although atopy is a common feature of childhood asthma, additional factors appear to contribute to severe, persistent disease expression, including early onset, chronic exposure to sensitized allergen in the home, and a dysregulated type 2 high immunopathologic condition.

Introduction

Natural history studies of allergic diseases and asthma are fundamental for predicting disease onset and prognosis. Such studies reveal a developmental "allergic march" in childhood, from the early onset of atopic dermatitis (AD) and food allergies in infancy, to asthma, to allergic rhinitis (AR), and to inhalant allergen sensitization in later childhood. Allergy and asthma of earlier onset and greater severity are generally associated with disease persistence. Therefore, allergy and asthma commonly develop during the early childhood years, the period of greatest immune maturation and lung growth. This highlights the importance of growth and development in a conceptual framework for allergy and asthma pathogenesis.

This chapter reviews the allergic march of childhood and its clinical manifestations: food allergies, AD, inhalant allergies, AR, and asthma. The natural history of anaphylaxis, an allergic condition not currently implicated in the allergic march, is also covered. Interventions that reduce the prevalence of allergy and asthma are reviewed toward the end of the chapter. The findings and conclusions presented in this chapter are largely based on long-term prospective (i.e., natural history) studies. Information on the epidemiology of allergic diseases in childhood can be found in Chapter 1 and discussion of the natural history and prevention of food allergy in Chapter 36.

Allergic March of Childhood

The allergic march of childhood refers to a common pattern of allergy and asthma development that begins in infancy, as follows:

- The highest incidence of AD and food allergies is in the first 2 years of life (Fig. 2.1). It is generally thought that infants rarely manifest allergic symptoms in the first month of life. By 3 months of age, however, AD, food allergies, and wheezing problems are common.
- This is paralleled by a high prevalence of food allergen sensitization in the first 2 years of life.[1] Early food allergen sensitization is an important risk factor for food allergies, AD, and asthma.
- Allergic airways diseases generally begin slightly later in childhood (see Fig. 2.1). Childhood asthma often initially manifests with a lower respiratory tract infection or bronchiolitis episodes in the first few years of life.
- AR commonly begins in childhood, although there is also good evidence that it often develops in early adulthood.[2,3]
- The development of AR and persistent asthma is paralleled by a rise in inhalant allergen sensitization. Perennial inhalant allergen sensitization (i.e., cat dander, dust mites) emerges between 2 and 5 years of age, and seasonal inhalant allergen sensitization becomes apparent slightly later in life (ages 3–5 years).

Early Immune Development Underlying Allergies

A paradigm of immune development underlies allergy development and progression in early childhood. Briefly, the immune system of the fetus is maintained in a tolerogenic state, preventing

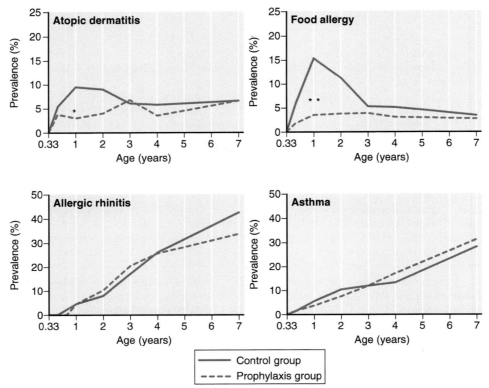

• **Fig. 2.1** Allergic march of early childhood. Period prevalence of atopic dermatitis, food allergy, allergic rhinitis, and asthma from birth to 7 years in prophylactic-treated (allergenic food avoidance) and untreated (control) groups (Kaiser Permanente; San Diego). *P ≤.05; **P <.01. (Data from Zeiger RS, Heller S. The development and prediction of atopy in high-risk children: follow-up at age seven years in a prospective randomized study of combined maternal and infant food allergen avoidance. J Allergy Clin Immunol 1995;95:1179–90; and Zeiger RS, Heller S, Mellon MH, et al. Effect of combined maternal and infant food-allergen avoidance on development of atopy in early infancy: a randomized study. J Allergy Clin Immunol 1989;84:72–89.)

adverse immune responses and rejection between the mother and fetus. Placental interleukin-10 (IL-10) suppresses the activation of fetal immune cells by mediators such as interferon-gamma (IFN-γ). IFN-γ down-regulates the production of proallergic cytokines, such as IL-4 and IL-13. The reciprocal relationship between these cytokines and the immune cells that produce them defines type 2 proallergic immune responses (i.e., IL-4, IL-13) and antiallergic "type 1" immune development (i.e., IFN-γ). Thus, the conditions that favor immune tolerance in utero may also foster allergic immune responses, such that newborn immune responses to ubiquitous ingested and inhaled proteins are type 2 biased.[4] Postnatally, encounters with these common allergenic proteins lead to the development of mature immune responses to them. The underlying immune characteristics of allergic diseases—allergen-specific memory type 2 lymphocytes and immunoglobulin E (IgE)—can be viewed as aberrant manifestations of immune maturation that typically develop during these early years and might have their roots in the inadequate or delayed development of regulatory immune responses that can inhibit them.

Total Serum Immunoglobulin E Levels

At birth, cord blood IgE levels are almost undetectable; these levels increase during the first 6 years of life. AD and allergic conditions are associated with elevated total serum IgE levels. Elevated serum IgE levels in infancy have also been associated with persistent

asthma in later childhood.[5] Similarly, high serum IgE levels in later childhood have been well correlated with bronchial hyper-responsiveness (BHR) and asthma.[6,7]

Allergen-Specific Immunoglobulin E

In two birth cohort (up to 5 years old) studies of IgG and IgE antibody development to common food and inhalant allergens, IgG antibodies to milk and egg proteins were detectable in nearly all subjects in the first 12 months of life, implying that the infant immune system sees and responds to commonly ingested proteins.[8,9] In comparison, food allergen–specific IgE (sIgE) (especially to egg) was measurable in approximately 30% of subjects at 1 year of age. Low-level IgE responses to food allergens in infancy were common and transient and sometimes occurred before introduction of the foods into the diet. In children who developed clinical allergic conditions, higher levels and persistence of food allergen sIgE were typical.

Of seasonal inhalant allergens, ragweed and grass allergen sIgGs were detectable in approximately 25% of subjects at 3 to 6 months of age and steadily increased to 40% to 50% by 5 years of age.[10,11] In comparison, allergen sIgE was detected in less than 5% of subjects from 3 to 12 months of age and increased in prevalence to approximately 20% by 5 years of age. Therefore, allergen sIgE production emerges in the preschool years and persists in those who develop clinical allergies.

Transient Wheezers and Persistent Asthma in Childhood

Approximately 80% of patients with asthma report disease onset before 6 years of age.[12] Indeed, preschool wheezing is common. Up to 50% of young children experience periods of recurrent wheezing and/or coughing in the first 6 years of life.[13] However, of all young children who experience recurrent wheezing, only a minority will go on to have persistent asthma in later life. The most common form of recurrent wheezing in preschool children occurs primarily with common respiratory viral infections (Box 2.1). The so-called transient early wheezers, who manifest wheezing episodes only in the first 3 years of life, are not at an increased risk of having asthma in later childhood. Transient wheezing is associated with airways viral infections, smaller airways and lung size, male gender, low birth weight, and prenatal environmental tobacco smoke (ETS) exposure.

Persistent asthma commonly begins and co-exists with the large population of transient wheezers (see Box 2.1 and Fig. 2.2).

• BOX 2.1   Key Concepts
Childhood Wheezing and Asthma Phenotypes

- *Transient early wheezing or wheezy bronchitis:* Most common in infancy and preschool years
- *Persistent allergy-associated asthma:* Most common phenotype in school-age children, adults, and elderly
- *Nonallergic wheezing:* Associated with bronchial hyperresponsiveness at birth; continues into childhood
- *Asthma associated with obesity, female gender, and early-onset puberty:* Emerges between 6 and 11 years of age
- *Asthma mediated by occupational-type exposures:* A probable type of childhood asthma in children living in particular locales, although not yet demonstrated
- *Triad asthma:* Asthma associated with chronic sinusitis, nasal polyposis, and/or hypersensitivity to nonsteroidal antiinflammatory medications (e.g., aspirin, ibuprofen); rarely begins in childhood

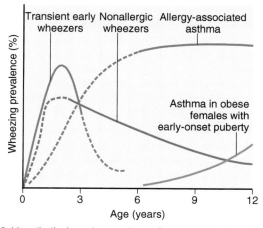

• Fig. 2.2 Hypothetical yearly prevalence for recurrent wheezing phenotypes in childhood (Tucson Children's Respiratory Study, Tucson, Arizona). This classification does not imply that the groups are exclusive. *Dashed lines* suggest that wheezing can be represented by different curve shapes resulting from many different factors, including overlap of groups. (Modified from Stein RT, Holberg CJ, Morgan WJ, et al. Peak flow variability, methacholine responsiveness and atopy as markers for detecting different wheezing phenotypes in childhood. Thorax 1997;52:946–52.)

Persistent asthma is strongly associated with allergy, which is evident in the early childhood years as clinical conditions (i.e., AD, AR, food allergies) and/or by testing for allergen sensitization to inhalant and food allergens (e.g., serum allergen sIgE, allergy skin testing). In particular, by the age of 3 years, recurrent wheeze associated with rhinovirus infection (i.e., rhinovirus susceptibility) and inhalant allergen sensitization are the strongest predictors for persistent asthma in the school age years, indicating the importance of these formative preschool years to long-term respiratory health.[14–17] Parental asthma is also a risk factor for persistent asthma.

Children with persistent asthma tend to improve with age from the lower to the middle-upper school years, with overall much less frequent severe exacerbations and 55% persisting versus 39% becoming "periodic" (i.e., years on and off with asthma) versus 6% "remitting" (i.e., no asthma for 4 years).[18,19] Persistent asthma in school-age children can be characterized as easy to control versus difficult to control, with a conventional guidelines-based approach to asthma management.[20] Children with difficult-to-control asthma have high burdens of asthma symptoms and exacerbations, especially in the fall, winter, and spring, and persistently lower spirometric lung function despite moderate to high levels of asthma controller medication use. Children with more severe asthma can be further characterized in two groups: (1) highly allergic (type 2-high) asthma, who are prone to severe exacerbations, have lower lung function, have greater BHR, and manifest many features of allergy, including allergic sensitization to most of a common panel of inhaled allergens; and (2) low/nonatopic asthma with a high burden of asthma symptoms.[21–23] Severity of childhood asthma also foreshadows asthma persistence into adulthood. The most common severe phenotype in children is consistent with a severe type 2-high phenotype in adults, with IL-13–induced epithelial gene expression, atopic airways inflammation, and exacerbation risk.[24]

Lung function generally matches the different phenotypes of childhood wheezing and asthma. In early life, transient wheezers had the lowest airflow measures in infancy, suggesting that they had the narrowest airways and/or the smallest lungs at birth.[13] Their reduced lung function improved significantly, but continued to be lower than normal through the age of 16 years, despite clinical resolution for most by the early school-age years.[19] In comparison, persistent wheezers may have normal lung function in the first few months of life but a significant decline in airflow measures by 6 years of age that persisted as lower than normal at age 16 years.[19] Children with difficult-to-control asthma have persistently lower lung function and BHR, especially those with the type 2-high severe phenotype.

Some children with BHR in early life are also more likely to have persistent asthma. Investigators of a birth cohort in Perth, Australia, found that BHR at 1 month of age was associated with lower lung function (i.e., forced expiratory volume in 1 second [FEV_1] and forced vital capacity [FVC]) and a higher likelihood of asthma at 6 years of age.[25] Interestingly, congenital BHR was not associated with total serum IgE, eosinophilia, allergen sensitization, or BHR at 6 years of age and was independent of gender, family history of asthma, and maternal smoking. In the Tucson Children's Respiratory Study (CRS), BHR measured at age 6 years predicted chronic and newly diagnosed asthma at the age of 22 years.[26]

Asthma From Childhood to Adulthood

A cohort of 7-year-old children with asthma living in Melbourne, Australia, was restudied for persistence and severity of asthma at

10, 14, 21, 28, 35, and 42 years of age. At 42 years of age, 71% of the patients with asthma and 89% of those with severe asthma continued to have asthma symptoms; 76% of the patients with severe asthma reported frequent or persistent asthma.[27] In comparison, 15% of those with mild wheezy bronchitis (i.e., wheezing only with colds at 7 years of age) and 28% of those with wheezy bronchitis (i.e., at least five episodes of wheezing with colds) reported frequent or persistent asthma. These observations—that many children with asthma experience disease remission or improvement in early adulthood but that severe asthma persists with age—are remarkably similar to those of several other natural history studies of childhood asthma into adulthood.[28-31]

Spirometric measures of lung function in the children in the Melbourne study initially revealed that patients with asthma (especially with severe asthma) had lung function impairment, whereas those with wheezy bronchitis (i.e., transient wheezing) had lung function that was not different from that of individuals without asthma. Over the ensuing years, these differences in lung function impairment between groups persisted in parallel, without a greater rate of decline in lung function in any group (Fig. 2.3).[27,32] Beginning from birth, in the Tucson CRS, low lung function in infancy also persisted through ages 11, 16, and 22 years.[33] However, some children with persistent asthma demonstrate progressive decline in lung function. In the longitudinal Childhood Asthma Management Program (CAMP) study, children with mild to moderate persistent asthma were followed from lower school through early adulthood.[34] Some developed lower lung function by reduced lung growth (primarily in the lower school years) and/or steeper rate of decline in early adulthood such that, by the age of approximately 26 years, 11% had spirometric lung function impairment consistent with chronic obstructive lung disease.[34,35] Risk factors for progressive decline in lung function included male gender, younger age, and hyperinflation; inhaled corticosteroid controller

therapy in childhood did not appear to mitigate lung function decline. These findings support the importance of the early childhood years in lung and asthma development. The establishment of chronic disease and lung function impairment in early life appears to predict persistent asthma and lung dysfunction well into adulthood; however, progressive decline in lung function can occur in some children during school-age and early adult years.

Risk Factors for Persistent Asthma

Biologic, genetic, and environmental risk factors for persistent asthma have been identified (Box 2.2). Globally, in the 56-nation International Study of Asthma and Allergies in Childhood, strong correlations between asthma prevalence and both allergic rhinoconjunctivitis and AD prevalence in different sites throughout the world suggest that allergy-associated asthma is the most common form of childhood asthma worldwide.[36] In children with recurrent cough or wheeze in early life, early manifestations of atopy and parental history of asthma are predictive risk factors for persistent asthma and lung dysfunction and form a commonly used Asthma Predictive Index (Fig. 2.4).[37-39] These and other asthma risk factors are reviewed later.

Allergy

Allergic disease and evidence of proallergic immune development in early life are significant risk factors for persistent asthma. Specifically, in the first few years of life, common clinical indicators of asthma risk include AD, AR, elevated total serum IgE, peripheral blood eosinophilia, food allergen sensitization (e.g., egg, milk, peanut), and especially perennial inhalant allergen sensitization.[13,37,40-42]

Inhalant Allergen Sensitization

Asthma in children is largely associated with inhalant allergen sensitization. For example, U.S. studies have found that 88% to

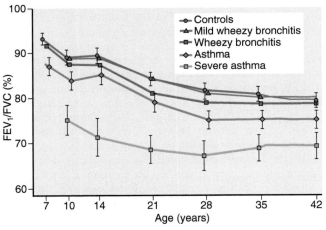

• **Fig. 2.3** Natural history of lung function from childhood to adulthood (Melbourne Longitudinal Study of Asthma, Melbourne, Australia). Subjects were classified according to their diagnosis at time of enrollment: nonwheezing control, mild wheezy bronchitis, wheezy bronchitis, asthma, and severe asthma. Lung function is represented as forced expiratory volume in 1 second (FEV₁) corrected for lung volume (FEV₁/(forced vital capacity [FVC] ratio). Mean values and standard error bars are shown. (Modified from Oswald H, Phelan PD, Lanigan A, et al. Childhood asthma and lung function in mid-adult life. Pediatr Pulmonol 1997;23:14–20; with data for age 42 years from Horak E, Lanigan A, Roberts M, et al. Longitudinal study of childhood wheezy bronchitis and asthma: outcome at age 42. BMJ 2003;326(7386):422–3.)

• BOX 2.2   Key Concepts
Risk Factors for Persistent Asthma

Allergy
- Atopic dermatitis
- Allergic rhinitis
- Elevated total serum immunoglobulin E levels (first year of life)
- Peripheral blood eosinophilia greater than 4% (2–3 years of age)
- Inhalant and food allergen sensitization

Lower Respiratory Tract Infections
- Rhinovirus, respiratory syncytial virus
- Severe bronchiolitis (i.e., requiring hospitalization)
- Pneumonia

Parental Asthma

Environmental Tobacco Smoke Exposure (Including Prenatal)

Gender
Males
- Transient wheezing
- Persistent allergy-associated asthma
Females
- Asthma associated with obesity and early-onset puberty
- "Triad" asthma (adulthood)

94% of school-age children with persistent asthma have inhalant allergen sensitization.[43,44] Early inhalant allergen sensitization (especially more than one) by 2 to 3 years of age increases the probability of asthma at age 7 to 8 years to more than likely.[14,16] Chronic exposure of sensitized children to inhalant allergens in early life worsens outcomes. The combination of sensitization to major indoor allergens (dog, cat, and/or mite) by the age of 3 years with higher levels of allergen exposure in the home has been strongly associated with persistent asthma and lower lung function into adolescence.[45] Natural history studies of asthma extending into adulthood continue to find allergy to be a risk factor for persistent asthma.[29,30] Asthma severity is strongly associated with high levels of inhalant allergen sensitization. For example, in U.S. inner cities, where exacerbation-prone asthma is more prevalent, the common phenotype of moderate to severe type 2 asthma is strongly associated with allergen sensitization to most common inhalant allergens (i.e., positive to 14/22 inhalant allergens or 64%).[21] The pathophysiology of how inhalant allergen sensitization drives and exacerbates asthma is also well understood: allergic immune responses to inhaled allergens cause airway inflammation and congestion and BHR and impair innate antiviral responses to common respiratory viruses (e.g., rhinovirus).[46] Thus, inhalant allergen sensitization strongly influences and predicts asthma development, persistence, severity, and exacerbations in children.

Lower Respiratory Tract Infections

Although common respiratory viruses have been associated with wheezing problems in children, the most common and strongest asthma exacerbation–associated respiratory virus in children is human rhinovirus (HRV).[47–49] HRV, a "common cold" virus, comprises more than 160 types classified in three species (A, B, and C).[50] HRV accounts for 40% to 70% of wheezing illnesses and asthma exacerbations in children.[51–53] People with asthma do not appear to be more susceptible to rhinovirus infection, but they are more likely to develop lower respiratory tract symptoms that are more severe and longer lasting.[54] In the Childhood Origins of Asthma (COAST) birth cohort study, 90% of children with

At least 4 wheezing episodes, plus:	
1 Major criterion	**or 2 Minor criteria**
Parental asthma	Allergic rhinitis
Eczema	Wheezing apart from colds
Inhalant allergen sensitization	Eosinophils ≥4%
	Food allergen sensitization

• **Fig. 2.4** Modified Asthma Predictive Index for children (Tucson Children's Respiratory Study, Tucson, Arizona). Through a statistically optimized model for 2- to 3-year-old children with frequent wheezing in the past year, one major criterion or two minor criteria provided 77% positive predictive value and 97% specificity for persistent asthma in later childhood. (Modified from Castro-Rodriguez JA, Holberg CH, Wright AL, et al. A clinical index to define risk of asthma in young children with recurrent wheezing. Am J Respir Crit Care 2000;162:1403–6; and Guilbert TW, Morgan WJ, Zeiger RS, et al. Atopic characteristics of children with recurrent wheezing at high risk for the development of childhood asthma. J Allergy Clin Immunol 2004;114:1282–7.)

rhinovirus-associated wheezing episodes by the age of 3 years had asthma at age 6 years, such that a rhinovirus-associated wheezing episode by age 3 years was a stronger predictor of subsequent asthma than aeroallergen sensitization (odds ratios [OR] 25.6 versus 3.4); the OR for both was 45.[17,55]

Although all strains of rhinovirus have been associated with asthma exacerbations, HRV-C has been more prevalent than other respiratory tract viruses or rhinovirus groups in preschool and lower school–age children.[56] How HRV-C causes severe exacerbations is particularly well understood and provides a prototypical example of a genetic susceptibility to a common environmental exposure underlying asthma development and exacerbations. The epithelial receptor for HRV-C is cadherin-related family member 3 (CDHR3).[57] A comprehensive genome-wide study replicated in five cohorts identified a specific *CDHR3* allele associated with recurrent, severe asthma exacerbations in children (i.e., requiring hospitalization).[58] A G-to-A transition mutation resulting in a single amino acid change from cysteine to tyrosine at CDHR3 position 529 increases airway epithelial expression of CDHR3, increases HRV-C binding and replication 10-fold, and increases cumulative risk of severe asthma exacerbations.[57,58] This example of genetic risk of asthma by HRV-C infection and exacerbation in young children further implicates the important role of virus-induced exacerbation in asthma development because exacerbations may contribute to progressive loss of lung function and increasing asthma severity over time.[59,60a]

Other common respiratory viral infections (e.g., respiratory syncytial virus, parainfluenza, metapneumovirus, influenza, adenovirus) are associated with wheezing episodes in children, although most are not linked to persistent asthma like HRV.[47] Respiratory syncytial virus (RSV) is the most common cause of severe bronchiolitis in young children and a concerning sentinel event for the development of persistent disease.[15,60b] In one longitudinal study, infants hospitalized with RSV bronchiolitis (most occurred by 4 months of age) were more likely to have asthma and lung dysfunction through the age of 13 years.[61] In other studies, infants experiencing RSV-associated lower respiratory tract infections were more likely to have wheezing symptoms at 6 years of age, but not at later ages (e.g., 13 years old).[17,47,62] Young children who had radiographic evidence of pneumonia or croup symptoms accompanying wheezing were more likely to have persistent asthma symptoms and lung function impairment at 6 and 11 years of age, suggesting that severity of pulmonary injury from the inciting viral infection portends persistent disease.[63,64]

Parental History of Asthma

Infants whose parents report a history of childhood asthma have lower lung function and are more likely to wheeze in early life,[65,66] in later childhood,[13,42] and in adulthood.[29] However, in a two-generation, longitudinal study in Aberdeen, Scotland, the children of well-characterized subjects without atopy or asthma were found to have a surprisingly high prevalence of allergen sensitization (56%) and wheezing (33%).[67] Similarly, in the German Multicentre Allergy Study (MAS), the majority of children with AD and/or asthma in early childhood were born to nonallergic parents.[68] For example, of the study's asthmatic children at 5 years of age, 57% were born to parents without an atopic history. Therefore, allergen sensitization and asthma seem to be occurring at high rates, even in persons considered to be at low genetic risk for allergy and asthma.

Gender

Male gender is a risk factor for both transient wheezing and persistent asthma in childhood.[13,42] This is generally believed to be caused by the smaller airways of young boys compared with girls.[69,70] Later in childhood, BHR and inhalant allergen sensitization are more prevalent in boys than in girls.[71,72] However, as children age into adulthood, asthma becomes more prevalent in women. From childhood to adulthood, female gender is a risk factor for greater asthma persistence, level of severity,[29] and BHR.[28] In later childhood, females also have a higher incidence of new-onset asthma. Female children who become overweight and have early-onset puberty are more likely to develop asthma in adolescence, an association not appreciated in males (see Fig. 2.2).[73] These observations are consistent with the gender "flip" in asthma prevalence—higher in males in childhood and in females by adulthood.[12]

Environmental Tobacco Smoke Exposure

ETS exposure is a risk factor for wheezing problems at all ages. Prenatal ETS exposure is associated in a dose-dependent manner with wheezing manifestations and decreased lung function in infancy and early childhood[74–76] and with asthma in school-age children.[16,77] Postnatal ETS exposure is associated with a greater likelihood of wheezing in infancy,[66] transient wheezing, and persistent asthma in childhood.[13] ETS exposure is a major determinant of asthma severity in school-age children that is independent of atopy.[77,78] Cigarette smoking also has been strongly associated with persistent asthma and asthma relapses in adulthood.[30]

ETS exposure is also associated with food allergen sensitization,[79] AR, hospitalization for lower respiratory tract infections, BHR, and elevated serum IgE levels.[80,81] In a 7-year prospective study, ETS exposure was associated with greater inhalant allergen sensitization and reduced lung function.[42]

Ambient Pollutant Exposures

Common air pollutants (e.g., particulate matter, nitrogen dioxide, sulfur dioxide, carbon monoxide, ozone) have been shown to play an important role in respiratory health and asthma morbidity in children.[82,83] Exposure to these air pollutants and proximal living to freeways and roadways (i.e., traffic-related pollutants) have been associated with worse asthma symptoms and lung function.[84–87] Indoor ambient tobacco smoke, nitrogen dioxide, and endotoxin exposure in urban homes and public schools have also been associated with greater asthma severity.[88–92] Since the Clean Air Act of 1970, significant control measures have been implemented in the United States to regulate and reduce ambient levels of these air pollutants. Significant reductions in these exposures have been associated with improved lung function and reduced bronchitic symptoms in children, especially those with asthma.[93,94]

Genetic susceptibility to common air pollutant exposures may influence the expression of asthma. For example, polymorphisms in the endogenous antioxidant glutathione S-transferase (GST) genes (e.g., *GST-M1* null) were associated with less asthma in children; these associations were strengthened when genetic GST susceptibility was combined with maternal smoking.[95–97] In a longitudinal birth cohort study, diesel exhaust particulate exposure was associated with persistent wheezing only in those children carrying a specific genotypic variant in *GST-P1* (valine at position 105).[98] In children with asthma, high ozone exposure was associated with lower lung function (forced expiratory flow [FEF]$_{25-75}$) only in those with a *GST-M1* null (i.e., deletion) genotype; antioxidant (vitamin C and E) supplementation abrogated ozone's effect on lung function in only *GST-M1* null asthmatic children.[99] These findings demonstrate how ordinary environmental exposures conspire with genetic susceptibilities to exert stronger effects on the development of asthma and allergy than either genes or environmental exposures alone.

It is important to note that asthma mediated by occupational-type exposures is often not considered in children, and yet some children are raised in settings where occupational-type exposures can mediate asthma in adults (e.g., on farms or with domestic animals in the home). For example, high endotoxin exposure causing asthma and progressive lung dysfunction in farmers, domestic animal workers, and cotton factory workers has also been associated with more wheezing in children living on farms with domestic animals and in early life.[100–103] Globally, it is common for children to be raised in homes with wood/coal/biomass burning for cooking and heat, which is a public health concern across ages (e.g., pneumonias, asthma, COPD, respiratory-related mortality). Children with these types of exposures are relatively understudied and likely contribute to the global burden of asthma.

Asthma-Protective and Allergy-Protective Environments

Locale and lifestyle differences may impart strong asthma- and/or allergy-protective effects. A compelling example is based on the protective influence of traditional Bavarian dairy farm life on allergy and asthma development in children.[104,105] Amish and Hutterite families in the United States are emigrant descendants of the Bavarian farmers who continue to lead a farming life and are of nearly identical genetic ancestry[106]; yet, the prevalence of asthma in Amish versus Hutterite schoolchildren is 5.2% versus 21.3%, and the prevalence of allergic sensitization is 7.2% versus 33.3%.[107,108] Although their genetic and lifestyle origins are the same, thematic environmental and immunologic differences between Amish and Hutterite children were observed. House dust endotoxin levels, a marker of bacterial burden, were much higher in homes of Amish children, presumably because of the Amish families' proximal living near their domestic animals, preferring to have their barns with their cows and horses attached to their homes, similar to traditional dairy farming lifestyles of their Bavarian counterparts and different from the modern, industrialized farming practices of Hutterites.[106] Aligning with this observation, peripheral blood samples from Amish children had more neutrophils, more monocytes with suppressive phenotype markers (i.e., lower human leukocyte antigen DR and higher inhibitory molecule immunoglobulin-like transcript 3), produced fewer cytokines when stimulated with endotoxin in vitro, and had higher expression of antimicrobial, innate immune genes. In this example, the microbe-rich environment of Amish children might prevent allergy and asthma development via innate antimicrobial and antiinflammatory pathways and may be similar to other asthma- and allergy-protective exposures that have been observed.

Microbial Exposures

Numerous epidemiologic studies have found that a variety of microbial exposures are associated with a lower likelihood of allergen sensitization, allergic disease, and asthma. This has led to a "hygiene" hypothesis, which proposes that the reduction of microbial exposures in childhood in modernized locales has led to the rise in allergy and asthma.[109] Microbes and their molecular components are thought to influence early childhood development by inducing antimicrobial type 1 and regulatory immune development and immune memory, thereby preventing the development of allergen sensitization and diseases while strengthening the immune response and controlling inflammation to common respiratory viral infections. A number of microbe-rich environmental circumstances in early life appear to have allergy- and/or asthma-protective effects, including being raised as the younger child in larger families or in daycare from an early age[110]; having more runny nose colds[111]; pet dog or cat ownership[112–114]; domestic animal exposure[115–117]; and, in U.S. inner cities, cockroach, mouse, and/or cats.[16,118] There is a notable paradox that cat, dog, cockroach, and mouse exposures in homes are associated with asthma persistence and severity in allergen-sensitized children while also having a protective influence on asthma and allergy inception.

Features of the potentially protective environmental microbiome may include greater abundance, diversity, and specific species; communities; and their functional influence on immune development. Higher house dust endotoxin levels have been associated with these exposures and also associated with less AD,[100,119,120] inhalant allergen sensitization,[101,121–123] AR, and asthma.[102,124] Allergy- and asthma-protective farming environments are associated with greater house dust endotoxin levels and greater microbial diversity.[104–106] Complementary immunologic studies reveal that higher house dust endotoxin levels were associated with increased proportions of T helper type 1 (T_H1) cells,[121] higher levels of IFN-γ from stimulated peripheral blood samples,[125,126] and immune down-regulation of endotoxin-stimulated blood samples.[102] In U.S. inner cities, house dust microbiome analysis identified hundreds of bacterial taxa that were more or less abundant in the homes of children with asthma.[16] Most of these bacterial taxa levels correlated with protective exposures (i.e., cat, dog, cockroach, and/or mouse); in particular, higher abundance of *Bifidobacterium* and *Brevundimonas* spp. in house dust partially mediated the association between higher cockroach allergen concentration and lower asthma risk.

The developing gastrointestinal (GI) microbiome rapidly evolves in early life and may also influence the development of allergy and asthma at critical time points in its evolution. Stool bacteria from newborns and infants who ultimately go on to develop allergic disease can be less diverse and have more clostridia and *Staphylococcus aureus,* whereas nonallergic infants had more enterococci, bifidobacteria, lactobacilli, and *Bacteroides* organisms.[127–131] In longitudinal birth cohort studies, more sophisticated molecular approaches to GI microbiome characterization at 1 month[132] or 3 months[132] of age showed compositional differences associated with subsequent atopy/asthma risk. At 1 month of age, lower relative abundance of certain bacteria (e.g., *Bifidobacterium, Akkermansia,* and *Faecalibacterium* spp.) and higher relative abundance of particular fungi (*Candida* and *Rhodotorula*) were found in infants who subsequently developed allergen sensitizations and asthma.[132] Their fecal metabolome was also enriched for proinflammatory metabolites, and ex vivo culture of human peripheral T lymphocytes with sterile fecal water from these high-risk infants increased the proportion of $CD4^+$ cells producing IL-4 and reduced the relative abundance of regulatory $CD4^+CD25^+FOXP3^+$ cells. In a different cohort, sampling at 3 months of age revealed lower abundances of genera

Faecalibacterium, Lachnospira, Rothia, and *Veillonella* in infants who subsequently developed the "atopy plus wheeze" phenotype at high risk for asthma.[133] Complementary immunologic studies revealed a protective effect of these four fecal bacterial genera on airway inflammation. Alterations in the gut microbiome of infants from dietary and environmental differences (e.g., breastfeeding, semisterile food, infections, antibiotic use, siblings, pets) may influence the developing immune system and allergy outcomes.

Conversely, some microbial exposures have been associated with the development of persistent asthma. Nasopharyngeal carriage of common respiratory pathogens (*Streptococcus pneumoniae, Moraxella catarrhalis, Haemophilus influenzae*) in infancy and in children with asthma in later childhood (*S. pneumoniae, M. catarrhalis*), was associated with asthma exacerbations, implicating these respiratory pathogens as coexposures in the pathogenesis of asthma persistence and exacerbations.[134,135]

Atopic Dermatitis

AD usually begins during the preschool years and persists throughout childhood. Two prospective birth cohort studies found the peak incidence of AD to be in the first 2 years of life (see Fig. 2.1).[42,136] Although 66% to 90% of patients with AD have clinical manifestations before 7 years of age,[137,138] eczematous lesions in the first 2 months of life are rare. Natural history studies of AD have reported a wide variation (35%–82%) in disease persistence throughout childhood.[138,139] The greatest remission in AD seems to occur between 8 and 11 years of age and, to a lesser extent, between 12 and 16 years.[138] Natural history studies of AD may have underestimated the persistent nature of the disease for reasons that include (1) AD definition—some studies have included other forms of dermatitis that have a better prognosis over time (i.e., seborrheic dermatitis)[140]; (2) AD recurrence—a 23-year birth cohort study found that many patients who experienced disease remission in childhood had an AD recurrence in early adulthood[138]; and (3) AD manifestation—it is generally thought that patients with childhood AD often evolve to manifest hand and/or foot dermatitis as adults.

Parental history of AD is an important risk factor for childhood AD. This apparent heritability complements studies revealing a high concordance rate of AD among monozygotic versus dizygotic twins (0.72 versus 0.23, respectively).[141] In a risk factor assessment for AD in the first 2 years of life, higher levels of maternal education and living in less crowded homes were risk factors for early-onset AD.[142] The environmental/lifestyle risk factors reported for AR and asthma are similar. A meta-analysis of prospective breastfeeding studies concluded that exclusive breastfeeding of infants with a family history of atopy for at least the first 3 months of life is associated with a lower likelihood of childhood AD (OR 0.58). This protective effect was not observed, however, in children without a family history of atopy.[143]

Initial AD disease severity seems predictive of later disease severity and persistence. Of adolescents with moderate to severe AD, 77% to 91% continued to have persistent disease in adulthood.[144] In comparison, of adolescents with mild AD, 50% had AD in adulthood. Food allergen sensitization and exposure in early childhood also contribute to AD development and disease severity. Food allergen sensitization is associated with greater AD severity.[42,145] Furthermore, elimination of common allergenic foods in infancy (i.e., soy, milk, egg, peanuts) is associated with a lower prevalence of allergic skin conditions up to the age of 2 years (see Fig. 2.1).[42]

AD severity	Initial examination			4 years later			
	Inhalant ± food	**Food only**		**Inhalant ± food**	**Food only**	**Asthma and/or AR**
Mild	15%	20%		31%	6%	15%
Moderate	18%	26%		52%	6%	32%
Severe	20%	45%		100%	0%	75%

• **Fig. 2.5** Atopic dermatitis *(AD)* in young children (2 months to 3 years of age) and allergen sensitization (to food and inhalant allergens), asthma, and allergic rhinoconjunctivitis *(AR)* 4 years later. At enrollment, AD severity was determined, and no subjects had AR or asthma. Four years later, 88% of subjects had a marked improvement or complete resolution of AD. However, all children with severe AD at enrollment were sensitized to inhalant allergens, and 75% had asthma and/or AR. (From Patrizi A, Guerrini V, Ricci G, et al. The natural history of sensitizations to food and aeroallergens in atopic dermatitis: a 4-year follow-up. Pediatr Dermatol 2000;17:261–5.[146])

Natural history studies have found early childhood AD to be a major risk factor for food allergen sensitization in infancy,[146] inhalant allergen sensitization,[146,147] and persistent asthma in later childhood.[13,37] In particular, severe AD in early childhood is associated with a high prevalence of allergen sensitization and airways allergic disease in later childhood (i.e., 4 years later; Fig. 2.5). Indeed, in young patients with severe AD, 100% developed inhalant allergen sensitization and 75% developed an allergic respiratory disease (mostly asthma) over 4 years. In contrast to severe AD, patients with mild to moderate AD were not as likely to develop allergen sensitization (36%) or an allergic respiratory disease (26%). More information on current concepts of barrier and immune dysfunction in AD and the role of food hypersensitivity can be found in Chapters 50 and XXX, respectively.

Allergic Rhinitis

Many people develop AR during childhood. Two prospective birth cohort studies reported a steady rise in total (i.e., seasonal and perennial) AR prevalence, reaching 35% to 40% by the age of 7 years.[42,148] Seasonal AR emerged after 2 years of age and increased steadily to 15% by age 7 years.[148]

AR also commonly begins in early adulthood. In a 23-year cohort study of Brown University students, beginning in their freshman year, perennial AR developed in 4.8% at 7 years and 14% at 23 years of follow-up.[2,3] The incidence increase for seasonal AR was substantially greater: 13% at 7 years and 41% at 23 years of follow-up.[2,3] Allergen skin test sensitization and asthma were prognostic risk factors for the development of AR.

AR persistence has been evaluated in adult patients. Three follow-up studies of adult patients with AR found a disease remission rate of 5% to 10% by 4 years[149] and 23% by 23 years.[2] In the 23-year follow-up study, 55% of the follow-up subjects reported improvement in rhinitis. Onset of disease in early childhood was associated with greater improvement.[2]

Anaphylaxis

Anaphylaxis in children can result from numerous possible exposures (e.g., foods, antibiotics, insulin, insect venoms, latex) and is sometimes anaphylactoid (a clinically similar but non–IgE-mediated reaction, such as occurs with radio-contrast media and aspirin/nonsteroidal antiinflammatory drugs) or idiopathic. In a retrospective medical records review of 601 cases, causes of anaphylaxis were determined in 41%: foods 22%, medications 11%, and exercise 5%. Episodes tended to become less frequent over time.[150] A history of AR or asthma is a risk factor for anaphylaxis to foods and latex.[151] Surprisingly, a history of asthma, pollenosis or food and/or drug allergy is a risk factor for anaphylactoid reactions to radio-contrast media, with a higher prevalence of adverse reactions to ionic versus nonionic contrast media observed.[152] In contrast, atopy is not a risk factor for anaphylaxis to insulin,[153] penicillin[154] or insect stings.[155] The natural history of anaphylactic reactions in children has been studied prospectively only for food-induced anaphylaxis (described previously) and bee sting anaphylaxis.

In a Johns Hopkins study examining the natural history of bee venom allergy in children, venom-allergic children with a history of mild generalized reactions were randomly assigned to venom immunotherapy or no treatment and then subjected to a repeat sting in a medical setting 4 years later.[156] Systemic allergic reactions occurred in 1.2% of the treated group and 9.2% of the untreated group. Moreover, systemic reactions that occurred were no more severe than the original incidents. In a smaller study of children and adults with venom hypersensitivity, repeat sting challenges, at least 5 years after the original incidents, induced no systemic reactions in those who originally presented with only urticaria/angioedema but did induce systemic reactions in 21% of those who originally had respiratory and/or cardiovascular complications.[157]

These studies suggest that insect sting anaphylaxis is often self-limited in children, with spontaneous remission usually occurring within 4 years. Children at greatest risk of persistent hypersensitivity include those with previous severe anaphylactic episodes. Conversely, those children with mild systemic reactions to bee stings are less likely to have an allergic reaction on re-sting, and any future anaphylactic episodes from bee stings are not likely to be severe. Finally, in a re-challenge study of subjects with no clinical response to a first sting challenge, 21% experienced anaphylaxis to the second challenge, and, of those, half developed symptomatic hypotension requiring epinephrine.[158]

Allergy and Asthma Prevention

Because allergies and asthma are highly prevalent conditions that usually begin in young children, prevention strategies often aim for early life. Besides peanut allergy prevention beginning in infancy,[159,160] well-proven approaches to allergy and asthma prevention are currently lacking. Yet scientifically strong lines of preventive investigation are ongoing and, in some circumstances, have led to ongoing prevention clinical trials in young children, with the potential for transformative success. Prevention of food allergy (Chapter 36) and asthma (Chapter 29) are fully addressed in other chapters.

When considering prevention strategies, it can be helpful to distinguish primary, secondary, and tertiary approaches to prevention of disease, because the basis of disease inception, development, and persistence/severity can differ, respectively. In this context, preventive interventions can be characterized as *primary* (preventing allergy/asthma inception by prenatal and/or postnatal interventions), *secondary* (e.g., preventing persistent asthma with interventions in toddler-age children), or *tertiary* (e.g., asthma exacerbation prevention).

Microbial Supplementation

Some studies suggest that oral probiotic supplementation in infancy may prevent atopy by promoting type 1 and/or regulatory immune development. The most commonly trialed so far have been probiotic/prebiotic dietary supplementations. A meta-analysis of six randomized controlled trials (RCTs) to prevent AD in children, usually beginning with maternal intake before birth, reported less AD in the probiotic-treated group.[161] Other clinical trials with lactobacillus or combined probiotics/prebiotics demonstrated reduced respiratory infection illnesses in young children.[162–164] A large RCT (N = 1018) of prebiotic/probiotic supplementation to prevent allergies found no significant differences in allergic sensitization, AD, AR, or asthma at 5 years of age; however, it significantly reduced the OR (0.47) of IgE-associated allergic disease in children delivered by cesarean section.[165] Differences in the specific probiotic strains used in the various clinical trials may contribute to the differences in findings among studies. A systematic review and meta-analysis of randomized clinical trials of an oral extract of different bacteria responsible for respiratory infections (Broncho-Vaxom) revealed a reduction in recurrent respiratory tract illnesses.[166] A National Institutes of Health (NIH)-sponsored RCT with Broncho-Vaxom in 6- to 18-month-old children to prevent early-onset asthma is underway.

Preventing the Allergic March

In addition to microbial supplementation as primary prevention of the allergic march, secondary prevention approaches are also being considered. Inhalant allergen sensitization in toddler-age children with recurrent preschool wheeze is a strong predictor and physiologic mediator of persistent asthma (discussed earlier); therefore, an NIH-sponsored RCT with anti-IgE (omalizumab) in high-risk toddlers is underway. Allergen-specific immunotherapy (AIT) has been studied to determine whether it can reduce the likelihood of asthma development in children with AR. An RCT found that a 3-year AIT course administered to children with birch and/or grass pollen AR reduced rhinoconjunctivitis severity, conjunctival sensitivity to allergen, and the likelihood of developing asthma at 2 and 7 years after AIT discontinuation.[167,168] AIT also prevents the development of new sensitizations to inhalant allergens.[169,170] These studies suggest that AIT may alter the allergic march of inhalant allergen sensitization and asthma, but the difficulties and risks of conventional AIT in children warrant careful consideration.

Early life elimination of allergenic foods (cow's milk, peanut, egg, fish)[42] and/or inhalant allergens[171–174] have not significantly prevented allergic disease or asthma. A multifaceted intervention from prebirth through infancy comprising pet, house dust, and ETS exposure avoidance; breastfeeding; and delayed introduction of solid foods significantly reduced asthma prevalence at age 7 years, without reducing AR, AD, allergen sensitization, or BHR.[175] A systematic review and meta-analysis of three multifaceted and six mono-faceted allergen reduction trials suggested that reduction in exposure to multiple indoor allergens, but not monoallergen interventions, modestly reduced the likelihood of asthma in children.[176]

Several conventional controller pharmacotherapies for allergic conditions or asthma have been tested in prevention trials in early life and were found not to be preventive, or only modestly so, including antihistamines (cetirizine),[177,178] inhaled corticosteroids (fluticasone),[179–182] and prenatal vitamin D supplementation.[183]

Numerous studies have investigated the potential of early breastfeeding as a protective influence against the development of allergy and asthma. Meta-analyses of prospective studies of exclusive breastfeeding for 4 or more months from birth have been associated with less AD and asthma (summary ORs of 0.68 and 0.70, respectively).[143,184] Although definitive proof of the preventive value of reducing or eliminating ETS exposure in infancy and childhood has been hindered by the difficulties in achieving long-term smoking cessation in RCTs, ETS exposure at all ages, from prenatal exposure of mothers to smoking in asthmatic adults, is associated with more wheezing problems and more severe disease. When considered with other health benefits of ETS exposure avoidance, this is strongly recommended.

Conclusions

Allergic diseases and asthma commonly develop in the early childhood years and can have lifelong implications. Although many allergy and asthma sufferers improve through later childhood and can even become disease-free, those with severe disease and some particular conditions (e.g., peanut allergy) are likely to have lifelong disease. Current paradigms of immune development, lung growth, and susceptibility to common exposures shape the understanding of disease pathogenesis and resilience and health. The systemic nature of these conditions is such that manifestations of one allergic condition are often risk factors for others (e.g., AD and allergen sensitization are risk factors for persistent asthma). In contrast, children raised in allergy- and asthma-protective environments provide insights and hope for future prevention.

Acknowledgment

Our sincere gratitude to our colleague, Dr. Lynn Taussig, for his previous authorship of this chapter and his legacy of natural history investigation in childhood asthma.

The reference list can be found on the companion Expert Consult website at http://www.expertconsult.inkling.com.

3

The Genetics of Allergic Disease and Asthma

JOHN W. HOLLOWAY

KEY POINTS

- Inherited genetic susceptibility plays an clear role in the aetiology of allergic disease such as asthma.
- Allergic diseases are complex genetic diseases arising from the combined effect of many genetic variants and their interaction with environmental exposures.
- The phenotype (observable disease characteristics) used is an essential component to designing and interpreting studies of the genetics of allergic disease.
- Genetic factors not only influence allergic disease susceptibility, but also influence the interaction of environmental factors with

atopy and allergic disease, disease severity, and response to treatment (pharmacogenetics).
- While there a genetic factors, for example those influencing atopy, that are common to multiple allergic diseases, there are also unique genetic risk factors for each disease.
- Epigenetic processes also play a role in allergic disease and are a mechanism whereby environmental exposure can have long term effects on allergic disease susceptibility and severity even after the environmental exposure is no longer present.

Introduction

Since the first report of linkage between chromosome 11q13 and atopy in 1989,[1] thousands of studies have been published on the genetics of asthma and other allergic diseases. Their aim has been to identify the genetic factors that modify susceptibility to allergic diseases, determine severity of disease in affected individuals, and affect the response to treatment. This recent expansion in our knowledge has provided intriguing insights into the pathophysiology of these complex disorders. In this chapter, we outline the approaches used to undertake genetic studies of common diseases such as atopic dermatitis (AD) and asthma and provide examples of how these approaches are beginning to reveal new insights into the pathophysiology of allergic diseases.

Why Undertake Genetic Studies of Allergic Disease?

Susceptibility to allergic disease is likely to result from the inheritance of many gene variants, but the underlying cellular defects are unknown. By undertaking research into the genetic basis of these conditions, these gene variants and their gene products can be identified solely by the anomalous phenotypes they produce. Identifying the genes that produce these disease phenotypes provides a greater understanding of the fundamental mechanisms of these disorders, stimulating the development of specific new drugs or biologic agents to both relieve and prevent symptoms. In addition, genetic variants also may influence the response to

therapy, and the identification of individuals with altered response to current drug therapies will allow optimization of current therapeutic measures (i.e., disease stratification and pharmacogenetics). The study of genetic factors in large longitudinal cohorts with extensive phenotype and environmental information allows the identification of external factors that initiate and sustain allergic diseases in susceptible individuals and the periods of life in which this occurs, with a view to identifying those environmental factors that could be modified for disease prevention or for changing the natural history of the disorder. For example, early identification of vulnerable children would allow targeting of preventive therapy or environmental intervention, such as avoidance of allergen exposure. Genetic screening in early life may eventually become a practical and cost-effective option for allergic disease prevention.

Approaches to Genetic Studies of Complex Genetic Diseases

What Is a Complex Genetic Disease?

The use of genetic analysis to identify genes responsible for simple mendelian traits such as cystic fibrosis[2] has become almost routine in the 30 years since it was recognized that genetic inheritance can be traced with naturally occurring DNA sequence variation.[3] However, many of the most common medical conditions known to have a genetic component to their cause, including diabetes, hypertension, heart disease, schizophrenia, and asthma, have much more complex inheritance patterns.

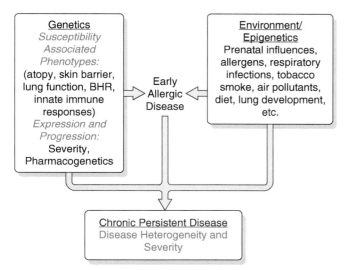

• **Fig. 3.1** Allergic disease such as asthma is due to a combination of both genetics and environmental exposures leading to early disease. Additional gene variants and further environmental exposures lead to chronic persistent disease with heterogeneous subtypes (e.g., mild versus severe asthma). *BHR,* Bronchial hyperresponsiveness. (Modified from Meyers DA, Bleecker ER, Holloway JW, et al. Asthma genetics and personalized medicine. Lancet Respir Med 2014;2(5):405–415.)

Complex disorders show a clear hereditary component; however, the mode of inheritance does not follow any simple mendelian pattern. Furthermore, unlike single-gene disorders, they tend to have high prevalence. Asthma occurs in at least 10% to 20% of children in some populations, and atopy is as high as 40% in some population groups[4] compared with cystic fibrosis at 1 in 2000 live Caucasian births. Characteristic features of mendelian diseases are that they are rare and involve mutations in a single gene that are severe, resulting in large phenotypic effects that may be independent of environmental influences. In contrast, complex disease traits are common and involve many genes, with mild mutations leading to small phenotypic effects with strong environmental interactions (Fig. 3.1).

How to Identify Genes Underlying Complex Disease

Before any genetic study of a complex disease can be initiated, a number of different factors need to be considered. These include (1) assessing the heritability of a disease of interest to establish whether there is indeed a genetic component to the disease in question, (2) defining the phenotype (or physical characteristics) to be measured in a population, (3) the size and nature of the population to be studied, (4) determining which genetic markers are going to be typed in the DNA samples obtained from the population, (5) how the relationships between the genetic data and the phenotype measures in individuals are to be analyzed, and (6) how these data can be used to identify the genes underlying the disease.

Inheritance

The first step in any genetic analysis of a complex disease is to determine whether genetic factors contribute at all to an individual's susceptibility to disease. The fact that a disease has been observed to "run in families" may reflect common environmental exposures, biased ascertainment, or a potential true genetic component. A number of approaches can be taken to determine whether genetics contributes to a disease or disease phenotype of interest, including family studies, segregation analysis, twin and adoption studies, heritability studies, and population-based relative risk to relatives of probands.[5,6]

Family studies involve estimation of the frequency of the disease in relatives of affected individuals, compared with unaffected individuals. Determining the relative contribution of common genes versus common environment to clustering of disease within families can be undertaken using twin studies in which the concordance of a trait in monozygotic and dizygotic twins is assessed. Monozygotic twins have identical genotypes, whereas dizygotic twins share, on average, only half of their genes. In both cases, they share the same childhood environment. Therefore, a disease that has a genetic component is expected to show a higher rate of concordance in monozygotic than in dizygotic twins. Another approach used to disentangle the effects of nature versus nurture in a disease is in adoption studies, in which, if the disease has a genetic basis, the frequency of the disease should be higher in biologic relatives of probands than in their adopted family.

Once familial aggregation with a probable genetic cause for a disease has been established, the mode of inheritance can be determined by observing the pattern of inheritance of a disease or trait and how it is distributed within families. For example, is there evidence of a single major gene and is it dominantly or recessively inherited? Segregation analysis is the most established method for this purpose. However, for complex diseases, it is often difficult to undertake segregation analysis because of the multiple genetic and environmental effects making any one model hard to determine. This has implication for the methods of analysis of genetic data in studies, because some methods, such as the parametric logarithm of the odds (LOD) score approach, require a model to be defined to obtain estimates of parameters such as gene frequency and penetrance (see page 18).

Phenotype

Studies of a genetic disorder require that a phenotype be defined, to which genetic data are compared. Phenotypes can be classified in two ways. They may be complex, such as asthma or atopy, and are likely to involve the interaction of a number of genes. Alternatively, intermediate phenotypes may be used, such as bronchial hyperresponsiveness (BHR) and eosinophilia for asthma and serum immunoglobulin E (IgE) levels and specific IgE (sIgE) responsiveness or positive skin prick tests to particular allergens for atopy. Together, these phenotypes contribute to an individual's expression of the overall complex disease phenotype but are likely to involve the interaction of fewer genetic influences, thus increasing the chances of identifying specific genetic factors predisposing toward the disease. Phenotypes also may be discrete or qualitative, such as the presence or absence of wheeze, atopy, and asthma, or quantitative. Quantitative phenotypes, such as blood pressure (millimeters of mercury [mm Hg]), lung function measures (e.g., forced expiratory volume in 1 second [FEV_1]) and serum IgE levels, are phenotypes that can be measured as a continuous variable. With quantitative traits, no arbitrary cut-off point has to be assigned (making quantitative trait analysis important) because clinical criteria used to define an affected or unaffected phenotype may not reflect whether an individual is a gene carrier. In addition, the use of quantitative phenotypes allows the use of alternative methods of genetic analysis that, in some situations, can be more powerful. More recently, cluster analysis has been used to identify individual phenotypic expressions of asthma in a population sample.[7-9] In many cases, phenotype choice represents a trade-off between greater specificity and sample size. Sophisticated phenotypes, such as clustering, have the potential to give important biologic insights into the role of genetic variation in specific aspects of disease pathophysiology, but simple phenotypes, such as self-reported or doctor-diagnosed asthma, are available in most studies facilitating meta-analysis and/or extremely large population samples.

Population

Having established that the disease or phenotype of interest does have a genetic component to its cause, the next step is to recruit a study population in which to undertake genetic analyses to identify the gene(s) responsible. The type and size of study population recruited depend heavily on a number of interrelated factors, including the epidemiology of the disease, the method of genetic epidemiologic analysis being used, and the class of genetic markers genotyped. For example, the recruitment of families is necessary to undertake linkage analysis, whereas association studies are better suited to either a randomly selected population or case-control cohort. In family-based linkage studies, the age of onset of a disease will determine whether it is practical to collect multigenerational families or affected sibling pairs for analysis. Equally, if a disease is rare, actively recruiting cases and matched controls will be a more practical approach than recruiting a random population that would need to be very large to have sufficient power. Increasingly, genetic analysis of complex disease is now being dominated by extremely large (>100,000) population cohorts for which genotypes and comprehensive phenotypes are available (e.g., the UK Biobank population).[10]

Genetic Markers

Genetic markers used can be any identifiable site within the genome (locus) where the DNA sequence is variable (polymorphic between individuals). The most common genetic markers used for linkage analysis are microsatellite markers comprising short lengths of DNA consisting of repeats of a specific sequence (e.g., CA_n). The number of repeats varies among individuals, thus providing polymorphic markers that can be used in genetic analysis to follow the transmission of a chromosomal region from one generation to the next. Single-nucleotide polymorphisms (SNPs) are the simplest class of polymorphism in the genome, resulting from a single base substitution (e.g., cytosine substituted for thymidine). SNPs are much more frequent than microsatellites in the human genome, occurring in introns, exons, promoters, and intergenic regions, with millions of SNPs now having been identified and mapped through initiatives such as the 1000 Genomes Project.[11] Another source of variation in the human genome that has been recognized to be present to a much greater extent than was previously thought are copy number variations (CNVs). CNVs are either a deletion or insertion of a large piece of DNA sequence; CNVs can contain whole genes and therefore are correlated with gene expression in a dose-dependent manner.[12] Sequencing of individual human genomes has revealed that non-SNP variation (which includes CNVs) made up more than 20% of all variation in individuals but involves more than 70% of all variant DNA bases in that genome.[13]

Approaches to Analysis

Linkage analysis involves proposing a model to explain the inheritance pattern of phenotypes and genotypes observed in a pedigree.[14] Linkage is evident when a gene that produces a phenotypic trait and its surrounding markers are coinherited. In contrast, those markers not associated with the anomalous phenotype of interest will be randomly distributed among affected family members as a result of the independent assortment of chromosomes and crossing over during meiosis. Whereas family-based analysis using linkage analysis was the mainstay of gene identification for monogenic diseases in the past, it has been superseded for analysis of common disease by the use of genome-wide association studies (GWASs) (for common variants) and next-generation sequencing of whole or partial (e.g., the protein-coding fraction or exome) individual genomes for rare variants.

Association studies do not examine inheritance patterns of alleles; rather, they are case-control studies based on a comparison of allele frequencies between groups of affected and unaffected individuals from a population. The odds ratio (OR) of the trait in individuals is then assessed as the ratio of the frequency of the allele in the affected population compared with the unaffected population. The greatest problem in association studies is the selection of a suitable control group to compare with the affected population group. Although association studies can be performed with any random DNA polymorphism, they have the most significance when applied to polymorphisms that have functional consequences in genes relevant to the trait (candidate genes).

It is important to remember with association studies that there are a number of reasons leading to an association between a phenotype and a particular allele, as follows:

- A positive association between the phenotype and the allele will occur if the allele is the cause of, or contributes to, the phenotype. This association would be expected to be replicated in other populations with the same phenotype, unless there are several different alleles at the same locus contributing to the same phenotype, in which case association would be difficult to detect, or if the trait was predominantly the result of different genes in the other population (genetic heterogeneity).
- Positive associations may also occur between an allele and a phenotype if that particular allele is in linkage disequilibrium (LD) with the phenotype-causing allele. That is, the allele tends to occur on the same parental chromosome that also carries the trait-causing mutation more often than would be expected by chance. LD will occur when most causes of the trait are the result of relatively few ancestral mutations at a trait-causing locus and the allele is present on one of those ancestral chromosomes and lies close enough to the trait-causing locus that the association between them has not been eroded away through recombination between chromosomes during meiosis. LD is the nonrandom association of adjacent polymorphisms on a single strand of DNA in a population; the allele of one polymorphism in an LD block (haplotype) can predict the allele of adjacent polymorphisms (one of which could be the causal variant).
- Positive association between an allele and a trait also can be artefactual as a result of recent population admixture. In a mixed population, any trait present in a higher frequency in a subgroup of the population (e.g., an ethnic group) will show positive association with an allele that also happens to be more common in that population subgroup.[15] Thus, to avoid

spurious association arising through admixture, studies should be performed in large, relatively homogeneous populations.

Historically, association studies were not well suited to whole genome searches in large mixed populations. Because LD extends over very short genetic distances in an old population, many more markers are needed to be typed to cover the whole genome. Therefore, genome-wide searches for association were more favorable in young, genetically isolated populations because LD extends over greater distances and the number of disease-causing alleles is likely to be fewer.

However, advances in array-based SNP genotyping technologies and haplotype mapping of the human genome[11,16] means GWASs have revolutionized the study of genetic factors in complex common disease.[17,18] For hundreds of phenotypes, from common diseases to physiologic measurements such as height and body mass index and biologic measurements such as circulating lipid levels and blood eosinophil levels, GWASs have provided compelling statistical associations for thousands of different loci in the human genome[19] and are now the method of choice for identification of genetic variants influencing physiologic or disease phenotypes.

Identify Gene

If, as in most complex disorders, the exact biochemical or physiologic basis of the disease is unknown, there are two main approaches to finding disease genes. One method is GWAS, using SNPs evenly spaced throughout the genome as an assumption-free approach to locate disease-associated genes involved in disease pathogenesis. Because GWASs use large data sets, often millions of SNPs to test for association, stringent genotype calling, quality control, population stratification (genomic controls), and statistical techniques have been developed to handle the analysis of such data.[20] Studies start by reporting single marker analyses of primary outcome; SNPs are considered to be strongly associated if the p-values are below the 1% false discovery rate or showing weak association above 1% but below the 5% false discovery rate. A cluster of p-values below the 1% false discovery rate from SNPs in one chromosomal location is defined as the region of maximal association and is the first candidate gene region to examine further, with analysis of secondary outcome measures, gene database searches, fine mapping to find the causal locus and replication in other cohorts/populations. It is unlikely that the SNP showing the strongest association will be the causal locus, because SNPs are chosen to provide maximal coverage of variation in that region of the genome and not on biologic function. Therefore, GWASs will often include fine mapping/haplotype analysis of the region with the aim of identifying the causal locus. If LD prevents the identification of a specific gene in a haplotype block, it may be necessary to use different racial and ethnic populations to locate the causative candidate gene that accounts for the genetic signal in GWASs.

Alternatively, candidate genes can be selected for analysis because of a known role for the encoded product of the gene in the disease process. Polymorphisms in the genetic region containing the gene are tested for association with the disease or phenotype in question. A hybrid approach is the selection of candidate genes based not only on their function, but also on their differential expression in disease-relevant tissue.

Once a gene has been identified, further work is required to understand its role in the disease pathogenesis. Further molecular genetic studies may help identify the precise genetic polymorphism that is having functional consequences for the gene's expression or function, as opposed to those that are merely in LD with the causal SNP. Often the gene identified may be completely novel, and cell and molecular biology studies will be needed to understand the gene product's role in the disease and to define genotype/phenotype correlations. Furthermore, by using cohorts with information available on environmental exposures, it may be possible to define how the gene product may interact with the environment to cause disease. Ultimately, knowledge of the gene's role in disease pathogenesis may lead to the development of novel therapeutics.

Allergy and Asthma as Complex Genetic Diseases

From studies of the epidemiology and heritability of allergic diseases, it is clear that these are complex diseases in which the interaction between genetic and environmental factors plays a fundamental role in the development of IgE-mediated sensitivity and the subsequent development of clinical symptoms. The development of IgE responses by an individual, and therefore allergies, is the function of several genetic factors. These include the regulation of basal serum immunoglobulin production, the regulation of the switching of immunoglobulin-producing B cells to IgE, and the control of the specificity of responses to antigens. Furthermore, the genetic influences on allergic diseases such as asthma are more complex than those on atopy alone, involving not only genes controlling the induction and level of an IgE-mediated response to allergen but also lung-specific or asthma-specific genetic factors that result in the development of asthma. This also applies equally to other clinical manifestations of atopy such as rhinitis and AD.

Phenotypes for Allergy and Allergic Disease: What Should We Measure?

The term *atopy* was originally used by Coca and Cooke[21] in 1923 to describe a particular predisposition to develop hypersensitivity to common allergens associated with an increase of circulating reaginic antibody, now defined as IgE, and with clinical manifestations such as whealing-type reactions, asthma, and hay fever. Today, even if the definition of *atopy* is not yet precise, the term is commonly used to define a disorder that involves IgE antibody responses to ubiquitous allergens and that is associated with a number of clinical disorders such as asthma, allergic dermatitis, allergic conjunctivitis, and allergic rhinitis.

Atopy can be defined in several ways, including raised total serum IgE levels, the presence of antigen sIgE antibodies, and/or a positive skin test to common allergens. Furthermore, because of their complex clinical phenotype, atopic diseases can be studied using intermediate or surrogate disease-specific measurements, such as BHR or lung function for asthma. As discussed earlier, phenotypes can be defined in several ways, ranging from subjective measures (e.g., symptoms), objective measures (e.g., BHR, blood eosinophils, or serum IgE levels), or both. It is a lack of a clear definition of atopic phenotypes that presents the greatest problem when reviewing studies of the genetic basis of atopy and atopic disease, with multiple definitions of the same intermediate phenotype often being used in different studies. Likewise, definition of disease status such as asthma can be problematic because this can be clinical (symptoms, parental or self-reports, doctor diagnosis), pharmacologic (bronchodilator reversibility, steroid responsiveness), or through intermediate physiologic measures (BHR, lung function).

The Heritability of Atopic Disease: Are Atopy and Atopic Disease Heritable Conditions?

In 1916 the first comprehensive study of the heritability of atopy was undertaken by Robert Cooke and Albert Vander Veer.[22] Although the atopic conditions they included, and those excluded (e.g., eczema), may be open for debate today, the conclusions nonetheless remain the same. There is a high heritable component to the development of atopy and atopic disease, and it is now more clearly understood biologically, owing to the inheritance of a tendency to generate sIgE responses to common proteins.

Subsequent to the work of Cooke and Van der Veer, the results of many studies have established that atopy and atopic disease such as asthma, rhinitis, and eczema have strong genetic components. Family studies have shown an increased prevalence of atopy and phenotypes associated with atopy among the relatives of atopic compared with nonatopic subjects.[23–25] In a study of 176 normal families, Gerrard and colleagues[26] found a striking association between asthma in the parent and asthma in the child, between hay fever in the parent and hay fever in the child, and between eczema in the parent and eczema in the child. These studies suggest that end-organ sensitivity, or which allergic disease an allergic individual will develop, is controlled by specific genetic factors, differing from those that determine susceptibility to atopy per se. This hypothesis is borne out by a questionnaire study involving 6665 families in southern Bavaria. Children with atopic diseases had a positive family history in 55% of cases compared with 35% in children without atopic disease (P <.001).[27] Subsequent researchers used the same population to investigate familial influences unique to the expression of asthma and found that the prevalence of asthma alone (i.e., without hay fever or eczema) increased significantly if the nearest of kin had asthma alone (11.7% versus 4.7%, P <.0001). A family history of eczema or hay fever (without asthma) was unrelated to asthma in the offspring.[27]

Numerous twin studies[28–34] have shown a significant increase in concordance for atopy among monozygotic twins compared with dizygotic twins and both twin and family studies have shown a strong heritable component to atopic asthma.[32,33,35–37] Using a twin-family model, Laitinen and colleagues[38] reported that in families with asthma in successive generations, genetic factors alone accounted for as much as 87% of the development of asthma in offspring and the incidence of the disease in twins with affected parents is 4-fold compared with the incidence in twins without affected parents. This indicates that asthma is recurring in families as a result of shared genes rather than shared environmental risk factors. This has been further substantiated in a study of 11,688 Danish twin pairs, suggesting 73% of susceptibility to asthma was the result of the genetic component. However, a substantial part of the variation in liability of asthma was the result of environmental factors; there also was no evidence for genetic dominance or shared environmental effects.[39]

Molecular Regulation of Atopy and Atopic Disease, I: Susceptibility Genes

Positional Cloning by Genome-Wide Linkage in Families

In the two decades after the first such study in 1989, many genome-wide linkage studies for atopy and atopic disorder susceptibility genes were undertaken. Multiple regions of the genome were observed to be linked to varying phenotypes, with differences between cohorts recruited from both similar and different populations.[40] This illustrates the difficulty of identifying susceptibility genes for complex genetic diseases. Different genetic loci show linkage in populations of different ethnicities and different environmental exposures. As mentioned earlier, in studies of complex disease, the real challenge has not been identification of regions of linkage but rather identification of the precise gene and genetic variant underlying the observed linkage. To date, several genes have been identified as the result of positional cloning using a genome-wide scan for allergic disease phenotypes, including *ADAM33*, *DPP10*, *HLAG*, *PHF11*, *PTDGR*, *NPSR1*, and *PLUAR* for asthma; *COL29A1* for AD; and *PCDH1* for BHR.[41]

Genes Identified by Genome-Wide Association Studies

Subsequent to positional cloning studies, improvements in technology enabled GWASs to be performed with great success in allergic diseases, such as asthma, eczema, and allergic sensitization. The GWAS catalog currently (2020) lists more than 1200 SNP associations in more than 100 studies for asthma, the most studied allergic disease,[19] with the largest GWASs conducted to date in more than 350,000 subjects in the UK Biobank population identifying more than 100 loci associated with asthma, rhinitis, and eczema.[42–44] Fig. 3.2 illustrates the results of one such GWAS to identify genes for severe asthma.

The first novel asthma susceptibility locus to be identified by a GWAS approach contained the *ORMDL3* and *GSDMB* genes on chromosome 17q12-21.1.[45] A total of 317,000 SNPs (in genes or surrounding sequences) were characterized in 994 subjects with childhood-onset asthma and 1243 without asthma, followed by replication in a further 2320 subjects that revealed five significantly associated SNPs. After gene expression studies, *ORMDL3* was found to be strongly associated with disease-associated markers ($P < 10^{-22}$ for rs7216389) identified by the GWAS.

Importantly, many subsequent studies have replicated the association between variation in the chromosome 17q21 region (mainly rs7216389) and childhood asthma in ethnically diverse populations.[46] A GWAS was conducted by the GABRIEL consortium[47] of 26,475 people confirmed the association between *GSDMB-ORMDL3* and childhood-onset asthma, implicating a number of genes involved in T_H2 activation, including *IL33*, *IL1RL1*, and *SMAD*. The loci associated with asthma were not associated with serum IgE levels.

However, subsequent studies have implicated gasdermin A (*GSDMA*) and post-glycosylphosphatidylinositol (GPI) attachment to proteins 3 (*PGAP3*) on either side of the core region as potentially independent asthma loci,[46] and one of the largest asthma GWASs to date identified the strongest association with rs2952156 in Erb-B2 receptor tyrosine kinase 2 (*ERBB2*) at least 180 kilobases from the previously recognized asthma-associated

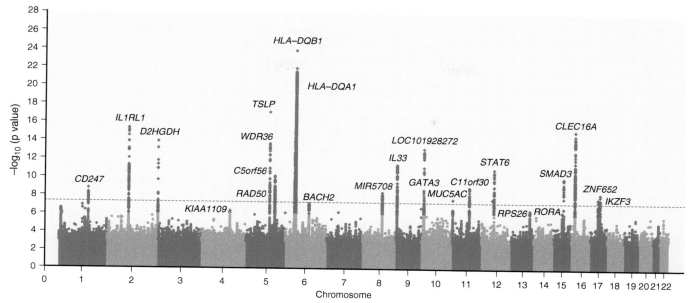

• **Fig. 3.2** Manhattan plot for analyses of risk of moderate to severe asthma. The *y*-axis shows the level of association between a single-nucleotide polymorphism (SNP) and the phenotype (–log10[p-value]) and the *x*-axis position in the genome. Each point represents the association of a single SNP with the outcomes. Data are for 5135 cases with moderate to severe asthma and 25,675 controls assessed for 33.8 million variants, and the *dotted line* indicates genome-wide significance ($p < 5 \times 10^{-8}$). Loci are labeled with the nearest gene for the 24 signals meeting genome-wide significance. (Reproduced from Shrine N, Portelli MA, John C, et al. Moderate-to-severe asthma in individuals of European ancestry: a genome-wide association study. Lancet Respir Med 2019;7(1):20–34.)

signals at the *GSDMB/ORMDL3* haplotype block.[48] Long-distance genomic interactions can mean that the gene within which the SNP is located is not necessarily the causal gene.[49,50] Therefore, it is important to remember that considerable work is still required to fully characterize this region of the genome before accepting *ORMDL3* as the causal gene through guilt by association because many genes in a region of LD will be associated with disease in a GWAS without, necessarily, being the causative gene. The extensive LD across this region in populations of European and Asian ancestry[48] make it difficult to definitively identify the asthma gene or genes within this region, especially because the asthma-associated 17q SNPs are associated with gene expression (expression quantitative trait loci [eQTLs]) for multiple nearby genes, *including GSDMA, ORMDL3, GSDMB,* and *PGAP3* in immune cells, lung cells, or both. This means that despite a decade or more of research into the 17q locus, it is still unclear which gene or genes underlie early-life wheezing and asthma pathogenesis, what are the functions of and the mechanisms by which the 17q genes affect asthma onset, and in which cell types (blood cells, airway cells, or both) are the expression of these genes most relevant to the 17q asthma-associated risk.[46] This illustrates the difficulty of translating genetic associations into deeper understanding of disease pathogenesis.

GWASs have also identified novel genes underlying blood eosinophil levels (and also associated with asthma),[51] occupational asthma,[52] total serum IgE levels,[53] and eczema.[54,55] Studies of other atopic disease have focused on serum IgE levels and/or allergic sensitization. Weindinger et al[53] identified a locus associated with the high-affinity IgE receptor (*FCER1A*) as strongly associated with both serum IgE and sensitization and confirming candidate gene findings of signal transducer and activator of

transcription 6 *(STAT6)* and the 5q31 region related to T_H2 cytokines. An Icelandic study showed an association between *IL1RL1* (the interleukin 33 [IL-33] receptor coding gene) and blood IgE levels.[51] A meta-analysis of GWASs into allergic sensitization that included a total of 16,170 sensitized individuals identified a total of 10 loci that are estimated to account for 25% of allergic sensitization and allergic rhinitis.[56] Of the 10 SNPs identified, 9 also showed a directionally consistent association with asthma. Associations were also identified with AD, albeit weaker than with asthma. The authors also investigated known susceptibility loci and found only weak associations with total IgE levels (*FCER1A* and human leukocyte antigen A *[HLA-A]*) and asthma (17q12-21 and *IL33*). This suggests that these loci do not increase asthma risk through allergic sensitization.[56] Subsequent studies have also shown that although there is considerable overlap in the loci associated with asthma, eczema, and hay fever, a number of SNPs have a significantly larger effect on one of these phenotypes than the others, suggesting that part of the genetic contribution to allergic disease is more phenotype specific[43,57] (Fig. 3.3).

Until recently there had been very little known of the genetic causes of AD, aside from filaggrin, which is described in more detail later. However, in the last decade GWASs have expanded this knowledge; a recent meta-analysis of AD studies by Paternoster and colleagues[55] of more than 15 million genetic variants in 21,399 cases and 95,464 controls from populations of European, African, Japanese, and Latino ancestry, followed by replication in 32,059 cases and 228,628 controls identified 31 loci associated with AD risk, including candidate genes with roles in both skin barrier formation and regulation of innate host defences and T cell function.[55] These associations add further evidence that AD arises from both epithelial and immune dysfunction, which is further

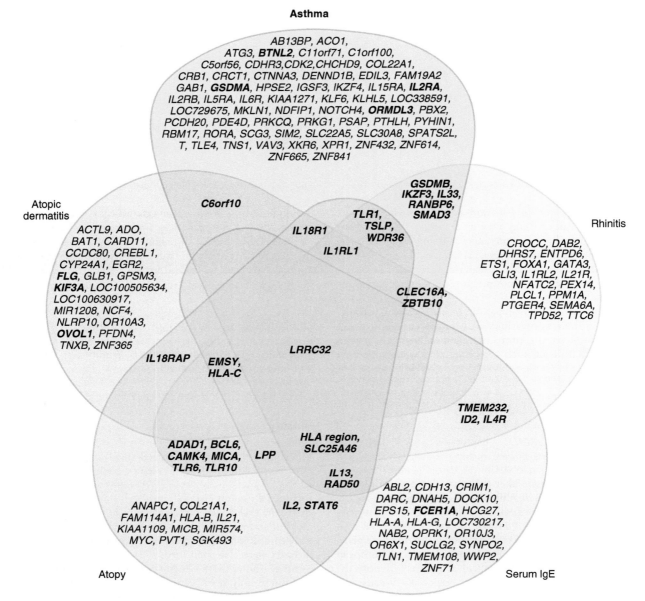

Asthma

AB13BP, ACO1,
ATG3, **BTNL2**, C11orf71, C1orf100,
C5orf56, CDHR3,CDK2,CHCHD9, COL22A1,
CRB1, CRCT1, CTNNA3, DENND1B, EDIL3, FAM19A2
GAB1, **GSDMA**, HPSE2, IGSF3, IKZF4, IL15RA, **IL2RA**,
IL2RB, IL5RA, IL6R, KIAA1271, KLF6, KLHL5, LOC338591,
LOC729675, MKLN1, NDFIP1, NOTCH4, **ORMDL3**, PBX2,
PCDH20, PDE4D, PRKCQ, PRKG1, PSAP, PTHLH, PYHIN1,
RBM17, RORA, SCG3, SIM2, SLC22A5, SLC30A8, SPATS2L,
T, TLE4, TNS1, VAV3, XKR6, XPR1, ZNF432, ZNF614,
ZNF665, ZNF841

Atopic dermatitis

ACTL9, ADO,
BAT1, CARD11,
CCDC80, CREBL1,
CYP24A1, EGR2,
FLG, GLB1, GPSM3,
KIF3A, LOC100505634,
LOC100630917,
MIR1208, NCF4,
NLRP10, OR10A3,
OVOL1, PFDN4,
TNXB, ZNF365

C6orf10

**GSDMB,
IKZF3, IL33,
RANBP6,
SMAD3**

*TLR1,
TSLP,
WDR36*

IL18R1

IL1RL1

Rhinitis

CROCC, DAB2,
DHRS7, ENTPD6,
ETS1, FOXA1, GATA3,
GLI3, IL1RL2, IL21R,
NFATC2, PEX14,
PLCL1, PPM1A,
PTGER4, SEMA6A,
TPD52, TTC6

**CLEC16A,
ZBTB10**

IL18RAP

**EMSY,
HLA-C**

LRRC32

**TMEM232,
ID2, IL4R**

**ADAD1, BCL6,
CAMK4, MICA,
TLR6, TLR10**

LPP

*HLA region,
SLC25A46*

*IL13,
RAD50*

IL2, STAT6

ABL2, CDH13, CRIM1,
DARC, DNAH5, DOCK10,
EPS15, **FCER1A**, HCG27,
HLA-A, HLA-G, LOC730217,
NAB2, OPRK1, OR10J3,
OR6X1, SUCLG2, SYNPO2,
TLN1, TMEM108, WWP2,
ZNF71

ANAPC1, COL21A1,
FAM114A1, HLA-B, IL21,
KIAA1109, MICB, MIR574,
MYC, PVT1, SGK493

Atopy

Serum IgE

• **Fig. 3.3** Overlapping sets of genes have been reported in genome-wide association studies for asthma, rhinitis, serum immunoglobulin E (IgE) levels, atopy, and atopic dermatitis, supporting a common genetic element within the mechanisms predisposing individuals toward different allergic disease phenotypes. Genome-wide association studies (GWASs) have also identified many genes in association with only one allergic disease phenotype; these most likely represent the tissue-specific component of each allergic disease (e.g., *FLG* in the epidermal barrier in atopic dermatitis). To date, more GWASs have been conducted analyzing genetic variants associated with asthma than with other allergic diseases. In the future it is likely that more risk variants for other allergic diseases will be identified. Genes reported in more than one GWAS are shown in bold font. The genes reported for SNPs detected to be significantly associated ($P \le 1 \times 10^{-5}$) with each allergic disease phenotype were obtained by searching the National Human Genome Research Institute GWAS catalog. (From National Human Genome Research Institute. GWAS catalog, <http://www.genome.gov/gwasstudies>.)

supported by the discovery of an AD-associated SNP adjacent to *C11orf30,* which was previously identified as a susceptibility locus for Crohn's disease, another disease of immune and epithelial dysfunction.[58]

Atopic rhinitis has been less well studied, but GWASs have identified loci in *C11orf30,*[59] mentioned previously; the HLA region, *MRPL4* and *BCAP*[60]; and loci associated with the phenotype asthma and hay fever.[57] Although, as noted earlier, studies of

multiple allergic disease phenotypes in the UK Biobank and other populations[43,57,61] have shown some distinctive association with rhinitis separate from asthma and eczema.

Genome-wide studies of food allergy have been undertaken, but these have been limited by relatively small sample sizes compared with the large-scale studies of asthma noted earlier (typically 1–2000 cases). However, in addition to association in the HLA region, other loci such as the clade B serpin (SERPINB) gene cluster at 18q21.3, the T$_H$2 cytokine gene cluster at 5q31.1, the filaggrin gene, and the *EMSY* (*C11orf30*) locus have been shown to be associated with food allergy to several allergens.[62–66]

In summary, these GWASs demonstrate the power of the genome-wide approach for identifying complex disease-susceptibility variants, and the number of loci will increase with the increasing availability of genomic data from extremely large population studies, such as national biobanks, and use of additional meta-analyses that combine information from individual studies with analysis of other asthma-related phenotypes such as disease severity,[67] and age of onset.[42,44,68] For other complex, chronic inflammatory diseases such as Crohn's disease and type 1 diabetes mellitus (which have been extensively studied using GWAS), the study results have not fully explained the heritability patterns. It is thought that the inability to find all of the genetic factors underlying disease susceptibility may be explained by limitations of GWAS, which include the presence of other variants in the genome not captured by the current generation of genome-wide genotyping platforms, analyses not being adjusted for gene-environment and gene-gene (i.e., epistasis) interactions, or epigenetic changes in gene expression.[71]

Current research is both expanding these known variants and confirming their associations with clinical phenotypes.[69] GWAS has now moved on from simple loci of association with a broad disease definition, such as asthma, and studies are now identifying particular regions associated with phenotypes of disease or subgroups. For example, Du and associates[70] identified *CRTAM* as associated only with asthma exacerbations in those with low vitamin D,[70] and another 2014 GWAS has identified *CDHR3* as being associated with severe asthma exacerbations.[71]

Although GWAS has not fully explained the heritability of asthma and atopic disease, geneticists remain optimistic, because it is thought that this "missing heritability" can be explained.[72] It is thought that this inability to find genes could be explained by both overestimations of actual heritability as a result of shared familial environment[73] and limitations of GWAS, such as insufficient power to detect variants of small effect, variants not screened for, or analyses not adjusted for gene-environment and gene-gene interactions or epigenetic changes in gene expression. One explanation for missing heritability, after assessing common genetic variation in the genome, is that rare variants (below the frequency of SNPs included in GWAS studies) of high genetic effect, or common CNVs may be responsible for some of the genetic heritability of common complex diseases.[74] Exome screening studies have already shown that rare variants may contribute to asthma and lung function.[75,76]

Candidate Gene/Gene Region Studies

A large number of candidate regions have been studied for both linkage to and association with a range of atopy-related phenotypes. In addition, SNPs in the promoter and coding regions of a wide range of candidate genes have been examined. Candidate genes are selected for analysis based on a wide range of evidence, for example, biologic function, differential expression in disease, involvement in other diseases with phenotypic overlap, affected tissues, cell type(s) involved, and findings from animal models. There are now more than 500 studies that have examined polymorphism in more than 200 genes for association with asthma and allergy phenotypes.[77,78] When assessing the significance of association studies, it is important to consider several things. For

example, was the size of the study adequately powered if negative results are reported? Were the cases and controls appropriately matched? Could population stratification account for the associations observed? In the definitions of the phenotypes, which phenotypes have been measured (and which have not)? How were they measured? Regarding correction for multiple testing, have the authors taken multiple testing into account when assessing the significance of association?

Genetic variants showing association with a disease are not necessarily causal because of the phenomenon of LD, whereby polymorphism A is not affecting gene function, but rather it is merely in LD with polymorphism B that is exerting an effect on gene function or expression. Positive association may also represent a Type 1 error; candidate gene studies have suffered from nonreplication of findings between studies, which may be due to poor study design, population stratification, different LD patterns between individuals of different ethnicity and differing environmental exposures between study cohorts. The genetic association approach also can be limited by underpowered studies and loose phenotype definitions.[79]

An Example of a Candidate Gene: Interleukin-13

Given the importance of T$_H$2-mediated inflammation in allergic disease and the biologic roles of *IL13*, including switching B cells to produce IgE, wide-ranging effects on epithelial cells, fibroblasts, and smooth muscle promoting airway remodeling and mucus production, *IL13* is a strong biologic candidate gene.[80] Furthermore, *IL13* is also a strong positional candidate. The gene encoding *IL13*, like *IL4*, is located in the T$_H$2 cytokine gene cluster on chromosome 5q31 within 12 kb of *IL4*,[81] with which it shares 40% homology. This genomic location has been extensively linked with a number of phenotypes relevant to allergic disease, including asthma, atopy, specific and total IgE responses, blood eosinophils, and BHR, including in subsequent GWAS studies.[47,48]

Asthma-associated polymorphisms have been identified in the *IL13* gene, including a single–base pair substitution in the promoter of *IL13* adjacent to a consensus nuclear factor of activated T cell binding sites. Patients with asthma are significantly more likely to be homozygous for this polymorphism, and the polymorphism is associated, in vitro, with reduced inhibition of IL-13 production by cyclosporin and increased transcription factor binding.[82] Hypotheses proposed to explain the association of this *IL-13* polymorphism and development of atopic disease include decreased affinity for the decoy receptor IL13Rα2, increased functional activity through IL13Rα1, and enhanced stability of the molecule in plasma.[83]

An amino acid polymorphism of *IL13* also has been described: R110Q (rs20541).[84–86] The 110Q variant enhances allergic inflammation compared with the 110R wild-type IL-13[87] by inducing STAT6 phosphorylation, CD23 expression in monocytes, and hydrocortisone-dependent IgE switching in B cells. It also has a lower affinity for the IL-13Rα2 decoy receptor and produced a more sustained eotaxin response in primary human fibroblasts expressing low levels of IL-13Rα2.[88]

IL13 polymorphism associations have been inconsistent, with some studies showing association with atopy in children[86,89] and others showing associations with asthma and not atopy.[87] Howard and colleagues[90] also showed that the −1112 C/T variant of *IL13* contributes significantly to BHR susceptibility ($P = 0.003$) but not to total serum IgE levels. Thus, it is possible that polymorphisms in *IL13* may confer susceptibility to airway remodeling in persistent asthma and to allergic inflammation in early life.

As discussed previously, positive association observed between an SNP and phenotype does not imply that the SNP is causal. *IL13* lies adjacent to *IL4,* an equally strong biologic candidate in which SNPs have shown association with relevant phenotypes,[91] and within the chromosome 5q31 gene cluster that is known to contain an asthma susceptibility gene. Therefore, association observed with *IL13* SNPs may simply represent a proxy measure of the effect of polymorphisms in *IL4* or another gene in the region. For example, a genome-wide association study of total IgE levels reported significant associations between polymorphisms in an adjacent gene, *RAD50,* and total serum IgE levels,[53] in a region containing a number of evolutionary conserved noncoding sequences that may play a role in regulating *IL4* and *IL13* transcription.[92] However, given the extensive biologic evidence for functionality and studies examining polymorphisms across the gene region showing independent effects of the *IL13* R110Q SNP, it is likely that the reported *IL13* associations are real.

Many studies have observed positive associations of specific genetic polymorphisms with differential response to environmental factors in asthma and other respiratory phenotypes.[93] *IL13* levels have been shown to be increased in children whose parents smoke,[94] and interaction between *IL13* –1112 C/T and smoking with childhood asthma as an outcome has been reported,[95] in addition to evidence for this same SNP modulating the adverse effect of smoking on lung function in adults.[96] Thus, differences in smoking exposure among studies may account for some of the differences in findings among studies. DNA methylation is affected by both genetic variants and environment, which may later determine disease risk. For example, Patil and associates[97] demonstrated that although rs20541 polymorphisms interacted with maternal smoking to determine methylation at the cg13566430 *IL13* promoter region methylation site, a relationship between the rs1800925 SNP in the *IL13* locus and the same cg13566430 methylation site affected lung function. This demonstrates the two-step model of environment and genetic variance affecting disease state, as shown in Fig. 3.3.[97]

An Example of a Candidate Gene: Interleukin-33

Since its identification in 2005, IL-33 has emerged as one of the most important cytokines in T_H2 differentiation, and its receptor, ST2, is an excellent marker of T_H2 cells.[98] IL-33 is a member of the IL-1 family and the *IL33* gene is located on chromosome 9 and is therefore separate from the chromosome 5q31 cluster of *IL13* and *IL4,* and not in LD with these genes. Its receptor is encoded by *IL1RL1* on chromosome 2, associated with the *IL1* gene cluster. *IL33* polymorphisms within two LD blocks have been identified in GWAS as associated with asthma. A number of polymorphisms also have been identified by candidate gene approaches and by both candidate gene studies and GWAS in the *IL1RL1* gene (IL-33 receptor).[98] The IL-33/IL1RL1 pathway has been implicated in the stimulation of type 2 innate lymphoid cells (ILC2s) that produce IL-4, IL-5, and IL-13 and thus may have a pivotal role in initiating the T_H2 phenotype in atopy and asthma. Indeed, *IL1RL1* polymorphisms have been shown to be associated with lower levels of *IL1RL1* transcription,[99] and a rare variant in *IL33* that affects mRNA splicing producing a truncated form of the protein, is associated with lower eosinophil counts and reduced risk of asthma.[100] Joint analysis of SNPs in the IL-33-IL1RL1 pathway in birth cohorts showed that polymorphisms are associated with asthma and specific wheezing phenotypes, suggesting that they affect development of wheeze and subsequent asthma through sensitization in early childhood.[101]

Any observed association of *IL13* or *IL33/IL1RL1* polymorphisms should have its effect reported in context by considering other variations in other relevant genes whose products may modulate its effects. For example, there are a number of other functional polymorphisms in genes encoding other components of the *IL4/IL13* signaling pathway (*IL4, IL13, IL4RA, IL13RA1, IL13RA2,* and *STAT6*) with synergistic effects.[102] Likewise, the *IL1RL1* locus is closely related to the IL-18 receptor gene (*IL18R1*), which has a complex LD structure. IL-18 is associated with T_H1 responses and cell adhesion.

The *IL13/IL33* polymorphism studies illustrate many of the difficulties of genetic analysis in complex disease. Replication is often not found among studies, and this may be accounted for by the lack of power to detect the small increases in disease risk that are typical for susceptibility variants in complex disease. Differences in genetic make-up,[103,104] in environmental exposure between study populations, and failure to strictly replicate[105] in either phenotype (IgE and atopy versus asthma and BHR) or genotype (different polymorphisms in the same gene) can all contribute to the lack of replication among studies. Furthermore, studies of a single polymorphism, or even a single gene in isolation, can oversimplify the complex genetic variants in asthma pathogenesis and the cross-talk among implicated cytokines, as shown by the roles of IL-13, IL-33, IL1RL1, and T_H2/ILC2 cells in asthma pathogenesis.

The observations regarding the association of *IL13* variants with allergic disease outcomes described previously also illustrate the difficulty of the functional genomic studies that are needed to understand the statistical association between phenotype and genetic variant, and this is despite the already extensive knowledge of the biologic function of IL-13 that existed before the associations were first reported, and indeed why IL13 was a candidate gene in the first place. When considering novel associations arising from GWAS studies, the first step is trying to identify the causative gene(s) and variant(s) underlying the association signal. Several approaches can be used for this, including assessment of the variant in different ethnic populations in whom there is different LD structure,[48] integrating with the ever-increasing public sources of data such as catalogs of association between genetic variants and gene expression (eQTL) in different tissues (e.g., the Genotype-Tissue Expression [GTEx] project), and epigenetic and regulatory features in the genome (e.g., the ENCylopedia Of DNA Elements [ENCODE]).

Animal models can provide insights into gene function when little is already known about the identified gene (e.g., by comparing physiologic responses in gene-knockout and wild-type mice). For example, a soluble form of the positionally cloned asthma gene *ADAM33,* when induced in utero or added ex vivo, causes remodeling of the airways, which enhances postnatal airway eosinophilia and BHR after subthreshold challenge with an allergen.[106] This also illustrates the difficulty of studying gene function in animal models because an *Adam33* knock-out mouse showed no differences in measurement of inflammatory outcomes in a well-established ovalbumin challenge model compared with wild-type animals.[107] Similarly, knock-out or overexpression studies in mice have provided insight into other asthma genes, including *ORMDL3* and *GSDMB,* and in identification of spontaneous airway hyperresponsiveness in these mice.[108] These and other functional studies of disease-susceptibility genes highlight the gap between gene identification and disease biology that will take considerable effort to close in order to realize benefits of studies of disease genetics on our understanding of pathogenesis and development of novel therapeutics.

Analysis of Clinically Defined Subgroups

One approach is to identify genes in a rare, severely affected subgroup of patients in whom disease appears to follow a pattern of inheritance that indicates the effect of a single major gene. The assumption is that mutations (polymorphisms) of milder functional effect in the same gene in the general population may play a role in susceptibility to the complex genetic disorder. One example of this has been the identification of the gene encoding the protein filaggrin as a susceptibility gene for AD.

Filaggrin

Filament-aggregating protein (filaggrin) has a key role in epidermal barrier function. The protein is a major component of the protein-lipid cornified envelope of the epidermis important for water permeability and blocking the entry of microbes and allergens.[109] In 2002 the condition ichthyosis vulgaris, a severe skin disorder characterized by dry flaky skin and a predisposition to AD and associated asthma, was mapped to the epidermal differentiation complex on chromosome 1q21. This gene complex includes the filaggrin gene *(FLG)*.[110] In 2006, Smith and colleagues reported that loss of function mutations in the filaggrin gene caused ichthyosis vulgaris.[111]

Noting the common occurrence of AD in individuals with ichthyosis vulgaris, these researchers subsequently showed that common loss of function variants (combined carrier frequencies of 9% in the European population[112]) were associated with AD in the general population.[113] AD in children is often the first sign of atopic disease, and these studies of filaggrin mutation have provided a molecular mechanism for the co-existence of asthma and dermatitis. It is thought that deficits in epidermal barrier function could lead to allergic sensitization by allergen exposure through the skin and start the atopic march in susceptible individuals.[114–116] Mechanistically, the role for filaggrin has been confirmed by analysis of the spontaneous recessive, mutant flaky tail gene *(Flt)* in mice, whose phenotype results from a frameshift mutation in the murine filaggrin gene *(Flg)* with enhanced cutaneous allergen priming and in allergen sIgE and IgG antibody responses.[117]

Molecular Regulation of Atopy and Atopic Disease, II: Disease-Modifying Genes

The concept of genes interacting to alter the effects of mutations in susceptibility genes is not unknown. A proportion of interfamilial variability can be explained by differences in environmental factors and differences in the effect of different mutations in the same gene. Intrafamilial variability, especially in siblings, cannot be so readily accredited to these types of mechanisms. Many genetic disorders are influenced by modifier genes that are distinct from the disease susceptibility loci.

Genetic Influences on Disease Severity

Very few studies of the heritability of IgE-mediated disease have examined phenotypes relating to severity. Sarafino and Goldfedder[30] studied 39 monozygotic twin pairs and 55 same-sex dizygotic twin pairs for the heritability of asthma and asthma severity. Asthma severity (as measured by frequency and intensity of asthmatic episodes) was examined in twin pairs concordant for asthma. Severity was significantly correlated for monozygotic pairs but not for dizygotic pairs, suggesting there are distinct genetic factors that determine asthma severity as opposed to susceptibility.

A number of studies have examined associations between asthma severity and polymorphisms in candidate genes but were initially hampered by the lack of clear, easily applied, accurate phenotype definitions for asthma severity that distinguish between the underlying severity and level of therapeutic control. For example, it has been suggested that β_2-adrenergic receptor polymorphisms could influence asthma severity, and the Arg16Gly polymorphism has been associated with measures of asthma severity.[118] However, it is not clear whether β_2-adrenergic receptor polymorphisms affect patients' responses to β_2 agonists or, regardless of their effects on treatment, these polymorphisms lead to more severe chronic asthma.[119] GWAS has identified *CDHR3* as being associated with severe asthma exacerbation in early childhood,[71] which subsequently has been shown to drive differentiation of ciliated bronchial epithelial cells and facilitate rhinovirus C infection.[120] A retrospective study of the Childhood Asthma Management Program (CAMP) cohort showed that variation in the gene encoding the low-affinity IgE receptor, *FCER2,* is associated with high IgE levels and increased frequency of severe exacerbations despite inhaled corticosteroid (ICS) treatment.[121] Most recently, Shrine and co-workers[122] undertook a GWAS comparing severe and mild asthma and identified 24 genome-wide significant signals of association with moderate-to-severe asthma, including several signals in innate or adaptive immune-response genes and in the *MUC5AC* region. Although there was substantial shared genetic architecture between mild and moderate to severe asthma, the *MUC5AC* signal was not associated with asthma when analyses included mild asthma.[122]

Genetic Regulation of Response to Therapy: Pharmacogenetics

Genetic variability may not only play a role in influencing susceptibility to allergy but may also modify its severity or influence the effectiveness of therapy. In asthma, patient response to drugs, such as bronchodilators, corticosteroids, and anti-leukotrienes is heterogeneous.[123,124] In the future, identification of such pharmacogenetic factors has the potential to allow individualized treatment plans based on an individual's genetic background. One of the most investigated pharmacogenetic effects has been the effect of polymorphisms at the gene encoding the β_2-adrenergic receptor, *ADRB2*, on the bronchodilator response to inhaled short- and long-acting β_2 agonists.

Clinical studies have shown that β_2-adrenergic receptor polymorphisms may influence the response to bronchodilator treatment. The two most common polymorphisms of the receptor are at amino acids 16 (Arg16Gly) and 27 (Gln27Glu).[125] Patients with asthma who carry the Gly16 polymorphism have been shown to be more prone to developing bronchodilator desensitization,[127] whereas children who are homozygous or heterozygous for Arg16 are more likely to show positive responses to bronchodilators.[128] Studies in vitro have shown that the Gly16 increases down-regulation of the β_2-adrenergic receptor after exposure to a β_2 agonist. In contrast, the Glu27 polymorphism appears to protect against agonist-induced down-regulation and desensitization of the β_2-adrenergic receptor.[129,130] In a genotype-stratified, randomized, placebo-controlled cross-over trial, Israel and colleagues[130] showed that during the run-in period, with minimum albuterol, patients with the Arg/Arg genotype had an increase in morning peak expiratory flow rate (PEFR). In contrast during randomized treatment, patients with the Gly/Gly genotype had an increase in morning PEFR during treatment with regularly scheduled albuterol compared with placebo, and patients with the Arg/Arg genotype had lower morning PEFR. The genotype-attributable treatment difference was −24 L/min (−37 to −12; P = .0003).[130]

In contrast to the possible effects on short-acting bronchodilators, pharmacogenetic analysis of β$_2$-adrenergic receptor polymorphisms have found no effect on response to long-acting β$_2$ agonist therapy in combination with corticosteroids.[131,132] These findings are difficult to explain in the light of the studies discussed linking the Gly16 allele with BHR, β$_2$ agonist effectiveness, and asthma severity but may indicate that the co-administration of corticosteroids abrogates the effect of variation of *ADRB2*. The complexity of the genotype by response effects observed for variation in *ADRB2* makes clinical application limited at this time. However, in contrast to studies in adults, in children an increased risk for exacerbations has been seen in Arg16 homozygotes. In a meta-analysis of data from 4226 children from five independent Caucasian and Latino populations showed an increased OR for asthma exacerbations of 1.52 (P = .0021) for each copy of the *Arg16* allele among children treated with ICSs plus long-acting β agonist (LABA).[133] Lipworth and associates[134] also showed in a prospective randomized trial of 5- to 18-year-old patients with asthma with the Arg16 homozygous genotype on ICSs, add-on montelukast compared with salmeterol significantly improved asthma symptoms, asthma-related school absence, and quality of life. Future studies are needed to establish whether prospective genotyping of this SNP would inform prescribing advice in children whose asthma is not well controlled on ICSs.

As well as variation in *ADRB2*, many candidate gene studies and several GWAS studies have been undertaken to identify variants associated with short-acting β agonist (SABA) responsiveness.[135] Although a number of variants have been associated with SABA responsiveness, the effect sizes are low and few have studied the effect on treatment response to LABAs. Future prospective genotype-stratified studies are necessary to confirm these associations and study the effect on LABA responsiveness.

Although glucocorticoid therapy is a potent antiinflammatory treatment for asthma, some patients with asthma are poor responders and clinical studies have shown that those with severe disease are more likely to have glucocorticoid resistance.[136] Numerous mutations in the glucocorticoid receptor gene that alter expression, ligand binding, and signal transactivation have been identified; however, these are rare and studies in asthma have not revealed an obvious correlation between any specific polymorphism in the glucocorticoid receptor gene and a response to corticosteroid treatment. However, a number of studies have examined variations in components of downstream signaling pathways or other related genes.[135] For example, Tantisira and colleagues[137] demonstrated that variation in the adenyl cyclase 9 gene predicts improved bronchodilator response after corticosteroid treatment and also identified variation in the *CRHR1* locus,[138,139] *TBX21*,[140] and *GLCCI1*[141] as potential markers for steroid responsiveness.

However, many of these findings have not been replicated. This could be because of the use of different clinical endpoints, heterogeneity in study groups (i.e., age, sex, and disease severity), and patterns of treatment.

Genetic polymorphism may also play a role in regulating responses to anti-leukotrienes. In part, this is mediated by polymorphism in both *ALOX5* and other components of the leukotriene biosynthetic pathway.[137] There is also a substantial overlap in the genetic modulation of response to the two classes of leukotriene

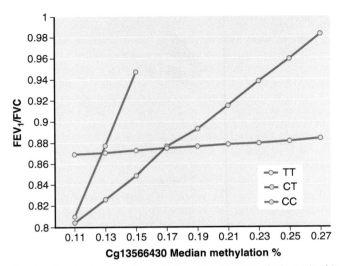

• **Fig. 3.4** Graph showing effect of interaction between single nucleotide polymorphism (SNP) at rs1800925 (*red, blue, and green lines* show different genotypes) and percentage methylation at cg13566430 on lung function (*FEV$_1$/FVC*). The modifying effect of genotype on the relationship between methylation and lung function demonstrates the interaction of early environment (methylation) and genetics (SNP).[97] *CC*, homozygous for the C allele; *CT*, heterozygous; *FVC*, forced vital capacity; *FEV$_1$*, forced expiratory volume in 1 second, *TT*, homozygous for the T allele.

modifier drugs (5-lipoxygenase inhibitors and cysteinyl leukotriene 1 receptor antagonists).[142] *ALOX5* polymorphisms also have been linked to asthma severity in children.[143]

The effect size of the genetic variants identified to date on treatment response are small, and/or there are no ready alternatives for therapy. Thus, although personalizing therapies based on genotypic profiling is now becoming a reality for some diseases, especially cancers, they are not yet applicable to allergic diseases such as asthma. However, the development of a number of biologic therapies, particularly for severe asthma, holds the promise of advancing personalized medicine approaches, including responder analyses based on pharmacogenetic parameters. For example, in a dose ranging study of a biologic (pitrakinra, a recombinant human IL-4 variant) inhibiting the IL-4/13 pathway, there was a significant dose-response effect on the primary endpoint of asthma exacerbation observed only in individuals with a specific *IL4RA* genotype, representing approximately one-third of the patient population.[144] Given that targeted biologic therapies are expensive, biomarkers such pharmacogenetic predictors of response, such as genotype, gene expression, and DNA methylation, could improve targeting of therapy to those who would most benefit, increasing efficacy and reducing the cost of prescribing to individuals who will not benefit.[135]

Epigenetics and Allergic Disease

The important role of epigenetics as a mechanism by which the environment can alter disease risk in an individual is being increasingly recognized. The term *epigenetics* refers to biologic processes that regulate gene activity but do not involve changes in the DNA sequence. Epigenetic processes include posttranslational modification of histones by acetylation and methylation, and DNA methylation (Fig. 3.4). Modification of histones, around which the DNA is coiled, alters the tightness with which the chromatin fiber is packed and affects the rate of transcription. DNA methylation involves the addition of

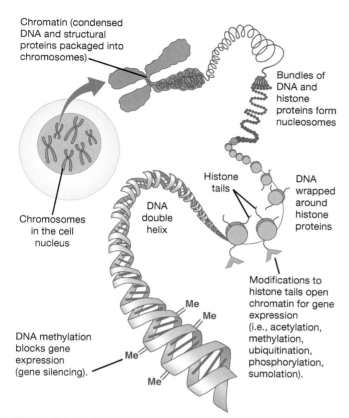

a methyl group to specific cytosine bases, altering gene expression. Increased DNA methylation in the promoter is typically associated with decreased gene expression, whereas within the body of the gene it is associated with increased gene expression, and around exon boundaries it can affect alternative splicing. DNA methylation patterns can be heritable across both cellular divisions (mitosis) and possibly across organismal generations (meiosis).[145] Epigenetic marks are altered by environmental exposures experienced by the individual, and these changes can last decades. Epigenetic profiles differ among individuals with and without allergic disease,[146–148] though it is important to note that this does not imply that they lie on the causal pathway, and in most cases these epigenetic changes can be consequences of allergic disease. Importantly, changes to histone modifications and DNA methylation can be induced by risk factors for allergy, such as tobacco smoke, cesarean birth, and maternal nutrition in early life.[149] This evidence strongly supports epigenetics as a mechanism by which the environment affects allergic disease risk and a mechanism by which gene-environment interaction can occur. Indeed, interactions between genetic variants and DNA methylation have been observed in asthma,[150,151] lung function,[97] (Fig. 3.5), and eczema.

However, in itself, environmentally induced epigenetic change to an individual's epigenome cannot explain the observed heritability of allergic disease; this would require the epigenetic change to be inherited through meiosis and the effect of exposure in one generation to lead to increased risk in subsequent generations. In humans, transgenerational effects have been observed in which the initial environmental exposure occurred in the F0 generation and changes in disease susceptibility were still evident in F2 (grandchildren).

What Can Genetics Studies of Allergic Disease Tell Us?

Greater Understanding of Disease Pathogenesis
- Identification of novel genes and pathways leading to new pharmacologic targets for developing therapeutics

Identification of Environmental Factors That Interact With an Individual's Genetic Make-Up to Initiate Disease
- Prevention of disease by environmental modification

Identification of Susceptible Individuals
- Early-life screening and targeting of preventive therapies to at-risk individuals to prevent disease

Targeting of Therapies
- Subclassification of disease on the basis of genetics and targeting of specific therapies based on this classification
- Determination of the likelihood of an individual responding to a particular therapy (pharmacogenetics) and individualized treatment plans

Observations such as grandmaternal and preconceptional paternal smoking increasing the risk of childhood asthma in their children and grandchildren support the concept that transgenerational epigenetic effects may be operating in allergic disease.[145] It is probable in the near future that the study of large prospective multigenerational birth cohorts will provide important insights into the role of epigenetic factors in the heritability of allergic disease.

Conclusions

The varying and sometimes conflicting results of studies to identify allergic disease susceptibility genes reflect the genetic and environmental heterogeneity seen in allergic disorders and illustrate the difficulty of identifying susceptibility genes for complex genetic diseases. This is the result of a number of factors, including difficulties in defining phenotypes and population heterogeneity, with different genetic loci showing association in populations of differing ethnicity and differing environmental exposure. However, despite this, there is now a rapidly expanding list of genes robustly associated with a wide range of allergic disease phenotypes.

This leads to the question of whether it possible to predict the likelihood that an individual will develop allergic disease. To an extent, clinicians already make some predictions of the risk of developing allergic disease through the use of family history, and this has been shown to have some validity.[152] However, at present, we are not in a position to use the rapidly accumulating knowledge of genetic variants that influence allergic disease progression in clinical practice. This simply reflects the complex interactions between different genetic and environmental factors required to initiate disease and determine progression to a more severe phenotype in an individual, meaning that the predictive value of variation in any one gene is low, with a typical genotype relative risk of 1.1 to 1.5.

However, it is possible that, as our knowledge of the genetic factors underlying disease increases, the predictive power of genetic testing will increase sufficiently to enable its use in clinical decision making (Box 3.1). For example, the development of polygenic risk scores for complex disease such as cardiovascular disease demonstrate the utility of polygenic risk profiling to identify groups of individuals at high risk, who could benefit from the knowledge of their susceptibility to disease.[153] Whether this is

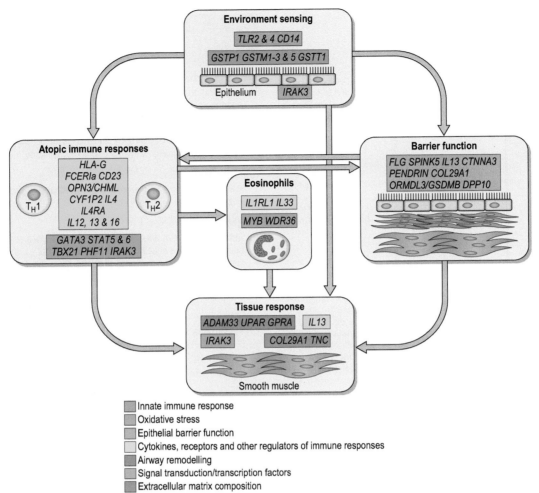

Environment sensing

TLR2 & 4 CD14

GSTP1 GSTM1-3 & 5 GSTT1

Epithelium | IRAK3

Atopic immune responses

HLA-G
FCERla CD23
OPN3/CHML
CYF1P2 IL4
IL4RA
IL12, 13 & 16

T_H1 | T_H2

GATA3 STAT5 & 6
TBX21 PHF11 IRAK3

Eosinophils

IL1RL1 IL33

MYB WDR36

Barrier function

FLG SPINK5 IL13 CTNNA3
PENDRIN COL29A1
ORMDL3/GSDMB DPP10

Tissue response

ADAM33 UPAR GPRA | IL13

IRAK3 | COL29A1 TNC

Smooth muscle

Innate immune response
Oxidative stress
Epithelial barrier function
Cytokines, receptors and other regulators of immune responses
Airway remodelling
Signal transduction/transcription factors
Extracellular matrix composition

• **Fig. 3.6** Susceptibility genes for allergic disease. A large number of robustly associated genes have been identified that predispose to allergic disease. These can be broadly divided into four main groups. *Group 1: Sensing the environment.* This group of genes encodes molecules that directly modulate the effect of environmental risk factors for allergic disease. For example, genes such as *TLR2*, *TLR4*, and *CD14* encoding components of the innate immune system interact with levels of microbial exposure to alter risk of developing allergic immune responses. Polymorphism of glutathione S-transferase genes (*GSTM1*, *-2*, *-3*, and *-5*, *GSTT1*, and *GSTP1*) have been shown to modulate the effect of exposures involving oxidant stress such as tobacco smoke and air pollution on asthma susceptibility. *Group 2: Barrier function.* The body is also protected from environmental exposure through the direct action of the epithelial barrier both in the airways and in the dermal barrier of the skin. A high proportion of the novel genes identified for susceptibility to allergic disease through genome-wide linkage and association approaches has been shown to be expressed in the epithelium. This includes genes, such as *FLG*, that directly affect dermal barrier function and are associated not only with increased risk of atopic dermatitis but also with increased atopic sensitization and inflammatory products produced directly by the epithelium, such as chemokines and defensins. Other novel genes, such as *ORMDL3/GSDMB*, are also expressed in the epithelium and may have a role in possibly regulating epithelial barrier function. *Group 3: Regulation of (atopic) inflammation.* This group of genes includes genes that regulate T_H1/ T_H2 differentiation and effector function such as *IL13*, *IL4RA*, *STAT6*, *TBX21* (encoding Tbet) and *GATA3* and genes such as *IRAK3* and *PHF11* that potentially regulate both atopic sensitization and the level of inflammation that occurs at the end organ location for allergic disease (airway, skin, nose, etc.). This also includes the genes associated with a range of allergic condition and the level of blood eosinophilia (*IL1RL1*, *IL33*, *MYB* and *WDR36*). *Group 4: Tissue response genes.* This group of genes appears to modulate the consequences of chronic inflammation, such as airway remodeling. They include genes such as *ADAM33* expressed in fibroblasts and smooth muscle and *COL29A1*, encoding a novel collagen expressed in the skin and linked to atopic dermatitis. It is important to recognize that some genes may affect more than one component; for example, *IL13* may regulate atopic sensitization through switching B cells to produce immunoglobulin E but also has direct effects on the airway epithelium and mesenchyme, promoting goblet cell metaplasia and fibroblast proliferation.

likely to improve on diagnostics using traditional risk factor assessment is a separate issue. Analyses of the power of genetic testing to predict risk of asthma demonstrate that, currently, the inclusion of common genetic variants has only a small effect on the ability to predict asthma development in childhood over and above clinical and environmental risk factors.[154] However, the identification of further risk factors and the development of better methods for incorporating genetic factors into risk models are likely to substantially increase the value of genotypic risk factors and may also provide a means for predicting progression to severe disease and targeting of preventive treatment in the future.

Whatever the future value of genetic studies of allergic disease in predicting risk, it is unlikely that this will be the area of largest impact of genetics studies on the treatment and prevention of these conditions. Rather, it is the insight the genetic studies have provided, and undoubtedly will continue to provide, into disease pathogenesis. It is clear from genetic studies of allergic disease that the propensity to develop atopy is influenced by factors different from those that influence atopic disease. However, these disease factors require interaction with atopy (or something else) to trigger disease. For example, in asthma, bronchoconstriction is triggered mostly by an allergic response to an inhaled allergen accompanied by eosinophilic inflammation in the lungs, but in some people who may have asthma susceptibility genes but not atopy, asthma is triggered by other exposures, such as toluene diisocyanate.[52] It is possible to group the identified genes into four broad groups (Fig. 3.6). First, there is a group of genes that are involved in directly modulating response to environmental exposures. These include genes encoding components of the innate immune system that interact with levels of microbial exposure to alter risk of developing allergic immune responses and detoxifying enzymes such as the glutathione S-transferase genes that modulate the effect of exposures involving oxidant stress, such as tobacco smoke and air pollution. The second major group that includes many of the genes identified through hypothesis-independent genome-wide approaches is a group of genes involved in maintaining the integrity of the epithelial barrier at the mucosal surface and signaling of the epithelium to the immune system after environmental exposure. For example, polymorphisms in *FLG* that directly affect dermal barrier function are associated not only with increased risk of AD but also with increased atopic sensitization. The third group of genes are those that regulate the immune response, including those such as *IL13, RAD50 IL4RA, STAT6, TBX21* (encoding Tbet), *FCER1A, HLA-G,* and *GATA3* that regulate T_H1/T_H2 differentiation and effector function, but also others, such as *IRAK3* and *PHF11,* that may regulate the level of inflammation that occurs at the end organ for allergic disease (i.e., airway, skin, nose, etc.). Finally, but not least, a number of genes appear to be involved in determining the tissue response to chronic inflammation, such as airway remodeling. They include genes such as *ADAM33* expressed in fibroblasts and smooth muscle and *COL29A1* encoding a novel collagen expressed in the skin and linked to AD.

Thus, the insights provided by the realization that genetic variation in genes regulating atopic immune responses are not the only, or even the major, factor in determining susceptibility to allergic disease, has highlighted the importance of local tissue response factors and epithelial susceptibility factors in the pathogenesis of allergic disease.[155] This is possibly the greatest contribution that

---

genetic studies have made to the study of allergic disease and the area in which the most impact in the form of new therapeutics targeting novel pathways of disease pathogenesis is likely to occur.

In conclusion, over the past 20 years, there have been many linkage and association studies examining genetic susceptibility to atopy and allergic disease resulting in the unequivocal identification of a number of loci that alter the susceptibility of an individual to allergic disease. Although research is needed to confirm previous studies and to understand how these genetic variants alter gene expression and/or protein function, and therefore contribute to the pathogenesis of disease, genetic studies have already helped change our understanding of these conditions. In the future, the study of larger cohorts and the pooling of data across studies will be needed to allow the determination of the contribution of identified polymorphisms to susceptibility and how these polymorphisms interact with each other and the environment to initiate allergic disease. Furthermore, it is now apparent that the added complexity of epigenetic influences on allergic disease needs to be considered. Despite these challenges for the future, genetic approaches to the study of allergic disease have clearly shown that they can lead to identification of new biologic pathways involved in the pathogenesis of allergic disease, the development of new therapeutic approaches, and the identification of at-risk individuals (Box 3.2).

The reference list can be found on the companion Expert Consult website at http://www.expertconsult.inkling.com.

4

Approach to the Child With Recurrent Infections and Molecular Diagnosis

CHARLOTTE CUNNINGHAM-RUNDLES

KEY POINTS

- Chronic/recurrent respiratory tract infections are common in children in general and more likely in those in daycare, those with young siblings, or those with allergy. However, chronic or recurrent infections also may be the presenting symptom of an underlying immune defect.
- Exclusion of other causes, such as cystic fibrosis, ciliary dyskinesia, and a swallowing disorder is important.
- Diagnosis of immunodeficiency in these cases is essential for optimal clinical management and best outcomes.

- The presenting features of immunodeficiency include chronic or recurrent infections, infections of unusual severity, infections caused by opportunistic pathogens, and autoimmune/inflammatory disorders.
- The types of infections and family history can guide the choice of screening laboratory tests.
- Mutation analyses can confirm the diagnosis and facilitate genetic counseling for the patients and for other family members.

Introduction

Overall Considerations

Recurrent or persistent infections are the most common manifestations of immunodeficiency; however, normal infants and children also have many infections, making it difficult in practice to decide if an immune defect is present.[1] Infections in normal children are also more likely when there are common exposures such as daycare, siblings of school age, or smoking caregivers.[2,3] Other common causes of recurrent infections include atopic disease or gastrointestinal reflux. The age of the child is also relevant; chronic otitis media is common in the first 2 years of life but decreases after this in frequency. Although bronchitis is common, it would be unusual for a child to have more than one episode of pneumonia in childhood, unless severe allergy or reflux is also present.[4]

Most children with recurrent infections have normal immunity; however, early recognition of immune defects in the allergy immunology practice is important, because appropriate treatment then can be launched, improving both quality of life and clinical outcomes. In general, the question of an immune deficit arises when infections are too numerous, too severe, or too long lasting. To attempt to put some specifics into this overall statement, some years ago the Jeffrey Modell Foundation proposed a list of warning signs, which have since been further amplified[5,6] (Box 4.1),

recognizing that with increasingly complex syndromes being described, a list of clinical presentations could never be inclusive.

Defects of the immune system may be primary, the result of genetic causes, or secondary, stemming from systemic conditions or intercurrent disease. Primary immune defects are inherited and commonly become evident in infancy or the first two decades of life, but it is important to remember that some immune defects do not manifest for some years after this (in adult life). Although the true incidence of primary immune defects is not known, estimates from a household survey were as high as 1 in 1200 live births.[7] To classify the primary defects, these are usually divided on the basis of the different immune systems affected: combined cellular (T and B) defects, less severe defects of T cells, defects of B cells, the phagocytic system, and complement. More recently, these divisions have been modified to include more complex disorders, including syndromes of immune dysregulation and immune defects that manifest with selected unusual infections as outlined later.[8] Secondary immune defects are more likely to be diagnosed later than infancy, with the most common global causes being malnutrition or human immunodeficiency virus (HIV) infection. Other systemic causes might include sickle cell disease, diabetes, or organ failure. Additional causes of chronic infections would be airway obstruction (e.g., eustachian tube dysfunction, tonsillar hypertrophy), cardiovascular disease, foreign body, exposure to infected pets, and so on.

• BOX 4.1 Overall Signs of Immunodeficiency

Overall Conditions
- Four or more new ear infections within 1 year
- Two or more serious sinus infections within 1 year
- Two or more months of antibiotics with little effect
- Two or more pneumonias within 1 year
- Failure to gain weight or grow normally (failure to thrive)
- Recurrent deep skin or organ abscesses
- Recurrent or resistant oral or cutaneous candidiasis
- Need for intravenous antibiotics and/or hospitalization to clear infections
- Two or more deep-seated infections (sepsis, etc.)
- Family history of immunodeficiency

Added Useful Clinical Considerations
- Infections with unusual microbial organism
- Lack of appropriate vaccinations
- Complications from a live vaccine (e.g., rotavirus, varicella, and bacillus Calmette-Guérin [BCG])
- Severe Epstein-Barr virus or other viral infection
- Shingles, measles, mumps, or rubella in an immunized child
- Chronic diarrhea
- Severe enteropathy
- Extensive skin lesions/nonhealing wounds

Severe Autoimmunity/Autoinflammatory Features
- Syndromic features (hypocalcemia/cardiac defects/absent thymic shadow, skeletal features suggestive of cartilage hair hypoplasia, etc.)
- Warts, molluscum contagiosum lesions that do not resolve

To determine whether an infant or child has an immune defect, the first approach includes a review of the medical and family history, followed by physical examination and targeted laboratory testing.

Medical and Family History

For a first step, it is important to consider the birth history and if there have been any infectious or toxic exposures. Second is to determine feeding history, food intolerances, and breastfeeding history. Next, one determines the numbers and types of illnesses that the child has experienced and over what length of time; the antibiotics prescribed, if any; responses to antibiotics; and if the child has missed school or other activities because of illnesses.[2] The results of cultures taken and results of blood tests or X-rays need to be collected. If illnesses have occurred, any complications such as hospitalizations, acute or chronic respiratory tract infections, weight loss, severe early-onset inflammatory bowel disease, the need for unusual medical procedures (e.g., mastoidectomy, abscess drainage, lymph node biopsy) are important to know.[1,3,9] The health of the other family members enters into this discussion as well and whether there has been travel or other exposures that might have an impact on the child's health. Complications that are unusual and would suggest that an immune defect might be present would be pneumonia leading to empyema or otitis media leading to mastoiditis. Shingles, measles, mumps, or rubella in an immunized child would be extremely uncommon and warrant an immune evaluation. However, it is also important to remember that infections in a patient with an immunodeficiency may not be severe or even progressive because of the rapid institution of antibiotic therapy; this is a common occurrence and may obscure this history. For this reason, many patients ultimately diagnosed with a primary immunodeficiency present with an infection history that is not easily distinguishable from that of a normal child.

In an allergy practice, rhinitis, asthma, and acute or chronic sinusitis are common issues. Patients with immune defects do not have symptoms different from those of others with allergic disease. It is important to note that primary immunodeficiencies and allergic disease can co-exist. A history of atopy with production of specific immunoglobulin E (IgE) makes some immune defects less likely, because the production of IgE suggests preserved T and B cell functions. However, the exceptions are important and include patients with selective IgA deficiency, common variable immunodeficiency (CVID), and DiGeorge syndrome. Children with both Wiskott-Aldrich and hyper-IgE syndrome are likely to have eczema. Males with X-linked immunodeficiency with polyendocrinopathy and enteropathy (IPEX) are also likely to have atopic disease. For these cases, additional clinical details can help distinguish these patients from other children with atopic disease. For Wiskott-Aldrich syndrome, these would be males with thrombocytopenia, eczema, immunodeficiency; for hyper-IgE syndrome, early-onset severe dermatitis, retained primary teeth, bone fractures, and pneumonia; for IPEX this would be males with food allergies, chronic diarrhea, and endocrinopathy, especially insulin-dependent diabetes.

Helping in the dissection of the medical history is a thorough review of the family history to seek relatives with frequent infections, unknown medical problems, autoimmunity, or malignancy. Parental consanguinity, the presence of family members with recurrent infections, early death, malignancy, or possibly autoimmune disease might of course suggest that a genetic illness may be identified. However, one must recognize that because of small family size and/or dispersed relatives, the lack of known family members with suggestive medical illnesses does not exclude a genetic defect in the child. A genetic defect also may not be at all obvious if there are very few males in the maternal lineage, in the case of de novo mutations, or in the presence of autosomal dominant defects with variable penetrance.

The type of infection, if known, can provide a clue to the type of immune defect that might be present; the most common defects, those of humoral immunity, are likelier to lead to respiratory tract infections with *Streptococcus pneumoniae, Haemophilus influenzae,* or mycoplasma infections. Gastrointestinal symptoms caused by *Giardia lamblia* commonly occur in patients with antibody defects such as CVID or selective IgA deficiency. T cell defects might be more likely to lead to viral infections or opportunistic infections such as *Mycobacterium avium-intracellulare* or *Pneumocystis jirovecii.* Deep infections or organ abscesses, especially with staphylococcal or gram-negative infections, are more suggestive of defects of the phagocytic system (neutropenia or chronic granulomatous disease). However, it should be recognized that recurrent staphylococcal infections may be rather common in childhood and may represent persistent colonization.[10] In complement deficiency, the more common medical infections are due to encapsulated bacteria. Often, in dissecting the medical history, in addition to the infections that have developed, additional medical complications experienced provide clues about the type of immune defect that might be present. For example, children with defects of antibody production may have had autoimmune disease (immune thrombocytopenia, hemolytic anemia) gastroenteritis with selected organisms, or have persistently enlarged cervical lymph glands or an enlarged spleen. Failure to thrive is common to most significant immune defects in childhood, but particularly this is characteristic of children with T cell defects. The more common infectious manifestations of each type of immune defect are outlined in Table 4.1.

TABLE 4.1	Patterns of Infections and Other Conditions in Primary Immunodeficiency	
	ILLNESSES	
Disorder	**Type of Infection**	**Other conditions**
Antibody defects	Sinopulmonary infections (*Streptococcus pneumoniae, Haemophilus influenzae,* or mycoplasma sp.) Gastrointestinal (enteroviruses, *Salmonella, Campylobacter, Giardia,* norovirus)	Autoimmune disease (thrombocytopenia, hemolytic anemia, neutropenia) Inflammatory bowel disease Lymphadenopathy, splenomegaly Otitis, mastoiditis
Cell-mediated immunity defects	Pneumonia *(Pneumocystis jirovecii), Mycobacterium avium-intracellulare* Severe Epstein-Barr infection Gastrointestinal disease (viruses, cytomegalovirus) Fungi of the skin, nails, mucous membranes	Failure to thrive Splenomegaly, lymphadenopathy
Defects of phagocytosis	Skin, liver, lymph nodes, abscesses (*Staphylococcus,* gram-negative bacteria, fungi)	Inflammatory bowel disease Granulomatous infiltrations
Defects of complement	Sepsis and other blood-borne encapsulated bacteria; meningitis, (*Streptococcus, Pneumococcus, Neisseria*)	Autoimmune disease (systemic lupus erythematosus, ANA+, glomerulonephritis)

Physical Examination

Recognizing that a child with a significant immune defect may still have a normal physical appearance, there are medical signs that the recurrent infections or other illness experienced may be due to a genetic immune defect. Growth patterns are foremost, because growth failure is often a key finding as children with chronic disease or immunodeficiency tend to have poor weight gain or loss, especially for the more severe immune defects. Weight, height, and head circumference need to be plotted and followed over time. Part of the physical examination is to determine if developmental milestones have been achieved, because in several of the syndromic immunodeficiencies (ataxia-telangiectasia and DiGeorge syndrome) there is a delay. For infants with cleft palate, history of hypocalcemia, and cardiac abnormalities, the diagnosis of DiGeorge syndrome (DGS) is likely.[11] Cervical lymphadenopathy, often with enlarged spleen, is more common in antibody defects such as CVID but may be seen in T cell defects as well. Small or apparently absent tonsils are often said to suggest X-linked agammaglobulinemia (XLA), but this is a soft sign and not often clinically useful. Whereas eczema and petechiae in males suggest Wiskott-Aldrich syndrome, severe facial and neck eczema with lymphadenopathy and possibly fungal skin or nail infections suggests hyper-IgE syndrome. Children with significant T cell dysfunction may have oral or nail candidiasis or molluscum contagiosum.

Types of Primary Immune Defects

Immune defects have been divided for about six decades on the basis of the different immune systems affected: combined cellular (T and B) defects, less severe defects of T cells, combined defects of B cells, the phagocytic system, and complement. However, with a dramatic increase in the numbers of recognized genetic immune defects, more complex disorders have been added to cluster defects for more readily understood categories. Now also included are a number of syndromes of immune dysregulation and immune defects that manifest with selected unusual infections. Although

not inclusive, a current outline of defects according to these new divisions, and some examples of each, are listed on Table 4.2. Particularly pertinent for the child with recurrent infections are the defects of intrinsic and innate immunity, in which selected organisms such as mycobacteria, encapsulated bacteria, herpes simplex, Epstein-Barr virus, or candida lead to severe or chronic disease.

The molecular causes of the majority of primary immunodeficiency diseases listed in Table 4.2 are known, but with one main exception. For most of the subjects with defects of antibody production, the most common type of immunodeficiencies, the molecular basis has not been clarified. This includes selective IgA deficiency, IgG subclass, specific antibody defects, and most cases of CVID. CVID has had some remarkable advances in the past decade but still about 70% of patients do not have a genetic diagnosis.[12] However, each year, new defects with characteristic clinical features are described. One of the main lessons that has been learned from these studies is that the same gene can lead to quite different clinical and immunologic outcomes, depending on the site of the mutation, the genetic background of the patient, and likely modifying genes.

Laboratory Studies

Screening Blood Tests

Screening blood tests for the evaluation of immune defects manifesting with infections are the first step and are outlined in Table 4.3.[13] A flow chart is included (Fig. 4.1), but more detailed flow charts, based on extended clinical phenotypes, have been published.[14] These are also available on free smart phone applications (https://play.google.com/store/apps/details?id=com.horiyasoft.pidclassification or https://itunes.apple.com/us/app/pid-phenotypical-diagnosis/id1160729399?mt=8). Complete blood count, including a white blood cell count, differential, and platelet counts, will show the absolute numbers of lymphocytes, neutrophils, and eosinophils based on age-related normal values. Lymphopenia (<1500 cells/mm^3) would be abnormal in a child with infections and would suggest further investigations, if not drug

TABLE 4.2   Types of Primary Immune Defects

Immunodeficiencies Affecting Cellular and Humoral Immunity

T⁻ B⁺ NK⁻ SCID	Common gamma chain (IL2RG, X-linked), JAK3
T⁻ B⁺ NK⁺ SCID	IL7α, T cell receptor defects, CD45, PNP deficiency
T⁻ B⁻ SCID	RAG1, RAG2 defects, adenosine deaminase deficiency

Combined Immunodeficiencies, Generally Less Severe

MHC class I and II defects; T cell receptor defects; DOCK8, IL21, and IL21R, and others

Combined Immunodeficiencies With Syndromic or Other Features

With thrombocytopenia	Wiskott-Aldrich syndrome
DNA repair defects	Ataxia telangiectasia, Nijmegen breakage syndrome; Bloom syndrome, dyskeratosis congenital, LIG-4
Hyper IgE syndromes	STAT3 loss of function, and others
Immuno-osseous dysplasias	Cartilage hair hypoplasia Schimke immuno-osseous dysplasia
Ectodermal dysplasia	IKBKG deficiency (NEMO)

Thymic Defects With Additional Congenital Anomalies

DiGeorge, velocardiofacial syndrome
CHARGE syndrome

Antibody Defects

Agammaglobulinemias	X-linked and autosomal forms of agammaglobulinemia
Hyper-IgM syndromes	X-linked and autosomal forms
IgG or IgA deficiency	IgG subclass and IgA deficiency
IgG, and IgA and or IgM deficiency	Common variable immunodeficiency

Diseases of Immune Dysregulation

Familial hemophagocytic lymphohistiocytosis	Perforin deficiency; UNC13D.
With hypopigmentation	Chediak-Higashi, Griscelli, Hermansky-Pudlak syndromes
With autoimmunity	Autoimmune polyendocrinopathy with candidiasis and ectodermal dystrophy, autoimmune lymphoproliferative syndrome
With defects of regulatory T cells	X-linked immune dysregulation, polyendocrinopathy enteropathy (IPEX), defects of CTLA4, STAT3
Leading to severe Epstein-Barr virus	X-linked autoimmune lymphoproliferative syndrome, XIAP deficiency, magnesium transporter 1 (MAGT1)
With colitis	IL-10 defects

Congenital Defects of Phagocyte Number or Function

Neutropenia	Elastase deficiency, HAX1 deficiency, and others
Defects of motility	Leukocyte adhesion deficiency
Defects of respiratory burst	Chronic granulomatous disease
Other nonlymphoid defects	GATA2 deficiency

Defects in Intrinsic and Innate Immunity

Mycobacterial disease	IL-12, IL-23, INF-g, STAT1 defects, and others
Warts	Epidermodysplasia verruciformis (EVER), hypogammaglobulinemia, infections, myelokathexis syndrome (WHIM)
Viral infections	STAT1, STAT2, IRF7, and others
Herpes simplex encephalitis	TLR3, UNC93B1
Fungal diseases	CARD9, IL17 defects, STAT1
Bacterial susceptibility	IRAK4, MYD88, IRAK1, and others

continued

TABLE 4.2	Types of Primary Immune Defects—cont'd
Complement Deficiency	
Classical pathway	C1q-C9 defects
Alternative pathway	Factors B, D, I, H, properdin, and others
Regulatory and membrane controls	Co-factor proteins

CHARGE defect, Disorder with coloboma, heart defects, atresia choanae (also known as choanal atresia), growth retardation, genital abnormalities, and ear abnormalities; *Ig,* immunoglobulin; *PNP,* purine nucleoside phosphorylase; *SCID,* severe combined immunodeficiency.

TABLE 4.3	Screening Tests for Immunodeficiency Disorders
Suspected Abnormality	**Diagnostic Tests**
Antibody	Quantitative immunoglobulins (IgG, IgA, IgM)
	Antibody responses to immunizations: tetanus, diphtheria, chickenpox, haemophilus, pneumococcal vaccines
Cell-mediated immunity	CBC: absolute lymphocyte count
	Lymphocyte panel: CD3, CD4, CD8
	T cells: CD45 RO/RA, percent and numbers
	T lymphocyte function in vitro: proliferation to mitogens and antigens
	Chromosome 22q
Complement	Total hemolytic complement (CH$_{50}$), alternative complement (AH$_{50}$)
Phagocytosis	CBC: absolute neutrophil count
	Neutrophil oxidative burst (dihydrorhodamine test by flow cytometer)

CBC, Complete blood count; *Ig,* immunoglobulin.

induced (steroids in particular). Lymphopenia is usually a feature of T cell defects, such as DiGeorge syndrome, or combined immunodeficiency disorders. Note that all infants born in the United States are now examined at birth by a DNA test that reflects the number of T cell excision circles (TRECS); deficiency or loss of TRECS suggests defective absent thymic development. When low TREC levels are detected, infants are referred to specialty centers to determine causes; among these are the severe combined immunodeficiency (SCID), DiGeorge syndrome, prematurity, idiopathic lymphopenia, and, as also has been reported, ataxia telangiectasia.[15] HIV testing is of course indicated in any patient with a suspected T cell defect, done using antibody titers or, preferably, polymerase chain reaction. Neutropenia most often occurs secondary to immunosuppressive drugs, infection, malnutrition, or autoimmunity but may be a primary problem (congenital or cyclic neutropenia). A cell count below 1500 per mm³ would be labeled as mild neutropenia, whereas counts below 1000/mm³ and 500/mm³ are designated as moderate and severe neutropenia, respectively; for these, further workup will be required.[16] Chronic neutrophilia might suggest a leukocyte adhesion defect (LAD). Thrombocytopenia would suggest consideration of Wiskott Aldrich in a male patient, but other causes are DiGeorge syndrome, CVID, and IgA deficiency. Examination of red blood cells can yield a clue about splenic function—in particular, positive findings on blood smear for Howell-Jolly bodies may be seen in peripheral blood in cases of splenic dysfunction or absence. For the general chemistries, a low serum calcium value might suggest DGS whereas a low serum protein (globulin fraction) value would suggest a humoral immune defect. Cultures of any infections, where possible; the respiratory tract; the throat; and abscesses are important. In screening tests, the inclusion of renal and liver function tests, electrolytes, glucose tests, and urine analysis are important in the assessment of every patient. For children with chronic sinopulmonary infections, one would want to consider if a sweat chloride test or a nasal ciliary biopsy could be appropriate. With these basic screening tests in hand, the next step is to examine the individual immune compartments.

Evaluation of Humoral Immunity

Determination of serum IgG, IgA, and IgM actually serves as a screening test for all immunodeficiencies. Not only are defects of immune globulin and antibody the most common congenital defects, but individuals with T cell defects are also likely to have abnormal levels and poor antibody production. The first test is quantitative serum immune globulins (not serum protein electrophoresis or immunoelectrophoresis), interpreted using age-related standards. This test does not examine function, so the next step is to determine the titers of antibody to common childhood vaccines: tetanus toxoid, diphtheria, pneumococcal, or *Hemophilus influenzae* polysaccharide/protein conjugate vaccines. Some children will respond well to protein vaccine antigens but not polysaccharide antigens, a form of immunologic immaturity that may or may not persist. Other children may produce normal antibody responses to vaccines but then the protective antibody level disappears 6 to 12 months after immunization—another sort of immune defect.[17] Selective deficiencies of IgG subclasses are known, but the significance, unless there are proven antibody defects, is unclear.[18] Although vaccine responses are essential in this evaluation, until the immunologic capabilities of the patient are clear, live viral vaccines should not be given.[19] Also commonly useful is the determination by flow cytometry of B cell numbers. If there is a lack of B cells in a patient with pan-hypogammaglobulinemia, the diagnosis of XLA in males or, less likely, an autosomal form of agammaglobulinemia can

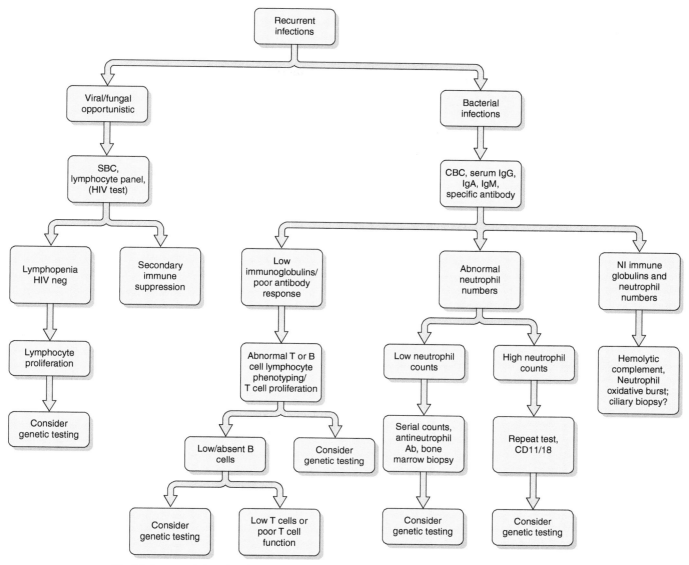

• **Fig. 4.1** A suggested workup for a child with recurrent infections using the medical history and screening tests as a guide. *CBC,* Complete blood count; *HIV,* human immunodeficiency; *Ig,* immunoglobulin;

be made. More recently, and of some clinical value, is the determination of memory B cell subsets; these examine the relative proportion of B cells that are activated and isotype switched, a marker of normal B cell capacity, but these studies do not substitute in the workup for actual documentation of functional antibody production.

Evaluation of high IgE levels deserves particular attention as children with high levels are commonly seen in allergy practice. For children with severe eczema, skin infections, and sometimes local abscesses that require drainage, a high serum IgE level might suggest the diagnosis of hyper-IgE syndrome. A scoring system used for older children and adults has been proposed,[20] but it works less well for young children who are not likely to display the characteristic facial features and in whom bacterial lung infections have not yet been a major feature. An additional scoring system for children has been proposed and a workflow suggested for this consideration.[21]

Evaluation of Cell-Mediated Immunity

Evaluation of defects of cell-mediated immunity starts with examination of the T cell compartment by flow cytometry on peripheral blood. As noted previously, infants with SCID and often DGS generally have decreased numbers of lymphocytes and thus low CD3, CD4, and CD8 T lymphocyte counts. Additional markers commonly used in flow cytometry to dissect the T cell phenotype are CD45RA (naïve) and CD45RO (memory) T cell subsets. CD45RA T cells are abundant in normal infancy but reduced in many immune deficient states. Further analysis of T cells might include expression of the α/β or γ/δ T cell receptor as perturbations suggest specific defects of T cell maturation. Although, as noted earlier, all newborns born after 2018 in the United States will have been screened for severe thymic defects, leading to the identification of infants with SCID and DiGeorge syndrome, in rare cases in which there are residual T cells and the congenital defect may be missed. For such infants, lymphocyte subset analyses need to be done.[15] The lack of a thymic shadow has been suggested as an indicator of thymic loss, but in practice a stressed infant will also have an X-ray suggesting thymic hypoplasia. If DGS is under consideration, fluorescence in situ hybridization to detect the 22q11 deletion is the preferred method. Knowing the numbers of T cells and subsets is a good start, but this does not reveal T cell functions. For this, one must assess in vitro proliferative response of T cells to mitogens (phytohemagglutinin A, concanavalin A) or, somewhat less useful in children, antigens (tetanus toxoid, candida).[22] Delayed-type hypersensitivity (skin testing) has been used, but with no standardized reagents and/or insufficient exposure to the antigens used the method is no longer particularly useful. An indirect marker for normal T cell function is antibody production to protein antigens; thus, the evaluation of vaccine responses can be helpful for this.

Evaluation of the Complement System

The most useful screening test for the complement deficiencies is the total serum hemolytic complement assay (CH_{50}), which depends on the functions of all of the components of the classical complement pathway, C1 through C9. A deficiency of any of these components will lead to an absent or very low CH_{50}.[23] In autoimmunity, consumption of complement components can also reduce the CH_{50} but does not eliminate it. Factor H, factor I, and properdin defects are quite rare but might be suspected if serum C3 level is low. Some laboratories also can test AH_{50}, which assesses the alternative pathway. A decreased AH_{50} test result suggests a deficiency in factor B, factor D, or properdin. A decrease in both CH_{50} and AH_{50} test results suggests deficiency in a shared complement component (from C3–C9). It is crucial to recall that a low CH_{50} is also very common in any sample that has not had proper handling or has been delayed in transit to the laboratory. Finally, sometimes measured but with no certain medical connection, mannose-binding lectin (MBL) is a serum protein that binds to numerous carbohydrates on microorganisms, ranging from viruses to parasites. Genetically about 5% of individuals can be found to be homozygous or compound heterozygous for mutations that lead to MBL "deficiency." In children some reports noted increased respiratory tract infections, but this was not the case in adults. Overall, there appears to be no reason to diagnose MBL deficiency in individual patients with infectious diseases.[24]

Evaluation of Phagocytic Cells

As for other immune functions, the evaluation of the phagocytic system includes determination of both numbers and function. First, a neutrophil count below 1500/mm³ would be labeled as mild neutropenia and counts below 1000/mm³ and 500/mm³ would be designated as moderate or severe neutropenia, respectively. In many cases the cause is known, such as medications, or it may be a viral infection or be caused by autoantibodies. Rarely the cause is a congenital neutropenia, autosomal dominant or recessive in inheritance.[16] As for causes, the diagnosis of cyclic neutropenia requires absolute neutrophil counts 2 to 3 times a week for 4 to 6 weeks. Severe congenital neutropenia is suggested if counts are less than 500 per/mm³ on several occasions. Here, bone marrow analysis is useful to exclude insufficient production or maturation arrest. Autoimmune neutropenia of infancy is accompanied by specific antineutrophil antibodies. High neutrophil counts suggest persistent infection or a lack of neutrophil migration because of leukocyte adhesion deficiency (LAD). When counts are normal but there is a suspicion of abnormal function, assessment of bactericidal activity is essential. For the most common of the congenital disorders, chronic granulomatous disease, the flow cytometric dihydrorhodamine (DHR) test measures the neutrophil oxidative metabolic response of neutrophils and can supply information about the residual oxidative capacity of the neutrophils.[25,26] The older nitroblue tetrazolium blue (NBT) test

has been used for decades, and although the test has been useful, it is difficult to apply in clinical medicine because it requires a fresh sample and experienced hands in a laboratory that still does this test.

Molecular Diagnosis

There are two main approaches to molecular diagnosis. In some cases the specific combination of clinical, family, and laboratory features will lead to an almost certain diagnosis, such as severe hypogammaglobulinemia with absent B cells in a male infant, which would be X-linked agammaglobulinemia. Here single gene testing may be the preferred and the most cost-effective route. In other cases, one could use a guide to molecular diagnostic testing in SCID because the pattern of T, B, and natural killer (NK) cell deficiency can suggest the type of defect (Fig. 4.2). However, in many cases, the clinical history is complex and the laboratory tests less clear cut; thus, a simple algorithm is not applicable. In these cases, a gene panel that includes a set of SCID genes can be used. For other immune defects, similar panels of genes targeting specific disease categories are available (e.g., antibody defects, inflammatory disease panels). Whole exome (or whole genome) sequencing is increasingly used, usually followed by the application of larger panels of 200 to 300 genes known to lead to primary immunodeficiency syndromes.[27,28] This method is particularly useful when unusual or complex phenotypes are present and unbiased genomic analyses are needed. These have been shown to be another highly successful method of either identifying or, more often, excluding these particular genes from consideration. In terms of overall frequency, autosomal recessive mutations have been more common than the autosomal dominant forms, but in the past few years the numbers of autosomal dominant defects have been increasing in numbers. However, with these one must remember that although "dominant," many of these have variable penetrance, making the family's genetic history not always easily deciphered. The results from large-scale genetic studies have also shown how one gene, with either gain or loss of function, can lead to completely different phenotypes. Examples of this are loss-of-function mutations in signal transducer and activator of transcription 1 (STAT1) that may lead to severe viral or mycobacteria diseases, whereas gain-of-function mutations cause chronic mucocutaneous candidiasis. Similarly, loss-of-function mutations in STAT3 produce hyper-IgE syndrome, whereas gain-of-function mutations produce both autoimmunity and lymphoproliferation. In general, for the more severe immune defects, determination of the genotype should be sought whenever possible to confirm the clinical diagnosis and direct therapy, for example, enzyme replacement therapy, bone marrow transplantation, or gene therapy. The genotype can be essential when it may provide critical prognostic information, for example, for patients with defects of DOCK8, in which there is a significant risk of malignancy. In other cases, identification of the causative genes can lead to a specific therapy, such as in patients with defects of CTLA4 or LRBA, in which a biologic agent (abatacept) has shown promise, or in defects of PI3kinase, which may be ameliorated by sirolimus. In all cases, knowing the genotype allows for genetic counseling and carrier testing, as well as prenatal or early postnatal diagnosis.

Treatment and Outcomes

Treatment of primary immunodeficiency is based on correction, to whatever extent possible, of the underlying immune

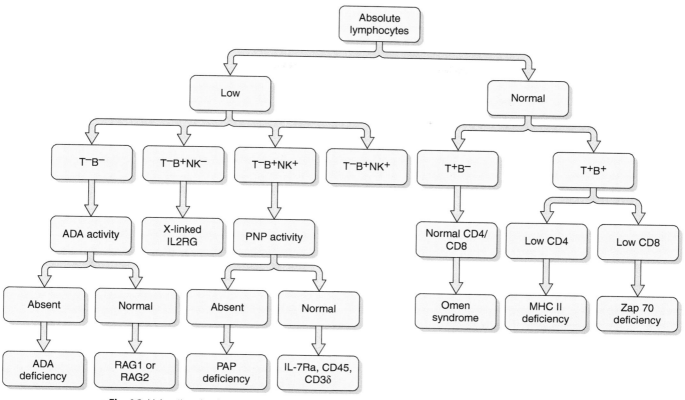

• **Fig. 4.2** Using the absolute lymphocytes count as a starting place to suggest the type of severe combined immunodeficiency (SCID) that may be present. *ADA,* Adenosine deaminase; *PNP,* purine nucleoside phosphorylase.

loss. The most common immune defects are those that lead to loss of antibody production; therefore, the mainstay of therapy will be immune globulin treatment by intravenous or subcutaneous routes. The doses are generally 400 to 600 mg/kg, given once a month, or with the same totals, but divided into injections weekly or biweekly. These products supply protective antibodies to the great majority of the organisms encountered and protection against the agents in common vaccines such as tetanus, diphtheria, measles, and varicella.[29] For all patients with immune defects, adequate treatment is essential to prevent infectious complications and organ damage. The outcomes of insufficient treatment of the respiratory tract, for example, are well known and include irreversible lung damage.[30] For severe cellular defects, stem cell transplantation or in some cases gene therapy[31,32] is required; with early diagnosis before invasive or persistent infections have occurred, successful restoration of immune function is likely.[15] Advances in this therapy have led to the use of lentiviral vectors to allow transmission of a corrected gene copy. If there is no appropriate donor match, hematopoietic stem cell transplantation can be done from a haploidentical family, using posttransplant cyclophosphamide, which reduces the risks of graft failure and

graft-versus-host disease.[33] Although stem cell transplants have been pioneered for SCID conditions, with the understanding that other genetic immune defects will lead to lifetime risks of infections, autoimmunity, and cancer, transplantation has been increasingly used for other immune defects, for example, the *DOCK8* defect.[34]

Conclusions

Recurrent or persistent infection is a major manifestation of primary immunodeficiency. Most children with recurrent infection have normal immunity; however, it is important to be vigilant in this population for unusually frequent or severe infections. The early involvement of a clinical immunologist in cases of suspected immunodeficiency is crucial because early investigation and treatment of a child with an underlying primary immunodeficiency can prevent significant end organ damage and improve survival and long-term outlook.

The reference list can be found on the companion Expert Consult website at http://www.expertconsult.inkling.com.

5

Primary Antibody Deficiency

PAUL J. MAGLIONE

KEY POINTS

- Primary antibody deficiency is the most common type of primary immunodeficiency and constitutes a range of immune deficit and clinical presentation.
- Clinicians must maintain an index of suspicion for primary antibody deficiency, and the diagnosis should be considered in those with a history of recurrent sinopulmonary infections.
- Immunoglobulin replacement therapy (by the intravenous or subcutaneous routes) and antibiotics form the backbone of management for primary antibody deficiency.

- Early recognition of primary antibody deficiency may help limit chronic medical complications.
- Some forms of primary antibody deficiency, such as selective immunoglobulin A (IgA) deficiency and IgG subclass deficiency, are relatively common and may not require treatment if found in asymptomatic individuals.

Introduction

The most common forms of primary immunodeficiency are those that predominantly impair antibody production, known collectively as primary antibody deficiency (PAD).[1] Antibodies are a vital aspect of humoral immunity and a fundamental component of the adaptive immune system. PAD results from absence of one or more immunoglobulin (antibody) isotypes and/or the ability to produce specific antibody responses against infection and vaccination. Although cellular immune defenses are often intact in PAD, some individuals with PAD have immune defects that extend beyond antibody deficiency. PADs account for more than half of primary immunodeficiency diagnoses, constituting a relatively broad group of disorders with varying scope of severity.[2,3] PAD typically predisposes to recurrent sinopulmonary infections, but chronic medical complications, including autoimmune, gastrointestinal (GI), and pulmonary disease, also occur and can be very challenging to manage.[4,5] Early recognition of PADs may help limit these complications. However, PAD diagnosis is typically delayed 5 years or more after symptoms are first reported, and this diagnostic delay is associated with development of chronic sequelae that increase morbidity and may affect survival.[6,7] It is also important to note that asymptomatic patients with reduced levels of immunoglobulin are occasionally found and may present a treatment dilemma. In this section, we will provide an overview of PAD diagnoses and cover diagnostic and therapeutic considerations to aid in the care of these patients.

Despite being the most common primary immunodeficiency, the genetic basis for most PAD cases is unknown and family history is rarely present.[8] Thus, in many cases, the etiology of PAD may be multifactorial and perhaps different between those with adult or pediatric onset. Evaluation of PAD is usually initiated because the patient reports frequent pneumonias or other respiratory bacterial infections (e.g., bronchitis, otitis media, or sinusitis). Recurrent sinopulmonary infections is the most common clinical presentation of such patients. Currently, there are no evidence-based guidelines to identify children who should be screened for PAD. Given the relatively low cost of quantitative immunoglobulin measurement but high burden of recurrent infections and potential complications for both medical care and patient morbidity, it is reasonable for pediatricians to have clinical suspicion for PAD in children with recurrent or particularly severe sinopulmonary infections.

The nature of antibody deficiency differs among the various forms of PAD and, accordingly, etiologies of immunodeficiency can be diverse as well. Some forms of PAD result from intrinsic defects of B cells, whereas others may be due to impairment of immune cells that promote or regulate antibody responses and do not affect B cells directly. Moreover, susceptibility to chronic, noninfectious complications vary among PAD diagnoses. Due to the important role of antibodies in protection against respiratory bacterial infection, the various PADs can all present with recurrence of these infections, including bronchiectasis, pneumonia, and sinusitis. Typical pathogens underlying sinopulmonary infections are similar to those without immunodeficiency and include *Haemophilus influenzae, Moraxella catarrhalis,* and *Streptococcus pneumoniae.* Heightened susceptibility to respiratory viral infections may also occur in PAD, particularly in those with chronic lung disease.[9] Appropriate usage of antibiotics and immunoglobulin replacement therapy (IRT) has reduced the incidence of severe infections, including pneumonia, and improved survival of patients with PAD.[10,11] Yet, certain complications faced by some

- Congenital agammaglobulinemia should be considered in children presenting with recurrent infections and severe agammaglobulinemia, but without profound T cell deficiency.
- Circulating B cells are usually profoundly reduced or absent.
- X-linked agammaglobulinemia (XLA) is the most common form of congenital agammaglobulinemia and may demonstrate a family history of affected boys.
- XLA can be diagnosed by demonstrating absence of Bruton's tyrosine kinase by flow cytometry (typically done using monocytes as B cells are often absent in patients with suspicion of this diagnosis).

patients with PAD occur and/or progress despite these interventions.[6] Many of these complications may not simply be the result of infection or inadequate IRT but instead result from immune dysfunction inherent in certain patients with PAD. With this overview of the similarities and differences among patients with PAD, we will now discuss the various forms of PAD encountered in clinical practice.

Congenital Agammaglobulinemia

Congenital agammaglobulinemia typically results in the most profound absence of antibody of all the forms of PAD. These patients are defined by severe reduction in all immunoglobulin isotypes. Congenital agammaglobulinemia is usually caused by genetic impairment of expression and/or signaling via the pre-B cell receptor, which arrests B cell development prematurely. Because there is usually an absence of B cells, the clinical evaluation can be notable for absence of palpable lymph nodes or tonsils and blood tests showing profound deficiency of circulating B cells. The most common form of congenital agammaglobulinemia, accounting for about 85% of patients, is X-linked agammaglobulinemia (XLA). Mutation of the Bruton's tyrosine kinase gene, *BTK,* which is carried on the X chromosome, causes XLA because it provides vital signals via the pre-B cell receptor during development (Box 5.1).[12] Although most patients with XLA have agammaglobulinemia (severe deficiency of all immunoglobulin isotypes), there are rare cases with less severe and more variable presentation.[13] In addition to XLA, there are autosomal recessive etiologies that account for approximately 15% of congenital agammaglobulinemia cases.[14] Like XLA, these rarer autosomal recessive etiologies affect genes involved in signaling through the pre-B cell receptor and consequently arrest B cell development in the bone marrow. Mutations in *IGHM, BLNK, CD79A, CD79B, IGLL1,* and *PIK3R1* have been reported as causes of autosomal recessive agammaglobulinemia.[15,16]

Children with congenital agammaglobulinemia typically present with recurrent bacterial infections after the first 6 months of life, coinciding with waning of maternal antibody acquired through the placenta. Approximately 60% of patients with congenital agammaglobulinemia develop recurrent sinopulmonary infections, but infections leading to arthritis, chronic conjunctivitis, gastroenteritis, meningitis, osteomyelitis, pyoderma, and sepsis are also reported.[17] Common bacterial pathogens of the respiratory tract, such as *H. influenzae* and *S. pneumoniae,* are most frequently found, but it is also thought that congenital agammaglobulinemia predisposes to certain viral infections, namely enteroviruses and hepatitis viruses. Perhaps because of their early clinical onset in

many cases, genetic etiologies are more commonly recognized in those with congenital agammaglobulinemia compared with other forms of PAD. Yet diagnostic delay is still significant in these cases, with the average age of diagnosis being 2.6 years in those with a family history of congenital agammaglobulinemia and 5.4 years in those without.[17]

Hyper–Immunoglobulin M Syndromes

The multiple types of hyper-IgM syndrome (HIGMS) are forms of PAD resulting from impaired switching of antibody isotypes. Under normal circumstances, immunoglobulins undergo class-switching from the IgD and IgM isotypes expressed on naïve B cells into IgA, IgG, and IgE on antigenic stimulation. Patients with HIGMS present with low levels of IgG and IgA along with normal or increased levels of IgM as a result of impairment of this immunoglobulin class–switching process. Patients with HIGMS have predisposition for autoimmunity, GI disease, and sinopulmonary infections.[18] The most common form of HIGMS, accounting for about 70% of cases, is due to mutations of *CD40LG,* which encodes CD40 ligand (CD40L) and is inherited on the X chromosome.[19] This form of HIGMS is sometimes referred to as type 1. A very rare form of autosomal recessive HIGMS affecting CD40 has been reported and can be referred to as type 3.[20] CD40:CD40L interaction is required for antibody isotype class switching and T cell activation of phagocytes, causing an immune defect that extends beyond antibody deficiency and is associated with a broader susceptibility to microbes, including infections with *Pneumocystis jirovecii* and cytomegalovirus.[21]

Despite IRT and antimicrobial prophylaxis, patients with X-linked HIGMS have heightened mortality risk, leading to use of hematopoietic stem cell transplant for many patients that has achieved encouraging results in those who have not developed liver disease.[22] In patients with X-linked HIGMS with liver disease, a combined hematopoietic stem cell and liver transplant may be advisable.[23] Although not impairing the CD40:CD40L interaction, mutation of *AICDA,* which encodes an enzyme vital to antibody isotype switching known as activation-induced cytidine deaminase, is the most common autosomal recessive cause of HIGMS. This form of HIGMS is referred to as type 2. Autosomal recessive mutation of *UNG,* which encodes uracil DNA glycosylase, also results in HIGMS with profound lymphoid hyperplasia, mimicking the phenotype of *AICDA* mutation–associated HIGMS and is referred to as type 5.[24] Those with HIGMS but without disease-causing mutations in the previously listed genes can be grouped into type 4. Some patients with common variable immunodeficiency (CVID) or monogenic causes of CVID-like syndromes, such as gain-of-function mutation in *PIK3CD,* can have elevated IgM levels with deficiency of isotype-switched immunoglobulins and thus mimic HIGMS.

Common Variable Immunodeficiency

CVID is thought to be the most common symptomatic primary immunodeficiency, with an estimated prevalence of about 1:25,000.[25] Patients with CVID have extensive heterogeneity of clinical presentation and genetic etiology, but all are unified by the defining laboratory characteristics of profoundly low levels of IgG and IgA or IgM, along with defective antibody responses, typically demonstrated by nonprotective antibody levels after vaccination.[26] CVID is not diagnosed before the age of 4 because of the possibility that the laboratory findings are due to transient hypogammaglobulinemia of infancy. Consistent with patients with other forms of PAD, patients with CVID typically present with recurrent sinopulmonary infections. Although common pathogens affecting patients with CVID include bacteria seen in those with other PADs, infections of atypical sites, such as the joints, with organisms such as *Mycoplasma* and *Ureaplasma,* also have been described.[27]

Contributing to the "variable" of CVID, these patients have heightened risk of autoimmunity; granulomatous inflammation; benign lymphoid hyperplasia in the GI tract, lungs, lymph nodes, and spleen; and increased incidence of malignancy, particularly lymphomas.[5] The fundamental defect causing CVID is impaired B cell differentiation into antibody-producing plasma cells and isotype-switched memory cells, but T cell abnormalities are also observed in about half of patients.[28,29] Although some genetic associations have been identified, the etiology of CVID is not known in the majority of cases. Broader application of genomics may allow for more frequent identification of genetic etiologies, which may be of particular importance because some of the monogenic CVID-like syndromes that will be discussed later can have usage of precision therapies as a key component of their management.[30]

In contrast to most other primary immunodeficiencies, CVID is commonly diagnosed in adulthood, typically between the ages of 20 and 40. The age of onset is variable, and pediatric diagnosis also occurs, though the diagnosis is not made until the fourth year of life, as previously mentioned. Although the mechanism for the late onset of CVID is not understood, evidence from study of monogenic causes of CVID indicate that B cell function can be lost gradually over time, such as is the case with heterozygous mutations of *IKZF1.*[31] Understanding the diverse pathogenic mechanisms leading to CVID is an active area of ongoing research efforts.

A number of monogenic immunologic syndromes have been described in patients with CVID. The monogenic forms of PAD usually manifest earlier than other forms in patients with CVID, often in childhood. Such patients include those with autosomal dominant cytotoxic T lymphocyte–associated protein 4 (CTLA-4) haploinsufficiency or autosomal recessive lipopolysaccharide-responsive and beige-like anchor (LRBA) protein deficiency.[32-34] CTLA-4 is an inhibitory checkpoint molecule up-regulated by activated T cells or constitutively expressed by regulatory T cells to inhibit cell proliferation, and LRBA helps maintain intracellular stores of CTLA-4.[35–37] Autoimmunity, GI inflammation, lymphoid hyperplasia, and lymphocytic infiltration of organs occur in these patients in addition to recurrent infections.

Patients with CTLA-4 or LRBA deficiency may develop progressive loss of circulating B cells and hyperactivation of effector T cells, suggesting that antibody deficiency could be resulting from immune exhaustion secondary to persistent immune activation. Similarly, activated phosphoinositide 3-kinase δ (PI3Kδ) syndrome is a CVID-like disorder with autoimmunity, lymphoproliferation, and recurrent infections, though the PAD may be limited to IgG_2 subclass deficiency.[38] PI3Kδ syndrome results from gain-of-function mutation in *PIK3CD,* which is expressed in lymphocytes and encodes the p110δ subunit of PI3K, causing excessive lymphocyte proliferation that leads to elevated effector to naïve lymphocyte ratio and resultant CD4+ T cell lymphopenia, reduced isotype-switched B cells, variably elevated levels of IgM along with hypogammaglobulinemia, IgG subclass deficiency, and/or poor immune responses to the pneumococcal vaccine.[38–40] Children with PI3Kδ syndrome can be distinguished

by a unique constellation of lymphadenopathy, lymphoid hyperplasia of mucosal surfaces, and increased susceptibility to Epstein-Barr virus and cytomegalovirus. Patients with CTLA-4 or LRBA deficiency and PI3Kδ gain-of-function have hyperactivation of the mTOR pathway; treatment with rapamycin can be beneficial both for inflammation-related complications and decreasing immune exhaustion. Moreover, targeted therapy with abatacept for CTLA-4 or LRBA deficiency and PI3K inhibition, such as with leniolisib, may be beneficial.[41,42]

Gain-of-function mutation of signal transducer and activator of transcription 3 (STAT3) cause an autosomal dominant syndrome result in PAD with early-onset, severe multiorgan autoimmunity, GI disease, and/or lymphocytic interstitial lung disease.[43–45] Notably, targeted inhibition of interleukin-6 (IL-6) receptor or STAT signaling may be of benefit for the treatment of these complications in patients with STAT3 gain of function.[46] Although diagnosis of genetic etiologies associated with CVID is exciting, it must be noted that diverse clinical presentations, antibody deficiency not meeting diagnostic criteria for CVID, variable penetrance, and variants of known significance occur and complicate interpretations.

Immunoglobulin G Subclass Deficiency and Specific Antibody Deficiency

Patients with recurrent infections and who have deficiency (<5th percentile) of one or more IgG subclasses measured on two separate occasions at least 1 month apart, but normal levels of total IgG, IgA, and IgM, have selective IgG subclass deficiency.[27] IgG subclass deficiency is frequently found in asymptomatic children, and its clinical significance in such patients is uncertain. There are four IgG subclasses, with IgG_1 the most prevalent in the blood and IgG_4 the most scarce under normal conditions. Those with impaired antibody response to polysaccharide vaccination, typically the unconjugated pneumococcal vaccine, but normal levels of immunoglobulins, including IgG subclasses, have specific antibody deficiency.[47] These patients typically experience recurrent bacterial infections of the respiratory tract.

Sometimes those with specific antibody deficiency against polysaccharide vaccination also have IgG_2 subclass deficiency, because IgG_2 is thought to be the predominant IgG subclass mediating immunity against carbohydrate antigens. IgG subclass deficiency and/or specific antibody deficiency are also associated with broader immunologic syndromes, such as Wiskott-Aldrich, ataxia-telangiectasia, and the monogenic immunologic syndromes discussed previously, such as PI3Kδ syndrome.[27,38,48–50] It is important to note that IgG against pneumococcal carbohydrate antigens may not reach maturity until the teenage years in some individuals, so caution must be taken when considering a diagnosis of specific antibody deficiency in children.[51,52]

Selective Immunoglobulin A Deficiency

Although most often asymptomatic, selective IgA deficiency (IgAD) is the most common primary immunodeficiency, occurring in about 1:600 throughout Europe and North America.[53] Children can be diagnosed with IgAD upon turning 4 years old and have absent serum IgA (<7 mg/dL) with IgG and IgM within the normal range.[54] Those with symptomatic IgAD typically have recurrent bacterial infections of the respiratory tract and heightened risk of allergy, autoimmunity, and GI disease.[55] IgG subclass

Differential Diagnosis of Recurrent Respiratory Tract Infections

Primary Antibody Deficiency
- Other primary immunodeficiencies with antibody deficiency (severe combined immunodeficiency, DiGeorge syndrome, Wiskott-Aldrich syndrome, many others)

Secondary Antibody Deficiency
- Complement deficiency
- Phagocyte defects (chronic granulomatous disease, leukocyte adhesion deficiency, neutropenia, others)
- Cystic fibrosis
- Ciliary dysfunction
- Eustachian tube or ostiomeatal obstruction
- Allergic rhinosinusitis

deficiency, particular the IgG_2 subclass, occurs with increased frequency in those with IgAD, as does impaired antibody response to pneumococcal polysaccharide vaccination.[56] Of interest, IgAD is more commonly found in families with CVID, and numerous studies have reported progression of IgAD to CVID.[57–59] Moreover, mutations in transmembrane activator and CAML interactor, a receptor involved in B cell activation and maturation, are found in both CVID and IgAD.[60,61] In the vast majority of patients with IgAD, the genetic etiology is unknown. There are two subclasses of IgA, IgA_1 and IgA_2, but the clinical significance of IgA subclass evaluation is unknown.

Transient Hypogammaglobulinemia of Infancy

During the first 6 months of life infants gradually lose maternal IgG while they build up their own IgG levels. A subset of infants have delay in the build-up of their IgG, resulting in a form of hypogammaglobulinemia known as transient hypogammaglobulinemia of infancy (THI). These children are diagnosed through demonstration of IgG that is two standard deviations below the mean for age in a child older than 6 months in whom alternative diagnoses have been excluded.[62] This form of antibody deficiency can persist until around the age of 5 but always resolves eventually. Although many with THI are asymptomatic, some develop recurrent and/or severe otitis, sinusitis, bronchitis, pneumonia, recurrent diarrhea, and, rarely, sepsis or meningitis. Symptomatic THI can be managed with prophylactic antibiotics or immunoglobulin replacement therapy, with continued surveillance of the immune system to determine when these treatments can be halted.

Differential Diagnosis

Secondary causes of antibody deficiency and other conditions that predispose to infections similar to PAD must be considered in the clinical evaluation of these patients. Box 5.2 lists the differential diagnosis of recurrent respiratory infections, the typical presentation of PAD. Except in cases of profound hypogammaglobulinemia, secondary antibody deficiency can be differentiated from PAD by the preservation of protective antibody levels against vaccination. Important causes of secondary antibody deficiency to consider include excessive loss of protein or lymphatic fluid, immunosuppression (particularly from the use of B cell–targeted therapies such as rituximab), malignancy (i.e., chronic

lymphocytic leukemia, lymphoma, or multiple myeloma), severe malnutrition, and occasionally usage of anticonvulsive agents (carbamazepine, levetiracetam, phenytoin, and possibly others). Upon ruling out secondary antibody deficiency, a diagnosis of PAD can be formally considered.

Medical conditions other than antibody deficiency can lead to recurrent respiratory infections and thus should be considered in the differential diagnosis for PAD. Both cystic fibrosis and ciliary dysfunction can predispose to sinopulmonary infections, but these patients usually do not have immunoglobulin deficiency. Allergic rhinosinusitis and eustachian tube or ostiomeatal obstruction are more common causes of persistent rhinosinusitis and/or otitis symptoms in children than PAD, and these patients will not have abnormal immunologic findings. Other primary immunodeficiencies can manifest much like PAD. Complement deficiency and phagocyte defects, such as chronic granulomatous disease, can result in respiratory infections, but can be differentiated from PAD through laboratory evaluation. Antibody deficiency may be a feature of combined or other severe primary immunodeficiencies; however, these patients often present with a wider range of infections and are characterized by broader immunologic defects on laboratory evaluation.

Evaluation

Fig. 5.1 is a flow chart outlining a recommended approach for evaluation of a patient with suspected PAD. This algorithm expects that severe defects of cellular immunodeficiency, such as chronic granulomatous disease and severe combined immunodeficiency (SCID), have already been ruled out, because patients suspicious for these diagnoses require rapid intervention. Likewise, diagnoses of malignancy and secondary causes resulting from immunosuppression are considered to be ruled out. The algorithm may have to be modified based on the individual characteristics of the patient being evaluated. We will discuss the stepwise approach to diagnosis of PAD using numbers corresponding to the specific step in the clinical evaluation.

Referencing the algorithm in Fig. 5.1, (1) patients 4 years of age or older can be considered for the diagnosis of PAD, given the high occurrence of THI in younger patients. The evaluation of PAD is initiated with (2) measurement of serum immunoglobulins, including IgG subclasses, antibodies to vaccination, and lymphocyte subset (B, T, and NK cell) enumeration. If both IgG (3) and T cells (4) are profoundly reduced, a diagnosis of combined immunodeficiency should be pursued (see Chapter 6). If IgG is profoundly reduced (3) but T cells are not (4), levels of B cells are informative, with low levels indicative of congenital agammaglobulinemia or some forms of CVID (10) and normal levels suggestive of CVID and HIGMS (11).

If IgG is not found to be profoundly reduced (3), levels of antibodies to vaccination (5) are useful to identify specific antibody deficiency, when levels are low (8). If specific antibodies to vaccines are not reduced (5) and IgG subclasses are reduced, IgG subclass deficiency should be considered for the diagnosis (12). If IgG subclasses are not reduced but IgA is, selective IgA deficiency should be considered for the diagnosis (14). If IgA is in the normal range, alternative diagnoses should be considered (15), including defects of cellular immunity such as complement deficiency (Chapter 7), chronic granulomatous disease (Chapter 11), cystic fibrosis, ciliary dysfunction, Eustachian tube or ostiomeatal obstruction, and allergic rhinoconjunctivitis (Chapter 17).

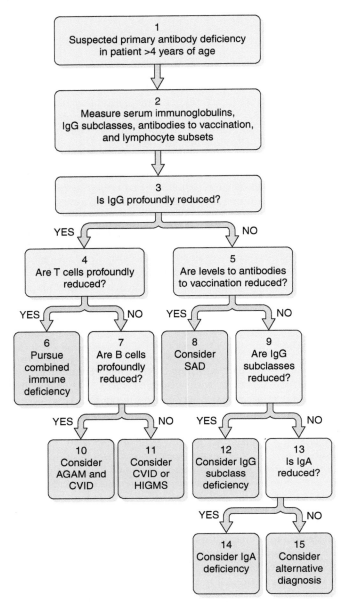

• **Fig. 5.1** Algorithm for evaluation of a patient with suspected primary antibody deficiency. *AGAM,* Congenital agammaglobulinemia; *CVID,* common variable immunodeficiency; *SAD,* specific antibody deficiency.

Treatment

The key therapeutic approaches for antibody deficiency are listed in Box 5.3. Mainstays of PAD management include antibiotics and IRT, but other considerations, such as infection avoidance and vaccination, often arise in discussion with patients and their families. Antibiotics can be used either in short courses to treat acute infections or for longer durations as prophylactic therapy. IRT functions as a form of passive immunity and comes in both intravenous and subcutaneous formulations. Intravenous immunoglobulin (IVIG) is typically dosed every 28 days, coinciding with the approximate half-life of IgG, but can be dosed more frequently if clinically warranted. Numerous formulations of subcutaneous IgG replacement exist, varying in terms of their concentration of IgG and presence of hyaluronidase, which allows for dosing every 4 weeks, as opposed to the standard weekly dosing or

---

• **BOX 5.3**   **Key Therapeutic Approaches for Antibody Deficiency**

Avoid Infection
- Practice appropriate personal and public hygiene

Treat Infections
- Standard doses of antibiotics, consider extended (double length) courses

Prevent Infections
- Antibiotic prophylaxis (see following table)
- Immunoglobulin replacement therapy (IRT) (see Chapter 10)
- Annual immunization against influenza (recombinant, not live, vaccine)

Antibiotic	Children	Adults
amoxicillin (consider with clavulanate)	10–20 mg/kg daily or bid	500 mg daily or bid
trimethoprim (TMP)/ sulfamethoxa-zole (dosing for TMP)	5 mg/kg daily	160 mg daily
azithromycin	10 mg/kg weekly or 5 mg/kg every other day	250 or 500 mg daily, or every Monday, Wednesday, Friday
clarithromycin	7.5 mg/kg daily or bid	500 mg daily or bid

dosing every 2 weeks of other subcutaneous formulations. IRT is designed to replace IgG; no products exist for substantial reconstitution of IgA or IgM. Intravenous and subcutaneous IRT are therapeutically equivalent, so selection of the administration method is based on the preferences and clinical considerations of the individual patient. More information regarding IRT is reviewed in Chapter 10.

Bacterial infections frequently occur in patients with PAD; therefore, antibiotic courses may be frequently used even after the initiation of IRT. Selection of antibiotic is shaped by site and severity of infection, allergy history, antibiotic sensitivity of the pathogen (if available), and even history of antibiotic use (to potentially limit resistance). Although a diagnosis of primary immunodeficiency does not warrant dose adjustment of antibiotics, a longer treatment course may be needed. Antibiotic prophylaxis can be useful to limit frequency of acute infections and should be considered in those in whom the form of PAD may not be severe enough to warrant IRT initially. However, if infections persist despite antibiotic prophylaxis, IRT should be considered. Suggested antibiotic prophylaxis regimens are included in Box 5.3. Depending on the seasonal occurrence of infections, antibiotic prophylaxis may be limited to certain times of year (such as the winter) or may need to be used year-round. Similarly, depending on the severity and course of antibody deficiency, necessity of antibiotic prophylaxis may need to be re-evaluated from time to time.

For patients with the diagnosis of agammaglobulinemia, CVID, or HIGMS, IRT is the standard of care.[27] For other forms of antibody deficiency, including IgG subclass deficiency, specific antibody deficiency, hypogammaglobulinemia not meeting the criteria for CVID, IgAD (with IgG subclass deficiency), transient hypogammaglobulinemia of infancy, or secondary antibody deficiency, IRT should be considered on a case-by-case basis. In general, for types of antibody deficiency in which IRT is not the standard of care, prophylactic antibiotics are tried first in those in whom infections are numerous.[63] Of importance, IRT is not likely to be beneficial in patients with IgAD without some evidence of significant IgG impairment, such as IgG subclass deficiency or specific antibody deficiency. Immunization against influenza with recombinant, not live, vaccine is advisable for all forms of PAD considering that IRT is not thought to offer protection against the latest influence strain, and the vaccine may stimulate protective T cell and/or residual antibody responses to the patient.

In some patients with PAD, infections continue despite IRT. It appears that IRT requirements vary among individuals, and thus some may need higher doses than others to achieve a satisfactory clinical response.[64] Additionally, the clinician may opt for antibiotic prophylaxis in addition to IRT for patients in whom an adequate clinical response cannot be achieved by IRT alone. Moreover, the use of antibiotic prophylaxis should be strongly considered in patients with PAD who are on IRT and have bronchiectasis or other chronic lung disease because this adjunct therapy may prevent disease progression.[65] As mentioned earlier, in patients with HIGMS resulting from defects of CD40 or CD40L, antimicrobial prophylaxis against *Pneumocystis* is required in addition to IRT.

Certain forms of PAD, particularly CVID and HIGMS, are complicated by autoimmunity, chronic inflammatory diseases affecting various organs, and malignancy at increased rates. These "noninfectious" complications are treated much the same as they would be in those without antibody deficiency. One special consideration is that B cell–targeted therapy may be more preferential in specific forms of PAD, such as CVID, because it appears more effective in these individuals than other patients and concerns of immunosuppression may be less given the use of IRT.[66] Although sometimes used in PAD, certain immunosuppressive agents, such as thioguanines, may increase the risk of malignancy, a noted concern given the already heightened risk of this complication in CVID. Moreover, broadly immunosuppressive agents may raise risk of infection in PAD because these patients already have immunocompromise at baseline and some, such as CVID and HIGMS, can have immune defects that expand beyond antibody deficiency. Judicious usage of immunosuppressive agents with close monitoring is imperative. Precision therapeutic approaches, as applied in some monogenic forms of PAD described previously, may be an important aspect of effective therapy that limits side effects.

Hematopoietic stem cell transplant (HSCT) is used for treatment of numerous types of primary immunodeficiency, particularly in young children, but is infrequently used in those with PAD. This may be due to the fact that B cell reconstitution is often poor after HSCT, and effectiveness of IRT makes the risk of the procedure too high to justify for most patients. Exceptions to this are HIGMS secondary to defects in CD40L or CD40, in which the severe cellular immune defect associated with the disorder justifies strong consideration of HSCT. For severe forms of CVID, including those with associated monogenetic etiologies as discussed earlier, HSCT has been done, though results have been mixed and the decision to undergo this procedure should be weighed heavily.[67] Patients with known monogenic defects for which targeted therapy exists may be candidates for precision medicine approaches, as previously discussed.

Conclusions

PAD is the most common form of primary immunodeficiency. Because PAD is the most likely form to be encountered by practicing physicians, basic understanding of PAD diagnosis and management is of significant importance. Recurrent sinopulmonary infections is the most common presentation of PAD, but many patients face other complications related to their immune defect, including autoimmune, GI, or lung disease. The etiology of PAD is not known in most cases and is varied when it is known, with both B cell intrinsic and extrinsic defects identified. Efficient diagnosis and appropriate usage of antibiotics and IRT are vital to the management of PAD.

Expanding application of genomics has led to identification of numerous etiologies of PAD and an expanding classification of monogenic forms of CVID and CVID-like syndromes. It is certain that in the coming years, etiologies and classification of PAD will only enlarge further. Certain genetic etiologies have been used to shape precision therapy of PAD complications, further emphasizing the impact of the genomic age on this field. It is likely that our understanding of PAD, and consequently our clinical management of these disorders, will continue to grow by leaps and bounds in the coming years.

Many unanswered questions relating to PAD remain. Although monogenic etiologies have been uncovered for some forms of PAD, will future efforts identify polygenic or other multifactorial causes of these primary immunodeficiencies? Will the advance of gene therapy approaches in the clinic expand to include PAD and make the use of IRT obsolete for some of these patients? How else might improved diagnostic and therapeutic technology enhance the care of PAD? Some of the oldest questions in the field remain, such as how, if at all, we should screen for antibody deficiency. Can better tests be developed to more definitively identify patients who require IRT among patients with hypogammaglobulinemia that is less severe than XLA and CVID but nonetheless symptomatic? The numerous recent advances in the field have been very encouraging, but much more work remains to be done.

The reference list can be found on the companion Expert Consult website at http://www.expertconsult.inkling.com.

6

T Cell Immunodeficiencies

LUIGI D. NOTARANGELO

KEY POINTS

- Defects of T cell development and/or function cause increased susceptibility to infections of bacterial, viral, and fungal origin and are often associated with autoimmune manifestations and malignancies.
- The most severe forms of these disorders, severe combined immunodeficiency (SCID), are fatal unless immune reconstitution is attained, typically with hematopoietic stem cell transplantation (HSCT) or in selected cases with gene therapy or enzyme replacement therapy.
- Newborn screening based on enumeration of T cell receptor excision circles (TRECs) permits early identification of SCID and

thereby allows adoption of therapeutic interventions aimed to reduce the risk of infection while preparing for HSCT, resulting in improved overall survival.
- Several forms of T cell immunodeficiency are associated with other hematopoietic and nonhematopoietic defects, whose severity may have a significant impact on prognosis and outcome.
- Hygiene measures, antimicrobial prophylaxis, regular immunoglobulin replacement therapy, and nutritional support are cardinal aspects of treatment for patients with T cell deficiencies, along with HSCT.

Introduction

T lymphocytes are an essential component of adaptive immunity. Through secretion of interleukin [IL]-2 they promote activation and proliferation of effector cells, and through cytolytic activity and secretion of T_H1 (interferon [IFN]-γ) and T_H17 (IL-17, IL-22) cytokines they mediate resistance to viruses, mycobacteria, and fungi. In addition, interaction of T_H2 cells with B lymphocytes and antigen-presenting cells and release of soluble mediators such as IL-4 promote T-dependent antibody responses and contribute to defense against extracellular pathogens. Consequently, defects in T cell development and/or function result in severe combined immunodeficiency (SCID), with increased susceptibility to severe infections from early in life.[1] Furthermore, impaired development and/or function of regulatory T (T_{REG}) lymphocytes, which play a crucial role in immune homeostasis, causes autoimmunity.

This chapter will discuss the etiology, clinical presentation, diagnostic approach, and main principles of treatment for congenital T cell disorders. For a more detailed discussion of hematopoietic stem cell transplantation (HSCT) and gene therapy, the reader is referred to Chapter 16.

Severe Combined Immunodeficiency

Etiology

SCID is a heterogeneous group of disorders that manifest with a distinct immunologic phenotype (Table 6.1). Molecular and cellular mechanisms responsible for SCID include the following:

- *Defects of lymphocyte survival:* Adenosine deaminase (ADA) deficiency, reticular dysgenesis
- *Signaling defects:* X-linked SCID, Janus-associated kinase 3 (JAK3) deficiency, IL-7R deficiency, CD45 deficiency
- *Defects of expression and signaling through the pre–T cell receptor (pre-TCR) and the TCR:* Defects of recombinase activating gene 1 (*RAG1*), *RAG2*, Artemis, Cernunnos, DNA ligase IV (*LIG4*), DNA protein kinase catalytic subunit (DNA-PKcs), defects of CD3 chains (CD3δ, CD3ε, CD3ζ), defect of TCRα constant (TRAC) chain, CD45 deficiency.

Hypomorphic mutations in these genes may allow for residual T cell development, with or without immune dysregulation. These conditions and other defects at later stages in T cell development will be discussed separately in this chapter (see "Other Combined Immunodeficiencies").

SCID Caused by Adenosine Deaminase Deficiency

ADA mediates conversion of adenosine into inosine and of deoxyadenosine into deoxyinosine. Deficiency of ADA, inherited as an autosomal recessive trait, accounts for 5% to 10% of all cases of SCID. Lack of ADA results in intracellular accumulation of deoxyadenosine and its phosphorylated metabolites, among which dATP is particularly toxic to lymphoid precursors.[2] Consequently, complete ADA deficiency is characterized by extreme lymphopenia (T– B– natural killer [NK]– SCID) and extra-immune manifestations (reflecting the housekeeping nature of the *ADA* gene) from early in life. However, partial defects of the enzyme may result in less severe clinical presentation (delayed or late-onset forms) that may even manifest in adulthood.[3]

Disease	Gene	Inheritance	CIRCULATING LYMPHOCYTES		
			T	B	NK
B⁻ SCID					
Reticular dysgenesis	AK2	AR	↓↓	N to ↓	↓
RAG deficiency	RAG1, RAG2	AR	↓↓	↓↓	N
Radiation-sensitive SCID	DCLRE1C (Artemis)	AR	↓↓	↓↓	N
	PRKDC	AR	↓↓	↓↓	N
	LIG4	AR	↓↓	↓↓	N
	NHEJ1	AR	↓↓	↓↓	N
ADA deficiency	ADA	AR	↓↓	↓	↓↓
T⁻ B⁺ SCID					
X-linked SCID	IL2RG	XL	↓↓	N	↓↓
JAK-3 deficiency	Jak-3	AR	↓↓	N	↓↓
IL-7Rα deficiency	IL7R	AR	↓↓	N	N
CD45 deficiency	CD45	AR	↓↓	N	↓
CD3δ, CD3ε, or CD3ζ deficiency	CD3D, CD3E, CD3Z	AR	↓↓	N	N
Coronin-1A deficiency	CORO1A	AR	↓↓ naïve	N	N
LAT deficiency	LAT	AR	N to ↓	N	N
Other combined immunodeficiencies					
Nucleoside phosphorylase deficiency	PNP	AR	↓↓	↓/N	↓/N
Omenn syndrome	RAG1, RAG2, DCLRE1C, LIG4, ADA, AK2	AR	Variable	↓↓	N
	IL7R, RMRP	AR	Variable	N	N
	IL2RG	XL	Variable	N	↓↓
	ZAP70	AR	↓(↓↓ CD8)	N	N
TCRα constant chain deficiency	TRAC	AR	↓(almost all T cells are TCRγδ⁺)	N	N
ZAP-70 deficiency	ZAP70	AR	↓(↓↓ CD8)	N	N
LCK deficiency	LCK	AR	N (↓↓ CD4 naïve)	N	N
RHOH deficiency	RHOH	AR	↓↓ naïve T cells	N	N
STK4 deficiency	STK4	AR	↓↓ naïve T cells	↓	N
ITK deficiency	ITK	AR	Progressive ↓	N	N
DOCK8 deficiency	DOCK8	AR	↓	↓Memory B	N
DOCK2 deficiency	DOCK2	AR	↓	N	N (but ↓ function)
Moesin deficiency	MSN	XL	N (but ↓ function)	↓	N
Transferrin receptor deficiency	TFRC	AR	N (but ↓ function)	↓Memory B	N
FCHO1 deficiency	FCHO1	AR	↓	N to ↓	N
Coronin-1A deficiency	CORO1A	AR	↓↓	N	N
BCL11B deficiency	BCL11B	AD	↓	N	N
STIM1 deficiency	STIM1	AR	N	N	N

TABLE 6.1   Genetic and Immunologic Features of Combined Immunodeficiency—cont'd

Disease	Gene	Inheritance	CIRCULATING LYMPHOCYTES		
			T	B	NK
ORA1 deficiency	*ORAI1*	AR	N	N	N
MAGT1 deficiency	*MAGT1*	XL	↓CD4	N	N (↓ function)
IL2RA deficiency	*IL2RA*	AR	↓	N	N
IL2RB	*IL2RB*	AR	↓	N	N
STAT5b deficiency	*STAT5B*	*AR*	↓	*N*	*N*
Human "nude" SCID phenotype	*FOXN1*	AR	↓↓	N	N
MALT1 deficiency	*MALT1*	AR	N (↓ function)	N	N
BCL10 deficiency	*BCL10*	AR	N (↓ function)	N	N
CARD11 deficiency	*CARD11*	AR	N (↓ memory T)	N (mostly transitional)	N
IKBKB deficiency	*IKBKB*	AR	N (↓ memory T)	N (↓↓ memory B)	N
RelB deficiency	*RELB*	AR	↓Naïve T	N	N
cRel deficiency	*c-REL*	AR	N (↓ memory T)	↓	↓
NIK deficiency	*MAP3K14*	AR	N (↓ function)	N	N
Activated PI3K-δ	*PI3KCD, PIK3R1*	AD	↓CD4, ↑ T$_{EMRA}$	↓	N
IL-21R deficiency	*IL21R*	AR	N	N (↓ function)	N
IL-21 deficiency	*IL21*	AR	N (N or ↓ function)	↓	
CD27 deficiency	*CD27*	AR	N	N (↓↓ memory B)	N
CD70 deficiency	*CD70*	AR	N (↓ function)	N (↓ memory B)	N
MHC class I deficiency	*TAP1, TAP2, TAPBP*	AR	↓(↓↓ CD8)	N	N
MHC class II deficiency	*CIITA, RFXANK, RFX5, RFXAP*	AR	↓(↓↓ CD4)	N	N
CTPS1 deficiency	*CTPS1*	AR	↓CD4	N (↓ memory B)	N
X-linked hyper-IgM syndrome	*CD40LG*	XL	N	N	N
ID with multiple intestinal atresia	*TTC7A*	AR	↓	↓	N
Cartilage hair hypoplasia	*RMRP*	AR	↓/N	N	N
Schimke syndrome	*SMARCAL1*	AR	↓	N	N
Wiskott-Aldrich syndrome	*WAS*	XL	Progressive ↓	N	N
WIP deficiency	*WIPF1*	AR	Progressive ↓	N	N
ARPC1B deficiency	*ARPC1B*	AR	N	N	N

AR, Autosomal recessive; *B,* B lymphocytes; *N,* normal; *NK,* natural killer lymphocytes; *T,* T lymphocytes; *XL,* X-linked.

Reticular Dysgenesis

This rare form of autosomal recessive SCID is characterized by severe lymphopenia and agranulocytosis, associated with sensorineural deafness.[4] The disease is caused by mutations of the *AK2* gene, encoding for adenylate kinase 2, which controls intramitochondrial levels of ADP. AK2 deficiency results in increased cell death in lymphoid progenitors and in myeloid precursors committed to neutrophil differentiation.[5]

X-Linked Severe Combined Immunodeficiency (SCIDX1, γ$_c$ Deficiency)

SCIDX1 is the most common form of SCID in humans, with an estimated incidence of 1:100,000 to 1:150,000 live births. Inherited as an X-linked trait, it is characterized by complete absence of both T and NK lymphocytes, with preserved number of B lymphocytes (T⁻ B⁺ NK⁻ SCID). The disease is caused by mutations in the *IL2RG* gene that encodes for the IL-2 receptor common γ chain (IL-2Rγ_c, γ_c).[6] The γ_c chain is constitutively expressed by T, B, and NK cells, myeloid cells, and other cell types, including keratinocytes. The γ_c protein is an integral component of various cytokine receptors, that is, IL-2R, IL-4R, IL-7R, IL-9R, IL-15R, and IL-21R. In all of these receptors, the γ_c is coupled with the intracellular tyrosine kinase JAK-3, which mediates signal transduction.[1] Lack of circulating T and NK cells in SCIDX1 males reflects defective signaling through IL-7R and IL-15R, respectively.

JAK-3 Deficiency

JAK-3 is a cytoplasmic tyrosine kinase that is physically and functionally associated with the γ_c in all of the γ_c-containing cytokine receptors.[1] Mutations of the *JAK3* gene result in a clinical and immunologic phenotype (i.e., T- B+ NK- SCID) that is undistinguishable from SCIDX1[7,8] but has an autosomal recessive pattern of inheritance.

IL-7Rα Deficiency

IL-7Rα deficiency results in an autosomal recessive form of SCID characterized by lack of circulating T lymphocytes, with a preserved number of B and NK cells (T- B+ NK+ SCID).[9] IL-7 is produced by stromal cells in bone marrow and in the thymus and provides survival and proliferative signals to IL-7R+ lymphoid progenitor cells.

T– B– SCID Caused by Defective VDJ Recombination

B and T lymphocytes recognize foreign antigens through specialized receptors, the immunoglobulin (Ig) and the T cell receptor (TCR), respectively. These receptors are encoded by variable/diversity/joining *(VDJ)* gene segments that undergo somatic rearrangement through a mechanism known as VDJ recombination.[10] This process is initiated when the lymphoid-specific RAG1 and RAG2 proteins recognize specific recombination signal sequences (RSS) that flank each of the *V, D,* and *J* gene elements and introduce a DNA double-strand break (dsb) in this region.[11] Subsequently, a series of ubiquitously expressed proteins (including Ku70, Ku80, DNA-PKcs, XRCC4, DNA ligase IV, Artemis, and Cernunnos/XLF) involved in recognition and repair of DNA damage mediate the final steps of the VDJ recombination process.

Defects of V(D)J recombination cause complete absence of both T and B lymphocytes, with preserved presence of NK cells (T- B- NK+ SCID). *RAG1* and *RAG2* mutations do not affect mechanisms of DNA dsb repair and hence are not associated with increased cellular radiosensitivity.[12] By contrast, defects of Artemis, LIG4, Cernunnos/XLF, or DNA-PKcs cause increased radiosensitivity, reflecting impaired dsb repair.[13] Of note, hypomorphic mutations in the *RAG1* and *RAG2* genes and in the Artemis-encoding *DCLRE1C* gene have been associated with variable clinical and immunologic phenotypes, ranging from Omenn syndrome (OS) to expansion of TCRγδ+ T cells to delayed-onset immunodeficiency with granuloma and/or autoimmunity.[14,15] Moreover, hypomorphic *DCLRE1C* mutations also predispose to lymphoid malignancies[16]; defects in LIG4, DNA-PKcs, and Cernunnos/XLF cause microcephaly and growth retardation.[17–19]

CD3/TCR Deficiencies

The CD3 complex consists of CD3γ, δ, ε, and ζ chains and is required to mediate signaling through the pre-TCR and the TCR. In humans, defects of the CD3 δ, ε, or ζ chains cause autosomal recessive T- B+ NK+ SCID.[20–22] In contrast, CD3γ deficiency is associated with a partial T cell lymphopenia and a variable clinical phenotype, often manifesting with autoimmunity.[23,24]

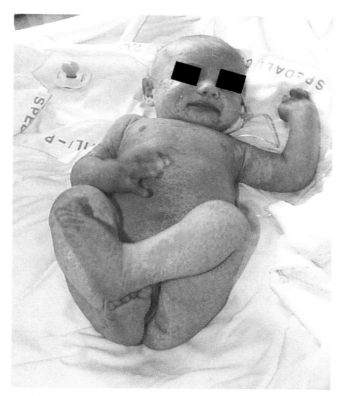

• **Fig. 6.1** Typical clinical features in an infant with Omenn syndrome. Note generalized erythroderma with scaly skin, alopecia, and edema.

CD45 Deficiency

Complete absence of the CD45 protein, a phosphatase that modulates signaling through the TCR/CD3 complex, causes a form of SCID with complete lack of T cells, with normal to increased B cell counts.[25,26]

Other Combined Immunodeficiencies

Omenn Syndrome and Other Conditions Associated With Hypomorphic RAG Mutations

Omenn syndrome (OS) is a combined immunodeficiency characterized by generalized erythroderma, lymphadenopathy, hepatosplenomegaly, respiratory infections, diarrhea, failure to thrive, hypoproteinemia with edema, and eosinophilia[27] (Fig. 6.1). IgE serum levels are often elevated, and T lymphocytes have an oligoclonal repertoire.

In most cases, OS is due to hypomorphic mutations in *RAG1* and *RAG2* genes[28]; however, it also may be caused by hypomorphic defects in other genes, including *DCLRE1C, IL7R, LIG4, RMRP, IL2RG, ADA, ZAP70,* and *AK2*.[29] Impaired thymic expression of AIRE, a transcription factor involved in expression and presentation of self-antigens, has been reported in patients with OS and may favor survival of autoreactive T cell clones.[30]

Patients with hypomorphic mutations in the *RAG1* and *RAG2* genes also may present with other clinical and immunologic phenotypes. Expansion of TCRγδ+ T cells has been frequently reported after cytomegalovirus (CMV) infection and may associate with autoimmunity (especially cytopenias).[31,32] In other cases, RAG deficiency may manifest with granulomatous lesions and/or autoimmunity.[14,15,33] The severity of the clinical phenotype of RAG deficiency correlates, at least in part, with the residual levels of recombination activity of the mutant protein.[34–36] However, environmental factors are also important, because patients with similarly severe mutations may present with distinct phenotypes.[36]

Nucleoside Phosphorylase Deficiency

Purine nucleoside phosphorylase (PNP) converts guanosine into guanine and deoxyguanosine to deoxyguanine. Autosomal recessive PNP deficiency causes accumulation of phosphorylated deoxyguanosine metabolites (and of dGTP in particular) that inhibit ribonucleotide reductase, the activity of which is essential to DNA synthesis. PNP deficiency is particularly deleterious to developing T lymphocytes and CNS cells, causing severe T cell lymphopenia and neurologic deterioration.[37] Autoimmune cytopenias, and autoimmune hemolytic anemia in particular, are frequently observed.[38]

TCRα Constant Chain (TRAC) Gene Defect

A homozygous splice-site mutation of the *TRAC* gene, causing loss of the transmembrane and intracytoplasmic domain, has been initially reported in two patients.[39] All T cells expressing CD3 at normal density co-expressed TCRγδ; an unusual population of CD3low T cells expressed TCRαβ at very low levels. In vitro lymphocyte proliferation to mitogens and antigens was decreased. In addition to increased susceptibility to infections (including chronic Epstein-Barr virus [EBV] infection), patients with TRAC deficiency also manifest immune dysregulation.[39]

Defects of TCR Signaling

Stimulation of T cells through TCR results in activation of the p56lck kinase, which mediates tyrosine phosphorylation of immunoreceptor tyrosine-based activation motifs (ITAMs) in the CD3γ, CD3δ, CD3ε, and CD3ζ chains. The ζ-associated protein of 70 kDa (ZAP-70) is then recruited to the CD3/TCR complex, allowing activation of downstream signaling molecules such as linker for activation of T cells (LATs) and SLP-76.[40] Autosomal recessive ZAP-70 deficiency is characterized by lack of CD8+ T cells; CD4+ T lymphocytes are present but nonfunctional.[41–43]

Deficiency of p56lck has been demonstrated in a child with recurrent infections and autoimmunity, associated with CD4+ T cell lymphopenia, oligoclonal T cell repertoire, and impaired T cell proliferation.[44]

Deficiency of the LATs, a transmembrane adaptor involved in signaling through the TCR, causes an autosomal recessive form of combined immunodeficiency characterized by severe recurrent infections since infancy, progressive lymphopenia, hypogammaglobulinemia, and lymphoproliferation with splenomegaly. Autoimmune cytopenias also have been reported.[45,46]

The Ras homolog family member H (RHOH) is a small GTPase that plays an important role in T cell activation. Bi-allelic loss-of-function variants of the *RHOH* gene cause marked reduction of naïve CD4+ T cells, restricted T cell repertoire, expansion of memory T cells, including TEMRA (CD8+ CD45RA+ CCR7- CD244+) cells, and impaired in vitro T cell proliferation.[47] The clinical phenotype includes warts, Burkitt's lymphoma, psoriatic-like skin rash, and lung granulomatous disease.

The serine/threonine kinase 4 (STK4) molecule is involved in intracellular signaling. Patients with STK4 deficiency show increased susceptibility to recurrent bacterial and viral infections (including warts and molluscum contagiosum), autoimmunity associated with severe reduction of naïve T cells, increased proportion of CD8+ TEMRA cells, restricted T cell repertoire, impaired proliferation to mitogens, increased apoptosis of T lymphocytes, and reduced number of memory B cells.[48–50]

The IL-2–inducible T cell kinase (ITK) is activated in response to TCR stimulation and participates in intracellular signaling. ITK deficiency is characterized by increased risk of infections (especially herpesviruses) and prominent immune dysregulation, associated with a reduced number of naïve CD4+ cells, defective T cell proliferation, and progressive hypogammaglobulinemia. There is an increased risk of EBV-driven lymphoproliferative disease, with frequent pulmonary involvement.[51,52]

DOCK8 Deficiency

The dedicator of cytokinesis 8 (DOCK8) protein plays an important role in intracellular signaling and cytoskeleton reorganization. Mutations of the *DOCK8* gene cause a severe autosomal recessive immunodeficiency, with increased incidence of skin abscesses, mucocutaneous candidiasis, and especially cutaneous viral infections, eczema, severe food allergy, and markedly elevated IgE levels and eosinophilia.[53,54] There is a high risk of human papillomavirus (HPV)-associated squamous cell carcinoma. Vascular thrombosis in the CNS, autoimmune cytopenias, and other autoimmune manifestations also have been reported. The immunologic phenotype is characterized by multiple abnormalities,[55] with a reduced number of naïve T cells, increased proportion of CD8+ TEMRA cells, and defective in vitro T cell proliferation to CD3/CD28 stimulation. Deficiency of TH17 cells accounts for the increased risk of candidiasis. Migration of T cells and dendritic cells to inflamed/infected tissues is defective. NK and NKT cell function is also compromised. Immunoglobulin levels are variable, although low serum IgM levels are frequently seen. B cell response to TLR9 activation is severely compromised. Antibody responses to T-dependent antigens may be initially normal but are not sustained over time. The disease has a dismal prognosis, but can be treated by HSCT.[56,57]

DOCK2 Deficiency

The DOCK2 molecule is also involved in intracellular signaling and cytoskeleton reorganization after engagement of the TCR, the B cell receptor, and various NK and G-protein coupled receptors. DOCK2 deficiency accounts for an autosomal recessive combined immunodeficiency with increased susceptibility to severe infections and death early in life, unless the disease is treated with HSCT.[58]

Moesin Deficiency

Moesin (MSN) is a member of the ezrin-radixin-moesin complex that links actin filaments to the plasma membrane. Mutations of the *MSN* gene are responsible for an X-linked combined immunodeficiency characterized by bacterial and viral infections, profound lymphopenia, hypogammaglobulinemia, and fluctuating neutropenia.[59] The disease can be identified with low T cell receptor excision circles (TRECs) levels during newborn screening for SCID. However, overall survival is not affected.[60]

Transferrin Receptor (TFRC) Deficiency

Intracellular iron plays an important role in hematologic and immune homeostasis. A homozygous missense mutation of the *TFRC* gene, affecting transferrin internalization and iron transport, was found to cause hypogammaglobulinemia, decreased T cell proliferative responses, and intermittent neutropenia and thrombocytopenia in affected individuals from a large consanguineous Kuwaiti family. HSCT cured the disease.[61]

FCHO1 Deficiency

The FCHO1 protein is involved in the initial stages of clathrin-mediated endocytosis. FCHO1 deficiency accounts for a combined immunodeficiency with recurrent and severe infections since the first years of life, associated with T cell lymphopenia. The disease is fatal unless treated by HSCT.[62]

Human "Nude" Phenotype (FOXN1 Defect)

FOXN1 is a transcription factor that controls development of thymic epithelial cells. Bi-allelic mutations of the *FOXN1* gene cause a severe T cell immunodeficiency with complete lack of CD8+ T cells, associated with alopecia.[63] Treatment is based on thymus transplantation.[64]

Coronin-1A Deficiency

Coronin-1A is an actin regulator that regulates T cell survival and migration. Mutations of the *CORO1A* gene cause immunodeficiency with increased risk of EBV lymphoproliferative disease, associated with profound naïve T cell lymphopenia, oligoclonal T cell repertoire, and severe reduction of invariant natural killer T (iNKT) cells and mucosa-associated invariant T (MAIT) cells.[65,66]

B Cell Lymphoma 11B (BCL11B) Deficiency

The *BCL11B* gene encodes for a transcription factor involved in hematopoietic cell differentiation. Heterozygous mutations of this gene cause a combined immunodeficiency with profound T cell lymphopenia, associated with hypotonia, dysmorphic features, and developmental delay. Low levels of TRECs are detected during newborn screening for SCID.[67]

Major Histocompatibility Complex Class II Deficiency

Lack of major histocompatibility complex (MHC) class II molecule expression on the surface of thymic epithelial cells results in an inability to positively select CD4+ thymocytes and, hence, in the very low number of circulating CD4+ lymphocytes. In addition, the ability to mount antibody responses is also impaired.

MHC class II deficiency has an autosomal recessive pattern of inheritance and may be caused by mutations in the *CIITA, RFXANK, RFX5,* and *RFXAP* genes, which encode for transcription factors that govern MHC class II antigen expression.[68–71]

Major Histocompatibility Complex Class I Deficiency

Human leukocyte antigen (HLA) class I molecules play an essential role in presenting antigenic peptides to cytotoxic T lymphocytes and in modulating the activity of NK cells. HLA class I molecules are composed of a polymorphic heavy chain, associated with β2-microglobulin (β2M). The assembly of HLA class I molecules occurs in the lumen of the endoplasmic reticulum (ER), where they are loaded with peptides derived from the degradation of intracellular organisms. These peptides are transported into the ER via transporters associated with antigen presentation (TAP) proteins.[72] TAP consists of two structurally related subunits (TAP1 and TAP2). In addition, the TAP-binding protein (TAPBP), tapasin, plays an important role in the loading process. Defects in TAP1, TAP2, or tapasin result in impaired peptide-HLA class I/β2M complex formation with reduced surface expression of HLA class I molecules. Patients with MHC class I deficiency have recurrent sinopulmonary infections and deep skin ulcers, associated with a reduced number of circulating CD8+ T cells.[73–75]

Deficiency of Calcium-Release Activated Channels and Magnesium Flux

Lymphocyte activation depends on calcium mobilization. In particular, TCR-induced activation results in release of Ca^{2+} from the ER stores. Depletion of these Ca^{2+} stores is sensed by the stromal interaction molecule 1 (STIM1) proteins, which oligomerize and bind to the calcium release-activating modulator 1 (ORAI1) proteins that form the pore of the Ca^{2+}-release activated channels (CRACs) located in the cell membrane, allowing Ca^{2+} entry. Mutations of the *STIM1* and *ORAI1* genes cause an autosomal recessive immunodeficiency with increased risk of infections, hypogammaglobulinemia, impaired antibody responses, and profoundly reduced in vitro T cell proliferation.[76–78] Autoimmune manifestations (especially cytopenias) are common, in particular in patients with STIM1 deficiency. Extra-immune manifestations include nonprogressive myopathy and ectodermal dysplasia.

Mutations of the X-linked magnesium transporter 1 *(MAGT1)* gene in humans cause immunodeficiency with increased susceptibility to viral and bacterial infections and to EBV-driven lymphoproliferative disease.[79,80] CD4+ T cell lymphopenia has been frequently observed. Expression of the NKG2D molecule on the surface of cytolytic T cells and NK cells is reduced, and NK cytolytic activity is impaired.[81] Defects of N-glycosylation have been observed in patient-derived cells.[82]

Immunodeficiency With Immune Dysregulation From Impaired Interleukin-2 Signaling

IL-2 signaling maintains peripheral immune homeostasis. Deficiencies of the α chain of the IL-2 receptor (IL-2Rα, CD25) and of the IL-2Rβ chain cause a similar phenotype, with immune dysregulation and lymphoproliferation, often associated with early-onset viral and bacterial infections, oral thrush and chronic diarrhea, and an increased rate of autoimmune cytopenias.[83–86]

Signal transducer and activator of transcription 5b (STAT5b) is a transcription factor that is activated in response to growth hormone (GH) and cytokines, including IL-2. STAT5b deficiency is characterized by short stature, GH insensitivity, and a variable degree of immunodeficiency and immune dysregulation.[87]

IL-21 Receptor Deficiency

Loss-of-function mutations of IL-21 receptor (IL-21R) have been reported in four patients with sclerosing cholangitis as a result of *Cryptosporidium* infestation, recurrent pneumonia, chronic diarrhea, and failure to thrive.[88] The proportion of switched memory B cells was reduced. T cell proliferation to mitogens was preserved, but proliferation to antigens was impaired. A similar phenotype also has been reported in patients with IL-21 deficiency.[89]

CD27 Deficiency

CD27 is a costimulatory molecule that interacts with CD70. Both *CD27* and *CD70* mutations are responsible for autosomal recessive forms of combined immunodeficiency with EBV lymphoproliferative disease, reduced T cell proliferation to mitogens and antigens, and progressive hypogammaglobulinemia.[90,91]

T Cell Defects With Impaired Nuclear Factor-κB Activation

The mucosa-associated lymphoid tissue 1 (MALT1), B cell lymphoma 10 (BCL-10), and caspase recruitment domain family, member 11 (CARD11) proteins form a complex that is activated in response to TCR stimulation, allowing nuclear translocation of nuclear factor κB (NF-κB). Autosomal recessive *MALT1* deficiency causes recurrent bacterial, viral, and fungal infections.[92] In spite of normal T and B lymphocyte count, proliferative responses to CD3 stimulation and antigens are decreased, and specific antibody responses are also impaired.

CARD11 deficiency causes increased susceptibility to opportunistic infections.[93,94] A reduced number of memory T cells and hypogammaglobulinemia with increased proportion of transitional B cells are present.

Mutations of the *IKBKB* gene, encoding for the IKKβ component of the IKK complex, cause early-onset infections and hypogammaglobulinemia.[95] Immunologic abnormalities included lack of memory T and B cells and of T$_{REG}$ lymphocytes, and defective in vitro T cell proliferation to CD3 stimulation.

RelB is a component of the noncanonical NF-κB signaling pathway. RelB deficiency accounts for an autosomal recessive combined immunodeficiency, characterized by recurrent infections, low proportion of naïve T cells, impaired T cell proliferative responses, and defective antibody responses.[96]

Deficiency of c-Rel has been reported in a child with a history of opportunistic infections, *Mycobacterium tuberculosis* infection, and impaired T and B cell activation.[97]

Mutations of the NF-κB–inducing kinase (NIK) impair activation of both canonical and noncanonical NF-κB signaling and are responsible for a combined immunodeficiency with B cell lymphopenia, hypogammaglobulinemia, reduced number of memory T cells, and impaired NK cell function.[98]

Immunodeficiency Resulting From Activating PI3K-δ Mutations

Phosphatidylinositol-3-OH kinases (PI3Ks) include a series of molecules that participate in cell signaling, enabling generation of PIP$_3$ from PIP$_2$, and activation of the mammalian target of rapamycin (mTOR) and protein kinase B (Akt). Heterozygous, gain-of-function mutations of the *PI3KCD* gene, encoding for the p110δ subunit of phosphatidylinositol-3-OH kinase (PI3K), cause increased susceptibility to recurrent respiratory tract infections, EBV lymphoproliferative disease (frequently associated with hepatosplenomegaly and lymphadenopathy), and CMV viremia.[99,100] A similar phenotype is also observed in patients with heterozygous mutations of the *PIK3R1* gene, encoding for the p85α regulatory subunit of PI3K, that unleash p110δ catalytic activity.[101,102] Reduction of naïve CD4+ cells, expansion of memory and T$_{EMRA}$ CD8+ cells, and decreased number of switched memory B cells have been reported. IgM serum levels are increased. Constitutive activation of Akt is associated with increased activation-induced cell death of lymphocytes. Treatment with rapamycin, an mTOR inhibitor, may reduce lymphoproliferation and organomegaly. Clinical trials using PI3K inhibitors have been started, with initial promising results.[103]

Cytidine 5' Triphosphate Synthase 1 (CTPS1) Deficiency

Autosomal recessive mutations of the *CTPS1* gene, involved in the synthesis of cytidine 5' triphosphate (CTP), cause early-onset viral and bacterial infections and an increased risk of EBV-driven non-Hodgkin B cell lymphoma, associated with CD4 lymphopenia, increased proportion of effector memory T cells, absence of iNKT and MAIT lymphocytes, impaired proliferation to mitogens and antigens, and reduced number of memory B cells.[104]

Differential Diagnosis of Severe Combined Immunodeficiency and Other Combined Immunodeficiencies

SCID and other combined immunodeficiencies are characterized by typical clinical signs (Box 6.1), with early-onset severe infections sustained by bacteria, viruses, and fungi, including opportunistic pathogens (such as *Pneumocystis jirovecii,* CMV), and growth failure[105] (Fig. 6.2). Skin manifestations (rash, generalized erythroderma, alopecia) are also common and may reflect the

---

• BOX 6.1   Clinical Pearls
Key Concepts Clinical and Laboratory Elements in the Diagnosis of SCID

Clinical Features
- Positive family history (X-linked, other siblings affected, parental consanguinity)
- Presentation early in life (within the first months of age)
- Severe respiratory infections (interstitial pneumonia)
- Protracted diarrhea
- Failure to thrive
- Persistent candidiasis
- Skin rash, erythroderma may be present

Diagnostic Criteria (Elaborated by the PIDTC)[109]
Typical SCID
- Absence or very low number of T cells (CD3+ T cells <300/μL), *AND*
- No or very low T cell function (<10% of lower limit of normal) as measured by response to phytohemagglutinin (PHA)
OR
- Cells of maternal origin present

Atypical (Leaky) SCID
- Presence of maternal lymphocytes tested and not detected
  AND either one or both of the following:
    1. <50% of lower limit of normal T cell function as measured by response to PHA or to anti-CD3/CD28 antibody
    2. Absent or <30% of lower limit of normal proliferative response to candida and tetanus toxoid antigens
  AND at least two of the following:
    1. Reduced number of CD3+ T cells (age ≤2 years: <1500 cells/μL; age >2 years ≤4 years: 800 cells/μL; age >4 years: <600 cells/μL)
    2. ≥80% of CD3+ or CD4+ T cells are CD45R0+
  AND/OR >80% of CD3+ or CD4+ T cells are CD62L−
  AND/OR >50% of CD3+ or CD4+ T cells express HLA-DR
  (at <4 years of age)
  AND/OR are oligoclonal T cells
    3. Hypomorphic mutation in *IL2RG* in males or homozygous hypomorphic mutation or compound heterozygosity with at least one hypomorphic mutation in an autosomal SCID-causing gene
    4. Low TRECs and/or the percentage of CD4+ CD45RA+ CD31+ or CD4+ CD45RA+ CD62L+ cells is below the lower limit of normal
    5. Functional testing in vitro supporting impaired, but not absent, activity of the mutant protein
  AND does not meet criteria for Omenn syndrome

Reticular Dysgenesis
- Absence or very low number of T cells (CD3+ cells <300/μL)
- No or very low T cell function (PHA response <10% of lower limit of normal)
- Severe neutropenia (absolute neutrophil count <200 cells/μL)
- Sensorineural deafness and/or absence of granulopoiesis at bone marrow examination and/or a deleterious *AK2* mutation

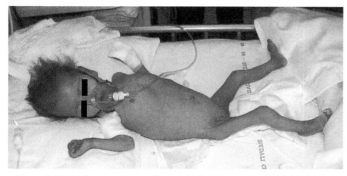

• **Fig. 6.2** Typical appearance of an infant with severe combined immunodeficiency (SCID). Note severe growth failure and respiratory distress.

presence of autoreactive T cell clones (such as in OS) or true graft-versus-host disease (GvHD) caused by transplacental passage of alloreactive maternal T lymphocytes.[106] Other manifestations of maternal T cell engraftment include liver dysfunction, cytopenia (as a result of bone marrow aggression), and eosinophilia.[106]

Typical clinical and laboratory features are present in some forms of SCID. Cupping and flaring of the ribs and liver dysfunction are often present in ADA deficiency.[107] Autoimmune hemolytic anemia and regression of psychomotor skills are observed in PNP deficiency.[38] Sensorineural deafness is part of reticular dysgenesis,[4] whereas microcephaly and growth abnormalities are seen in patients with defects of DNA repair.[17–19] Alopecia is observed in patients with FOXN1 deficiency.[63] Nonprogressive myopathy is a characteristic feature of CRAC channel defects. Severe food allergy is common in DOCK8 deficiency. Autoimmunity is a hallmark of IL-2RA, IL-2RB, STAT5B deficiencies, and defects of Ca^{2+} signaling (especially STIM1), but is also frequently seen in patients with *RAG* mutations.

SCID is a medical emergency. Therefore, all infants with a possible diagnosis of SCID need to be carefully and rapidly evaluated by means of appropriate laboratory assays (see Box 6.1 and later discussion) and careful family history. The differential diagnosis includes other conditions with increased risk of infections (congenital heart disease, pulmonary defects, cystic fibrosis, HIV infection, and other secondary immune deficiencies). For patients with generalized erythroderma secondary to OS or maternal T cell engraftment, the differential diagnosis includes severe allergy; ichthyosis; X-linked immunodeficiency with polyendocrinopathy and enteropathy (IPEX); and Netherton's syndrome.

Evaluation and Management

A correct diagnosis of SCID should be established as soon as possible to offer an optimal perspective on treatment. TRECs are a by-product of V(D)J recombination and are present in newly generated T lymphocytes. No or low levels of TRECs are detected in infants with SCID, and universal newborn screening for SCID based on enumeration of TRECs in dried blood spots collected at birth is currently performed in the entire United States.[108] However, confirmation of SCID requires additional tests. Severe lymphopenia is observed in most infants with SCID, but a normal (or nearly normal) number of lymphocytes may be seen in some forms of combined immunodeficiency (OS, MHC class II deficiency, ZAP-70 deficiency) or in infants with maternal T cell engraftment. In most cases, enumeration of total (CD3+) T lymphocytes, CD4+ and CD8+ T cell subsets (including number of naïve T cells), B (CD19+) lymphocytes, and NK (CD16/56+) cells

will reveal the diagnosis of SCID and also orient toward specific gene defects. Early in life the vast majority of T lymphocytes are naïve T cells (CD45RA+); by contrast, patients with OS or with maternal T cell engraftment show an increased proportion of activated/memory (CD45R0+) T cells. Moreover, in vitro lymphocyte proliferation to mitogens is markedly reduced in patients with SCID, including those with maternal T cells. Selective deficiency of CD4+ lymphocytes may suggest MHC class II deficiency, whereas deficiency of CD8+ T cells is observed in ZAP-70 deficiency and in MHC class I deficiency.

Measurement of enzymatic ADA and PNP activity and of dATP and dGTP levels in red blood cells is important to reach a final diagnosis of ADA or PNP deficiency.

Distinguishing typical SCID from atypical forms of the disease has important implications. Patients with persistence of autologous, partially functioning T cells typically require use of chemotherapy in preparation for HSCT, whereas no conditioning is strictly required in babies with SCID. The Primary Immune Deficiency Treatment Consortium (PIDTC) has identified criteria to distinguish SCID from atypical forms of the disease.[109]

Ultimately, mutation analysis represents an important diagnostic tool to confirm the diagnosis of SCID and related disorders (see Table 6.1).

Treatment

Optimal treatment of SCID is based on HSCT, as discussed in greater detail in Chapter 16. Before HSCT, infants with SCID need to be protected from infections (Box 6.2). Prophylactic trimethoprim-sulfamethoxazole (TMP-SMX) is effective in preventing *P. jirovecii* pneumonia (PJP). Regular administration of intravenous immunoglobulins (IVIGs), reinforcement of hygiene measures, and nutritional support may help improve the health status of infants with SCID while waiting for HSCT. Blood products need to be irradiated because alloreactive T cells contained in the transfusion would invariably cause rapidly fatal GvHD.

Alternative therapeutic approaches are available in selected cases. Patients affected with ADA deficiency who do not have an HLA-identical donor may be treated with weekly intramuscular injections of polyethylene glycol–conjugated ADA (PEG-ADA).[110]

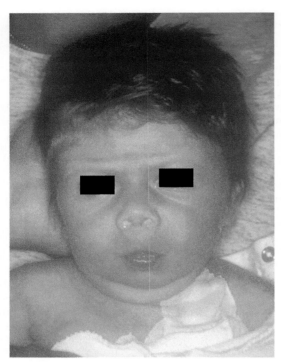

• **Fig. 6.3** Facial dysmorphic features in an infant with DiGeorge syndrome. Note hypertelorism, enlarged nasal root, anteroverted nostrils, low-set ears, and micrognathia.

Gene therapy has been highly successful in patients with ADA deficiency[111,112] and is currently considered first-line treatment equal to HSCT from matched sibling donors.[110] Initial attempts of gene therapy for X-linked SCID using retroviral vectors had shown good immune reconstitution[113,114]; however, 5 of 20 patients had developed leukemic proliferation as a result of insertional mutagenesis.[115,116] Improved safety, with no occurrence of leukemia, has been observed with use of self-inactivating (SIN) retroviral[117] and more recently SIN-lentiviral[118,119] vectors. Furthermore, inclusion of reduced-intensity chemotherapy in the preparative regimen facilitates attainment of humoral immune reconstitution.[118,119]

DiGeorge Syndrome

DiGeorge syndrome (DGS) is characterized by thymic hypoplasia, hypoparathyroidism with consequent hypocalcemia, congenital heart disease (especially interrupted aortic arch type B or truncus arteriosus), and facial dysmorphisms (i.e., micrognathia, hypertelorism, antimongoloid slant of the eyes, and ear malformations) (Fig. 6.3).[120] Feeding problems, microcephaly, speech delay, and neurobehavioral problems (including bipolar disorders, autistic spectrum disorders, and schizophrenia) are frequently observed.[120] The majority of patients have a partial monosomy of the 22q11 region of chromosome 22. Most patients have a residual thymus and a milder immunodeficiency (partial DGS), whereas approximately 1% of the patients show complete absence of the thymus and extreme T cell lymphopenia (complete DGS).[120] In some cases, patients with complete DGS may develop a variable number of oligoclonal, activated, and functionally anergic T lymphocytes. This phenotype is also referred to as complete atypical DGS and may manifest clinically with skin erythroderma and lymphadenopathy, resembling OS.[120] Patients with DGS who have low TRECs at birth may be more prone to viral infections.[121]

Heart defects should be treated aggressively. Hypocalcemia requires supplementation with calcium and vitamin D. If a significant immune defect is present, prophylaxis of PJP with TMP-SMX is indicated. Live attenuated vaccines can be safely administered to patients with partial DGS who have good cellular immunity; however, these vaccines are contraindicated in patients with complete DGS. Thymic transplantation is the treatment of choice for patients with complete (typical or atypical) DGS and results in good (75%) long-term survival and immune reconstitution.[121,122]

Syndromes With Significant T Cell Deficiency

Cartilage Hair Hypoplasia

Cartilage hair hypoplasia (CHH) is an autosomal recessive disease characterized by short-limbed dwarfism, light-colored hypoplastic hair, and a variable degree of immunodeficiency, associated with an increased occurrence of bone marrow dysplasia, malignancies, and Hirschsprung's disease. The disease is caused by mutations of the gene encoding for the untranslated RNA component of the ribonuclease mitochondrial RNA processing (RMRP) complex.[123]

The majority of patients with CHH have a limited susceptibility to bacterial and viral infections; however, some may present with severe infections early in life and show an immunologic phenotype of SCID, OS, or selective CD8⁺ lymphocytopenia, which may require HSCT.[124]

Schimke Syndrome

Schimke syndrome is an autosomal recessive disease characterized by dwarfism with progressive renal failure, facial dysmorphisms, lentigines, and immunodeficiency and increased occurrence of bone marrow failure and early-onset atherosclerosis.[125] The syndrome is caused by mutations of the *SMARCAL1* gene that encodes for a chromatin remodeling protein.[125] T cell lymphopenia is common and may occasionally be severe enough to cause SCID. Recurrent bacterial, viral, or fungal infections are seen in almost half of the patients.

Combined Immunodeficiency With Multiple Intestinal Atresias

This autosomal recessive disease is caused by mutations of the tetratricopeptide repeat domain 7A *(TTC7A)* gene,[126] resulting in increased Ras homolog family member A (RHOA) signaling and disruption of intestinal epithelial apicobasal polarity.[127] Profound lymphopenia and hypogammaglobulinemia are present in most patients, causing increased susceptibility to early-onset bacterial and opportunistic infections.[128] Overall, the disease has a dismal prognosis. Surgical resections are needed to treat the intestinal atresias, and small bowel transplantation may be required. HSCT may cure the immunodeficiency, but a high mortality rate has been observed.[129]

Immunodeficiency Syndromes With Defective DNA Repair

Ataxia-telangiectasia (AT) is an autosomal recessive disorder characterized by telangiectasia, progressive ataxia, recurrent respiratory tract infections, and increased susceptibility to tumors.[130] The disease is caused by mutations of the *ATM* gene, which encodes for a large protein that participates in the repair of DNA breakage and controls cell cycle and cellular apoptosis.[131]

Nijmegen breakage syndrome (NBS) is another cellular radio-sensitivity syndrome, characterized by microcephaly, growth retardation, bird-like facies, and increased susceptibility to infections and tumors. The disease is caused by mutations of the *NBS1* gene, which encodes for nibrin.[132]

A subgroup of patients with an AT-like disorder have been identified in whom the defect was in the *hMRE11* gene, which encodes for another component of the DNA repair machinery that associates with nibrin.[133]

Patients with AT have increased serum levels of alpha-fetoprotein (AFP), and development of reciprocal chromosomal translocations (mostly involving chromosomes 7 and 14) in a fraction of T lymphocytes is common. Laboratory investigations in patients with AT, AT-like disease, or NBS show progressive reduction of the T cell number (particularly the CD4+ subset) with impaired in vitro proliferative response to mitogens. Low TREC levels at birth may be seen in patients with AT[134]; therefore, this condition must be included in the differential diagnosis of disorders that may be identified through newborn screening for SCID.

At present, there is no definitive cure for AT and NBS. Use of prophylactic antibiotics, chest physiotherapy, and administration of IVIGs may decrease the risk of infections, but the prognosis remains poor and infections and tumors are the main causes of death.[130] Exposure to ionizing radiation should be avoided, if possible.

Wiskott-Aldrich Syndrome and Other Related Disorders

Wiskott-Aldrich syndrome (WAS) is an X-linked disorder characterized by eczema, congenital thrombocytopenia with small platelets, and immunodeficiency (Fig. 6.4). The *WAS* gene is located on the X chromosome and encodes for a protein involved in cytoskeleton reorganization in hematopoietic cells.[135] Most patients with typical WAS have mutations that impair expression and/or function of the WAS protein (WASP). However, some missense mutations are associated primarily with isolated X-linked thrombocytopenia (XLT), although progression to typical forms of WAS can be observed with age.[136]

The immunodeficiency of WAS may manifest as recurrent bacterial and viral infections, autoimmune manifestations, and increased occurrence of tumors (leukemia, lymphoma). Immunologic laboratory abnormalities include lymphopenia (particularly among CD8+ lymphocytes), impaired in vitro proliferation to immobilized anti-CD3, reduced serum IgM with increased levels of IgA and IgE, and inability to mount effective antibody responses, especially to T-independent antigens.[135] Analysis of intracellular WASP expression by flow cytometry may assist in the diagnosis; absence of the protein is most often associated with a severe clinical phenotype, whereas patients with XLT tend to show residual protein expression that is usually associated with missense mutations in exons 1 and 2 of the gene.[136] Somatic reversion, leading to WASP expression in a proportion of cells (mostly in T lymphocytes), has been observed in several patients, but its implications on the evolution of the clinical phenotype are unclear.[137]

The mainstay of treatment of WAS is HSCT, but promising results have been reported with gene therapy using a lentiviral vector (see Chapter 16). Administration of IVIGs, regular antibiotic prophylaxis, topical steroids to control eczema, and vigorous immune suppression for autoimmunity are the hallmarks of conservative treatment. Splenectomy may be indicated in the

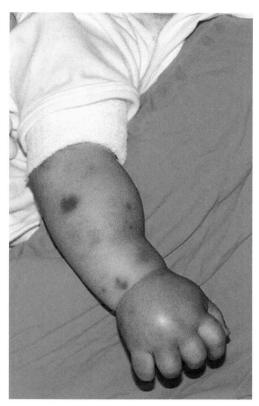

• **Fig. 6.4** Severe vasculitis and petechiae in a child with Wiskott-Aldrich syndrome.

case of severe and refractory thrombocytopenia; however, it carries the risk of overwhelming sepsis. Gene therapy can restore immune function, but the effects on the platelet count are less consistent.[138,139]

Mutations of WASP-interacting protein (WIP) cause an autosomal recessive disease with a similar phenotype.[140] ARPC1B is a component of the ARP2/3 complex that controls actin polymerization. Mutations of the *ARPC1B* gene cause an autosomal recessive combined immunodeficiency with severe infections, inflammation, and allergy.[141]

Hyper-IgM Syndromes Resulting From CD40 Ligand (CD40L) or to CD40 Deficiency

CD40 ligand (CD40L, CD154) is a cell surface molecule predominantly expressed by activated CD4+ T lymphocytes. Interaction of CD40L with its counter-receptor CD40 (expressed by B and dendritic cells, macrophages, endothelial cells, and some epithelial cells) is essential for germinal center formation, terminal differentiation of B lymphocytes and effective defense against intracellular pathogens. Mutations in the *CD40LG (TNFSF5)* gene, mapping at Xq26, result in X-linked hyper-IgM syndrome (HIGM1), characterized by an increased occurrence of bacterial and opportunistic infections, chronic diarrhea (often sustained by *Cryptosporidium*), liver/biliary tract disease, and susceptibility to liver and gut tumors.[142]

Presentation early in life with opportunistic infections (PJP) requires differential diagnosis with SCID and other forms of severe T cell defects. The typical immunoglobulin profile (undetectable or very low serum IgG and IgA, with normal to increased IgM) may also be observed in common variable immunodeficiency or in autosomal recessive hyper-IgM caused by defects in the *AID, UNG,* or *CD40* genes. Neutropenia is a common finding. The diagnosis of HIGM1 is made based on the demonstration of defective expression of CD40L (but not of other activation markers) on the surface of T cells after in vitro activation and is eventually confirmed by mutation analysis.[142]

Treatment is based on regular use of IVIGs, prophylactic TMP-SMX, and use of sterile/filtered water to prevent *Cryptosporidium* infection. Monitoring of liver and biliary tract morphology and function by ultrasound scanning, measurement of appropriate laboratory parameters of liver and biliary tract function, and, when indicated, liver biopsy are also advised. Severe neutropenia may be treated with recombinant granulocyte colony-stimulating factor. In spite of these measures, the long-term prognosis is poor because of severe infections and liver disease. The only curative approach is HSCT, and improved outcome has been reported in recent years, especially if transplantation is performed before development of lung problems or *Cryptosporidium* infection.[143]

Conclusions

Irrespective of the specific definitive diagnosis, all forms of T cell immunodeficiencies are characterized by significant morbidity and some of them also by high early-onset mortality rates, emphasizing the critical role played by T lymphocytes in ensuring effective immune defense mechanisms and in maintaining homeostasis. Consequently, it is a primary physician's responsibility to perform accurate clinical and laboratory evaluation of patients with a putative T cell immunodeficiency. Whereas clinical history and physical examination may disclose the diagnosis in some forms of T cell immunodeficiency (e.g., WAS, AT, and CHH), laboratory evaluation is most often required to provide a definitive diagnosis. In spite of the heterogeneity of this group of disorders, simple laboratory assays (total lymphocyte count and subsets distribution, in vitro proliferative responses) are usually sufficient to confirm the suspicion. It is noteworthy that some forms of T cell immunodeficiencies (SCID in particular) represent true medical emergencies and warrant prompt and accurate evaluation and treatment by HSCT. Based on recent experience, it is likely that gene therapy may be successfully applied in a broader group of disorders in the near future.

Helpful Websites

Online Mendelian Inheritance in Man (OMIM); website (www.ncbi.nlm.nih.gov/omim/)

European Society for Immune Deficiencies (ESID); website (www.esid.org/)

Jeffrey Modell Foundation; website (www.jmfworld.com/)

Immune Deficiency Foundation; website (www.primaryimmune.org)

Primary Immune Deficiency Treatment Consortium (PIDTC); website (https://www.rarediseasesnetwork.org/cms/pidtc)

United States Immunodeficiency Network (USIDNET); website (usidnet.org)

The complete reference list can be found on the companion Expert Consult website at http://www.expertconsult.inkling.com.

The reference list can be found on the companion Expert Consult website at http://www.expertconsult.inkling.com.

7

Complement Deficiencies

KATHLEEN E. SULLIVAN

KEY POINTS

- Systemic lupus erythematosus and neisserial infections are the common phenotypes seen in allergy immunology practices.
- The total serum hemolytic complement assay (CH_{50}) and alternative pathway hemolytic assay (AH_{50}) tests measure the

intactness of the classical and alternative pathways and represent logical starting points for evaluation.
- Management of infection risk and autoimmunity are critically important.

Introduction

An increased susceptibility to infection is a prominent clinical expression of most of the complement deficiency diseases. The activation of the complement system by microorganisms generates opsonic activity (C3b), anaphylatoxic activity (C4a, C3a, and C5a), chemotactic activity (C5a), and bactericidal activity (C5b, C6, C7, C8, and C9), all critical for host defense (Table 7.1). The opsonic function of C3b renders the pathogen more easily phagocytosed and is the most central function of complement. Other common phenotypes seen in allergy immunology practices are systemic lupus erythematosus (SLE) and atypical hemolytic uremic syndrome (aHUS).

Clinical Settings in Which Complement Deficiency Should Be Considered

Complement is often assessed as part of a "humoral" evaluation for recurrent infection, but infections related to complement deficiency are quite different from those associated with antibody deficiencies (Box 7.1) (Fig. 7.1). Sinopulmonary infections are not the best predictor of complement deficiencies. Systemic infections represent a key indicator for a complement assessment. Complement deficiencies are common among patients with systemic neisserial infections, and thus routine screening is worthwhile.[1-3] The prevalence of complement deficiencies among patients with a single episode of meningococcal sepsis has varied from 5% to 15%. The prevalence is as high as 40% if the patient has had recurrent meningococcal sepsis, has an infection with an uncommon serotype, or has a positive family history of meningococcal systemic infections.[4-7] Chronic meningococcemia is an uncommon disease that appears to be enriched in people with terminal complement deficiencies. Analyses of patients with systemic infections with encapsulated organisms generally has led to the conclusion that recurrent systemic infections with encapsulated organisms is associated with a rate of complement deficiency of 11%.[8] All of the detected complement deficiencies were C2

deficiency, which is enriched in Caucasian populations. Thus, the types of deficiencies and the frequency may be different in other populations. Among young adults with a first invasive bacterial infection, 19% had an immunodeficiency, and in this cohort 10% were found to have a complement deficiency.[9] From these studies, it is suggested that an otherwise healthy person with an invasive infection with encapsulated bacteria should have an immunologic assessment. Certainly people with a history of recurrent invasive

TABLE 7.1	Functions of Complement Components
Components	**Functions**
C4a, C2a, C3a	Anaphylatoxins, histamine release
C3b	Opsonin, costimulation of B cells
C5a	Chemotaxis
C5, C6, C7, C8, C9	Membrane attack complex, lysis

• BOX 7.1 Common Phenotypes of Complement Deficiencies

- Systemic lupus erythematosus
- Invasive infections with encapsulated bacteria
- Neisserial infections
- Early-onset atherosclerosis
- Thrombotic microangiopathies
  - Atypical hemolytic uremic syndrome
  - Preeclampsia and HELPP syndrome
  - Macular degeneration
- Periodontal Ehlers-Danlos syndrome
- Autoinflammation
- Membranoproliferative glomerulonephritis

TABLE 7.2   Founder Effects in Complement Deficiencies

Deficiency	Frequency	Population
C7	1:400	Israeli Moroccan Jews
C9	1:1000	Japanese
C6	1:1400	African Americans
C2	1:10,000	Caucasians

bacterial infections with no clear predisposition, should have an immunologic assessment that includes complement analyses. In this setting, a total serum hemolytic complement assay (CH_{50}) represents the best approach.

The other phenotype for which data are emerging is that of early-onset SLE. In adult cohorts of patients with SLE, the frequency of complement deficiency is about 1%. Universal testing of patients with SLE may make sense because these patients have a higher risk of cardiac events and infection. Although not often done on a systematic basis in the United States, there may be benefit to considering the cost benefit of detection of adult complement-deficient persons. Among early-onset cases of SLE, complement deficiencies have been detected in 9% of those with onset before 18 years of age,[10] 6% of cases with onset younger than 12 years of age,[11] 13% of those with onset before 6 years of age,[10] and 80% of those cases with onset before 5 years of age.[12] There appears to be a clear gradient of epidemiologic association with the strongest association of complement deficiencies with the earliest age of onset, although the precise frequencies vary by population and detection strategy.

Two last phenotypes are not associated with infection or autoimmunity. C1 inhibitor (C1-INH) deficiency is well known to most practicing allergists as a picture of recurrent angioedema in the absence of urticaria or other signs of an atopic trigger. This is inherited in autosomal dominant fashion, and therefore there is often but not universally a positive family history. The last phenotype is that of aHUS. There is a broad range of complement regulatory mutations associated with predisposition to this condition.

Collectively, the epidemiologic associations with complement deficiencies leads to recommendations for complement evaluation for patients with neisserial infections outside of an epidemic, recurrent invasive infections with encapsulated organisms, and early-onset SLE (Box 7.2). Diagnosis of underlying genetic susceptibility to aHUS usually relies on a sequencing approach, and there are several recommendations for assessment. In considering specific complement deficiency states, it can be useful to recognize founder effects, in which specific mutations may be enriched (Table 7.2). Information on deficiencies of each specific component are given in capsule form in the following text for easy reference and in Table 7.3.

Cascade Component Deficiencies

C1q Deficiency

C1q plays a critical role in activation of the classical pathway and the generation of the biologic activities of C3 and C5 through C9. In addition, recent studies have shown that C1q recognizes apoptotic cells and targets them for clearance.[13,14] Individuals with deficient C1q have markedly reduced serum total hemolytic activity and C1 functional activity. In most affected individuals, C1q protein level is also markedly reduced, but in some patients a dysfunctional immunoreactive protein is produced. There is a founder effect in Turkey.[15–18]

Clinical Expression

The most prominent clinical manifestation of C1q deficiency is early-onset SLE. Patients with C1q deficiency carry the highest risk (>90% prevalence) of SLE among the complement deficiencies.[19–21] Those with C1q deficiency have impaired clearance of the immune complexes and apoptotic cells and fail to tolerize B cells properly. The age of onset of SLE is nearly always prepubertal, and the disease tends to be severe. [22] Anti–double-stranded (ds) DNA antibodies may be negative.

Nearly one-third of patients with C1q deficiency have significant bacterial infections, and 10% have died of infections.[19–21] C1q, almost uniquely among complement components, is produced in substantial amounts by hematopoietic cells, and hematopoietic stem cell transplantation has been effective as a curative treatment.[23]

C1r/C1s Deficiency

C1r and C1s are closely linked on chromosome 12 and encode highly homologous serine proteases. C1q, after it binds to an immune complex, activates C1r, which in turn activates C1s. It is C1s that cleaves C4 and C2, resulting in the assembly of the C3 cleaving enzyme C4b2a. Patients with C1r deficiency have a markedly reduced CH_{50} and C1 functional activity.[21] Deficiency of C1r or C1s leads to reduced levels of the other, suggesting that neither is stable in the absence of the other.

Clinical Expression

The most common clinical expression of C1r/s deficiency has been SLE.[19–21] Some patients have also presented with glomerulonephritis or bacterial infections. A 2016 report of periodontal Ehlers-Danlos syndrome associated it with heterozygous truncating mutations, but it is yet unclear if that is due to a specific mutation effect.[24]

C4 Deficiency

The fourth component of complement (C4) is encoded by two closely linked genes (*C4A* and *C4B*) located within the major histocompatibility complex (MHC) on chromosome 6. There are four amino acid differences between them. Because C4 is encoded by two distinct genes, patients with complete

TABLE 7.3 Clinical Characteristics of Inherited Complement Deficiency Diseases

Component	Inheritance	Major Clinical Expression
Classical Pathway		
C1q, C1r, C1s, C4, C2	Autosomal recessive	SLE and bacterial infections with encapsulated organisms, one report of periodontal Ehlers-Danlos syndrome in C1r and C1s deficiency
C3	Autosomal recessive	Glomerulonephritis, severe bacterial infections HUS can be due to heterozygous gain-of-function mutations
Terminal Components		
C5, C6, C7, C8, C9	Autosomal recessive	Neisseria
Regulatory Proteins		
C1 inhibitor	Autosomal dominant	Angioedema
Factor B	Autosomal dominant gain-of-function	aHUS
Factor H	Variable	Infections and aHUS
Factor I	Variable	Infections and aHUS (two reports of autoinflammatory conditions)
MCP	Variable	aHUS
Properdin	X-linked recessive	Neisseria
Factor D	Autosomal recessive	Neisseria

aHUS, Atypical hemolytic uremic syndrome; *HUS,* hemolytic uremic syndrome; *SLE,* systemic lupus erythematosus.

C4 deficiency are homozygous deficient at both loci *(C4A*Q0, C4B*Q0/C4A*Q0, C4B*Q0).*[25,26] Copy number variation at this locus is extremely high, and serum levels of C4 track with the number of inherited copies of C4. Approximately 13% to 14% of the population is heterozygous for C4A deficiency and 15% to 16% heterozygous for C4B deficiency, with the corresponding frequencies for homozygous-deficient individuals being 1% and 3%. Individuals who have *complete* C4 deficiency are homozygous deficient for *both* C4A and C4B), have a very low CH_{50}, and have markedly reduced levels of C4 protein and functional activity.

Clinical Expression

Patients with complete C4 deficiency may present with SLE and/or an increased susceptibility to infection. The onset of SLE is usually early in life and is characterized by prominent cutaneous features such as photosensitive skin rash, vasculitic skin ulcers, and Raynaud's phenomenon. Anti-DNA titers may be absent.[22] Patients with complete C4 deficiency also have an increased susceptibility to bacterial infections, and most deaths in these patients are the result of infection.

The prevalence of homozygous C4A deficiency in patients with SLE is thought to be increased, and it may modify the phenotype.[27-32] In contrast to individuals with homozygous C4A deficiency, individuals with homozygous C4B deficiency lack the C4 isotype that interacts most efficiently with polysaccharides. There is an increased prevalence of homozygous C4B deficiency in children with bacteremia and/or bacterial meningitis.[33,34]

C2 Deficiency

The second component of complement (C2) is encoded by a gene within the MHC on chromosome 6. C2, like C4, plays a critical role in generating the biologic activities of C3 and the terminal components, C5 through C9. Patients with C2 deficiency usually have a very low CH_{50} and less than 1% of the normal levels of C2 protein and function.[35] The majority of C2-deficient individuals (>95%) are Caucasian and have the same molecular genetic defect, a 28–base pair (bp) deletion, which causes premature termination of transcription.[36,37] The gene frequency of this deletion is between 0.05 and 0.007 in individuals of European descent, which translates into a prevalence of homozygotes of approximately 1:10,000.[37,38]

Clinical Expression

Patients with C2 deficiency manifest many of the typical clinical features of lupus, although photosensitive cutaneous lesions are more common.[39,40] They also have a lower prevalence of anti-DNA antibodies than other patients with SLE, but the prevalence of anti-Ro and anti-La antibodies is higher.[22] Unlike in C1 and C4 deficiencies, the lupus is not necessarily more severe than typical SLE, and the age of onset is more variable.

An increased susceptibility to infection is also a prominent clinical presentation of C2 deficiency. The infections are usually caused by encapsulated pyogenic organisms such as *Pneumococcus, Streptococcus,* and *Haemophilus influenzae* and are blood-borne, such as sepsis, meningitis, arthritis, and/or osteomyelitis. Infection is the leading cause of death.[39,40] A phenomenon described in 2005 in C2 deficiency that is likely true in other early component deficiencies is the accelerated atherosclerosis that significantly contributes to mortality.[40]

C3 Deficiency

Whether activated by the classical or alternative pathway, C3 is cleaved into two fragments of unequal sizes. The larger fragment, C3b, is an opsonin and also forms part of the classical and alternative pathway enzymes that activate C5 and generate the membrane attack complex. Both the AH_{50} and CH_{50} will be very low in complete C3 deficiency. The mutations responsible for C3 deficiency in humans have been diverse; however, there is a relatively common deletion of 800 bps found among Afrikaans-speaking South Africans (gene frequency of 0.0057).[41,42]

Clinical Expression

Patients with C3 deficiency have very severe infections.[43] Patients tend to present in very early childhood with invasive infections with *pneumococcus, H. influenzae,* and *meningococcus.* Localized infections such as pneumonia and sinusitis also have been reported. Some patients have had arthralgias and vasculitic skin rashes (similar to serum sickness) associated with active infection.

Most patients have had membranoproliferative glomerulonephritis. True SLE is less common in C3 deficiency than in the other early component deficiencies. The membranoproliferative

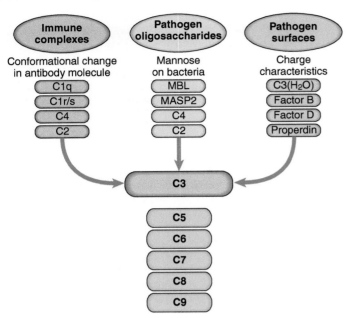

• **Fig. 7.1** The complement cascade. The classical pathway *(blue)* is activated primarily by antibody while the mannose-binding lectin *(MBL) (green)* and alternative pathways *(orange)* are activated directly by pathogens. In each case, the activation arm leads to cleavage of C3 and deposition of C3b onto the surface of the pathogen, where it can act as an opsonin and costimulate B cells.

glomerulonephritis in C3 deficiency[43] is characterized by electron dense deposits in both the mesangium and subendothelium of the capillary loops. Immunofluorescent studies have revealed the presence of immunoglobulins in the kidney, and circulating immune complexes may be present in the serum.

C5 Deficiency

When C5 is activated, it is cleaved into two fragments of unequal size. The smaller fragment, C5a, is a potent chemotactic fragment, and the larger, C5b, initiates assembly of the membrane attack complex, C5b through C9, and is critical for bactericidal activity (Fig. 7.1).

Clinical Expression

The most common clinical expression of C5 deficiency is an increased susceptibility to systemic neisserial infections.[19,20]

C6 Deficiency

C6 participates in the formation of the membrane attack complex. The usual form of C6 deficiency is characterized by very low levels (<1%) of serum C6 and a very low CH_{50}. Another form of C6 deficiency, subtotal C6 deficiency (C6SD), is characterized by 1% to 2% of the normal levels of C6 and levels of total hemolytic activity that are reduced but present.[44] The most common mutation causing C6 deficiency is a single base-pair deletion at position 879.[45,46] C6SD is the result of a loss of the splice donor site of intron 15 and results in a truncated C6 that can support some lytic activity.[44]

Clinical Expression

C6 deficiency is one of the most common complement deficiencies. Among African Americans in the United States, it is reported to be as common as 1:1600 individuals (0.062%).[47] It is thought to be uncommon among individuals of European descent. C6 deficiency is associated with systemic neisserial infections.

C7 Deficiency

C7 participates in the formation of the membrane attack complex. Patients who are deficient in C7 have markedly reduced CH_{50} and C7 levels.

Clinical Expression

The most prominent clinical manifestation of C7 deficiency is an increased susceptibility to systemic neisserial infections. A few patients have presented with SLE, rheumatoid arthritis, pyoderma gangrenosum, and scleroderma, but it is unclear whether these are related to the C7 deficiency.

C8 Deficiency

C8 comprises three different polypeptide chains (α, β, and γ), which are encoded by separate genes *(C8A, C8B, and C8G)*. The α and γ chains are covalently linked to form one chain (C8 α–γ), which is joined to the C8 β chain by noncovalent bonds. C8 is an integral part of the membrane attack complex C5b-9. There are two forms of C8 deficiency, and each is inherited as an autosomal recessive trait. In one form, patients lack the C8 β subunit, whereas in the other form, the α–γ subunit is deficient.[48,49] In either form, the CH_{50} level is usually zero.

C8β is more common among individuals of European descent, and C8 α–γ deficiency is more common among individuals of African descent. Approximately 86% of C8 β-null alleles are the result of C-to-T transition in exon 9, which results in the generation of a premature stop codon.[49,50] Only a limited number of patients with C8 α–γ deficiency have been examined, and in most instances an intronic mutation alters the splicing of exons 6 and 7 of the C8A chain and creates an insertion that generates a premature stop codon.[51]

Clinical Expression

Systemic neisserial infections have been the predominant clinical presentation of C8 deficiency.[51]

C9 Deficiency

Patients with C9 deficiency have markedly reduced levels of both C9 antigen and functional activity. However, the hemolysis of antibody-sensitized erythrocytes can occur and is not dependent on C9. Therefore, patients with C9 deficiency have some hemolytic activity, although it is reduced to between one-third and half of the lower limit of normal.[52–55] C9 deficiency is common in Japan. A nonsense mutation in exon 4 has a gene frequency of 1:1000 in Japanese populations.[53,56]

Clinical Expression

Individuals with C9 deficiency have an increased susceptibility to systemic neisserial infections, although the susceptibility appears to be mitigated by the residual bactericidal activity in individuals with C9 deficiency individuals.[57,58]

Mannose-Binding Lectin Deficiency

Mannose-binding lectin (MBL) deficiency is quite common, with 2% to 7% of people having MBL deficiency.[59] There are structural polymorphisms that destabilize the higher order complexes and several promoter mutations that compromise production. The mutations/polymorphisms exist in haplotypes of varying severity.

Clinical Expression

MBL deficiency has, at most, a modest effect on infection susceptibility. Similarly, it represents a modest risk factor or disease modifier in autoimmune diseases such as SLE or rheumatoid arthritis. The high frequency in the general population suggests that the effect size, if any, is small.

Mannose-Binding Lectin-Associated Serine Protease 2 (MASP2) Deficiency

Mutations and polymorphisms in mannose-binding lectin-associated protease 2 (MASP2) are common and have variable effects on function.[60] Although originally described in a patient with recurrent pneumonia and ulcerative colitis, subsequent studies have not identified an increased susceptibility to infection.[61–63]

Regulatory Component Deficiencies

C1 Esterase Inhibitor Deficiency

C1 esterase inhibitor (C1-INH) binds covalently to C1r and C1s, leading to dissociation of the C1 macromolecular complex and inhibition of the enzymatic actions of C1r and C1s. Genetically determined C1 esterase inhibitor deficiency is inherited as an autosomal dominant trait. In the most common form (type I), accounting for approximately 85% of the patients, the sera of affected individuals are deficient in both C1-INH protein (5% to 30% of normal) and C1-INH function.[64,65] In the other less common form (type II), a dysfunctional protein is present in normal or elevated concentrations, but the functional activity of C1-INH is markedly reduced.[66,67] Mutations causing C1-INH deficiency are diverse. C1-INH function is usually 30% to 50% of normal. C4 levels are usually reduced below the lower limit of normal, both during and between attacks, because of the uncontrolled cleavage by C1s.

C1-INH is the major inhibitor of kallikrein and C1, and therefore, diminished levels of C1-INH lead to unregulated activation of the classical pathway and kallikrein after exposure to a mild trigger (Fig. 7.2).[68–70] Complement anaphylatoxins are thought to play a minor role in the process, and bradykinin is the major mediator of the angioedema.[71] There are now known phenocopies of C1-INH deficiency, including mutations affecting factor XII and plasminogen.

Clinical Expression

C1-INH deficiency is responsible for most cases of the clinical disorder of hereditary angioedema (HAE).[72] Attacks involving the subcutaneous tissue may involve an extremity, the face, or the genitalia. In some instances, there may be changes just preceding the edema such as subtle mottling, a transient serpiginous erythema, or frank erythema marginatum.[73] The edema usually expands outward from a single site and may vary in size from a few centimeters to the involvement of a whole extremity. The lesions are characteristically nonpruritic. There may be a feeling of tightness in the skin because of the accumulation of subcutaneous fluid. Attacks usually progress for 1 to 2 days and resolve over an additional 2 to 3 days in the absence of treatment.

Attacks involving the upper respiratory tract represent a significant cause of morbidity and occasionally death. In one series published in 1976, pharyngeal edema had occurred at least once in nearly two-thirds of the patients.[65] Laryngeal edema, accompanied by hoarseness and stridor, occurs and progresses to respiratory

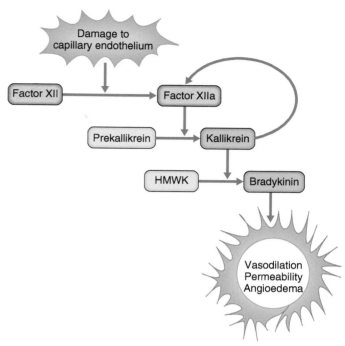

• Fig. 7.2 The role of C1 inhibitor in angioedema. The edema in C1 inhibitor deficiency is due primarily to activation of bradykinin. Factor XII (Hageman factor) is activated by exposure to damaged capillary vessels. Kallikrein performs two roles: it acts to cleave bradykinin from high molecular weight kininogen (HMWK) and enhance factor XIIa activation in a feed-forward loop.

obstruction. This is a life-threatening emergency. In fact, in that same series, tracheotomies had been performed in 1 of every 6 patients with HAE.[65] Today, with improved treatment, this is becoming less common.

Symptoms in the gastrointestinal tract are related to edema of the bowel wall and may include anorexia, dull aching of the abdomen, vomiting, and, in some cases, crampy abdominal pain. Abdominal symptoms are often prominent in childhood and can occur in the absence of concurrent cutaneous or pharyngeal involvement. In some instances, abdominal symptoms may be the only symptoms the patient has ever had, leading to difficulty in diagnosis.[74]

Although the onset of symptoms occurs in more than half of the patients before adolescence, in some patients their first symptoms do not occur until they are well into adult life. In just over half of the patients, no specific event can be clearly identified as initiating attacks, although infection, trauma, anxiety, or stress are frequently cited. Dental extractions and tonsillectomy can initiate edema of the upper airway, and cutaneous edema may follow trauma to an extremity. A potential source of diagnostic confusion is the association of HAE with SLE, presumably because the secondary reduction of C4 predisposes to SLE. These patients can be quite difficult to diagnose and manage.

Factor H Deficiency

Factor H deficiencies have two distinct phenotypes that seldom occur together in the same patient. aHUS in factor H deficiency is thought to be the result of an inability to protect fenestrated endothelium in the glomerulus from complement-mediated damage.[75] The thrombotic microangiopathy of factor H deficiency can manifest as aHUS or HELLP syndrome (hemolysis, elevated liver enzymes, low platelets), in pregnancy.[76] A mild form of factor H deficiency causes macular degeneration for the same reason. Management of aHUS acutely uses the same modalities as for typical HUS; however, eculizumab, an antibody directed at C5, has gradually become integrated into medical care.

Neisserial infections are also seen in patients with factor H deficiency. The infections arise because of unregulated consumption of C3.[43,77,78] HUS-associated mutations are not always or even often associated with demonstrable defects in typical complement assays such as AH_{50} and CH_{50}. Neisseria-associated mutations often lead to a diminished level of C3.

Factor H–Related Genes

There are five genes encoding factor H–related proteins. These genes, CFHR1-5, exhibit copy number variation and frequent mutation. The precise function of these proteins is not known, although they interact with factor H and bind Neisseria. Deletions of CFHR1 and CFHR3 are associated with thrombotic microangiopathy and often have an autoantibody-mediated mechanism.[79,80] A point mutation in CFHR5 is associated with a mild nephropathy common in Cyprus.[81] Variants in these genes also appear to be increased in macular degeneration.

Factor I Deficiency

Factor I is a serine protease that cleaves C3b to produce iC3b, an inactive cleavage product that cannot function in the C3-cleaving enzyme of the alternative pathway. Two phenotypes are clearly associated with factor I deficiency: aHUS and susceptibility to Neisseria. There are two reports of autoinflammatory conditions in people who were found to have factor I deficiency. The mutations associated with infection and aHUS are distinct, and the aHUS mutations also can be seen in preeclampsia and HELLP syndrome.[76] HUS-associated mutations do not always lead to altered AH_{50}.

Membrane Co-factor Protein (CD46) Deficiency

Membrane co-factor protein is a widely expressed membrane-bound glycoprotein that inhibits complement activation on host cells. Deficiencies of membrane co-factor protein (MCP) are associated with aHUS, although the presentation is usually later and milder than in patients with factor H or factor I deficiencies.[82–85] MCP mutations account for approximately 10% of all cases of aHUS. MCP is expressed on renal tissues, and therefore, renal transplantation can be successful. Traditional complement analyses are normal.

Properdin Deficiency

Properdin is the only gene of the complement system that is encoded on the X chromosome. Properdin stabilizes the alternative pathway C3 and C5 convertases by extending the half-lives of the C3 and C5 converting enzymes. Protein may be absent or reduced in the serum depending on the specific mutation. The AH_{50} may be normal to extremely low.

Clinical Expression

Approximately 50% of the patients described with properdin deficiency have had systemic meningococcal disease.[19,20,86] Isolated cases of SLE and discoid lupus also have been seen in properdin-deficient patients, but this may represent ascertainment bias.

Factor D Deficiency

Neisserial infections are seen in factor D deficiency.[19,20,87] Systemic streptococcal infections also have been seen. Other complement levels are typically normal in factor D deficiency; however, there is almost no ability to activate the alternative pathway.

CD55 (DAF) Deficiency

CD55 is a membrane-bound protein that regulates both classical and alternative pathway activation on the surface. Congenital CD55 deficiency is associated with protein-losing enteropathy. Somatic mutations can lead to acquired loss of CD55 in paroxysmal nocturnal hemoglobinuria (PHN).

Management of Genetically Determined Complement Deficiencies

Prevention of Infectious Diseases

Two strategies have been attempted to reduce susceptibility to infections and/or modify the clinical course of the infections in patients with genetically determined deficiencies of complement. One strategy is to immunize these patients against common bacterial pathogens such as pneumococcus, H. influenzae, and meningococcus. Data support the use of repeated meningococcal vaccination to mitigate the risk of infection for patients with terminal complement component deficiencies.[88] Guidelines should be consulted because recommendations change frequently as new vaccines become available, and there are specific recommendations about the sequence of vaccines because nonconjugated vaccine administration can interfere with subsequent conjugated vaccine responses.[88–90]

A second strategy in the prevention of infection is the use of prophylactic antibiotics. Because patients with complement deficiencies have a high risk of recurrent episodes of blood-borne infections and because immunizations may not afford them complete protection, some patients have been placed on antibiotic prophylaxis. Any recommendation for antibiotic prophylaxis must be viewed in the context of the emergence of antibiotic resistance among bacteria. A related strategy is to offer emergency antibiotics for those who travel or live far from medical care. This strategy requires strong counseling that medical care must be sought. The antibiotics are not intended to supplant medical care.

Management of Autoimmune Disorders

Regardless of the disorder, autoimmune conditions are most often treated with the same immunosuppressive agents and antiinflammatory medications as one would use in a complement-sufficient patient. Most autoimmune disorders are associated with an increased risk of atherosclerosis in their own right, and the early complement component deficiencies appear to add to that risk. Therefore, aggressive management of cardiac risk factors is advisable. The one alternative approach is the use of hematopoietic stem cell transplantation for C1q deficiency. The outcomes for conventionally treated patients with C1q deficiency are poor, and further exploration of the role of transplantation in this setting is desirable.

Management of Angioedema

Attenuated androgens such as oxandrolone or danazol are highly effective[91,92] and act by increasing transcription of the normal allele of SERPING1.[93] However, because of their androgenic effects and newer drugs with high efficacy, their use has declined significantly. C1-INH concentrate is approved for use as both prophylaxis and treatment.[94,95] Twice-weekly intravenous administration and cost for prophylaxis will be barriers for some patients, but it is widely used for acute episodes. Recently approved is a subcutaneous form of C1-INH that can be self-administered as prophylaxis. C1-INH is widely used as a presurgical prophylaxis. Ecallantide and icatibant are also available as treatment for acute episodes and are given as subcutaneous injections on demand. Icatibant is designed for home administration, and ecallantide is designed to be given with healthcare supervision. A recently approved kallikrein inhibitor given as a subcutaneous injection every 2 weeks, lanadelumab-flyo, is available for children over 12 years of age and adults.

Management of angioedema also requires education of the family and cautions against estrogen-containing birth control pills, undue exposure to trauma, and use of angiotensin-converting enzyme inhibitors.[96] All of these can precipitate episodes. Acute attacks can be emergencies, and patients should have an action plan that includes contingencies for airway involvement. Epinephrine, antihistamines, and corticosteroids are of no proven benefit in C1-INH deficient patients. Fresh frozen plasma (FFP) has some advocates; however, clinical data on its use are limited, and there is a theoretical concern of providing substrate for additional activation of the deleterious pathways.[97]

Management of HUS

As is done for thrombotic thrombocytopenia purpura (TTP), most patients with aHUS receive apheresis and FFP replacement for acute episodes.[82,83] Factor H replacement may be of benefit, and FFP may be used to replace factor H. In the case of MCP deficiency, in which the affected protein is membrane-bound, it is less clear that pheresis and FFP would provide benefit, but it could potentially act to clear inciting agents or complement activation products. Eculizumab, a C5 inhibitor, has been approved as treatment for aHUS resulting from complement deficiencies.[98] The appropriate use of eculizumab in this setting is still being defined. For patients with factor H or factor I deficiency and end-stage renal disease, renal transplantation is not recommended. In contrast, renal disease in MCP does not recur in the transplanted kidney.

Secondary Complement Deficiencies

Secondary complement deficiencies are relatively common. Any pathologic process that results in activation of the complement cascade or interferes with the synthesis of complement components, such as liver disease, can result in a secondary complement deficiency (Table 7.4). These conditions are of high clinical importance, and multiple studies have demonstrated an increased risk of infection in settings with complement consumption.

Impaired synthesis

Newborn

In full-term infants, the levels of most components of either the classical or alternative pathways are 50% to 80% of adult levels.[99] However, C8 and C9 are more severely depressed, with levels in full-term newborn infants as low as 28% and 10%, respectively, of maternal levels.[100,101]

Cirrhosis

Patients with cirrhosis have decreased serum concentrations of C3, C4, and total hemolytic activity as a result of diminished synthesis.[102] There is a correlation between the low levels of C3 and a predisposition to spontaneous bacterial peritonitis and mortality in cirrhosis.[103]

TABLE 7.4	Common Secondary Causes of Low Complement Studies	
Impaired synthesis (Usually low CH50 and AH50)	Cirrhosis or other liver synthetic disease
	Immaturity
Classical pathway activation (Low CH_{50}, AH_{50} variable, low C3 and C4)	Systemic lupus erythematosus, Sjögren's, other systemic autoimmune diseases
	Hemolytic anemia
	Cryoglobulinemia
	Vasculitis
	IgG4 disease
Alternative pathway activation (Low AH_{50}, CH_{50} variable, low C3 with normal C4)	Typical C3 nephritic factor

Malnutrition

Malnutrition, both kwashiorkor and marasmus, is associated with decreased levels of serum total hemolytic complement activity and most of the individual components of complement, such as C3 and C5.[104,105] The degree of the decrease in complement components, such as C3, correlates strongly with serum albumin.

Protein Loss

Nephrotic Syndrome

Loss of complement proteins in the urine, particularly factor B,[106] contributes to the increased susceptibility to infection.

Consumption of Complement Components

C3 Nephritic Factors

Membranoproliferative glomerulonephritis type II (dense deposit disease) is associated with a variety of autoantibodies directed at C3 convertases. The distinction between membranoproliferative glomerulonephritis types relies on the immunofluorescent analysis of biopsy samples. Types I and III are due to chronic antigen and immune complex deposition, and type II is caused by dysregulation of the alternative pathway of the complement cascade. Over 80% of patients with membranoproliferative glomerulonephritis have a C3 nephritic factor. Rarely, these autoantibodies may be clinically silent. A subset is associated with lipodystrophy. The most typical C3 nephritic factor is directed at the alternative pathway convertase and prolongs its activity. C3 is consumed, and this leads to a low AH_{50} and CH_{50}. Different autoantibodies can affect different convertases and include additional components. C3 nephritic factors are identified in reference laboratories through a mixing approach.

Autoimmune Disease

SLE is a systemic disorder in which immune complexes are generated. These activate the complement cascade, leading to consumption of individual components such as C3 and C4. The activation and consumption of the complement system typically

- Classical pathway and alternative pathway cascade component deficiencies are associated with a CH_{50} or AH_{50} of zero or nearly zero (with the exception of C9 deficiency).
- A very low CH_{50} and AH_{50} implies a defect in the terminal components.
- A very low CH_{50} with normal AH_{50} localizes the defect to C1, C4, or C2.
- Moderately low CH_{50} and AH_{50} levels can be due to regulatory component deficiencies, poor sample handling, consumption, impaired synthesis, or immaturity.
- C4 levels track with the copy number of C4 genes

precedes clinical flare, and the degree of hypocomplementemia, specifically levels of C3 and C4, generally reflects the degree of clinical activity.[107–110] Although complement activation as a result of the circulating immune complexes is particularly characteristic of lupus, it also has been described in other autoimmune diseases in which autoantibodies are pathologic. Development of antibodies to C1q occurs in SLE, in which it is associated with a high rate of renal disease and can occur as an isolated condition referred to as hypocomplementemic urticarial vasculitis (HUVS). This condition has a characteristic rash but can involve any organ. The antibodies to C1q lead to very low classical pathway component levels and CH_{50}.

Poststreptococcal Glomerulonephritis

Recovery of Complement Levels Can Be Protracted

Serum Sickness. Serum sickness is the consequence of immune complex formation in response to the administration of drugs (e.g., penicillin, cefaclor, and minocycline), foreign proteins (e.g., antithymocyte globulin, therapeutic monoclonal antibodies, or antivenoms), or, in some instances, infections.[111,112] Although rash, fever, and arthralgia/arthritis are the most common clinical findings, severe cases may progress to renal involvement.[113] Immune complexes are present in the circulation early in the process. Most cases have significant hypocomplementemia.[114,115]

Sepsis. Acute bacterial sepsis may be associated with transient hypocomplementemia characterized by low levels of C3 and C4 and low total hemolytic activity (CH_{50}).[116] The hypocomplementemia is most commonly found in patients who have some degree of cardiovascular compromise and is strongly correlated with the severity of the shock and morbidity. Viral sepsis can also drive consumption.

Cardiopulmonary Bypass, Extracorporeal Membrane Oxygenation, and Hemodialysis

Cardiopulmonary bypass, extracorporeal membrane oxygenation, and hemodialysis bring the patient's blood in contact with artificial surfaces or membranes. As a result, there may be activation of the complement system, generation of biologically

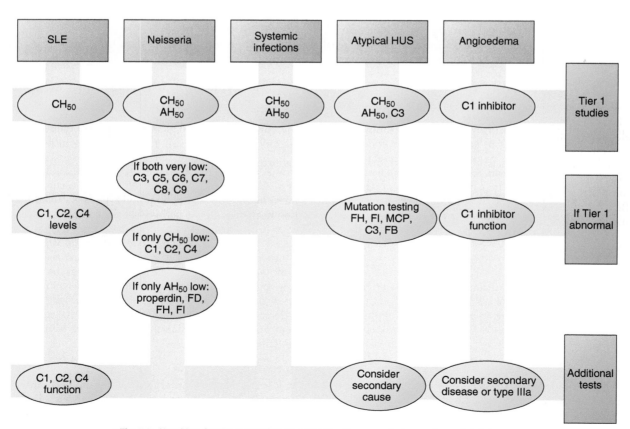

• **Fig. 7.3** Algorithm for the evaluation of patients with suspected complement deficiency.

active cleavage products, and consumption of complement components. A number of studies have suggested that the generation of these anaphylatoxins is responsible for the generalized inflammatory response that follows cardiopulmonary bypass (postperfusion syndrome) and hemodialysis (pulmonary neutrophil sequestration).[117]

Paroxysmal Nocturnal Hemoglobinuria

PNH is characterized by recurrent episodes of hemoglobinuria secondary to intravascular hemolysis and is associated with acquired somatic mutations of PIG-A or PIG-T in a clone of bone marrow progenitor cells.[118,119] PNH can be associated with complement dysfunction. Inherited CD59 deficiency has been associated with a PNH-like syndrome.[120] PNH today is usually diagnosed on the basis of flow cytometry for CD55 and CD59 on multiple hematopoietic lineages.

Eculizumab Treatment

Eculizumab blocks C5 and therefore leads to blockade of both AH_{50} and CH_{50} functions in vivo, and this extends to laboratory assessment.[121]

Laboratory Assessment of Complement

The CH_{50} result reports the dilution of serum capable of lysing 50% of antibody-coated sheep cells, and the AH_{50} reports the dilution of serum capable of lysing 50% of rabbit red cells. The CH_{50} measures the intactness of the classical pathway from C1 through C9, and the AH_{50} measures the intactness of the alternative pathway from factor B through C9. A plate-based assay is available widely in Europe and offers advantages in terms of stability of assay components, ease of use, and throughput.[122] With the exception of C9 deficiency, genetic deficiencies of all the cascade components lead to a CH_{50} or AH_{50} of zero or near zero. For a finding of low levels of CH_{50} or AH_{50}, the tests should be repeated and appropriate handling of the serum should be ensured. Complement components are consumed quickly once blood has been drawn. Other causes of low, but not absent, CH_{50} results are complement consumption resulting from infection or autoimmune disease. Less common, but more medically important are the regulatory protein defects leading to consumption of C3, such as factor D, factor H, and factor I deficiency. C9 deficiency also leads to a reduction in both the CH_{50} and AH_{50} (Fig. 7.3). Nephritic factors (antibodies to complement components) can lead to a chronically low CH_{50}, AH_{50}, or both. Box 7.3 offers useful clinical pearls for the interpretation of laboratory results.

Once an abnormal CH_{50} or AH_{50} has been confirmed, nephelometry is used to define the serum levels of certain components (C3 and C4 primarily) and enzyme-linked immunosorbent assays (ELISAs) are available for certain other components. Individual component functional assays are not widely available but are available through reference laboratories. Once the specific diagnosis is established, the management path becomes clearer.

Conclusions

Complement represents a bridge between innate and adaptive immunity. It is important for the phagocytosis of immune complexes, opsonization of bacteria, lysis of bacteria, solubilizing immune complexes, and elimination of apoptotic cells. Complement deficiencies often manifest as either susceptibility to recurrent infections or susceptibility to autoimmune/immune complex–mediated diseases. Deficiencies of early components of the classical complement cascade (C1, C2, C4, and C3) are associated with both autoimmune/immune complex diseases and susceptibility to infections. Deficiencies of components of the alternative pathway (factor H, factor I, factor D, and properdin) and of late components of the complement system C5 to C9 are associated with susceptibility to infections, primarily neisserial infections in the case of deficiency of C5 through C9. The diagnosis of a complement component deficiency must be entertained in all cases with recurrent severe bacterial infections, particularly in the face of elevated or upper range levels of serum immunoglobulins and adequate antibody titers. The diagnosis of a deficiency in the early components of the classical complement cascade must be entertained in cases of SLE with a history of significant infection or early-onset SLE, and defects in regulatory proteins should be sought in cases of aHUS. A diagnosis of C1-INH deficiency must be considered in cases of nonpruritic angioedema in the absence of urticaria, particularly in the presence of a similar family history and in cases precipitated by trauma. Fortunately, treatment and education regarding risk can be life-saving.

Acknowledgments

Jerry Winkelstein's wisdom and passion for complement are gratefully acknowledged. He co-authored the original version of this chapter.

The reference list can be found on the companion Expert Consult website at http://www.expertconsult.inkling.com.

8

Defects of Innate Immunity

SERGIO D. ROSENZWEIG, STEVEN M. HOLLAND

KEY POINTS

- White blood cells (lymphoid or myeloid) can suffer from quantitative or functional congenital disorders.
- The type of cells or mechanisms that are mainly affected will define the spectrum of infectious diseases a particular patient will suffer.
- The pathophysiology, clinical manifestations, and diagnostic

approaches on classic innate immunity defects (e.g., neutropenias, chronic granulomatous disease, leukocyte adhesion deficiency, and mucocutaneous candidiasis among other syndromes) are discussed.
- Recently recognized genetic diseases (e.g., IRF8, ISG15, and some forms of mucocutaneous candidiasis) are presented.

Introduction

This chapter focuses on neutrophils and monocytes and disorders that arise from their quantitative or functional defects. Mature neutrophils develop in the bone marrow from a myeloid stem cell over 14 days, during which time proliferation, differentiation, and maturation take place. Mature neutrophils, with their load of primary, secondary, and tertiary granules, are released into the bloodstream, where they stay 6 to 10 hours before exiting by diapedesis. In tissues, they may work in ways that are primarily phagocytic, bactericidal, or fungicidal or in the removal of damaged tissue. Neutrophil disorders can be divided into quantitative (increase or decrease) and functional (failures in specific metabolic or interactive pathways). Quantitative disorders include neutrophilia (>7000 neutrophils/μL in adult patients) and neutropenia (mild: <1500 neutrophils/μL, moderate: 500 to 1000 neutrophils/μL, severe: <500 neutrophils/μL). With very few exceptions (e.g., chronic idiopathic neutrophilia, leukocyte adhesion deficiencies [LADs], myeloproliferative diseases), neutrophilia depends on causes extrinsic to the neutrophils (e.g., acute or chronic infection, steroids, epinephrine). On the other hand, the causes of neutropenia are multiple and can be intrinsic or extrinsic to neutrophils or their progenitors (Box 8.1). Neutropenia usually falls into categories of decreased production, increased destruction, or a combination of the two.

Qualitative myeloid disorders include defects in motility (i.e., adhesion, chemotaxis), defects in phagocytosis, defects of granule synthesis and release, and defects in killing (see Box 8.1).

A neutrophil disorder should be suspected in patients with recurrent, severe, bacterial, or fungal infections, especially those caused by unusual organisms (e.g., *Chromobacterium violaceum*) or in uncommon locations (e.g., liver abscess; Table 8.1). Viral and parasitic infections are typically not increased in these patients.

Initial laboratory evaluation should take into account the clinical presentation to direct where the defect is likely to be. Some

assays, such as repeated white blood cell (WBC) counts with differentials or microscopic evaluation of neutrophils, are relatively simple and can readily exclude neutropenia or some granule defects. Flow cytometry requires a careful consideration of which markers to examine. Functional assays, such as oxidative burst testing, phagocytosis, or chemotaxis are the most challenging because so few laboratories perform them routinely (Table 8.2). We will consider some of the clinical, diagnostic, and management aspects of a few of the best characterized myeloid disorders.

Severe Congenital Neutropenia

Severe congenital neutropenia (SCN) comprises a heterogeneous group of disorders that share the common characteristics of bone marrow granulocytic maturation arrest at the promyelocyte or myelocyte stage, severe chronic neutropenia (<200 neutrophils/μL), and increased susceptibility to acute myeloid leukemia.[1,2]

In 1956 Kostmann[3] described a Swedish kindred with SCN inherited in an autosomal recessive pattern. Klein and colleagues[4] identified homozygous mutations in the antiapoptotic molecule HAX1 in patients with autosomal recessive SCN, which was confirmed to be the cause in the original Kostmann pedigree, as well. Some patients with HAX1 deficiency also have cognitive problems and/or epilepsy.[5]

Among patients with SCN, single allele mutations in the granulocyte colony-stimulating factor (G-CSF) receptor (GCSFR, 1p35-p34.3) have been associated with the development of acute myeloid leukemia.[6] However, not all patients with SCN develop mutations in the G-CSF receptor, indicating that these mutations are somatic mutation epiphenomena that occur in the setting of SCN but do not cause it.[7] Autosomal recessive mutations in the glucose-6-phosphatase catalytic subunit 3 (G6PC3) also cause congenital neutropenia along with cardiac and urogenital malformations.[8]

• BOX 8.1 Neutrophil Disorders
Causes

Neutrophilia
- Usually depends on causes *extrinsic* to the neutrophils (e.g., acute or chronic infection, steroids)

Neutropenia
- Caused by defects *intrinsic* to the neutrophils or their progenitors (severe congenital neutropenia, cyclic neutropenia, neutropenia associated to other well-defined syndromes [e.g., Schwachman's syndrome, Fanconi's syndrome, dyskeratosis congenita, Chédiak-Higashi syndrome, reticular dysgenesis, WHIM syndrome])
- Caused by defects *extrinsic* to the neutrophil or their progenitors (splenomegaly, infections, drugs, immune mediated, metabolic diseases, nutritional deficiencies, bone marrow infiltration)

Motility Disorders
- Adhesion: Leukocyte adhesion deficiency 1, 2, or 3
- Chemotaxis: Leukocyte adhesion deficiency 1, 2, or rac2; localized juvenile periodontitis, neutrophil β-actin deficiency, secondary to extensive burns, secondary to alcohol consumption

Phagocytosis Disorders
- Leukocyte adhesion deficiency 1 (complement-mediated only), secondary to antibody deficiencies, complement deficiencies, mannose-binding protein deficiency

Disorders of Granule Formation and Content
- Chédiak-Higashi syndrome, specific granule deficiency

Microbicidal Disorders
- Chronic granulomatous disease, myeloperoxidase deficiency, glucose-6-phosphate dehydrogenase deficiency, glutathione pathway deficiencies

---

Horwitz and colleagues[9] and Dale and colleagues[10] found that 22 of 25 patients with dominant or spontaneous SCN had heterozygous mutations in the gene encoding neutrophil elastase (*ELA2* or *ELANE,* 19p13.3). Interestingly, mutations in this same gene are also responsible for cyclic neutropenia. *ELANE* mutations are responsible for more than 50% of SCN cases in Caucasian patients.[11]

The clinical manifestations of SCN appear promptly after birth: 50% of affected infants are symptomatic before the first month of life and 90% within the first 6 months; omphalitis, upper and lower respiratory tract infections, and skin and liver abscesses are common. Subcutaneous recombinant G-CSF (5 μg/kg/day) has dramatically changed the prognosis of these patients.[1,2] Since the advent of recombinant G-CSF, reductions in the number of infections and hospitalization days and an increase in life expectancy have been described.[1,2]

Devriendt and colleagues[12] described a family with an X-linked form of SCN (XLN) caused by mutations in the Wiskott-Aldrich syndrome protein (WASP). In contrast to the WASP mutations that produce classic Wiskott-Aldrich syndrome or X-linked thrombocytopenia, most of which are caused by mutations resulting in reduced WASP transcription or translation, the mutation causing XLN (p.Leu270Pro) creates a constitutively active mutant protein.

Two families with heterozygous mutations in *GFI1* and congenital neutropenia and monocytosis have been described.[13] *GFI1* mutations act in a dominant-negative way; that is, inheritance is autosomal dominant. Reticular dysgenesis is an autosomal

recessive severe combined immunodeficiency characterized by early myeloid arrest, neutropenia, lymphopenia, and sensorineural loss (see Chapter 6).

Cyclic Neutropenia/Cyclic Hematopoiesis

Cyclic neutropenia/cyclic hematopoiesis is inherited as an autosomal dominant trait and characterized by regular cyclic fluctuations in all hematopoietic lineages. However, clinical manifestations are almost exclusively associated with variations in neutrophils. Neutrophil counts cycle on an average of every 21 days (range 14–36 days), including periods of severe neutropenia (<200/μL) that last from 3 to 10 days.[14,15] Mutations in *ELANE* (neutrophil elastase 2, 19p13.3) have been identified in all pedigrees analyzed.[10,11] Most patients have manifestations of neutropenia in early childhood. Oral ulcerations, gingivitis, lymphadenopathy, pharyngitis/tonsillitis, and skin lesions are the most frequent findings. Early loss of permanent teeth as a consequence of chronic gingivitis and periapical abscesses is common.[16] Bone marrow aspirates obtained during periods of neutropenia show maturation arrest at the myelocyte stage or bone marrow hypoplasia.[17]

G-CSF improves peripheral neutrophil counts and decreases morbidity in patients with cyclic neutropenia. Infections and hospitalizations appear to naturally lessen with age.[16]

Large granular lymphocytosis (LGL) deserves special mention as a cause of adult-onset cyclic or sustained neutropenia. This disease is due to increased and usually clonal expansion of CD8 or NK cells with a tropism for neutrophils and sometimes other marrow elements. This diagnosis is suspected in an adult with new-onset neutropenia and is confirmed by identification of clonal CD8 cells infiltrating bone marrow, often in lymphoid aggregates.[18]

Warts, Hypogammaglobulinemia, Infections, and Myelokathexis (WHIM) Syndrome

Myelokathexis (from the Greek, meaning "retained in the bone marrow") is a congenital disorder with severe chronic neutropenia. Unlike other forms of congenital neutropenia, bone marrow aspirates from patients with myelokathexis show myeloid hypercellularity with increased numbers of granulocytes at all stages of differentiation. A significant number of patients with myelokathexis also have warts, hypogammaglobulinemia, and infections of varying severity. Most patients with WHIM have heterozygous deletions affecting the chemokine receptor CXCR4.[19] Enhanced CXCR4 activity delays release of mature neutrophils from the bone marrow, resulting in peripheral neutropenia.[20,21] Recurrent sinopulmonary infections are frequent. Memory B cells are also depressed in this disease, in part accounting for their humoral defects.[22] During episodes of infection, neutrophil counts typically increase compared with baseline levels. Steroids, subcutaneous epinephrine, intravenous endotoxin, and G-CSF and granulocyte-macrophage colony-stimulating factor (GM-CSF) can mobilize mature neutrophils from WHIM bone marrow. Sustained therapy with G-CSF or GM-CSF increases the number of neutrophils in the peripheral blood and decreases the number of infections. Plerixafor (Mozobil), a small molecule that binds and blocks CXCR4 and is used for hematopoietic stem cells mobilization for transplantation also has been shown to have a beneficial effect in patients with WHIM.[23,24]

TABLE 8.1	**Infections and White Blood Cell Defects** *Features Highly Suspicious of Phagocyte Disorders: (A) Severe Infections, (B) Recurrent Infections, (C) Infections Caused by Specific Microorganisms, (D) Unusually Located Infections*						
(A) SEVERE INFECTIONS		**(B) RECURRENT INFECTIONS**		**(C) SPECIFIC INFECTIONS**		**(D) UNUSUALLY LOCATED INFECTIONS**	
Type of Infection	Diagnosis to Consider	Site of Infection	Diagnosis to Consider	Microorganism	Diagnosis to Consider	Site of Infection	Diagnosis to Consider
Cellulitis	Neutropenia, LAD, CGD, HIES	Cutaneous	Neutropenia, CGD, LAD, HIES	*Staphylococcus epidermidis*	Neutropenia, LAD	Umbilical cord stump	LAD
Colitis	Neutropenia, CGD	Gums	LAD, neutropenia, neutrophil motility disorders	*Serratia marscecens, Chromobacterium violaceum, Nocardia, Burkholderia cepacia, Granulibacter bethesdensis*	CGD	Liver abscess	CGD
Osteomyelitis	CGD, MSMD pathway defects	Upper and lower respiratory tract	Neutropenia, HIES, functional neutrophil disorders	*Aspergillus*	Neutropenia, CGD, HIES	Gums	LAD, neutropenia, neutrophil motility disorders
		GI tract	CGD, MSMD pathway defects (*Salmonella* spp.)	Nontuberculous mycobacteria, BCG	MSMD pathway defects, SCID, CGD		
		Lymph nodes	CGD, MSMD pathway defects (mycobacteria)	*Candida*	Neutropenia, CGD, MPO, STAT1 GOF		
		Osteomyelitis	CGD, MSMD pathway defects				

CGD, Chronic granulomatous disease; *CMC,* chronic mucocutaneous candidiasis; *GOF,* gain of function; *HIES,* hyper-IgE syndrome; *LAD,* leukocyte adhesion deficiency; *MPO,* myeloperoxidase deficiency; *MSMD,* Mendelian susceptibility to mycobacterial diseases; *SCID,* severe combined immunodeficiency.

Immune-Mediated Neutropenias

Alloimmune Neonatal Neutropenia

Alloimmune neonatal neutropenia (ANN) is produced by the transplacental transfer of maternal antibodies against NA1 and NA2, two isotypes of the immunoglobulin receptor FcγRIIIb, causing destruction of neonatal neutrophils.[25-29] If the mother does not express FcγRIIIb on her own neutrophils, she may elaborate antibodies against paternally encoded FcγRIIIb expressed on fetal neutrophils. These complement-activating antineutrophil antibodies can be detected in 1 in 500 live births, making the potential incidence of ANN high. This disease should be considered in the evaluation of all infants with neutropenia, with or without infection. Antibody-coated neutrophils in ANN are phagocytosed in the reticuloendothelial system and removed from the circulation, leaving the neonate neutropenic and prone to infections. Omphalitis, cellulitis, and pneumonia may be the presenting infections within the first 2 weeks of life. The diagnosis can be made by detection of neutrophil-specific alloantibodies in maternal serum. Parenteral antibiotics (even in the absence of other signs of sepsis) and G-CSF should be included in the initial management of ANN. As expected, ANN tends to spontaneously improve with the waning of maternal antibody levels, but this process may take months.[29]

Primary and Secondary Autoimmune Neutropenia

Autoimmune neutropenia (AIN) is a rare disorder, caused by peripheral destruction of neutrophils and/or their precursors by autoantibodies present in patient serum or mediated by large granular lymphocytes (LGL, CD3+/CD8+/CD57+ T cells) in the bone marrow. AIN can be either primary or secondary. When the neutropenia is an isolated clinical entity, it is primary AIN, and when associated with another disease, it is secondary AIN.

Primary Autoimmune Neutropenia

Primary AIN is the most common cause of chronic neutropenia (absolute neutrophil count <1500/μL lasting at least 6 months) in infancy and childhood. There is a slight female predominance, and it has been reported in about 1:100,000 live births, 10 times more frequent than SCN. Antibodies directed against different neutrophil antigens can be detected in almost all patients. Approximately one-third of these autoantibodies are anti-NA1 and anti-NA2 isoforms of FcγRIIIb (the same targets recognized in ANN). Almost 85% of these antibodies are immunoglobulin G (IgG). Other antigens toward which autoantibodies can be found are CD11b/CD18 (Mac-1), CD32 (FcγRII), and CD35 (C3b complement receptor). The average age at diagnosis for primary AIN is 8 months. The majority of patients present with either skin or

TABLE 8.2	Laboratory Evaluation of Patient With Suspected Neutrophil Disorder*	
Test	**If Normal, It Excludes . . .**	
White blood cell count and differential (repeated)	All forms of neutropenia	
Neutrophil morphologic evaluation	Specific granule deficiency; Chédiak-Higashi syndrome	
Flow cytometry		
CD18	LAD 1 (complete)	
CD15s (sialyl Lewis^x)	LAD 2	
Dihydrorhodamine (DHR) oxidation	CGD (MPO deficiency, severe G6PD deficiencies and glutathione pathway deficiencies have abnormal DHR oxidation as well)	
STAT1 phosphorylation	Complete IFNGR1, IFNGR2 deficiency	
STAT4 phosphorylation	Complete IL-12Rβ1 and TYK2 deficiency	
Bone marrow aspirate		
Neutrophil maturation	Severe congenital neutropenia; cyclic neutropenia	
Neutrophil retention	WHIM syndrome	
Nitroblue tetrazolium reduction	CGD (severe G6PD deficiencies and glutathione pathway deficiencies have abnormal NBT reduction as well)	

*Patients should be evaluated considering their familial history, physical examination, and associated comorbid factors.

CGD, Chronic granulomatous disease; *G6PD*, glucose-6-phosphate dehydrogenase; *IL*, interleukin; *LAD*, leukocyte adhesion deficiency; *MPO*, myeloperoxidase; *STAT*, signal transducer and activator of transcription; *WHIM*, warts, hypogammaglobulinemia, infections, and myelokathexis.

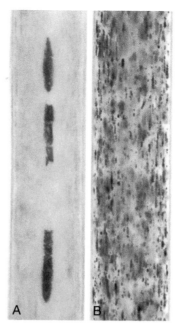

• **Fig. 8.1** Pigment distribution in hair. Normal hair (A) shows opacity typically located in the cortex of the hair shaft. In Chédiak-Higashi syndrome (B) small aggregates of clumped melanin are haphazardly distributed all along the hair shaft. (20× magnification.)

upper respiratory tract infections. Infrequently, some patients may have severe infections, such as pneumonia, meningitis, or sepsis. The diagnosis may be incidental, because patients may remain asymptomatic despite low neutrophil counts. Monocytosis is also frequent. Neutrophil counts are usually less than 1500/μL, but the majority of patients have more than 500 neutrophils/μL at the time of diagnosis. The neutrophil count may increase 2-fold to 3-fold during severe infections and return to neutropenic levels after resolution. Bone marrow findings may be normal or hypercellular. The cause of this disease remains unknown. Detection of granulocyte-specific antibodies is key to the diagnosis of primary AIN and may require repeated testing.[30]

AIN is usually a self-limited disease. The neutropenia remits spontaneously within 7 to 24 months in 95% of patients, preceded by the disappearance of autoantibodies from the circulation. Symptomatic treatment with antibiotics for infections is usually sufficient. Treatment for severe infections or in the setting of emergency surgery often now includes G-CSF.[30]

Secondary Autoimmune Neutropenia (Secondary AIN)

Secondary AIN can be seen at any age but is more common in adults and has a more variable clinical course. Various systemic and autoimmune diseases such as systemic lupus erythematosus, Hodgkin's disease, LGL proliferation or leukemia, Epstein-Barr

virus infection, cytomegalovirus infection, human immunodeficiency virus (HIV) infection, and parvovirus B19 infection have been associated with secondary AIN.[30] These patients are also predisposed to the development of other autoimmune problems. Antineutrophil antibodies typically have pan-FcγRIII specificity, rather than specificity to the FcγRIII subunits, making the resulting neutropenia more severe. Anti-CD18/11b antibodies have been detected in a subset of patients. Secondary AIN responds best to therapy directed at the underlying cause.[30]

Defects of Granule Formation and Content

Chédiak-Higashi Syndrome

Chédiak-Higashi syndrome (CHS) is a rare and life-threatening autosomal recessive disease, characterized by oculocutaneous albinism, pyogenic infections, neurologic abnormalities, and a relatively late-onset hemophagocytic lymphohistiocytosis (HLH)-like "accelerated phase." The disease is caused by mutations in the lysosomal trafficking regulator gene *CHS1*.[31,32] Patients show hypopigmentation of the skin, iris, and hair because of giant and aberrant melanosomes (macromelanosomes). Hair color is usually light brown to blonde, with a characteristic metallic silver-gray sheen. Under light-microscopy, CHS hair shafts show pathognomonic small, irregular aggregates of clumped pigment spread throughout the shaft (Fig. 8.1).[33–35]

Giant azurophil granules formed from the fusion of multiple primary granules are seen in neutrophils, eosinophils, and basophils. Mild neutropenia secondary to intramedullary destruction is also common. Progressive neuropathy of the legs, cranial nerve palsies, seizures, intellectual disability, and autonomic dysfunction are also common.

The accelerated phase, one of the main causes of death in CHS, is clinically indistinguishable from other hemophagocytic syndromes, with fever, hepatosplenomegaly, lymphadenopathy, cytopenias, hypertriglyceridemia, hypofibrinogenemia, hemophagocytosis, and tissue lymphohistiocytic infiltration. Etoposide, steroids, and intrathecal methotrexate (when the CNS is involved) have been effective treatments. However, without successful bone marrow transplantation, the accelerated phase usually recurs.

Neutrophil-Specific Granule Deficiency

Neutrophil-specific granule deficiency is a rare, heterogeneous, autosomal recessive disease characterized by the profound reduction or absence of neutrophil-specific granules and their contents.[36] In several cases a homozygous, recessive mutation was found in C/EBPε.[37] However, not all cases have mutations in C/EBPε, suggesting genetic heterogeneity.

Bilobed neutrophils are common (e.g., pseudo–Pelger-Huët anomaly), eosinophils may be unapparent in peripheral smears, and there is increased susceptibility to pyogenic infections of the skin, ears, lungs, and lymph nodes. Neutrophils have very low specific granule contents (e.g., lactoferrin) and low to absent defensins, a primary granule product. Hemostasis abnormalities, caused by reduced levels of platelet-associated high molecular weight von Willebrand factor, platelet fibrinogen, and fibronectin, have been reported.[38]

Aggressive diagnosis of infection, prolonged and intensive therapy, and early use of surgical excision and debridement are necessary. Unrelated bone marrow transplantation corrected neutrophil-specific granule deficiency (C/EBPε mutation negative) in a 13-month-old patient with intractable diarrhea and severe infections.[39]

Defects of Oxidative Metabolism

Chronic Granulomatous Disease

Chronic granulomatous disease (CGD) predisposes to recurrent life-threatening infections caused by a small subset of bacteria and fungi and exuberant granuloma formation resulting from defects in the nicotinamide adenine dinucleotide phosphate (NADPH) oxidase.[40] The NADPH oxidase exists as a heterodimeric membrane-bound complex embedded in the walls of secondary granules and four distinct cytosolic proteins. These structural components are referred to as *phox* proteins (*ph*agocyte *ox*idase). The secondary granule membrane complex is also called cytochrome b_{558}, composed of a 91-kd glycosylated β chain (gp91phox) and a 22-kd nonglycosylated α chain (p22phox), which together bind heme and flavin. The cytosol contains the structural components p47^{phox}, p67^{phox}, and the regulatory components p40^{phox} and RAC. On cellular activation the cytosolic components p47^{phox} and p67^{phox} associate with p40^{phox} and RAC, and these proteins combine with the cytochrome complex (gp91^{phox} and p22^{phox}) to form the intact NADPH oxidase. Superoxide is formed and, in the presence of superoxide dismutase, is converted to hydrogen peroxide, which, in the presence of myeloperoxidase (MPO) and chlorine, is converted to bleach. It has been postulated that production of reactive oxygen species is most critical for microbial killing through the activation of certain primary granule proteins inside the phagosome.[41] This hypothesis for NADPH oxidase–mediated microbial killing suggests that the reactive oxidants are most critical as intracellular signaling molecules, leading to activation of other pathways rather than exerting a microbicidal effect per se.

Mutations in six genes involved in NADPH oxidase have been found to cause CGD. Mutations in the X-linked gp91phox

TABLE 8.3	Prevalence of Infection by Site in 268 Patients With Chronic Granulomatous Disease Followed at the National Institutes of Health*
Type of Infection (Most Frequent Microorganisms Isolated)	**Total (N = 268) No. (%)**
Pneumonia (*Aspergillus* spp., *Staphylococcus* spp., *Burkholderia cepacia*, *Nocardia* spp.)	233 (87)
Liver abscess (*Staphylococcus* spp., *Serratia* spp., *Aspergillus* spp., *Burkholderia* spp.)	85 (32)
Suppurative adenitis (*Staphylococcus* spp., *Aspergillus* spp., *Burkholderia* spp., *Serratia* spp., *Nocardia* spp.)	67 (25)
Osteomyelitis (*Serratia* spp., *Aspergillus* spp., *Nocardia* spp., *Staphylococcus* spp.)	7 (2)
Bacteremia/fungemia (*Burkholderia cepacia*, *Serratia* spp.)	5 (2)
Cellulitis (*Serratia marcescens*, *Staphylococcus* spp., *Aspergillus* spp., *Nocardia* spp., *Burkholderia* spp.)	68 (25)

*These data include patients on variable prophylactic regimens and are meant to portray the natural history of disease over four decades of follow-up.

Modified from Marciano BE, Spalding C, Fitzgerald A, et al. Common severe infections in chronic granulomatous disease. Clin Infect Dis 2015;60(8):1176–83.

account for about two-thirds of cases; the remainder are autosomal recessive, and there are no autosomal dominant cases of CGD.[40] p40^{phox} deficiency is somewhat distinct in that it has high rates of colitis with very low rates of infection; the diagnostic dihydrorhodamine (DHR) assay is intermediate in p40^{phox} deficiency and may lead to some diagnostic difficulty.[42,43] A protein that stabilizes the co-expression of the gp91^{phox} and p22^{phox} complex in the endoplasmic reticulum has been recently identified (essential for reactive oxygen species), EROS, encoded by *CYBC1*.[44] The frequency of CGD in the United States is higher than 1:200,000. Clinically, CGD is quite variable but the majority of patients are diagnosed as toddlers and young children.[45] Infections, granulomatous lesions, or colitis may be the usual first manifestations. The lung, skin, lymph nodes, and liver are the most frequent sites of infection (Table 8.3). The majority of infections in CGD in North America are caused by only five organisms: *Staphylococcus aureus*, *Burkholderia cepacia* complex, *Serratia marcescens*, *Nocardia spp.*, and *Aspergillus spp.*[45] Trimethoprim-sulfamethoxazole (TMP-SMX) prophylaxis has reduced the frequency of bacterial infections, especially of staphylococcus. On prophylaxis, staphylococcal infections are essentially confined to the liver and cervical lymph nodes.[45] Staphylococcal liver abscesses encountered in CGD are dense, cáseous, and difficult to drain, and previously required surgery in almost all cases.[46] However, recognizing the simultaneous infection susceptibility and dysregulated inflammatory response in CGD, combined steroid and antibiotic therapy has obviated the need for surgery in almost all cases and leads to better outcomes and better survival.[47,48]

The gastrointestinal (GI) (Fig. 8.2A) and genitourinary (see Fig. 8.2B) tracts are frequently affected by inflammatory and granulomatous manifestations in patients with CGD. GI inflammatory manifestations may eventually occur in up to half of patients with CGD.[49] Abdominal pain is the most common

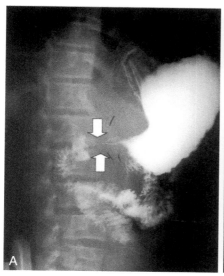 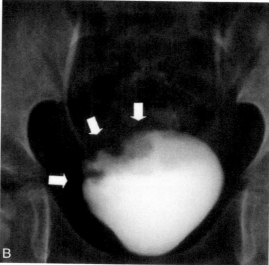

• **Fig. 8.2** Gastrointestinal and genitourinary obstructive lesions in chronic granulomatous disease. (A) High-grade obstruction of the gastric outlet in a 17-year-old boy with gp91phox-deficient chronic granulomatous disease (CGD) (arrows). He had early satiety, weight loss, and intermittent vomiting for several weeks. He improved rapidly on steroid therapy. (B) Extensive bladder granuloma formation in the superior aspect of the bladder in a 3-year-old boy with gp91phox-deficient CGD (arrows). Note the mildly dilated ureter on the obstructed side. This child presented with dysuria and right hydronephrosis that responded promptly to steroids.

GI symptom; diarrhea, nausea, and vomiting also occur. Colonic granulomatous lesions mimicking Crohn's-like inflammatory bowel disease (IBD), oral ulcers, esophagitis, gastric outlet obstruction, villous atrophy, intestinal strictures, fistulae, and perirectal abscesses also occur. The extraintestinal manifestations of Crohn syndrome (i.e., pyoderma, arthritis) are typically absent.

Most CGD-associated IBD manifestations are responsive to steroids. Prednisone (1 mg/kg/day for several weeks followed by progressive tapering) usually resolves the symptoms. Unfortunately, relapses occur in nearly 70% of patients.[47] Low-dose maintenance prednisone may control symptoms without an apparent increase in serious infections. Sulfasalazine, mesalazine, 6-mercaptopurine, azathioprine, and cyclosporine are effective second-line treatment options. The use of tumor necrosis factor–alpha (TNF-α)-blocking antibodies in severe cases of IBD in patients with CGD have been associated with symptom control in anecdotal reports, but there were also severe infections with typical CGD pathogens.[50] Therefore, intensified prophylaxis and vigilance for intercurrent infections are needed in the setting of these potent immunosuppressives. Bone marrow transplantation is generally curative for CGD IBD.

Genitourinary strictures and granulomas occur in up to 18% of patients with CGD, mostly in patients with gp91^{phox} and p22^{phox} deficiency.[51] Steroid therapy similar to that used for GI manifestations usually controls these complications.[52,53]

Inflammatory retinal involvement is found in up to 24% of patients with X-linked CGD. Interestingly, this has also been detected in three female carriers of X-linked CGD. These lesions are typically nonprogressive and asymptomatic and need no specific treatment. However, two patients with CGD needed enucleation for painful retinal detachments.[54,55] These retinal lesions have been found to have bacterial DNA within them, but the importance of this finding is unclear because they rarely change after discovery and are usually not symptomatic.[56]

Autoimmune disorders such as idiopathic thrombocytopenic purpura and juvenile rheumatoid arthritis are more frequent in patients with CGD than in the general population.[45,57,58] Discoid and systemic lupus erythematosus occur in patients with CGD and female X-linked CGD carriers.

The X-linked carriers of gp91phox have one population of phagocytes that produces superoxide and one that does not, giving carriers a characteristic mosaic pattern on DHR testing. Infections are not usually seen in these female carriers unless the superoxide-producing neutrophils are less than 20%, in which case these carriers are at risk for CGD-type infections.[45,59]

The diagnosis of CGD is usually made by DHR oxidation but can be done by direct measurement of superoxide production, ferricytochrome c reduction, chemiluminescence, or nitroblue tetrazolium (NBT) reduction. The DHR assay is preferred because of its relative ease of use, its ability to distinguish X-linked from autosomal patterns of CGD, and its sensitivity to even very low numbers of functional neutrophils.[60,61] Of note, several other conditions, such as glucose-6-phosphate dehydrogenase (G6PD) deficiency, MPO deficiency, and synovitis, acne, pustulosis, hyperostosis, and osteitis (SAPHO) can also affect the respiratory burst and give DHR patterns that can be confused with CGD.[62,63]

Male sex, earlier age at presentation, and increased severity of disease suggest X-linked disease, but the precise gene defect should be determined in all cases for the purposes of genetic counseling, prognosis, and the emerging gene correction approaches. Autosomal recessive forms of CGD (mostly p47phox deficient) have a significantly better prognosis than X-linked disease.[64]

Prophylactic TMP-SMX (5 mg/kg/day based on TMP in two doses) reduces the frequency of major infections from about once every year to once every 3.5 years.[65] It reduces staphylococcal and skin infections without increasing the frequency of serious fungal infections in CGD.[65] Itraconazole prophylaxis prevents fungal infection in CGD (100 mg/day for patients <13 years or <50 kg; 200 mg/day for those ≥13 years or ≥50 kg).[66] IFN-γ also reduces

TABLE 8.4	Leukocyte Adhesion Deficiency Syndromes			
Leukocyte Adhesion Deficiency (LAD)	Type 1 (LAD1)	Type 2 (LAD2 or CDG-IIc)	Type 3 (LAD3)	RAC2 Deficiency (Dominant Negative)
OMIM*	116920	266265	612840	602049
Inheritance pattern	Autosomal recessive	Autosomal recessive	Autosomal recessive	Autosomal dominant
Affected protein(s)	Integrin β2 common chain (CD18)	Fucosylated proteins (e.g., sialyl-Lewis^x, CD15s)	KINDLIN 3	RAC2
Neutrophil function affected	Chemotaxis, tight adherence	Rolling, tethering	Chemotaxis, adhesion	Chemotaxis, superoxide production
Delayed umbilical cord separation	Yes (severe phenotype only)	Yes	Yes	Yes
Leukocytosis/ neutrophilia	Yes	Yes	Yes	Yes

OMIM, Online Mendelian Inheritance in Man.

the number and severity of infections in CGD by 70% compared with placebo, regardless of the inheritance pattern of CGD, sex, or use of prophylactic antibiotics.[67] Therefore, our current recommendation is to use prophylaxis with TMP-SMX, itraconazole, and IFN-γ (50 μg/m^2) in CGD. Because the differential diagnosis for a given process in these patients includes bacteria, fungi, and granulomatous processes, a microbiologic diagnosis is critical. Leukocyte transfusions are often used for severe infections, but their efficacy is anecdotal, and they carry the risk of alloimmunization to blood products, which may complicate bone marrow transplantation.[68a]

Winkelstein and colleagues[68b] reported that mortality in the United States from the 1970s through 1990s was approximately 5% per year for the X-linked form of the disease and 2% per year for the autosomal recessive varieties. The accumulated European experience from 1954 to 2003 found that patients with autosomal recessive CGD had an average life expectancy of 50 years whereas patients with X-linked CGD had an average life expectancy of close to 38 years.[69] Mortality in CGD correlates with noncirrhotic portal hypertension and progressive damage of the hepatic microvasculature. Local or systemic infections, in addition to drug-induced liver injury, may be underlying conditions that affect liver disease. A history of liver abscess, alkaline phosphatase elevations, and platelet decrease over time were individually associated with mortality in patients with CGD.[70]

Successful hematopoietic stem cell transplantation (HSCT) provides a cure for CGD. Gungor and colleagues[71] reported on 56 pediatric and adult European patients with CGD transplanted with stem cells from matched siblings or matched unrelated donors, even in the setting of active inflammatory and infectious complications. They had an overall success rate of 93% with modest toxicity.

Vectors providing normal *phox* genes can reconstitute NADPH oxidase activity in CGD cells. CGD gene therapy has been hampered by retroviral-mediated myeloproliferative disease and poor persistence of transduced cells.[72,73] However, newer protocols are using lentiviral vectors to avoid leukemogenesis and mild bone marrow ablation to permit more definitive engraftment.[74,75] Therefore, with HSCT being highly successful and as gene therapies become available, we think that all cases of CGD should at least have HSCT or gene therapy considered, because these hold the greatest promise of long-term prevention of morbidity and mortality and the living of a normal life.

Myeloperoxidase Deficiency

MPO deficiency is the most common primary phagocyte disorder. It is an autosomal recessive disease with variable expressivity: 1:4000 individuals have complete MPO deficiency, and 1:2000 have a partial defect.[76] MPO catalyzes the conversion of hydrogen peroxide to hypohalous acid. In the MPO-deficient patients who have had clinical findings, infections caused by *Candida* strains were the most common: mucocutaneous, meningeal, and bone infections and sepsis have been described.[77–80] Diabetes mellitus appears to be a critical co-factor for *Candida* infections in the context of MPO deficiency. A definitive diagnosis is established by sequencing of the MPO gene, neutrophil/ monocyte peroxidase histochemical staining, or specific protein detection. There is no specific treatment for MPO deficiency; diabetes should be sought and controlled, and infections should be treated.

Leukocyte Adhesion Deficiency, Type 1 (LAD1)

LAD1 is an autosomal recessive disorder produced by mutations in the common β2 chain (CD18) of the β2 integrin family (ITGB2, 21q22.3; Table 8.4).[81] Each of the β2 integrins is a heterodimer composed of an α chain (CD11a, CD11b, or CD11c), noncovalently linked to the common β2 subunit (CD18). The α-β heterodimers of the β2 integrin family include CD11a/CD18 (lymphocyte-function–associated antigen-1 [LFA-1]), CD11b/ CD18 (macrophage antigen-1, Mac-1, or complement receptor-3 [CR3]), and CD11c/CD18 (p150,95 or complement receptor-4 [CR4]). CD18 is required for normal expression of the α-β heterodimers. Therefore, mutations resulting in failure to produce a functional β2 subunit lead to either very low or no expression of CD11a, CD11b, and/or CD11c, causing LAD1.81.

The severe phenotype of LAD1 is caused by less than 1% of normal expression of CD18 on neutrophils, whereas the moderate phenotype shows 1% to 30% of normal expression.[82] However, patients with normal β2 integrin expression but without functional activity also have been described. Therefore, expression of CD18 alone is not sufficient to exclude the diagnosis of LAD1; functional assays must be performed if the clinical suspicion is high.[82,83]

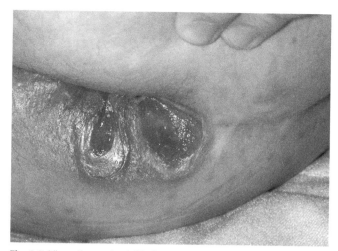

• **Fig. 8.3** Ulcerative perirectal lesion in an 18-year-old boy with leukocyte adhesion deficiency 1 (LAD1). No pus was seen, and there was poor inflammation in the surrounding tissues.

Patients with the severe phenotype of LAD1 characteristically have delayed umbilical stump separation and omphalitis; persistent leukocytosis (>15,000/μL) even in the absence of infection; and severe, destructive gingivitis and periodontitis with associated loss of dentition and alveolar bone. Recurrent infections of the skin, upper and lower airways, bowel, and perirectal area are common and usually caused by *S. aureus* or gram-negative bacilli, but not by fungi. Infections tend to be necrotizing and may progress to ulceration (Fig. 8.3). Typically, no pus is seen in these lesions, and there is almost complete absence of neutrophil invasion. Aggressive medical management with antibiotics and neutrophil transfusions, and prompt surgery when indicated, are required. Impaired healing of infectious, traumatic, or surgical wounds is also characteristic of LAD1. Scars tend to acquire a dystrophic "cigarette-paper" appearance. Patients with the moderate phenotype tend to be diagnosed later in life, have normal umbilical separation, have fewer life-threatening infections, and live longer. However, leukocytosis, periodontal disease, and delayed wound healing are still common.[82]

Flow cytometry of LAD1 blood samples shows reduction (moderate phenotype) or near absence (severe phenotype) of CD18 and its associated molecules CD11a, CD11b, and CD11c on neutrophils and other leukocytes. LAD1 patients show diminished neutrophil migration in vivo and in vitro.[71] Complement-mediated phagocytosis is severely impaired because of the absence of the complement receptor CD18/CD11b (CR3/Mac-1). Interestingly, one mechanism for severe periodontitis in LAD1 is that tissue macrophages produce interleukin-23 (IL-23) in response to tissue neutropenia, leading to local IL-17 production and inflammation. This severe inflammatory response can be blocked with resolution of the periodontal disease.[84]

Somatic reversion of the mutation has been reported in LAD1 involving cytotoxic T lymphocytes.[85] However, HSCT is the only definitive treatment.[86] Gene therapy studies in LAD1 are provocative, but not yet clinically available.[87]

Leukocyte Adhesion Deficiency, Type 2 (LAD2) or Congenital Disorder of Glycosylation Type IIc (CDG-IIc)

LAD2, or CDG-IIc, is a very rare autosomal recessive inherited disease in which fucose metabolism is primarily affected because of mutations in the guanosine diphosphate (GDP)-fucose transporter gene, *FUCT1*[88,89] (see Table 8.4). Lack of the GDP-fucose

transporter leads to a lack of expression of sialyl-Lewis[x] and other fucosylated proteins, impairing leukocyte rolling, adhesion, and other pathways. The clinical phenotype is characterized by infections of the skin, lung, and gums; leukocytosis; poor pus formation; and intellectual disability, short stature, distinctive facies, and the Bombay (hh) blood phenotype. The frequency and severity of infections tend to decline with time.[90] Fucose supplementation has had variable results in patients with LAD2.[91,92]

Leukocyte Adhesion Deficiency, Type 3 (LAD3)

LAD3 deficiency (previously known as LAD1 variant) resembles LAD1 on the one hand, but it is associated with a syndrome similar to Glanzmann's thrombasthenia (a β3 integrin–related bleeding disorder) on the other. These patients present in infancy with severe bleeding and infections. Mortality is high, even with stem cell transplantation. LAD3 is due to mutations in *FERMT3*, the gene encoding kindlin-3, a molecule responsible for β1, β2, and β3 integrin activation in leukocytes and platelets.[93,94]

RAC2 Deficiency

Ambruso and colleagues[95] and Williams and colleagues[96] reported a male patient with an autosomal dominant negative mutation in the Rho GTPase *RAC2* gene (*RAC2*, see Table 8.4). This molecule is critical to the regulation of the actin cytoskeleton and superoxide production. The patient had delayed umbilical cord separation, perirectal abscesses, failure to heal surgical wounds, and absent pus in infected areas despite neutrophilia. Chemotaxis and superoxide production were impaired. In addition, the patient's neutrophils showed defective azurophilic granule release and impaired phagocytosis. He was cured by bone marrow transplantation. A second case was identified through newborn screening for T cell excision circles (TRECs), although is still unclear why TRECs are low in RAC2 deficiency.[97] More recently Hsu and colleagues[98] and Lougaris and colleagues[99] identified autosomal dominant gain of function mutations in RAC2 that lead to a distinct syndrome with later disease manifestations, abnormal neutrophil morphology, and predominantly lymphoid features but also associated with low TRECs in the newborn period.

Syndromes With Susceptibility to Environmental Mycobacteria

The mononuclear phagocyte is crucial for protection against intracellular infections and for antigen presentation, for lymphocyte stimulation, lymphocyte proliferation, cytokine production, and response. Transcription factors binding to the GATA sequence are critical for early hematopoiesis of myeloid and lymphoid cells and for normal vessel development.[100] Mycobacteria infect macrophages leading to the production of IL-12p70, a heterodimer of IL-12 p40, and IL-12p35. IL-12 stimulates T cells and natural killer (NK) cells through its cognate receptor (IL-12Rβ1 and IL-12Rβ2) to phosphorylate signal transducer and activator of transcription 4 (STAT4) and produce interferon-gamma (IFN-γ). IFN-γ acts through its heterodimeric receptor (IFNγR1/IFNγR2) to phosphorylate STAT1 and turn on interferon-responsive genes as interferon response factor 8 (IRF8) and interferon stimulated gene 15 (ISG15) (Fig. 8.4).[101,102] In response to diverse signals, NF-κB essential modulator (NEMO) mediates the activation of the central transcription factor NF-κB. This transcription factor is therefore central to both immune and somatic pathways.[103]

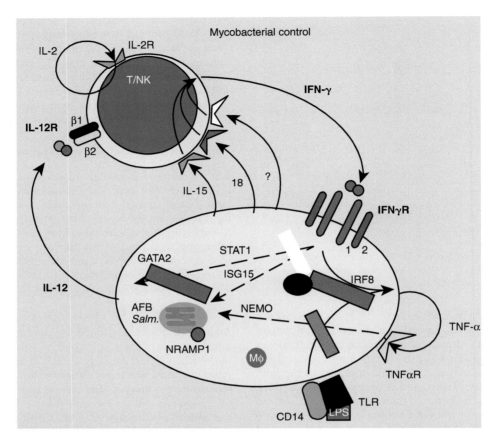

• **Fig. 8.4** Schematic representation of the interferon-γ/interleukin-12 pathway. Ingested pathogens such as acid-fast bacilli *(AFB)* or salmonella *(salm.)* stimulate interleukin-12 *(IL-12)* production by macrophages *(MΦ)*. Acting through its cognate IL-12 receptor, composed of the IL-12 receptor β1 chain *(IL-12Rβ1)* and the IL-12 receptor β2 chain *(IL12Rβ2)*, IL-12 stimulates T and natural killer *(NK)* cells to produce interferon-γ *(IFN-γ)* and interleukin-2 *(IL-2)*. Homodimeric IFN-γ binds to the interferon-γ receptor complex *(IFN-γR)*. Interferon-γ receptor 1 *(IFN-γR1)* is the binding chain, whereas interferon-γ receptor 2 *(IFN-γR2)* is necessary to transmit the signal intracellularly through the signal transduction and activator of transcription 1 *(STAT1)*. The mechanisms by which IFN-γ stimulates intracellular microorganism killing are not fully understood but are likely to be numerous (e.g., up-regulation of major histocompatibility complex expression and IL-12 production, enhancing of antigen processing and reactive oxygen species production, reducing the phagosomal pH). IFN-γ also stimulates tumor necrosis factor-α *(TNF-α)* production. TNF-α, acting through the TNF-α receptor *(TNF-αR)*, also shows effects against intracellular infections. Patients with mutations in the NF-κB essential modulator *(NEMO)*, a protein critical in the TNF-α signaling pathway, have enhanced susceptibility to mycobacterial disease and other infections. IL-12 is not the only cytokine that stimulates IFN-γ production: interleukin-15 *(IL-15)*, interleukin-18 *(IL-18)*, and probably other factors have the same effect. The lack of mycobacterium-induced ISG15 secretion by leukocytes—granulocytes in particular—reduces the production of IFN-γ by lymphocytes, including natural killer cells, probably accounting for the enhanced susceptibility to mycobacterial disease. IRF8 is critical for the development of monocytes and dendritic cells and for antimycobacterial immunity. Lipopolysaccharide *(LPS)* stimulation through the CD14/Toll-like receptor 2 (TLR2) complex can also stimulate IL-12 production.

Patients with defects in *GATA2, IL12B, IFNGR1, IFNGR2, IL12RB1, STAT1, NEMO, IRF8,* and *ISG15* have been identified through their susceptibility to mycobacteria and other intracellular infections, including *Salmonella* infection.[101,102,104,105] Superoxide also has a role in the killing of mycobacteria, as reflected in the higher rates of tuberculosis in CGD and bacillus Calmette-Guérin (BCG) infection in two families with unusual mutations in the *CYBB* gene.[106]

Haploinsufficiency for GATA2 leads to a late-onset immunodeficiency characterized by disseminated mycobacteria and viral (i.e., human papillomavirus [HPV], herpesviruses) infections often associated with diminished monocytes, B cells, and NK cells in peripheral blood along with hypoplastic myelodysplasia.[107]

Patients with autosomal recessive mutations leading to abolition of IFNγR1, IFNγR2, or STAT1 expression or function present early in life, especially if they receive BCG vaccination. In contrast, patients with an autosomal dominant mutation in *IFNGR1* as a result of a recurrent 4-base deletion (named 818del4) have only partial inhibition of receptor function. Patients with dominant *IFNGR1* mutations may present before the age of 7 with pulmonary nontuberculous mycobacterial infection but then characteristically go on to develop recurrent nontuberculous osteomyelitis.

Patients with mutations in IL-12p40 or IL-12Rβ1 and those with dominant negative *STAT1* mutations usually have less severe phenotypes. In IL-12Rβ1 deficiency the risk of nontuberculous mycobacterial infection wanes after age 12.[108] IRF8 defects are quite rare. One homozygous child had severe BCG infection with myeloproliferation, and two others with dominant negative IRF8 mutations developed mild but recurrent disseminated BCG.[101] The three patients reported with ISG15 defects had disseminated BCG shortly after vaccination but were eventually responsive to therapy.[102]

NEMO is encoded by a gene *(IKBKG)* on the X-chromosome; thus, hypomorphic NEMO mutations cause disease in hemizygous males (hypomorphic mutations are mostly asymptomatic in females). Hemizygous males may have a complex phenotype, including hypohidrotic ectodermal dysplasia, immunodeficiency, and, rarely, lymphedema with osteopetrosis. Almost 40% of males with hypomorphic mutations in NEMO develop mycobacterial infections, mostly with environmental organisms.[109] In heterozygous females, amorphic NEMO mutations are associated with *incontinentia pigmenti.*[110]

Flow cytometry is very efficient in detection of IFNGR1 defects, because this protein is expressed on all nucleated cells all the time. In the case of the autosomal dominant IFNGR1 deficiency (818del4), the protein is overabundant on the cell surface and therefore very easy to detect.[111] In contrast, detection of IFNγR2 and IL-12Rβ1 often requires cell culture and proliferation. Detection of intracellular phosphorylated STAT1 after IFNγ stimulation, or phosphorylated STAT4 after IL-12 stimulation, is an indirect means of demonstrating functional integrity of the IFNγ and IL-12 receptors, respectively.[112,113] Direct detection of IL-12p40 or IL-12 p70 can be used for the diagnosis of patients who are deficient in IL-12 p40. Demonstrating defects in STAT1 requires research techniques.

Treatment of infection in these patients poses special problems. For the patients with complete IFNγR defects, IFN-γ is of no help. However, in patients with autosomal dominant IFNγR1 deficiency, IL-12 defects, or IL-12R defects, IFN-γ is usually effective. However, approximately 30% of those with IL-12Rβ1 deficiency die, suggesting complex modifying factors.[114] Bone marrow transplantation for IFNγR defects is highly successful and should be considered at the earliest opportunity, preferably before disseminated mycobacterial disease occurs. Long-term prophylaxis against environmental mycobacterial infections with a macrolide such as azithromycin or clarithromycin seems advisable.

Hyper-IgE Syndrome (HIES; Job's Syndrome)

Hyper-IgE (HIES or Job's) syndrome is due to heterozygous autosomal dominant negative mutations in STAT3 and characterized by elevated serum IgE, eczema, recurrent skin and lung infections, and somatic features, including characteristic facies, scoliosis, and fractures[115–117] (Table 8.5). Almost all human mutations found thus far allow the production of full-length mutant STAT3 protein, which exerts dominant negative effects.

A newborn rash is usually the first manifestation of Job's syndrome. About one-fifth have the rash at birth, and one-quarter develop it in the first week of life. Mucocutaneous candidiasis is common, typically as oral thrush, vaginal candidiasis, or onychomycosis; systemic *Candida* infections are very rare.[115] Cutaneous "cold" abscesses are common and secondary to *S. aureus* infections. Antistaphylococcal antibiotics or topical antiseptics, such as bleach baths, are effective.

Recurrent pneumonias caused by *S. aureus, Streptococcus pneumoniae,* and *Haemophilus influenzae* typically start in childhood, with a paucity of symptoms. Pneumatoceles and bronchiectasis form during the healing process and usually persist once the infection has cleared. These anatomic abnormalities predispose

TABLE 8.5	Clinical Characteristics of Job's Syndrome

Clinical Findings in Job's Syndrome	Percentage (%)
Eczema	100
Peak IgE >2000 IU/mL	97
Eosinophilia	93
Recurrent pneumonias	87
Characteristic face	83
Mucocutaneous candidiasis	83
Pneumatoceles	77
Retained primary teeth	72
Pathologic fractures	71
Focal brain hyperintensities	70
Scoliosis (older than 16 years, >10 degrees)	63

IgE, Immunoglobulin E.

the patient to gram-negative bacterial (typically *Pseudomonas*) and fungal (typically *Aspergillus* or *Scedosporium* spp.) infections. The large cysts often become secondarily infected and may bleed, sometimes fatally. On the other hand, thoracic surgery can be complicated by poor healing of the remaining lung, often resulting in persistent air leak.[118] Antimicrobial prophylaxis to prevent *S. aureus* skin and lung infection (e.g., TMP-SMX) may be broadened if gram-negative lung infections occur. Antifungal prophylaxis to prevent pulmonary aspergillosis remains attractive but unproved, but it is highly effective in treating and preventing mucocutaneous candidiasis.

Scoliosis, osteopenia, minimal trauma fractures, hyperextensibility, degenerative joint disease, craniosynostosis, and Chiari 1 malformations also occur frequently but seldom need surgical correction.[119] The general mechanism underlying bone abnormalities is unknown, and the role of bisphosphonates in treating the osteoporosis and minimal trauma fractures in HIES is undefined.

In childhood and adolescence, most patients with Job's syndrome develop characteristic facial features, including facial asymmetry, broad nose, and deep-set eyes with a prominent forehead. Most patients retain some, if not all, of their primary teeth past the age of normal primary dental exfoliation; at times, layers of both primary and secondary teeth co-exist.[115,119] Vascular abnormalities are common in Job's syndrome, including coronary artery aneurysms,[120] dilations and tortuosities, carotid artery berry aneurysms, and early-onset magnetic resonance imaging T2-weighted hyperintensities (unidentified bright objects).[121] As reported in other primary immunodeficiency diseases affecting lymphocytes, both Hodgkin's and non-Hodgkin's lymphomas are significantly increased in Job's syndrome.[122]

DOCK8 deficiency is an autosomal recessive syndrome with IgE elevation, severe eczema, and recurrent skin and lung infections. However, in distinction to Job's syndrome, DOCK8 deficiency is characterized by cutaneous viral infections (molluscum contagiosum, herpes simplex, HPV) and severe allergic diathesis.[123–125] Severe eczematoid rashes start early in life, although not necessarily in the newborn period. Unlike Job's syndrome, pneumonias secondary to *S. aureus, H. influenzae, Proteus mirabilis, Pseudomonas aeruginosa,* and *Cryptococcus* spp. typically heal without pneumatocele formation. DOCK8 deficiency lacks the somatic features of Job's syndrome.

TYK2 deficiency is another autosomal recessive syndrome occasionally associated with IgE elevation and infection susceptibility. The few cases identified suggest that TYK2 deficiency is more involved in mycobacterial susceptibilty.[126,127]

Mucocutaneous Candidiasis

Candida spp. are commonly found on mucosal surfaces, where they are commensal. The innate response to candida appears to depend heavily on the production of IL-17 by dedicated Th17 lymphocytes. Accordingly, those mutations that affect IL-17–producing T cells are strongly associated with mucocutaneous candidiasis.[128] Candida sensing at the cellular level seems to depend on the surface receptor dectin-1 and its signal transduction pathway including CARD9.[129] Mutations in dectin-1 also have been identified, but their etiologic role in severe mucocutaneous candidiasis is hard to assign because of the common occurrence of some of these mutations.[130] Dominant negative mutations in STAT3 (Job's syndrome) lead to impaired Th17 production and mucocutaneous candidiasis.[116,117] More surprising is the discovery that dominant gain-of-function mutations in *STAT1* are the most common underlying cause of severe mucocutaneous candidiasis, apparently through the oversignaling of IFNγ.[131–133] These syndromes are critical to consider, because homozygous recessive CARD9 deficiency can be associated with severe dermatophyte infections and fungal brain infections.[134] Gain-of-function *STAT1* mutations can be associated with disseminated coccidioidomycosis, disseminated histoplasmosis, and progressive multifocal leukencephalopathy.[135]

Conclusions

Various defects of phagocytes have been elucidated over the last several decades. Despite the fact that profound neutropenia predisposes patients to most members of the bacterial and fungal kingdoms, metabolic defects in neutrophils and monocytes have relatively narrow spectra of infection. Some of these disorders have almost pathognomonic infection profiles (e.g., CGD, IFN-γ/IL-12 pathway defects). We have now put genetic faces to some of the names of these puzzling diseases. The simple recognition of genes and pathways should not be confused with careful and complete understanding of mechanism. The latter, despite all the complex diagrams, remains elusive (Boxes 8.2 and 8.3). Although we have been very successful at identifying rare and flagrant defects affecting white cells that lead to severe infections, the more subtle defects that cause recurrent staphylococcal infections, hydradenitis, and infections in diabetes, to name only a few of the vexing problems that frequently confront the clinical immunologist, remain to be determined. Careful study of the known pathways, assiduous following of the ramifications of those pathways to the points at which they merge with new pathways, and conscientious characterization of clinical phenotypes will lead to the discovery of these remaining immune defects. In the process we will gain new insights into exactly how we remain so remarkably healthy in the face of so many daily microbial challenges.

The reference list can be found on the companion Expert Consult website at http://www.expertconsult.inkling.com.

• **BOX 8.2** **Key Concepts**

White Blood Cell Defects: Evaluation and Management

- Patients with white cell defects usually present early in life with recurrent bacterial or fungal infections.
- Certain infections, such as *Burkholderia cepacia, Nocardia* spp., *Aspergillus* spp., or environmental mycobacteria should always prompt an inquiry into the possibility of an underlying immune defect.
- Specific infection locations, such as omphalitis or osteomyelitis should raise the suspicion of immune abnormalities.
- Abnormal aspects of host response, such as lack of fever, local inflammation, or pus, should immediately alert the clinician to the possibility of a white cell defect.
- It is better to perform the right test once than the entire battery of immune defect tests several times. Careful consideration of the clinical and microbiologic presentation usually indicates the right path to pursue.
- There is no substitute for the right drug, and that requires knowing the pathogen. Because the spectrum of infection in these diseases may range over several microbiologic kingdoms, empirical therapy is to be discouraged in favor of firm diagnoses.
- Prophylactic antibiotics, antifungal agents, and cytokines are highly successful in treating chronic granulomatous disease and appear to be useful in some other immunodeficiencies as well.
- Genetic testing should be pursued for all defects thought to be inborn. The expanding knowledge of genotype-phenotype relationships suggests that not all defects, even those within the same gene, are created equal.

• **BOX 8.3** **Therapeutic Principles**

- In general, attenuated or inactivated viral vaccines are not contraindicated in individuals with primary phagocyte disorders, because antiviral cell-mediated immunity is intact.
- Bacille Calmette-Guérin (BCG) vaccination should be avoided in individuals with chronic granulomatous disease (CGD) or mendelian susceptibility to mycobacterial diseases (MSMD) pathway defects, and in their newborn close relatives, until the defect is ruled out.
- Mulching and gardening should be avoided by individuals with increased susceptibility to *Aspergillus* infections, such as patients with CGD, Job's syndrome, or neutropenia.
- Patients with white blood cell defects often fail to mount a normal inflammatory response, so clinicians and parents must keep a high index of suspicion for asymptomatic or hyposymptomatic infection.
- Standard recommendations for duration of therapy of infections are based on experience in normal people. In the patient with a white cell defect, the host contribution to resolution of infection may be relatively small, resulting in a need for longer or more intensive antibiotic or antifungal therapy.
- When infections are necrotizing or poorly responsive to antibiotic therapy, surgery may be needed, even in situations in which it would not be needed in unaffected individuals (e.g., lymphadenitis in CGD often needs operative removal).
- Obtain experienced expert advice whenever possible.

9

Congenital Immune Dysregulation Disorders

TROY R. TORGERSON, JOAO BOSCO OLIVEIRA

KEY POINTS

- Patients with immune dysregulation typically have autoimmunity, autoinflammation, or nonmalignant lymphoproliferation as the dominant clinical features of disease.
- The gastrointestinal tract, skin, lungs, and hematopoietic system (red blood cells and platelets) are common targets of autoimmunity in immune dysregulation disorders.
- Many patients with immune dysregulation also may have recurrent or unusual infections.
- For most immune dysregulation disorders, identification of a

pathogenic mutation in a causative gene is the most definitive way to confirm a diagnosis.
- There is significant phenotypic overlap among immune dysregulation disorders, so performing broad-based genetic testing with a targeted multigene panel, whole exome sequencing, or whole genome sequencing is recommended.
- Treatment needs to address both major aspects of disease—immune dysregulation and infections—to optimize clinical outcomes and prevent permanent organ damage.

Introduction

Primary immunodeficiency disorders (PIDDs) were initially described in patients with recurrent or severe infections. The availability of antimicrobials to treat and prevent infections in these patients led to longer survival and, with this, the realization that some of these patients may also develop autoimmunity. This was, however, usually a minor feature of disease compared with the recurrent infections. In contrast, approximately 20 years ago, a new class of immunodeficiency caused by defects in genes that encode molecules required for regulation of immune responses was characterized. The regulatory molecules encoded by these genes control the activation state of immune cells and regulate their growth and survival. Unlike in traditional PIDDs, patients harboring defects in these genes typically present with immune-mediated pathologic conditions, including autoimmunity, autoinflammation, and nonmalignant lymphoproliferation. This chapter will discuss congenital disorders that affect central deletion of autoreactive T cells in the thymus and those that have an impact on other mechanisms involved in the maintenance of tolerance in the periphery. In all of these disorders the clinical phenotype includes autoimmunity together with other manifestations, including infections.

Autoimmune Polyendocrinopathy, Candidiasis, Ectodermal Dystrophy

Autoimmune polyendocrinopathy, candidiasis, and ectodermal dystrophy (APECED; OMIM #240300) is the prototype of defective central T cell immune tolerance. This disorder is caused by mutations in the gene encoding the autoimmune regulator (AIRE). Originally, the disorder was diagnosed clinically when patients developed two of the three characteristic clinical features: parathyroid dysfunction, adrenal insufficiency, and chronic mucocutaneous candidiasis (CMC). It is now diagnosed by identification of mutations in the AIRE gene. The extent of organ-specific autoimmune disease present in APECED is now known to be much broader than originally appreciated, with pulmonary autoimmunity, type 1 diabetes, gonadal failure, pernicious anemia, autoimmune hepatitis, and cutaneous manifestations now known to be prominent features of the disease.[1–3]

Genetics and Immunopathogenesis

AIRE is a DNA-binding transcriptional regulator that plays a key role in ectopic expression of tissue-specific antigens in the thymus. Murine studies have shown that AIRE-mediated self-antigen expression in thymic medullary epithelial cells (mTECs) plays an important role in negative selection of autoreactive T cells and in positive selection of thymically derived regulatory T (tT_{REG}) cells.[4–6] Evaluation of T_{REG} cells in patients with APECED demonstrated a decreased percentage of $CD4^+CD25^{high}$ T_{REG} cells and decreased FOXP3 protein expression in these cells compared to those in normal individuals.[7] Furthermore, isolated tT_{REG} cells from APECED patients had a decreased ability to suppress proliferation of effector T cells in vitro compared with those from healthy controls.[7]

In addition, patients with APECED often develop a broad range of pathogenic, tissue-specific autoantibodies directed toward parathyroid, adrenal, ovarian, lung, gut, and other antigens.[8–10] In addition, neutralizing autoantibodies against type I interferons (α and ω), interleukin-17 (IL-17), and IL-22 have been identified in many patients with APECED.[11–13]

Diagnosis and Treatment

A definitive diagnosis of APECED is made by sequencing of the *AIRE* gene. The disease is most commonly inherited in an autosomal recessive manner, but autosomal dominant inheritance also has been described with particular mutations.[14,15]

In a prospective study of APECED performed at the National Institutes of Health (NIH), it was found that interstitial pneumonitis is a more prominent and debilitating feature of the disease than previously recognized, affecting approximately 40% of patients. The pneumonitis often starts early in the course of the disease and may actually predate the other, more classic clinical features of APECED.[1] Further studies demonstrated that pulmonary immune infiltrates are a mixture of both T and B cells with an enrichment of neutrophils in the airways. A small pilot study showed clinical efficacy of a treatment regimen combining B cell depletion (anti-CD20 monoclonal antibody [mAb]) with azathioprine to suppress autoreactive T cell expansion.[16] This was supported by studies in *Aire*$-/-$ mice demonstrating a significant role for B cells and autoantibodies in pathogenesis of the disease.[17,18]

Other therapies for APECED have focused largely on symptomatic treatment, including calcium supplementation, steroid replacement, and the management of diabetes and other endocrinopathies. Mucocutaneous candidiasis can be particularly problematic because it causes significant morbidity and increases the risk of oral malignancies. In some cases, the candidal species develop reduced sensitivity to azole antifungals over time, complicating management.[19]

X-Linked Immune Dysregulation, Polyendocrinopathy, and Enteropathy

X-linked immunodeficiency with polyendocrinopathy and enteropathy (IPEX) syndrome (#OMIM 304930) is the prototype of defective peripheral immune tolerance. The basic clinical triad of IPEX includes autoimmune enteropathy, early-onset endocrinopathy, and dermatitis (Box 9.1).[20–24] The enteropathy typically manifests early in life as watery diarrhea, frequently resulting in malnutrition and failure to thrive. Type 1 diabetes is the most common endocrinopathy, but clinical and/or laboratory evidence of thyroiditis is also common. Eczema is the most common dermatitis in IPEX, but erythroderma, psoriasiform dermatitis, and pemphigus nodularis also have been observed.[25–27]

> **• BOX 9.1** | **Key Concepts**
> *Immunopathogenesis of IPEX Syndrome*
>
> - Enteropathy: Severe watery diarrhea caused by autoimmune enteropathy
> - Endocrinopathy: Type 1 diabetes and thyroiditis caused by autoimmunity to pancreas and thyroid
> - Autoimmunity: Absence of functional regulatory T cells
>
> *IPEX,* X-linked immunodeficiency with polyendocrinopathy and enteropathy.

In addition to the IPEX triad, most patients with IPEX have other associated autoimmune disorders, including autoimmune cytopenias, nephropathy, or hepatic disease.[20,21] These conditions contribute substantially to the morbidity of patients with IPEX and increase the risk of death from disease. The initial patients described with IPEX had severe, early-onset disease and typically died before 2 years of age with malnutrition, electrolyte imbalance, or infection if not treated with aggressive immunosuppression.[27] Now it is recognized that at least 50% of patients have a milder form of disease that may have a somewhat older age of onset and a more diverse clinical presentation.[21]

Genetics and Immunopathogenesis

IPEX is caused by mutations in the forkhead DNA-binding protein FOXP3, which is expressed by CD4+CD25+ regulatory T cells and is required for T_{REG} development.[28–32] Under quiescent conditions, FOXP3 expression is restricted primarily to T_{REG} cells; however, it also can be inducibly expressed in a large percentage of human T cells on activation.[33–36] FOXP3 originally was shown to be a transcriptional repressor acting on key cytokine genes[33–36]; however, genome-wide screening approaches suggest that FOXP3 also can function as a transcriptional enhancer.[37,38]

Most pathologic mutations in FOXP3 cluster in three important functional domains of the protein: the C-terminal forkhead DNA-binding domain, the leucine zipper, and the N-terminal repression domain.[39] Studies suggest that FOXP3 physically and functionally interacts with other transcription factors, including nuclear factor of activated T cells (NFAT), nuclear factor kappa-light-chain-enhancer of activated B cells (NF-κB), acute myeloid leukemia 1 (AML-1)/runt-related transcription factor 1 (RUNX1), and the retinoic acid receptor–related orphan receptors RORα and RORγt to modulate gene transcription at key cytokine promoters.[40–42]

Diagnosis and Treatment

In patients with clinical features of IPEX, a definitive diagnosis can be made by sequencing of the *FOXP3* gene. Ideally, sequencing should include analysis of copy number variants in the gene and the 3′ noncoding region of the gene where mutations in the mRNA polyadenylation signal account for approximately 5% of affected kindreds with IPEX. Because of the phenotypic overlap with a growing number of IPEX-like clinical syndromes caused by mutations in other genes, broad-based genetic testing by either whole exome sequencing or a gene panel is recommended as opposed to single-gene sequencing. Flow cytometry to investigate the presence of $CD4^+CD25^{high}FOXP3^+$ T_{REG} cells can be used as an adjunctive tool but is not good for screening and is rarely diagnostic (Fig. 9.1).

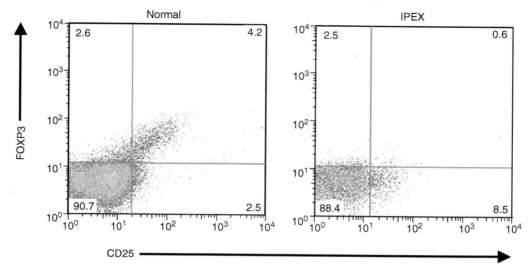

• **Fig. 9.1** Absence of FOXP3+ regulatory T cells in X-linked immunodeficiency with polyendocrinopathy and enteropathy *(IPEX)*. Peripheral blood mononuclear cells (PBMCs) from a normal individual and a patient with IPEX were fixed, permeabilized, and stained for the presence of CD4, CD25, and FOXP3. After gating on the CD4+ T cell population, two-dimensional analysis demonstrates the absence of CD25+FOXP3+ regulatory T cells in the PBMCs of a patient with IPEX syndrome as a result of a mutation in the polyadenylation site of the *FOXP3* gene.

From a clinical laboratory standpoint, the most consistent abnormality among patients with IPEX is markedly elevated immunoglobulin E (IgE), with IgA also modestly elevated in more than 50% of patients.[21] There are no consistent abnormalities in absolute lymphocyte numbers, and T cells usually proliferate normally in vitro.

Adoptive transfer studies in mice have demonstrated that the CD4+ T cells from an affected, Foxp3-deficient male are capable of recapitulating the disease phenotype in a recipient with lymphopenia.[43] Treatment of IPEX has therefore focused primarily on suppression of unregulated, autoaggressive T cells using cyclosporin A, tacrolimus (FK506), or sirolimus (rapamycin).[18,23,44,45] These are often combined with corticosteroids and/or other immunomodulatory agents, including methotrexate or azathioprine.[44,46] In cases in which there is evidence for pathogenic autoantibodies, rituximab (anti-CD20) has proved effective.[26] Immunosuppression can stabilize active disease, but, ultimately, virtually all patients develop breakthrough symptoms and fail immunosuppressive therapy.[47] Currently, hematopoietic stem cell transplantation (HSCT) is the only potentially curative therapy available.[20,21,48–50] Rapid diagnosis and definitive treatment, before the development of irreversible organ damage, is the ideal approach.

STAT1 Gain-of-Function Disease

The signal transducer and activator of transcription (STAT) family of DNA-binding proteins are critical mediators of cytokine and growth factor signaling in cells. STAT1 is the primary transcription factor activated by interferons, so it plays a major role in normal immune responses, particularly to viral, mycobacterial, and fungal pathogens. Autosomal dominant mutations in STAT1 that lead to increased functional activity of the protein have been identified and are most consistently associated with CMC. These gain-of-function (STAT1-GOF; #OMIM 614162) mutations

have been associated with other infections (e.g., dimorphic yeast, mycobacteria) and with IPEX-like autoimmunity.[51–53] The broad spectrum of clinical manifestations can delay diagnosis in some patients.

In addition to IPEX-like autoimmunity and CMC, many patients develop recurrent respiratory infections and bronchiectasis, herpesviral infections (herpes simplex virus [HSV] and varicella-zoster virus [VZV]), short stature with growth-hormone insufficiency, and arterial aneurysms (cardiac and central nervous system).[52] Unlike in IPEX, patients with STAT1-GOF mutations often have more humoral immune dysfunction, including poor vaccine responses, and many patients require treatment with immunoglobulin replacement therapy.

Genetics and Immunopathogenesis

STAT1-GOF disease is caused by heterozygous missense mutations in the *STAT1* gene, all of which cause increased STAT1 activity. Many of the mutations cause increased phosphorylation and/or delayed dephosphorylation of STAT1.[51] In most patients, the percentage of IL-17–secreting T helper type 17 (T_H17) cells in the CD4+ T cell population is reduced but not absent, possibly contributing to the susceptibility to CMC. The mechanism of susceptibility to autoimmunity in this disorder is, however, less clear. T_{REG} cells are present in normal to near-normal numbers and have been reported to be functional.[52]

Diagnosis and Treatment

Sequencing of the *STAT1* gene remains the gold standard for diagnosis of STAT1-GOF disease. Treatment needs to address both the autoimmune and infectious issues of the disease. CMC typically requires chronic or intermittent antifungal therapy by both the topical and systemic routes. Based on the observation that most mutations cause an increased pool of tyrosine-phosphorylated

STAT1 after cellular activation by cytokines, patients have been treated with Janus kinase (JAK) inhibitors (JAKinibs) to correct this in a targeted way.[54,55] Early anecdotal results suggest that JAKinibs can be highly effective at treating the autoimmunity but may cause increased risk of adverse outcomes in patients who already have invasive infections.[56] HSCT may hold promise in some patients with STAT1-GOF disease but outcomes are mixed. In an international compilation of HSCT outcomes in STAT1-GOF disease, 16 patients with STAT1-GOF disease who underwent transplantation were identified but overall survival was only 40%. Notably, the rate of primary or secondary graft failure was high (58%), suggesting that this disorder may pose unique challenges for HSCT that are not yet well understood.[57]

Defects in Interleukin 2 Signaling

Murine models with defects in IL-2 signaling demonstrate that ongoing IL-2 stimulation is required to sustain Foxp3 expression in T_{REG} cells. T_{REG} lacking the ability to respond to IL-2 as a result of defects in the IL-2 receptor or downstream signaling pathways (Fig. 9.2) exhibit decreased competitive fitness because they are unable to become activated and expand in vivo.[58] As a result of T_{REG} dysfunction, humans with defects in IL-2 signaling develop immune dysregulation with IPEX-like clinical features. Because IL-2 also plays a key role in expansion of effector T cells, these patients often have some degree of T cell lymphopenia and, as a result, are susceptible to viral pathogens such as cytomegalovirus (CMV) (see Fig.9.2).

CD25 Deficiency

Similar to IPEX, patients with CD25 deficiency (OMIM #606367) typically develop severe, chronic diarrhea and villous atrophy in infancy.[59–61] Most of the patients also have significant dermatitis, including eczema, pemphigus nodularis, and psoriasiform dermatitis, and a subset have developed early-onset endocrinopathies, including type 1 diabetes and thyroiditis.[59,61] In addition, patients typically develop autoantibodies and have hepatosplenomegaly, lymphadenopathy, and lymphocytic infiltrates in various organs indicative of ongoing immune dysregulation.[59,62] Unlike IPEX, serum IgE levels are usually only mildly elevated or normal.[59,61]

Despite the similar features of immune dysregulation, CD25 deficiency is significantly different from IPEX from the standpoint of infectious susceptibility. Virtually all described patients have had early-onset, recurrent CMV infections, and most had problems with persistent thrush, candidal esophagitis, chronic gastroenteritis, *Pseudomonas,* and staphylococcal and Epstein-Barr virus (EBV) infections.[59,63]

Genetics and Immunopathogenesis

CD25 deficiency is inherited in an autosomal recessive manner, so all described patients have mutations on both alleles of the gene leading to absence of CD25 protein on the surface of activated T cells and T_{REG}.[59,63] Studies in CD25-deficient mice have demonstrated that T_{REG} cell development is normal and that the cells exhibit normal suppressive function in vitro. However, the cells are not normal because survival, maintenance, and competitive fitness of mature T_{REG} cells in vivo is significantly abnormal, resulting in immune dysregulation.[58,64,65] This has proved difficult to study in humans, but it is assumed that a similar mechanism is at play.

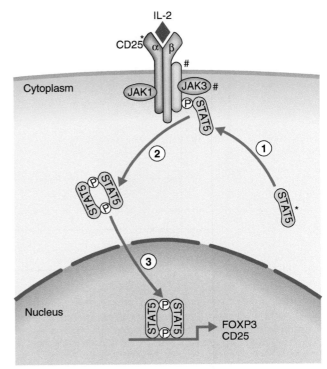

• **Fig. 9.2** The role of CD25 and STAT5b in the interleukin 2 (IL-2) signaling pathway. The illustration demonstrates the relative positions of CD25 and STAT5 (marked by *) in the IL-2 signaling pathway. Binding of IL-2 to the IL-2 receptor (made up of an α-chain [CD25], a β-chain, and a γ-chain [γc]) causes cross-phosphorylation of receptor chains on tyrosine by receptor-associated JAK1 and JAK3 kinases. Unphosphorylated STAT5 binds to phosphotyrosine residues on the activated receptor using its SH2 domain (1). STAT5 is then phosphorylated on tyrosine by the JAK kinases and released from the receptor, where it dimerizes through binding of the SH2 domain on one subunit to the phosphotyrosine residue on the adjacent subunit and vice versa (2). Dimerized STAT5 accumulates in the nucleus, where it directly binds to specific sites in the FOXP3 and CD25 promoters causing sustained expression of these two proteins in regulatory T cells (3). In contrast to deficiency in CD25 and STAT5B, which causes an IPEX-like phenotype, mutations in the IL-2 receptor γ chain or in JAK3 (both marked with #) cause a phenotype of severe combined immunodeficiency (SCID).

Diagnosis and Treatment

The most definitive approach to make a diagnosis of CD25 deficiency is through identification of pathogenic mutations in the *IL2RA* gene. It is possible, however, that novel mutations may be identified that are not clearly pathogenic. In these cases, flow cytometry to evaluate whether activated T cells express normal CD25 may be useful. To date, all identified patients were found to have no CD25 expression on the surface of their T cells, suggesting that flow cytometry could potentially be used as an alternative screening tool.

Because of the features of this syndrome that are similar to those of severe combined immunodeficiency (SCID), one patient underwent a successful bone marrow transplant from a matched sibling donor and has done well.[62,63] It is possible, however, that patients may respond to IL-2 therapy via the remaining low-affinity IL-2 receptor; the T cell proliferative defect was corrected in one patient ex vivo with high-dose IL-2 or IL-15.

- Growth abnormalities: Dwarfism as a result of growth hormone insensitivity (growth hormone levels normal but insulin-like growth factor 1 levels very low)
- Autoimmunity: IPEX-like enteropathy plus other autoimmunity (particularly pulmonary) as a result of low regulatory T cell numbers
- Immunodeficiency: Mild to moderate T and natural killer cell deficiency associated with recurrent/chronic viral and fungal infections

IPEX, X-linked immunodeficiency with polyendocrinopathy and enteropathy.

STAT5B Deficiency

STAT5 is the main transcription factor activated by IL-2 and related cytokines. Deficiency of the STAT5B subunit in particular (OMIM #245590) causes a rare autosomal recessive disorder that includes features of immunodeficiency and immune dysregulation.[66-68] Most patients suffer from recurrent varicella virus, herpesvirus, and *Pneumocystis jirovecii* infections as a result of T cell and natural killer (NK) cell lymphopenia (see Fig. 9.2).[66,68] The immune dysregulation features include chronic, early-onset diarrhea, eczema, and lymphocytic interstitial pneumonitis (Box 9.2).[66-68]

In addition, STAT5B is the primary transcription factor activated by the human growth factor receptor, so patients also have growth abnormalities, including dwarfism, prominent forehead, saddle nose, and a high-pitched voice.[69]

Genetics and Immunopathogenesis

Mice lacking STAT5B have a marked increase of activated T cells in the periphery and splenomegaly with a significant reduction in the number of Foxp3+ T$_{REG}$ cells in thymus and spleen.[70-72] Humans with STAT5B deficiency were found to have significantly fewer CD4+CD25^{high} cells than normal controls, FOXP3 expression was decreased, and the cells had no in vitro suppressive activity.[66,73] In addition, decreased CD25 expression (~20% of normal) was observed after T cell activation and is thought to synergize with the underlying STAT5B mutation to effectively abrogate IL-2 signals required for the maintenance of FOXP3 expression and T$_{REG}$ function. Interestingly, signaling pathways required for IL-2–induced expression of other effector molecules, such as perforin, remained intact in STAT5B-deficient T cells.[73]

Diagnosis and Treatment

Diagnosis of STAT5B deficiency should be suspected in patients with the overt physical features of dwarfism combined with a significant cellular immunodeficiency. Patients typically have normal serum growth hormone levels but very low insulin-like growth factor 1 (IGF-1) levels.[70,71] Immunologically, patients generally have low NK cell numbers and modest T cell lymphopenia.[71,73] Sequencing of the *STAT5B* gene is the gold standard for confirming a diagnosis.

Treatment of patients with STAT5B deficiency typically consists of antimicrobial prophylaxis to prevent opportunistic infections in addition to managing the immune dysregulation symptoms. Immunosuppression is tricky because of the risk of aggressive immunosuppression in the setting of a significant cellular immunodeficiency. There are no published reports of bone marrow transplantation (BMT) for STAT5B deficiency, although

murine studies demonstrate that BMT corrects the immune defects in mice lacking Stat5a/5b, suggesting that this could correct the immunodeficiency and dysregulation but not the growth abnormalities.[74]

Autoimmune Lymphoproliferative Syndrome

The typical clinical course in autoimmune lymphoproliferative syndrome (ALPS; OMIM #601859) begins within the first 5 years of life with nonmalignant, noninfectious peripheral lymphadenopathy.[75-77] In a review of a large number of ALPS cases the median age of onset was 3 years, with only 7% of the patients presenting later in life.[77] Lymphadenopathy and/or splenomegaly is commonly the initial manifestation in 69% of the patients and will eventually develop in all patients (Fig. 9.3). Hepatomegaly is found in about half of the cases. Despite being impressive, the lymphoproliferation tends to improve over time, and after the age of 20 years as many as 66% of the patients will have had complete remission of these manifestations, and the remaining patients will have seen an improvement. Because of the propensity for malignant transformation of the expanded lymphocytes, ongoing lymphoma surveillance in these patients should include careful attention to changes in lymph node size or appearance of new focal or generalized lymphadenopathy associated with concomitant systemic symptoms such as fever, drenching night sweats, and weight loss.

About a quarter of the patients present with an autoimmune disease, most often immune thrombocytopenic purpura or Coombs'-positive hemolytic anemia, in addition to the lymphoproliferation. Up to 72% of patients develop autoimmune manifestations by the age of 30. Most present with autoimmune cytopenias (52%) at a median age of 5 years. Autoimmune hemolytic anemia is the most frequent event, followed by autoimmune thrombocytopenia. Some patients (20%) also develop autoimmune diseases affecting other organs, such as autoimmune hepatitis, glomerulonephritis, uveitis, encephalomyelitis (Guillain-Barré syndrome), aplastic anemia, vasculitis, pancreatitis, angioedema, and alopecia. Unlike the lymphoproliferation, however, autoimmune disorders tend to persist in over 60% of patients, mostly requiring continuous or intermittent immunosuppressive therapy.

Only a minority (<5%) of patients present with pure autoimmunity or lymphoma as the initial manifestation of ALPS. Recurrent infections are not common but also can occur, mostly as a result of neutropenia and/or blockage of nasopharyngeal passages because of lymphadenopathy. A life-threatening ALPS manifestation is the dramatically increased incidence of lymphoma with germline *FAS* mutations. The increased relative risk is 149 for Hodgkin's disease and 61 for non-Hodgkin's lymphomas (Box 9.3).[77]

The laboratory findings in ALPS are summarized in Box 9.4. Immunophenotyping reveals expansion of α/β double-negative T (DNT) cells, often together with lymphocytosis. Other frequent abnormalities include an expansion of HLA-DR+ and a decrease in the CD25+ T cells plus very low numbers of CD20+CD27+ (memory) B cells.[78] A polyclonal increase in serum immunoglobulins is often observed, usually involving IgG and/or IgA. Autoantibodies directed against platelets and neutrophils not linked to the degree of cytopenias and antiphospholipid antibodies are present in 70% to 80% of patients.[78] IL-10 is markedly elevated in the serum of patients with ALPS that is, at least in part, from the α/β DNT cells and circulating monocytes.[79] More recently,

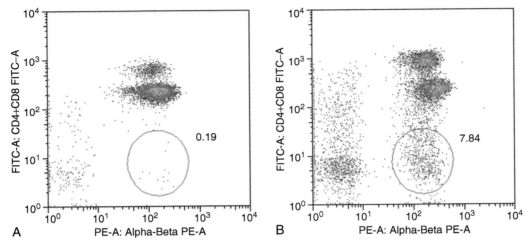

• **Fig. 9.3** Double-negative T cells in autoimmune lymphoproliferative syndrome (ALPS). Flow cytometric evaluation of peripheral blood from a control patient (A) and a patient with ALPS (B) demonstrating the increase of mature lymphocytes expressing the T cell receptor α/β (x-axis), that lack CD4 and CD8 co-receptor expression (y-axis) in ALPS.

• BOX 9.3   Key Concepts
Immunopathogenesis of Autoimmune Lymphoproliferative Syndrome

- Lymphadenopathy: Persistence of lymphocytes that normally would die
- Autoimmunity: Failure to eliminate autoreactive lymphocytes
- Lymphoma: Inability to eliminate lymphocyte oncogenic mutations

---

• BOX 9.4   Laboratory Findings in Autoimmune Lymphoproliferative Syndrome

Immunologic
- Lymphocytes
  - Increase: α/β double-negative T cells, CD8 T cells, B cells
  - Decrease: CD4/CD25 T cells, CD27+ B cells
- Immunoglobulins: Increased IgG, IgA, and IgE
- Cytokines: Increased levels of serum interleukin 10 (IL-10), IL-18
- Increased soluble FAS ligand
- Autoantibodies: Directed at blood cells

Hematologic
- Lymphocytosis
- Anemia
- Thrombocytopenia
- Neutropenia
- Eosinophilia

Chemistry
- Increased vitamin B_{12} level

---

elevated serum IL-18, soluble FAS ligand gene (*FASLG*), and vitamin B_{12} levels have been found. In the presence of elevated α/β DNT cells, these biomarkers strongly correlate with the presence of *FAS* mutations.[80,81] Histologically, the enlarged lymph nodes in ALPS show follicular hyperplasia and marked paracortical expansion with infiltrating α/β-DNT cells, immunoblasts, and plasma cells.[82]

Genetics and Immunopathogenesis

The majority of patients with ALPS have germline heterozygous *FAS* mutations, with most affecting the intracellular domains of the gene (~73%) and a smaller number affecting the transmembrane domains (~6%) and extracellular domains (~21%).[75,77,83] The site of the mutation has a direct impact on the development of disease manifestation with mutations in the intracellular *FAS* domains correlating with higher penetrance and more severe clinical manifestations.[84] The intracellular mutations typically act in a dominant negative manner, whereas extracellular mutations not affecting the preligand assembly domain usually result in haploinsufficiency.[85,86]

Somatic *FAS* mutations, detected primarily in α/β DNT cells, have been described in a number of patients with sporadic ALPS.[87,88] A minority of patients with ALPS do not have germline or somatic *FAS* mutations. Evaluation of the gene encoding FASLG identified two patients with typical findings of ALPS associated with heterozygous mutations, and homozygous *FASLG* mutations have been found in a limited number of patients with a severe ALPS phenotype.[89–90] Likewise, a small number of patients have been demonstrated to have a defect in the intracellular apoptotic protein, caspase 10 (Fig. 9.4).[91] Recent work has identified somatic *NRAS* and *KRAS* mutations in patients with some ALPS features that are associated with an intrinsic pathway apoptotic abnormality. This group of patients is now classified separately as RAS-associated autoimmune leukoproliferative disease (RALD).[92–94]

Diagnosis and Treatment

The diagnostic triad for ALPS is nonmalignant, noninfectious lymphoaccumulation; defective lymphocyte apoptosis; and increased levels of α/β DNT cells (Box 9.5). Flow cytometric evaluation of peripheral blood lymphocytes is necessary to evaluate for increased levels of α/β DNT cells (see Box 9.4). The assessment of FAS-mediated lymphocyte apoptosis or identification of a *FAS* mutation (or other ALPS-associated genetic defect) is required to establish this diagnosis. Mutation analysis is commonly performed currently through genetic panels, using next-generation

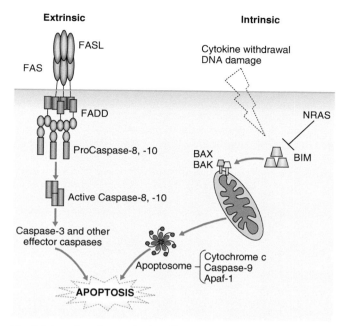

• **Fig. 9.4** Lymphocyte apoptosis pathways. Lymphocytes have two main pathways of apoptosis, regulated either by surface receptors of the tumor necrosis factor (TNF) superfamily (extrinsic pathway) or proteins of the BCL-2 family (intrinsic pathway). The majority of patients with autoimmune lymphoproliferative syndrome (ALPS) have a defect in the extrinsic pathway involving FAS, but some with ALPS also have been reported with a defect in the intrinsic pathway.

• **BOX 9.5 Key Concepts**
Diagnostic Criteria for Autoimmune Lymphoproliferative Syndrome*

Required Criteria
1. Chronic (>6 months), nonmalignant, noninfectious lymphadenopathy and/or splenomegaly
2. Elevated CD3+ TCRαβ+CD4−CD8− DNT cells (>1.5% of total lymphocytes or >2.5% of CD3+ lymphocytes) in the setting of normal or elevated lymphocyte counts

Accessory Criteria
Primary
1. Defective lymphocyte apoptosis in two separate assays
2. Somatic or germline pathogenic mutation in FAS, FASLG, or CASP10

Secondary
1. Elevated plasma sFASL levels (>200 pg/mL), plasma IL-10 levels (>20 pg/mL), serum or plasma vitamin B_{12} levels (>1500 ng/L) or plasma IL-18 levels >500 pg/mL
2. Typical immunohistologic findings as reviewed by a hematopathologist
3. Autoimmune cytopenias (hemolytic anemia, thrombocytopenia, or neutropenia) with elevated IgG levels (polyclonal hypergammaglobulinemia)
4. Family history of a nonmalignant/noninfectious lymphoproliferation with or without autoimmunity

A definitive diagnosis is based on the presence of both required criteria plus one primary accessory criterion. A probable diagnosis is based on the presence of both required criteria plus one secondary accessory criterion.

CASP10, Caspase 10; *DNT*, double-negative T cells; *FASLG*, FAS ligand gene; *IgG*, immunoglobulin G; *IL*, interleukin; *ng*, nanogram; *pg*, picogram; *sFASL*, serum FAS ligand; *TCR*, T cell receptor.
Based on First International ALPS Workshop 2009.

sequencing. If the patient has typical ALPS clinical findings with elevated biomarkers, including DNT cells, purification of α/β DNT cells for *FAS* sequencing to exclude somatic mutations is recommended.

ALPS management is aimed to (1) control autoimmune cytopenias (avoiding splenectomy) and (2) monitor for lymphoma.[95] The most important aspect of caring for patients with ALPS is the medical treatment of the chronic autoimmune multilineage cytopenias, because these frequently cause substantial morbidity. In recent studies, 59% to 74% of patients required medical and/or surgical treatment at some point in life, with the median age of onset of immunosuppression varying from 5.6 to 7.5 years.[76,77] Initial management for ALPS-related autoimmune cytopenias is similar to that for sporadic cytopenias in other patient populations. For autoimmune hemolytic anemia (AIHA) or immune thrombocytopenia, this includes the use of parenteral high-dose methylprednisolone (5–30 mg/kg per day for 1–2 days), followed by oral prednisone (1–2 mg/kg per day) that is tapered slowly over months. High-dose intravenous immunoglobulin (1–2 g/kg) may be considered for concomitant use with pulse-dose corticosteroids for severe AIHA. Some patients with autoimmune neutropenias who experience associated infection may be treated with low-dose granulocyte colony-stimulating factor (G-CSF 1–2 mg/kg administered subcutaneously two to three times per week).

As second-line therapy in patients with refractory autoimmune cytopenias requiring chronic corticosteroid therapy or unresponsive to first-line agents, mycophenolate mofetil (MMF) and sirolimus are the most effective agents. MMF has been shown over the past 10 years to be an effective corticosteroid-sparing agent that maintains adequate blood cell counts and reduces the need for other immunosuppressive agents or splenectomy in over 80% of patients.[96–98] However, it has little effect on the lymphoproliferation and depletion of DNTs. Despite this drawback, it should be considered the second-line drug of choice in patients with ALPS with mild to moderate lymphoproliferation and autoimmune cytopenias.

For patients with more severe autoimmune disease and clinically significant lymphoproliferation, sirolimus has become the agent of choice. Several studies have demonstrated the high efficacy of this drug, with complete or near-complete responses in 94% to 100% of treated patients.[96,99,100] These include improvements in autoimmune disease, lymphadenopathy, and splenomegaly within 1 to 3 months of drug use. Responses were also durable, with follow-up of almost 10 years. In addition, there was normalization of known biomarkers, including DNTs and serum levels of vitamin B_{12}, IL-10, and serum FAS ligand (sFASL).[100] A suggested treatment algorithm for autoimmune cytopenias associated with ALPS is given in Fig. 9.5.

Spleen guards, made of fiberglass by an occupational therapist familiar with such devices, should be considered for patients with ALPS with massive splenomegaly to help reduce the risk of traumatic splenic rupture. Practice of contact sports such as football or ice hockey is discouraged.

Sepsis postsplenectomy is the main cause of death in ALPS.[77] All patients who are asplenic should be treated with long-term antibiotic prophylaxis against pneumococcal sepsis, using penicillin V. Patients with ALPS frequently are unable to produce or maintain protective antibodies directed against polysaccharide antigens after vaccination, because of defects in memory B cell function.[101] Nevertheless, these patients should be vaccinated against encapsulated organisms such as pneumococcus, meningococcus, and

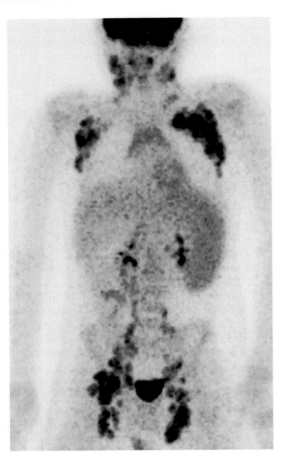

• **Fig. 9.5** Lymphoid accumulation in autoimmune lymphoproliferative syndrome (ALPS). Positron emission tomography demonstrating increasing fluorodeoxyglucose uptake on cervical, axillary, and inguinal lymph nodes and an enlarged spleen in ALPS.

Haemophilus influenzae type b. Patients who have undergone surgical splenectomy are encouraged to wear medical alert bracelets or necklaces or carry wallet cards warning about their risk for sepsis. On confirmation of a diagnosis of ALPS, patients should undergo counseling aimed at specifically addressing the risks associated with this condition.

Most importantly, the increased risk of lymphomas and other malignancies should be discussed, and patients should be encouraged to seek further evaluation for any sudden and persistent fluctuations in lymph node or spleen size.[77] Serial positron emission tomography studies and biopsies may be necessary in these patients to rule out malignant transformation. In patients with ALPS with intracellular *FAS* death domain mutations, the risk of lymphoma should be particularly emphasized.

Prognosis

The overall prognosis and outcome in most patients with ALPS are good, but the mortality and morbidity vary widely depending on disease severity. Most patients are expected to live a normal lifespan with few clinical complications. Lymphoproliferation tends to improve in most patients over time, especially after adolescence, but autoimmunity persists in over half of them, requiring chronic immunosuppression.[76,77] Patients with mutations affecting the intracellular domain of the FAS protein have more severe disease and are at increased risk for Hodgkin's and non-Hodgkin's B cell

lymphomas. A large cohort of patients with ALPS-FAS showed a 6% to 10% incidence of lymphoma with a median age of presentation of 17 years, and other reports relate a 15% risk before the age of 30.[76,77] Patients with mutations affecting the extracellular domain of FAS have been reported to develop lymphomas, extending the spectrum of at-risk patients.[77] ALPS-associated lymphomas appear to be as amenable to chemotherapy as sporadic lymphomas and should be managed as such.

Although lymphoma is the most feared complication in ALPS, the most lethal complication is postsplenectomy sepsis. In a 2011 series, 6 of 90 patients with ALPS died over a 25-year follow-up period: four of postsplenectomy infection, one of aplastic anemia, and one of a stroke.[76] In the NIH ALPS cohort, the most common cause of death was also postsplenectomy infection.[77] Based on these data, splenectomy is strongly discouraged in ALPS.

RAS-Associated Autoimmune Leukoproliferative Disorder

In 2007 the first patient with an ALPS-like phenotype caused by a somatic mutation in *NRAS* was described.[92] The patient had persistent splenomegaly, slightly elevated DNTs, autoimmune autoantibodies, and a history of lymphoma, but no mutations in known ALPS genes. He also had features not seen in typical ALPS, such as a history of significant leukocytosis early in life, persistent monocytosis, and lymph node histology not compatible with ALPS, as a result of the lack of DNT infiltration in the paracortical area. Later, additional patients with an ALPS-like disease were also found to have heterozygous dominant activating mutations in *NRAS* or *KRAS*. The disease was then identified as RALD.[92,93,102]

Patients with RALD have several clinical and laboratory features that overlap with those of ALPS. The age at diagnosis can vary between 1 and 47 years, and they present with a generally mild degree of peripheral lymphadenopathy, significant splenomegaly, and autoimmunity, including AIHA, immune thrombocytopenic purpura, and neutropenia. In some patients, a history of recurrent mild upper and lower respiratory tract infections and skin rashes with histiocytic infiltration can be elicited.[103] Unlike in ALPS, patients with RALD have a transient or persistent elevation in granulocytes and monocytes. Some patients with RALD have a clinical and laboratory phenotype very similar to that of juvenile myelomonocytic leukemia (JMML) early in life, with marked hepatosplenomegaly and monocytosis.[104] Unlike patients with JMML, the clinical outcome is usually chronic and benign. However, at least one case of progression to full JMML years after a RALD diagnosis has been described.[105] More recently a patient with a somatic mutation in *KRAS* and a mixed phenotype of Rosai-Dorfman and systemic lupus erythematosus was described, expanding the phenotype of this entity.[106]

Immunophenotyping in RALD reveals mild to no elevation in DNTs and an expansion of B cells. Total lymphocyte numbers are normal to modestly decreased. In contrast, absolute or relative monocytosis is noted in all patients. Autoantibodies are typically detected, including antinuclear antibody; rheumatoid factor; and antiphospholipid, anticardiolipin antiplatelet, antineutrophil, and/or anti–red cell antibodies. Unlike in patients with ALPS, serum sFASL and vitamin B_{12} are normal, as they are in vitro FAS-induced apoptosis. By contrast, in patients with RALD the T cells are resistant to IL-2 withdrawal–induced cell death, pointing to a fundamentally different apoptotic defect in RALD.[92,93,102] The histopathologic findings include nonspecific polyclonal plasmacytosis with reactive secondary follicles but without the typical paracortical expansion caused by DNT cells in ALPS. Given the small number of patients diagnosed to date, it is not known if these patients are at increased risk for hematologic malignancy. However, there are reports of patients developing lymphoma and at least one patient who developed full-blown JMML years after a diagnosis of RALD.[105]

Genetics and Pathophysiology

All patients with RALD known to date harbor somatic, gain-of-function mutations in *KRAS* or *NRAS,* which are present only in blood cells. Germline RAS pathway mutations have been described as causing the related Costello (*HRAS*), Noonan (*PTPN11, KRAS, SOS1, NRAS*), and cardiofaciocutaneous syndromes (*KRAS, BRAF, MEK1,* and *MEK*).[107]

The RAS genes (*NRAS, KRAS,* and *HRAS*) encode 21-kd proteins that are members of the superfamily of small guanosine triphosphate (GTP)-binding proteins, which have diverse intracellular signaling functions, including control of cell proliferation, growth, and apoptosis. RAS activity differs when bound to GTP versus guanosine diphosphate (GDP).[108] The conversion from a GTP- to a GDP-bound state is catalyzed by a weak intrinsic GTPase activity, which is greatly enhanced on interaction of RAS with GTPase activating proteins (GAPs). The *NRAS* and *KRAS* mutations seen in patients with RALD disrupt the interaction of RAS with the GAPs, diminishing its GTPase activity and locking the molecule in an "on" position. This permanent activation state increases cell signaling through the RAS–extracellular signal-related kinase (ERK) pathway, inducing phosphorylation and destruction of the proapoptotic protein BIM.[109] Consequently, the cells become resistant to certain kinds of apoptotic stimuli, such as growth-factor (IL-2) withdrawal. Interestingly, previous work suggested that adequate RAS signaling is also important for B cell selection, potentially explaining the multiple antibody-mediated autoimmune manifestations seen in these patients.[110]

Protein Kinase C Delta Deficiency

A patient with an ALPS-like condition with lymphadenopathy, splenomegaly, multiple autoantibodies, and elevated IgG was found to have a homozygous loss of function mutation in the gene encoding protein kinase C delta *(PKCδ).*[111] The mutation resulted in ex vivo B cell hyperproliferation and the lymph node histology of intense follicular hyperplasia and progressive transformation of germinal centers. Both of these findings mirror the *PKCδ* knock-out mouse model. The defect also altered NK cell function, causing chronic EBV infection. Flow cytometry demonstrated expansion of CD5+CD20+ B cells and mild elevation of α/β DNT cells that were not present in the lymph nodes. This patient responded to rapamycin therapy with marked decrease in splenomegaly and hyperglobulinemia. An additional report identified a second patient with a homozygous loss of function *PKCδ* mutation who presented with a somewhat different clinical phenotype.[112] Additionally, three children from one consanguineous family have been reported with homozygous loss of function *PKCδ* mutations linked to mendelian systemic lupus erythematosus.[113] Taken together, these findings suggest that *PKCδ* plays a central role in B cell tolerance and prevention of self-reactivity.

Conclusions

In recent years, identification of the genetic defects linked to patients with congenital systemic autoimmunity has led to the definition of a new class of PIDD in which the defect affects the regulatory compartment of the immune system. Lessons learned from these disorders have clarified aspects of thymic selection, T_{REG} function, FAS-mediated apoptosis, and intrinsic apoptosis–mediated via RAS proteins. There are a number of unresolved issues that include defining other contributing genetic and/or environmental factors and clarifying the basis for the specific patterns of autoimmunity seen in these disorders. Studying these experiments of nature will continue to be a fertile field of investigation over the coming years as we strive to uncover the basic mechanisms of immune tolerance.

The reference list can be found on the companion Expert Consult website at http://www.expertconsult.inkling.com.

10

Immunoglobulin Therapy

ELENA E. PEREZ, MARK BALLOW

KEY POINTS

- Immune globulin, administered by intravenous or subcutaneous route, is indicated as replacement therapy in patients with antibody immunodeficiency disorders.
- Dosing intravenous immunoglobulin (IVIG) to target higher immunoglobulin G troughs (http://nimblebooks.tnq.co.in/EL-SEVIER/app.html 700–1000 mg/dL) may be associated with decreased rate of infections and improved pulmonary outcomes in patients with primary immunodeficiency.
- IVIG is not a generic drug, and IVIG products are not interchangeable. Product differences may lead to differences in

tolerability and side effects for individual patients.
- Minor side effects of IVIG are common. Serious adverse effects, though relatively rare at standard replacement doses of IVIG, may include hemolysis, thromboembolic events, and acute renal failure.
- Many mechanisms for the effects of IVIG on immune modulation have been described. These mechanisms are not mutually exclusive and most likely work in concert, depending on the dose of IVIG administered and the specific inflammatory disease process.

Introduction

Primary immunodeficiency is the original indication for immunoglobulin replacement therapy approved by the U.S. Food and Drug Administration (FDA). The goal of this therapy in patients with primary immunodeficiency is to provide adequate antibodies to prevent infections and long-term complications, especially pulmonary disease. Patients with recurrent infections resulting from profound hypogammaglobulinemia and/or defective antibody production may be candidates for immunoglobulin replacement therapy,[1] with either intravenous immunoglobulin (IVIG) or subcutaneous immunoglobulin (SCIG). It is very important to evaluate the ability of the patient to produce specific antibodies to polysaccharide or protein antigens before treatment to confirm the primary immunodeficiency diagnosis. The uses approved by the FDA for IVIG as replacement or adjunct therapy in patients with immunodeficiency, recurrent infections, or autoimmune and inflammatory disorders are shown in (Box 10.1).

Practical tip for the office setting: For patients suspected to have a primary antibody deficiency, confirm the diagnosis of antibody deficiency before initiation of gamma globulin replacement therapy. Measurement of quantitative immunoglobulin G (IgG), IgA, IgM, and specific antibody responses before and after vaccinations such as tetanus, diphtheria, and pneumococcus is required to assess antibody level and function and justify therapy with gamma globulin.

Preparation of Intravenous Immunoglobulin

IVIG is made from pooled donated plasma from 10,000 to 60,000 donors and contains a broad spectrum of antibodies with biologic activity against infectious pathogens. It contains at least 90% intact monomeric IgG with a normal ratio of IgG subclasses and is free of aggregates. The biologic activity of the IgG is maintained, especially for Fc-mediated function, and it contains no infectious agents or other potentially harmful contaminants. Although there is no standardization for the titer of specific antibodies against common organisms such as *Streptococcus pneumoniae* and *Haemophilus influenzae,* each lot must contain adequate levels of antibody to certain pathogens, such as measles. Specific antibodies in IVIG products may vary slightly from manufacturer to manufacturer and from lot to lot, but they are generally comparable.[2] Some products containing very low amounts of IgA may be beneficial in some IgA-deficient patients with antibodies to IgA to minimize the risk of possible anaphylactic reactions,[3] though the role of anti-IgA antibodies in causing anaphylaxis to IVIG is a subject of controversy.[4]

The half-life of antibodies in the IVIG product varies depending on the isotype and the subclass of the antibody. Total IgG has a half-life of approximately 17 to 30 days.[5,6] However, the half-life of IgG3 is much shorter (7.5–9 days)[6,7] compared with those of IgG1 and IgG2, which have a half-life of approximately 27 to 30 days. Generally, it should take about 3 months after beginning monthly IVIG infusions or a dosage change to reach equilibration (steady state).[2] (Box 10.2).

Almost all products available today in the United States are liquids, either 5% or 10%, and are FDA approved for intravenous and/or subcutaneous administration. Two liquid 20% products and one 16.5% product are suitable only for administration by the subcutaneous route (Table 10.1). Incubation at low pH or treatment with solvent and detergent, pasteurization, depth filtration, and nanofiltration are important steps for viral removal and inactivation.

U.S. Food and Drug Administration–Approved Uses of Intravenous Immunoglobulin Therapy in Patients With Immunodeficiency Disorders, Infection, and Inflammatory Processes

1. Primary immunodeficiency disease or primary antibody immunodeficiency: Replacement therapy to prevent and/or control infection
2. Idiopathic thrombocytopenic purpura (ITP): Indicated to prevent and/or control bleeding
3. Kawasaki disease: Indicated for the prevention of coronary artery aneurysms
4. B cell chronic lymphocytic leukemia (CLL): Indicated for patients with hypogammaglobulinemia to reduce and/or prevent recurrent bacterial infections
5. Bone marrow transplantation: To decrease the risk of infection, interstitial pneumonia, and acute graft-versus-host disease
6. Pediatric HIV-1 infection: To decrease the frequency and severity of bacterial infections
7. Chronic inflammatory demyelinating polyneuropathy (CIDP): To improve neuromuscular impairment and for maintenance therapy to prevent relapse
8. Multifocal motor neuropathy: To improve neuromuscular impairment and for maintenance therapy to prevent relapse

• BOX 10.2 Features of Intravenous Immune Serum Globulin (IVIG)

- Cold ethanol fractionation (Cohn fraction II)
- Greater than 95% IgG; greater than 90% monomeric IgG
- Traces of other immunoglobulins (e.g., IgA and IgM, and serum proteins)
- Addition of an amino acid to stabilize IgG from aggregation
- Intact Fc receptor biologic function
  - Opsonization and phagocytosis
  - Complement activation
- Normal half-life for serum IgG
- Normal proportion of IgG subclasses
- Broad spectrum of antibodies to bacterial and viral agents

Dosage

The recommended dose for IVIG as replacement therapy is generally 400 to 600 mg/kg/month given every 4 weeks in patients with primary immunodeficiency (Box 10.3). A higher dose of immunoglobulin can lead to higher peak and trough levels of serum IgG.[8] On average, peak serum IgG levels increase approximately 250 mg/dL[8] and trough levels increase 100 mg/dL[9] for each 100 mg/kg of IVIG infused.

Multiple studies since the 1980s have demonstrated improved efficacy of the currently recommended dose range of IVIG over lower doses previously tried with respect to reduced days of fever and need for antibiotics, improved pulmonary function, decreased incidence of pneumonia, and hospitalized days.[10–13] Historically, IgG trough levels greater than 500 mg/dL have been shown to prevent severe bacterial infections. However, a study performed in 1999 on 22 patients with primary hypogammaglobulinemia and pulmonary abnormalities treated with IVIG showed that despite adequate trough serum IgG levels (>500 mg/dL), patients still had silent and asymptomatic pulmonary changes.[14] Another retrospective study of the clinical features and outcomes of 31 patients with X-linked agammaglobulinemia (XLA) receiving replacement

IVIG therapy between 1982 and 1997 treated with doses greater than 250 mg/kg every 3 weeks (median trough level of 700 mg/dL) showed a decreased incidence of bacterial infections requiring hospitalizations (0.4 versus 0.06 per patient per year); however, complications of sinusitis, bronchiectasis, obstructive pulmonary disease, and enteroviral meningoencephalitis still occurred.[15] The authors suggested that maintaining a higher serum IgG level, for example, greater than 800 mg/dL, may improve pulmonary outcome in patients with XLA. Targeting of higher IgG trough levels has since been demonstrated to improve outcomes in patients with hypogammaglobulinemia who are on IVIG therapy. Across all included studies in a meta-analysis of studies evaluating trough IgG levels and pneumonia incidence in patients with primary immune deficiency with hypogammablogulinemia, pneumonia incidence progressively declined with increasing trough IgG, with trough levels of 1000 mg/dL associated with one-fifth the incidence of pneumonia seen with trough levels of 500 mg/dL.[16]

There is emerging evidence that ideal trough levels to prevent infection may vary considerably from patient to patient. The concept of the biologic IgG level as the minimum serum IgG level that protects an individual patient with immunodeficiency against recurrent bacterial infections and bronchiectasis has been proposed.[17] This level is anticipated to be somewhere in the age-matched normal reference range but is unique for the individual patient.[17] This concept of individualized IgG trough is further supported by another study,[18] which showed that patients with common variable immunodeficiency (CVID) required a wide range of trough IgG levels, from 500 to 1700 mg/dL, to prevent recurrent infection. Patients with X-linked agammaglobulinemia required IgG troughs between 800 and 1300 mg/dL to prevent infection.[18]

Pulmonary abnormalities are among the most important factors associated with morbidity and mortality in patients with humoral primary immunodeficiencies. Therefore, periodic pulmonary function testing and judicious use of high-resolution chest computed tomography should be used to monitor for adequate control or prevention of pulmonary complications of humoral immunodeficiency.

Administration

In patients with primary immunodeficiency the replacement dose of IVIG is generally 400 to 600 mg/kg/month. The dose, manufacturer, and lot number should be recorded for each infusion to perform look-back procedures for adverse events or other consequences. It is crucial to record all side effects that occur during the infusion. It is also recommended to monitor liver and renal function tests periodically, approximately every 6 months. Antigen detection for hepatitis B and polymerase chain reaction (PCR) for hepatitis C should be performed, if clinically indicated.

There are several routes of administration of immunoglobulin.

Intravenous Administration

Early IVIG preparations caused rate-related side effects in 50% of patients.[19] Newer preparations are generally more tolerable, but significant side effects such as thrombosis have been associated with higher rates of infusion. Manufacturers recommend starting rates of 0.5 to 1 mg/kg/min and increasing incrementally up to rates between 3.3 and 12 mg/kg/min depending on the product and as stated in the package insert.[20–24] The FDA recommends that for patients at risk of renal failure, such as with preexisting renal insufficiency, diabetes, age older than 65 years, volume depletion, sepsis, or paraproteinemia and use of

TABLE 10.1   Commercially Available Intravenous Immunoglobulin Preparations in the United States

Brand (Manufacturer)	Manufacturing Process/Antiviral Inactivation	pH	Additives	Parenteral Form and Final Concentrations	IgA Content µg/mL	Approved Method of Administration
Asceniv (ADMA Biologics)	Modified classic Cohn Method 6/Oncley Method 9 fractionation procedure solvent/detergent treatment, 5 nm virus filtration	4.0–4.6	Glycine Polysorbate 80	10% liquid	<200	Intravenous
Bivigam (Biotest Pharmaceuticals Corp.)	Cohn-Oncley cold ethanol fractionation, ultrafiltration, solvent/detergent treatment	4.0–4.6	No sugars—stabilized with glycine	10% liquid	≤200	Intravenous
Flebogamma DIF (Grifols Therapeutics, Inc.)	Cohn-Oncley cold ethanol fractionation, ion exchange chromatography; PEG precipitation, heat pasteurization; pH 4 treatment, solvent detergent treatment; double nanofiltration	5–6	5% D-sorbitol	5% or 10% liquid	<50 (5% solution <100 (10% solution)	Intravenous
Gammagard S/D (Takeda)	Cohn-Oncley cold ethanol fractionation, ion exchange chromatography; solvent detergent treatment	6.4–7.2	2% glucose (5% solution)	Lyophilized powder 5% or 10%	<2.2 (5% solution)	Intravenous
Gammaplex (Bio Products Laboratory)	Kistler and Nitschmann fractionation, DEAE-Sephadex chromatography, Solvent/detergent treatment, CM-Sepharose chromatography, nanofiltration, low pH incubation	4.8–5.1	5% D-sorbitol	5% liquid	<10	Intravenous
Octagam (Octapharma USA, Inc.)	Cohn-Oncley cold ethanol fractionation, ion exchange chromatography, ultrafiltration, solvent/detergent treatment	5.1–6.0	Maltose 100 mg/mL	5% liquid	≤200	Intravenous
Panzyga (Octapharma/Pfizer)	Cold ethanol fractionation, solvent/detergent treatment, ion exchange chromatography, nanofiltration (20 ion-exchange nanofiltration (20 nm)	4.5–5.0	Glycine	10% liquid	100	Intravenous
Privigen (CLS Behring)	Cold ethanol fractionation, octanoic acid fractionation, anion exchange chromatography; pH 4 treatment, nanofiltration, depth filtration	4.8	No sugars, stabilized with L-proline	10% liquid	≤25	Intravenous
Gammagard Liquid (Takeda)	Cohn-Oncley cold ethanol fractionation, ion exchange chromatography; solvent detergent treatment, nanofiltration, low pH incubation	4.6–5.1	No sugars—stabilized with glycine	10% liquid	37	Intravenous and subcutaneous
Gammaked (Kedrion Biopharma, Inc.)	Cohn-Oncley cold ethanol fractionation, caprylate chromatography, anion exchange chromatography, low pH incubation, double depth filtration	4.0–4.5	No sugars—stabilized with glycine	10% liquid	46	Intravenous and subcutaneous
Gamunex-C (Grifols Therapeutics, Inc.)	Cohn-Oncley cold ethanol fractionation, caprylate chromatography, anion exchange chromatography, low pH incubation, double depth filtration	4.0–4.5	No sugars—stabilized with glycine	10% liquid	46	Intravenous and subcutaneous

Continued

TABLE 10.1 Commercially Available Intravenous Immunoglobulin Preparations in the United States—cont'd

Brand (Manufacturer)	Manufacturing Process/Antiviral Inactivation	pH	Additives	Parenteral Form and Final Concentrations	IgA Content µg/mL	Approved Method of Administration
Cutaquig (Octapharma)	Cold ethanol fractionation, ultrafiltration and chromatography; pH 4 treatment, solvent/detergent (S/D)	5.0 – 5.5	Maltose	16.5% liquid	≤600	Subcutaneous
Cuvitru (Takeda)	Modified Cohn-Oncley cold ethanol fractionation, cation and anion exchange chromatography, solvent/detergent treatment, 35-nm nanofiltration, low pH incubation at elevated temperature	4.6 – 5.1	Glycine	20% liquid	80	Subcutaneous
Hizentra (CLS Behring)	Cold ethanol fractionation, octanoic acid fractionation, anion exchange chromatography; pH 4 treatment, nanofiltration	4.6–5.2	No sugar, stabilized with L-proline	20% liquid	≤50	Subcutaneous
Xembify (Grifols)	Cold ethanol fractionation, caprylate precipitation and filtration, and anion-exchange chromatography, low pH treatment	4.1–4.8	Glycine polysorbate	20% liquid	Not reported	Subcutaneous
Hyqvia (Takeda)	Cohn-Oncley cold ethanol fractionation, ion exchange chromatography; solvent detergent treatment, nanofiltration, low pH incubation	4.6–5.1	Glycine	10% liquid	37	Subcutaneous with hyaluronidase

From manufacturers' package inserts and product publications.

IgA, Immunoglobulin A; *PEG*, polyethylene glycol.

• BOX 10.3 Clinical Pearls

- Because of the half-life of intravenous immunoglobulin (IVIG), waiting to check immunoglobulin G (IgG) levels until 3 months after initiation of IVIG or change in dose is advised for an accurate determination of steady-state trough level.
- For every 100 mg/kg of IVIG dose increase, expect the trough to increase by approximately 100 mg/dL.
- High-dose IVIG is useful for various autoimmune and inflammatory disorders and is generally defined as 1 to 2 g/kg/dose divided over 2 to 5 days.

---

nephrotoxic drugs or for patients at risk of thromboembolic complications, the dose should be gradually increased to a more conservative 3 to 4 mg/kg/min maximum.

Subcutaneous Immunoglobulin Administration

The subcutaneous route for immunoglobulin replacement therapy was first reported as safe, well tolerated, and effective in achieving adequate serum IgG levels in 1980[25] and was successfully used in several studies[26,27] but required a slow rate of infusion (1–2 mL/hr). Rapid subcutaneous infusion was studied more extensively in the 1990s and was demonstrated to be well tolerated and efficacious and resulted in fewer systemic side effects than IVIG.[28–31] A meta-analysis of SCIG versus IVIG efficacy and safety studies demonstrated a trend toward better infection control with SCIG (though not achieving statistical significance), along with improved patient quality of

life and decreased systemic adverse events compared with IVIG therapy.[32] Higher and more stable trough levels have been seen with the subcutaneous administration of immunoglobulin, alleviating the fatigue and general constitutional symptoms patients have on IVIG toward the end of their 3 to 4 weeks dosing interval. These qualities have made SCIG a viable alternative to IVIG for many patients, especially those with significant systemic adverse effects with IVIG.

When immunoglobulin is administered via the subcutaneous route, the dose is absorbed into the circulation and redistributed to the peripheral tissues more slowly than when given by the intravenous route.[33] SCIG infusions (100 mg/kg/week of a 16.5% preparation) reach steady state after 6 months if given weekly or in 1 week if patients are first loaded with IVIG or given daily subcutaneous infusions for 5 days before their maintenance weekly SCIG.[34]

In the United States, two 20% and one 16.5% immunoglobulin products for subcutaneous use are available and several 10% liquid products have both intravenous and subcutaneous indications (see Table 10.1). The monthly dose of one 10% product may be infused subcutaneously into one or two sites, with the addition of hyaluronidase before infusion. The FDA required a dose adjustment in SCIG licensing studies such that the weekly SCIG dose results in a total serum IgG exposure (area under the curve [AUC] of serum IgG versus time) equivalent to that of previous IVIG treatment.[35] Based on this AUC calculation, SCIG prescribing information recommends product-specific dosage increases of 37% to 53% when transitioning patients from IVIG to SCIG.[20,21,36] However, Berger and colleagues[37] have shown that all U.S.-licensed SCIG products have a similar bioavailability: 66.7% ± 1.8% of IVIG. They suggest that decreased bioavailability is a basic property of SCIG rather than the result of any manufacturing process or product concentration and that dose adjustments are not necessary when switching from one SCIG product to another.[37]

Several studies from the European Union, in which a 1:1 conversion from IVIG to SCIG is standard, suggest that a dose adjustment from IVIG to SCIG may not be necessary to achieve good clinical outcomes.[38,39] In contrast, Haddad and colleagues[40] found that patients receiving SCIG doses that were 1.5 times higher than their previous IVIG doses had significantly lower rates of nonserious infections, hospitalization, antibiotic use, and missed work/school activity compared with patients who received SCIG doses identical to previous IVIG doses. When switching a patient from IVIG to SCIG, making a dosage decision based on trough serum IgG levels and the clinical response to therapy is preferable to taking only pharmacokinetic measures into consideration.[35]

The technique of administering SCIG can be taught to most patients or caregivers to facilitate home self-administration. Infusions may be given daily to weekly or biweekly at one to six sites, depending on the total amount infused and the amount that can be accommodated in a single site (a function of body mass index). Infusion sites are usually on the abdominal wall and inner thigh. Other sites may include posterior upper arms, flanks, or above the buttocks. The rate of infusion of the various SCIG products is set initially at 15 to 20 mL/site/hr and subsequently may be increased up to 25 to 30 mL/site/hr, if no adverse reactions occur.[41]

Side Effects

Rate-Related Adverse Reactions (IVIG)

Most adverse reactions of IVIG are related to the rate of administration. Common adverse events include tachycardia, chest tightness, back pain, arthralgia, myalgia, hypertension or hypotension, headache, pruritus, rash, and low-grade fever (Box 10.4). More serious reactions include dyspnea, nausea, vomiting, circulatory collapse, and loss of consciousness. Patients with more profound immunodeficiency or patients with active infections have more severe reactions. Some of these reactions have been shown to be related to the complement-fixing activity of IgG aggregates in the IVIG.[42] In addition, the formation of oligomeric or polymeric IgG complexes can interact with Fc receptors and trigger the release of inflammatory mediators.[43] These adverse reactions occurred with lower frequency (10%–15%) and with less severity in more recent preparations of IVIG. These reactions most commonly occur in newly diagnosed patients with hypogammaglobulinemia and in patients who have chronic underlying infections such as sinusitis and bronchitis. One possible cause is the binding of the infused antibodies to pathogen component antigens of the underlying chronic infection or inflammatory process. In a large prospective study of 459 antibody-deficient patients,[44] of 13,508 infusions, the reaction rate was only 0.8%. There were virtually no severe reactions (0.1%).

Common reactions to IVIG, including fatigue, myalgia, and headache, may be delayed and may last several hours after the infusion. Slowing the infusion rate or discontinuing therapy until symptoms subside may diminish the reaction. Pretreatment with a nonsteroidal antiinflammatory agent, such as ibuprofen (10 mg/kg/dose), acetaminophen (15 mg/kg/dose), diphenhydramine (1 mg/kg/dose), and/or hydrocortisone (6 mg/kg/dose, maximum 100 mg)[9,42,45] 1 hour before the infusion may prevent adverse reactions. If the patient continues to have adverse effects from IVIG despite pretreatment and rate change, the physician should consider changing the route of administration to subcutaneous.

• **BOX 10.4** **Adverse Effects of Intravenous Immunoglobulin Administration**

Common
- Chills
- Headache
- Backache
- Myalgia
- Malaise/fatigue
- Fever
- Pruritus
- Rash, flushing
- Nausea, vomiting
- Tingling
- Hypotension or hypertension
- Fluid overload

Relatively Uncommon (Multiple Reports)
- Chest pain or tightness
- Dyspnea
- Severe headaches
- Aseptic meningitis
- Renal failure

Rare (Isolated Reports)
- Anaphylaxis
- Arthritis
- Thrombosis/cerebral infarction
- Myocardial infarction
- Acute encephalopathy
- Cardiac rhythm abnormalities
- Coagulopathy
- Hemolysis
- Neutropenia
- Alopecia
- Uveitis
- Noninfectious hepatitis
- Hypothermia
- Lymphocytic pleural effusion

Potential (No Reports)
- Prion disease
- HIV infections
- Parvovirus B19

Aseptic meningitis can occur with large doses, rapid infusions, and in the treatment of patients with autoimmune or inflammatory diseases.[46–49] Interestingly, this adverse reaction rarely occurs in immunodeficient patients.[45] Symptoms, including headache, stiff neck, and photophobia, usually develop within 24 hours after completion of the infusion and may last 3 to 5 days. Spinal fluid pleocytosis occurs in most patients.[46,47,49] Long-term complications are minimal.[49] The cause of aseptic meningitis is unclear, but migraine has been reported as a risk factor and may be associated with recurrence despite the use of different IVIG preparations and slower rates of infusion.[46]

Renal Adverse Effects

Acute renal failure is a rare but significant complication of IVIG treatment. Histopathologic findings of acute tubular necrosis, vacuolar degeneration, and osmotic nephrosis are suggestive of osmotic injury to the proximal renal tubules. In one study, 55% of the cases were in patients treated for idiopathic thrombocytopenic purpura (ITP), and less than 5% involved patients with primary immunodeficiency.[50] This complication may relate to the higher doses of IVIG used in ITP. The majority of the cases were treated successfully with conservative treatment, but deaths were reported in 17 patients who had serious underlying conditions. Reports suggest that IVIG products using sucrose as a stabilizer may carry a greater risk of this renal complication. Because of this, the infusion rate for sucrose-containing IVIG should not exceed 3 mg/kg/min in general, or 2 mg/kg/min in patients at risk of renal dysfunction or thromboembolic events. Risk factors for this adverse reaction include preexisting renal insufficiency, diabetes mellitus, dehydration, age older than 65, sepsis, paraproteinemia, and concomitant use of nephrotoxic agents. For patients at increased risk, monitoring blood urea nitrogen and creatinine before starting the treatment and periodically thereafter is necessary. If renal function deteriorates, the product should be changed to a non–sucrose-containing IVIG or to SCIG. There is no longer a commercial sucrose containing Ig product in the United States.

Anaphylactic Reactions

Anaphylactic reactions to IVIG infusions are relatively rare.[44] IgE and IgG antibodies to IgA have been reported to cause severe reactions in IgA-deficient patients receiving intravenous gamma globulin preparations.[3,51,52] Because of these concerns, the prescribing information for current gamma globulin products includes either a precaution or contraindication to usage in IgA-deficient patients. Several studies have shown that these patients who have reacted to conventional IVIG preparations could then go on to tolerate IVIG preparations containing very low concentrations of contaminating IgA.[3,53] However, other studies have described patients with anti-IgA antibodies tolerating IgA-containing IVIG preparations without reaction.[54,55] Therefore, the clinical significance of anti-IgA antibodies and the role that these antibodies play in cases of anaphylaxis to IVIG products remain controversial.

Thromboembolic Events

All human immunoglobulin products currently licensed in the United States carry an FDA warning of the risk of thrombosis with this class of products.[56] Local thromboses at infusion sites, deep vein thrombosis, pulmonary embolism, myocardial infarctions, transient ischemic attacks, and stroke have been reported after IVIG infusion.[57–60]

Risk factors for the development of IVIG-related thrombosis include advanced age, prolonged immobilization, hypercoagulable conditions, history of thrombosis, supplemental estrogens, indwelling central vascular catheters, hyperviscosity, and cardiovascular risk factors.[56,57,60,61]

It has been suspected that these thrombotic complications were due to platelet activation and/or increased serum viscosity in patients receiving large doses of IVIG.[62–64] One IVIG product's increased risk for thromboembolic events has been shown to be due to high levels of activated factor XI (FXIa).[65] Concerns over FXIa-related thrombosis have led to changes in manufacturing techniques, removal of factor XI/XIa using an adsorbent during the manufacturing process, and use of the thrombin-generation assay to monitor procoagulant activity of immunoglobulin products.[65]

Hemolytic Adverse Reactions

Because IVIG preparations are prepared from a large number of donors, IgG isohemagglutinins (antibodies against A/B blood group antigens) are present in these preparations. In non-O blood type recipients, anti-A and anti-B antibodies from the IVIG may react with red blood cells to cause asymptomatic Coombs' positivity or, less commonly, clinically significant hemolytic reactions, especially in those receiving high cumulative doses of immunoglobulin.[66–68] Clinically significant hemolysis is very rare in licensing studies of IVIG for primary immunodeficiency, using doses of 400 to 800 mg/kg. Currently all immunoglobulin products licensed in the European Union and United States are required to contain anti-A and anti-B titers that are 1:64 or less by the direct agglutination test.[69] Despite this, current products meeting these regulations are still implicated in cases of hemolysis, and strategies to address this issue are being pursued by the FDA.[69] Some manufacturers have instituted steps such as the use of adsorbents to lower titers of anti-A and anti-B.[70,71]

Infectious Complications

Hepatitis C virus (HCV) infection in patients receiving IVIG products was initially reported in experimental lots in Europe and the United States. HCV infection usually occurred in clusters associated with contaminated lots[72,73] and specific manufacturing procedures. However, routine screening of plasma donors for hepatitis C RNA by reverse transcriptase polymerase chain reaction (RT-PCR) and the addition of a viral inactivation process in the final manufacturing step, such as treatment with a solvent/detergent and/or pasteurization, has practically eliminated the risk of transmission of HCV and other viruses. Other innovative steps have been incorporated during the manufacturing process that include viral inactivation and viral removal stages. Some of the more common processes include solvent/detergent treatment of the final IVIG product to destroy potential lipid-envelope viruses, incubation at low pH, pasteurization, caprylate treatment, and viral removal steps with depth filtration and nanofiltration. In aggregate, these steps lead to a potential removal of 10 to 20 $\log_{10}$ reduction values (depending on the virus).[74,75] Thus, today's IVIG products are considered safe from a number of potential viral pathogens that were of concern in the early and mid-1990s. However, one potential group of pathogens that are still of potential concern are prions, which can cause transmissible spongiform encephalopathy, a fatal degenerative disease of the brain.[76] IVIG manufacturers have recognized prion-mediated disease as a potential problem and have initiated testing and IVIG purification and treatment steps (e.g., nanofiltration) to address this issue.[77]

Reactions to Subcutaneous Immunoglobulin

In general, the SCIG route has been remarkably free from severe systemic reactions.[20,21,36,78] In contrast, the majority of patients do experience local site reactions at some point during SCIG therapy, with symptoms of swelling, soreness, warmth, redness, induration, pruritus, and/or bruising. Most of these local reactions last for less than 48 hours, and the severity and frequency of local reactions decrease as the patient continues SCIG therapy.[79–81] The FDA warning of the risk of thrombosis with this class of products is also listed for SCIG products.

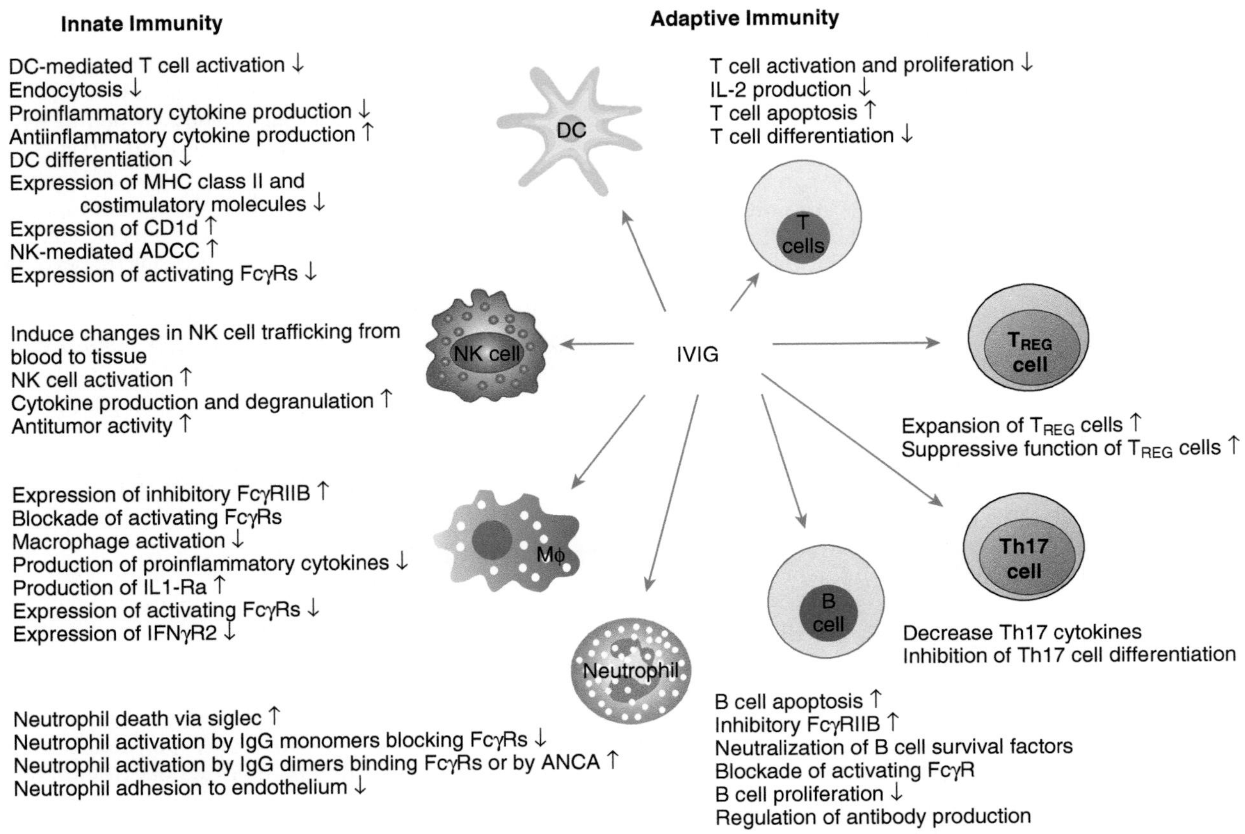

Innate Immunity

Adaptive Immunity

DC-mediated T cell activation ↓
Endocytosis ↓
Proinflammatory cytokine production ↓
Antiinflammatory cytokine production ↑
DC differentiation ↓
Expression of MHC class II and
 costimulatory molecules ↓
Expression of CD1d ↑
NK-mediated ADCC ↑
Expression of activating FcγRs ↓

T cell activation and proliferation ↓
IL-2 production ↓
T cell apoptosis ↑
T cell differentiation ↓

Induce changes in NK cell trafficking from
blood to tissue
NK cell activation ↑
Cytokine production and degranulation ↑
Antitumor activity ↑

Expansion of T$_{REG}$ cells ↑
Suppressive function of T$_{REG}$ cells ↑

Expression of inhibitory FcγRIIB ↑
Blockade of activating FcγRs
Macrophage activation ↓
Production of proinflammatory cytokines ↓
Production of IL1-Ra ↑
Expression of activating FcγRs ↓
Expression of IFNγR2 ↓

Decrease Th17 cytokines
Inhibition of Th17 cell differentiation

Neutrophil death via siglec ↑
Neutrophil activation by IgG monomers blocking FcγRs ↓
Neutrophil activation by IgG dimers binding FcγRs or by ANCA ↑
Neutrophil adhesion to endothelium ↓

B cell apoptosis ↑
Inhibitory FcγRIIB ↑
Neutralization of B cell survival factors
Blockade of activating FcγR
B cell proliferation ↓
Regulation of antibody production

• **Fig. 10.1** Mechanisms of action of intravenous immunoglobulin *(IVIG)* on the immune modulation of various components of the innate and adaptive immune systems. *DC,* Dendritic cell; *MΦ,* macrophage; *NK,* natural killer; *MHC,* major histocompatibility complex; *ADCC,* antibody-dependent cellular cytotoxicity; *ANCA,* antineutrophil cytoplasmic antibody; *siglec,* sialic acid–binding immunoglobulin-type lectin. (Modified from Tha-In T, Tha-In T, Metselaar HJ, et al. Patients treated with high-dose intravenous immunoglobulin show selective activation of regulatory T cells. Trends Immunol 2008;29(12):608–15; and Ballow M. The IgG molecule as a biological immune response modifier: mechanisms of action of intravenous immune serum globulin in autoimmune and inflammatory disorders. J Allergy Clin Immunol 2011;127(2):315–23.)

Intravenous Immunoglobulin as an Immune-Modulating Agent in Patients With Autoimmune or Inflammatory Disorders

Since the first report on the use of IVIG in childhood ITP,[82] IVIG has been used for the treatment of a variety of inflammatory and autoimmune disorders.[83] Several mechanisms have been postulated for the immunomodulatory effects of IVIG. These include the effects of immunoglobulin on Fc or Fab receptors and on the innate and adaptive arms of the immune system[84–87] (Fig. 10.1). In the past 10 years newer studies have raised more questions regarding our full understanding of the mechanism(s) of action that impart the antiinflammatory effects of IVIG, and murine models may not always be extrapolated to humans. IVIG is used clinically as an immune-modulating agent in a variety of disorders, including chronic inflammatory demyelinating polyneuropathy, multifocal motor neuropathy, ITP, dermatomyositis, toxic epithelial necrolysis, Kawasaki disease, and Guillain-Barré, among others. Different antiinflammatory mechanisms of action are postulated to provide therapeutic clinical effects in these distinct disorders. This body of work is beyond the scope of this chapter and is reviewed elsewhere.[85–126]

• **BOX 10.5** **Practical Tips for the Office Setting**

- Optimize immunoglobulin G trough levels individually for best clinical response, generally with trough levels greater than 800 mg/dL for best clinical outcomes.
- Rate-related side effects with intravenous immunoglobulin infusion can be avoided with slower infusion rates, especially in patients with risk factors, including older age, kidney disease, diabetes, sepsis, or conditions increasing the risk of thrombosis.

Conclusions

Immunoglobulin replacement is the mainstay of treatment for patients with primary humoral immunodeficiency. The goal of the treatment is to provide a broad spectrum of antibodies to prevent infections and chronic complications. The usual dose for immune replacement is 400 to 600 mg/kg/month, but this may vary individually, and higher doses may be required during active infection. A serum trough level greater than 500 mg/dL has been shown to be effective in the prevention of severe infections. However, studies have suggested that even higher doses and achieving IgG trough levels of 700 to 1000 mg/dL may be desirable.[16,17]

• BOX 10.6   Therapeutic Principles of Intravenous Immunoglobulin (IVIG) Treatment in Patients With Primary Immunodeficiency

- Initial dosage: 400 to 600 mg/kg every 4 weeks for replacement therapy.
  - Some patients may benefit from trough levels of 700 to 1000 mg/dL.
  - Adjust the dose and/or dosing interval depending on clinical response.
  - Record manufacturer, lot number, and dose with each infusion.
- Equilibration takes several months even when dosage changes made.
  - Check trough levels if patient continues to have infections or before dose change.
  - May be useful to determine adherence in patients on subcutaneous immunoglobulin.
  - Treat the patient and not the "numbers" (e.g., trough level).
- For patients with systemic adverse effects or poor venous access, the subcutaneous route may be a better option.
- Immunoglobulin replacement therapy is indicated as continuous replacement therapy for primary immunodeficiency. Treatment should not be interrupted once a definitive diagnosis has been established.
- Site of care. The decision to infuse IVIG in a hospital, hospital outpatient, community office, or home-based setting must be based on clinical characteristics of the patient.
- IVIG is not a generic drug, and IVIG products are not interchangeable. A specific IVIG product needs to be matched to patient characteristics to ensure patient safety. A change of IVIG product should occur only with the active participation of the prescribing physician.

Monitor

- Complete blood count with differential; liver and renal function tests every 6 to 12 months.
- Nucleotide testing for viral pathogens (e.g., hepatitis C) when indicated.
- Pulmonary function testing, diffusion capacity testing as indicated, chest x-ray, high-resolution chest tomography (initially if there is a history of lung disease and thereafter as indicated; may enhance patient's risk of malignancy).

Data from the Primary Immunodeficiency Committee of the American Academy of Allergy, Asthma and Immunology, <www.aaaai.org/practice-resources/practice-tools/ivig-toolkit.aspx>

SCIG has also gained acceptance as an alternative route for the administration of replacement therapy in patients with immunodeficiency. Generally, IVIG replacement therapy is considered safe in the majority of patients. Side effects are usually mild and treatable by premedication (Box 10.5). Improvements in good manufacturing practices; closer screening of plasma donors; testing of the source plasma with sensitive nucleic acid assays, such as PCR; and additional viral inactivation steps have made IVIG a better and safer plasma-derived product. The majority of the use of IVIG therapy is in patients with autoimmune disorders. The use of IVIG in these patient groups has not only led to a new treatment modality but also has enhanced our understanding of the disease pathogenesis and the mechanisms by which IVIG modulates the immune and inflammatory processes (Box 10.6).

The reference list can be found on the companion Expert Consult website at http://www.expertconsult.inkling.com.

11

Hematopoietic Stem Cell Therapies

DONALD B. KOHN

KEY POINTS

- Hematopoietic stem cell transplantation (HSCT) can correct many primary immune deficiencies (PIDs) by providing a normal source of stem cells that produce functional leukocytes to replace the defective cells, thereby restoring immunity.
- Best outcomes are obtained when using matched sibling donor bone marrow, although results using matched unrelated donors, adult or umbilical cord blood, or haploidentical (parental) donors continue to improve.
- Multiple factors affect outcomes, including the choice of pretransplant conditioning regimen used to facilitate engraftment, the source of donor hematopoietic stem cells, the general health of the recipient, including comorbidities of the specific PID being treated, and presence or absence of intercurrent infections.
- Early clinical trials of gene therapy—autologous transplantation with genetically corrected hematopoietic stem cells done in the 1990s using murine retroviral vectors—showed significant immune reconstitution. However, there was a high incidence of vector-related leukoproliferative complications in some studies.
- More recent trials using lentiviral vectors have yielded greater efficacy and safety than the prior trials, further improving outcomes for gene therapy for several PIDs.

Introduction

Many forms of primary immune deficiency (PID) result from mutations of genes involved in the production, function, or survival of leukocytes. Therefore, these PIDs can be treated by hematopoietic stem cell transplantation (HSCT) using allogeneic cells from related or unrelated donors, providing patients with a new source of genetically normal leukocytes. The first successful clinical allogeneic bone marrow transplants (BMT) were performed in 1968 for a patient with severe combined immunodeficiency (SCID), resulting in sustained reconstitution of immunity that has lasted now for several decades.[1] Since that time, allogeneic HSCT has become the standard of care for patients with SCID and is often used for patients with other severe, life-threatening forms of PID (e.g., Wiskott-Aldrich syndrome [WAS], chronic granulomatous disease [CGD], hemophagocytic lymphohistiocytosis [HLH]). Patients with less severe PIDs generally are not treated with HSCT, especially those primarily affecting production of antibodies that can be treated with immunoglobulin replacement therapy.

The major barriers to allogeneic HSCT are immunologic. In solid organ transplantation, a recipient's T cells can reject the organ donor's cells. Graft rejection is less of a problem in recipients with severe immunodeficiency, such as patients with SCID who lack functional T lymphocytes. However, in some forms of SCID that retain active function of some components of the immune system (e.g., natural killer [NK]+ SCIDS), a significant risk for graft rejection remains. In most PIDs other than SCID, transplant recipients need partial or essentially complete ablation of their endogenous immune and hematopoietic systems to achieve enduring engraftment of donor HSCs. Definition of optimal pretransplant conditioning regimens remains one of the major areas of ongoing discovery in the field.

Graft-versus-host disease (GvHD) is the flipside of graft rejection and is mostly limited to the HSCT setting and only rarely encountered in solid organ transplantation.

Alloreactive T cells from the donor that are given in relatively high numbers with the allogeneic bone marrow or mobilized peripheral blood stem cells (PBSCs) can, in effect, reject the recipient's tissues, especially the skin, gastrointestinal (GI) tract, and liver. GvHD can be severe, chronic, and even fatal; complications increase in frequency and severity with increasing degree of mismatch between the donor and the recipient. Efforts to prevent or suppress GvHD, by administration of immunosuppressive medications or by depleting the donor's mature T lymphocytes from the graft often result in prolonged immunodeficiency that poses high risks for opportunistic infections, especially beyond the infancy period, when patients may bear latent herpesviruses, BK virus, or adenovirus. Important advances are occurring in graft engineering and GvHD prophylaxis that are improving outcomes and allowing less well-matched donors to be used with greater success.

Severe Combined Immune Deficiency

SCID is the most severe of the PIDs, with inherited absence of T and B cell function (and, variably, NK activity). In the absence of medical intervention, infants with SCID have a high rate of early mortality from infections. SCID is a clinical phenotype that may result from defects in any one of more than a dozen genes (Box 11.1). The clinical research associated with the treatment of human SCID has produced many of the major advances in the field of HSCT (Box 11.2).

The goal of HSCT for SCID is to restore full immunity (T, B, and NK cell function) to provide normal resistance to infection and responses to therapeutic vaccines. Ideally, the treatment should bring minimal toxic side effects from chemotherapy or GvHD. The critical clinical issues to be determined in the treatment of patients with SCID with HSCT mainly concern determining the donor/stem cell source; deciding about the use of conditioning and, if it is used, which agent; and the timing of when to perform the HSCT.

One life-changing advance has been the advent of screening of newborns for SCID.[2] Thymic recombination excision circles (TRECs, produced during T cell receptor gene rearrangement) can be quantified by polymerase chain reaction in dried blood spots taken in the neonatal period and used to identify those with severe T lymphopenia. These patients are referred to a diagnostic center for definitive immunologic testing, allowing SCID to be recognized early in life before the acquisition of severe infections that can greatly increase risks from transplantation.

On diagnosis, the patient with SCID requires care by specialists experienced in the management of severely immunocompromised patients. It is essential to recognize the emergent nature of immediately instituting proper care for patients with SCID to allow them to come to definitive treatment with the lowest risks of acquiring infections. Treatment should include implementation of antibiotic prophylaxis for *Pneumocystis jirovecii* and yeast and other fungi and regular administration of immunoglobulin.[3] Most centers recommend cessation of breastfeeding, which may transmit cytomegalovirus (CMV), at least unless it can be determined that the mother is CMV sero-negative. Isolation from potentially infectious people is important, although it is not clear if this is best done in the hospital or at home. Decisions about the optimal place for a patient with SCID to be until transplantation require consideration of the specific family situation, such as if there are young siblings in the home attending daycare, the distance the family lives from the medical center, and the ability of the family to comply with strict isolation measures. During the pretreatment phase, live vaccines should not be administered to the patient or family members. These precautions can be alleviated as the immune system reconstitutes.[3]

Patients With Severe Combined Immunodeficiency With Matched Sibling Donors

When transplantation was first performed for patients with SCID, it was done using bone marrow collected from a matched sibling donor (MSD) that was infused intravenously without any preconditioning.[1] This approach remains the standard of care to the present time for those patients with SCID with a medically eligible MSD. Allogeneic HSCT can be curative for SCID when bone marrow from an MSD is used, with most centers reporting greater than 90% to 95% long-term survival.[4–6] Sufficient engraftment of either long-lived multipotent stem cells or at least T lymphoid precursors occurs in the absence of preconditioning to support long-term T cell immunity and in many cases B cell function for humoral immunity (Fig. 11.1). There is some concern that there is only minimal sustained stem cell engraftment without conditioning and that immunity may wane over decades, although most of these patients remain well. The use of pretransplant conditioning for patients with SCID receiving MSD transplants is sometimes discussed to produce more enduring and broad immunity, but rarely if ever used.

Patients With Severe Combined Immunodeficiency Lacking a Matched Sibling Donor

A major area of ongoing research over the past decades has been the best approaches to the majority of patients with SCID who lack an MSD. Options for these patients include haploidentical family donors, matched unrelated donors (MUD), and, as will be discussed in a subsequent section, autologous gene therapy.

Haploidentical Transplants

HSCT from human leukocyte antigen (HLA)-mismatched donors (e.g., a haploidentical/haplodisparate parent, sibling, or child) carries a significant risk of severe GvHD, because the donor's T cells contained in the graft would react against the nonshared HLA proteins (such as those inherited from the other parent). To prevent this, several methods to deplete T lymphocytes from bone marrow or PBSC to limit GvHD risks have been developed since the mid-1970s (Box 11.3). Using such approaches to deplete T

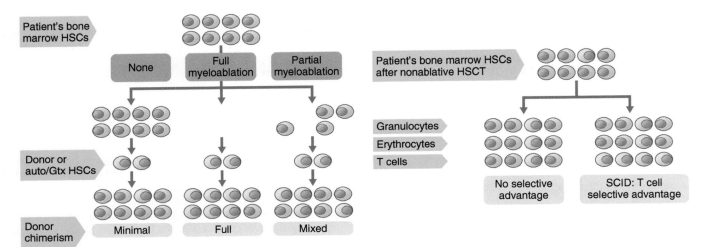

• **Fig. 11.1** Outcome after hematopoietic stem cell transplant *(HSCT)* with full, partial, or no myeloablative conditioning. If hematopoietic stem cells *(HSCs)* are transplanted from an allogeneic donor or as gene-corrected *(Gtx)* autologous cells with no pretransplant conditioning, only minimal chimerism of donor cells will occur *(lower left)*. If full myeloablation is given, essentially complete donor cell chimerism may be achieved *(lower middle)*. If partial myeloablation is administered, as has been done in some gene therapy clinical trials, mixed chimerism will be achieved with a significant fraction of donor or gene-corrected cells engrafted *(lower right)*.

• **BOX 11.3** **Methods for T Cell Depletion of Donor Bone Marrow**

- In vivo polyclonal antibodies (ALG, ATG)
- In vivo targeting of alloreactive donor T cells with posttransplant cytotoxic agents (methotrexate, cyclophosphamide)
- Soybean agglutinin/E-rosette with sheep red blood cells
- Counterflow centrifugation elutriation
- Cell fractionation by density gradients
- Monoclonal antibodies (anti-CD2, -CD3, -CD4, -CD5, -CD6, -CD7,-CD8, -CD52, -TcR$\alpha\beta$, -CD45RA)
- Stem cell enrichment (e.g., select CD34$^+$, CD34$^+$/CD38$^-$, CD34$^+$/CD90$^+$, CD34$^+$/CD133$^+$)

---

cells, marrow from parental donors has been frequently used for patients with SCID who lack an HLA-matched donor; 60% to 80% of patients with SCID have realized long-term survival.[5,6] The lower success rate with haploidentical donor transplants compared with MSD may reflect the morbidity and mortality associated with (1) the increased risks of graft rejection and/or GvHD; (2) the T cell depletion that is used to prevent GvHD, which slows immune reconstitution and prolongs the period of increased susceptibility to infections; and (3) the adverse effects secondary to the possible use of chemotherapy to make space in the marrow of engraftment and eliminate residual immunity.

Initial approaches to achieve depletion of alloreactive donor T cells used a variety of cell fractionation methods, as listed in Box 11.3. Subsequently, techniques commonly used involved direct depletion of all T cell populations (anti-CD3) or enrichment for hematopoietic stem and progenitor populations (anti-CD34) with negative selection against more mature blood cells of all lineages. The profound T cell depletion of the grafts led to reduced rates of GvHD, but often at the cost of increased risks for infections, especially from DNA viruses (CMV, Epstein-Barr virus [EBV], adenovirus, human herpesvirus-6 [HHV-6], BK, etc.). The ideal is to remove potentially alloreactive T cells but leave behind T cells reactive against viral infections, regulatory T

cells that may inhibit GvHD, and other T cell populations that may facilitate engraftment. Newer approaches currently under study include the selective depletion of specific T cell populations, often T cell receptor alpha/beta (TcR$\alpha\beta$)/CD19$^+$ cells to preserve antiviral TcR$\gamma\delta^+$ T cells in the graft and remove donor B cells that may harbor EBV or adding back specific mature cell populations, such as T regulatory cells that may mitigate GvHD, antiviral cytotoxic T lymphocytes, chimeric antigen receptor (CAR) T cells, NK populations, and so on.

One of the continuing controversies about the optimal approach to haploidentical HSCT for SCID concerns the necessity, or lack thereof, of pretransplant conditioning with chemotherapy or other immunosuppressive medications to facilitate long-term engraftment of donor HSCs. Conditioning generally involves a combination of cytoreductive agents, such as busulfan or melphalan, immunosuppressive drugs, such as the chemotherapeutic agents cyclophosphamide or fludarabine; and serotherapies, such as anti-thymocyte globulin (ATG) and Campath. Treosulfan is another cytoreductive agent that has been widely used in Europe for conditioning for PIDs with reduced hepatotoxicity in the leukemia setting; it is of limited availability in the United States but has been used successfully for a variety of PIDs.[7]

Studies from the Primary Immune Deficiency Treatment Consortium (PIDTC) found that initial survival was better in infants with SCID who were not receiving conditioning. But immunologic recovery was less robust in the unconditioned patients compared with those who received conditioning, with a significantly higher percentage of unconditioned patients not recovering full humoral immunity and thus requiring life-long immunoglobulin replacement therapy. There were also higher needs for repeat transplants or "boosts" in the unconditioned patients.[5,6] However, the acute and long-term toxicities of the chemoablative regimens may lead to increased morbidity and mortality in the initial period, especially in patients with preexisting unresolved infections, and may cause long-term growth, endocrine, and neurocognitive abnormalities.[8,9] A critical goal in the field is the development of non–chemotherapy-based conditioning methods that are effective and safe (see later).

Matched Unrelated Donor Transplants

Historically, less has been done using adult or cord blood MUD for transplantation in patients with SCID who do not have an HLA-MSD. HSCT using MUD adult bone marrow or PBSC or umbilical cord blood carries increased risks of GvHD, compared with the use of marrow from an MSD.[5] The frequency of severe GvHD in MUD marrow, PBSC, and cord blood HSCT is in the range of 20% to 40%. In addition, HSCT with cord blood has a risk of engraftment failure between 10% and 20%. These increased complications are likely to be due to more mismatches for non-HLA (minor) antigens.

Generally, full cytoablation and GvHD prophylaxis (i.e., post-transplant immune suppression) are used to prevent graft rejection or GvHD with MUD donors. MUD transplants performed without conditioning may restore T cell immunity but generally do not result in significant long-term donor stem cell engraftment; thus, long-term B cell and NK function is often poor.[10]

Approach to Infants With Severe Combined Immunodeficiency Diagnosed by Newborn Screening

Newborn screening for SCID has radically changed the presentation of these patients who now are routinely identified in the first week or two of life, while still asymptomatic. The approach to transplantation in these infants with SCID diagnosed early is the subject of a prospectively designed clinical trial comparing pretransplant conditioning regimens of differing intensities to define the minimal amounts of chemotherapy needed to ensure engraftment and full immune reconstitution ("C-SIDE"–NCT03619551). As the first prospective clinical trial designed to compare different transplant approaches for SCID, the results may inform the approach to these patients and demonstrate the potential for future rationally designed studies to define optimal treatments for PIDs.

Timing of Hematopoietic Stem Cell Transplant Performance

Several studies have found that for patients with SCID treated early in life (e.g., younger than 3.5 months of age), outcomes are good with any of these donor hematopoietic stem cell (HSC) source options. In general, patients with SCID should be transplanted as soon as is clinically possible once a suitable donor/stem cell source is identified, before infections may be acquired or progress. One reason to delay HSCT is to wait for patients diagnosed by newborn screening to be out of infancy to potentially decrease risks from the conditioning. There is a general concern about administering even reduced-intensity conditioning in the neonatal period, primarily because of concerns for neurotoxicity to the developing brain.

It is preferable to perform transplantation in patients with SCID who have acquired a severe infection after that infection is eradicated. However, it may be difficult to eliminate infections such as CMV or adenovirus in the absence of restored immunity. Recently introduced antiviral drugs against DNA viruses may lead to better efficacy before transplant. Antiviral cytotoxic T cells grown from partially matched donors that are then banked are becoming increasingly more available from research and commercial sources and can eliminate or control some viral infections before immune reconstitution from the HSCT.[11,12] Early

indicators of poor immune reconstitution, such as low CD4 count at 6 months, may lead to consideration of a boost, that is, administration of additional donor stem cells without conditioning or even a second transplant with some type of conditioning preparative regimen.[13]

Specific Severe Combined Immunodeficiency Genotypic Forms

Because SCID is rare and may be caused by various genetic defects, few studies have analyzed the outcome of HSCT in specific genotype forms of SCID.[14] The specific gene defect causing SCID may lead to different outcomes in terms of survival and immune reconstitution and may require genotype-specific approaches to conditioning.[13,15] Patients with defects of V(D)J recombination resulting from the *RAG1* and *RAG2* genes, *DCLRE1C* (Artemis), DNA PKcs *(PRKDC)*, *NHEJ1* (Cernunnos), and other DNA repair proteins and gene mutations have the lymphocyte phenotype of T– B– NK+ SCID. In the absence of effective nonhomologous end-joining DNA repair, which uses the products of these genes, T and B cells cannot rearrange their respective T and B cell receptor genes and T and B cells are not produced, whereas NK cell production and function is normal.

In addition, SCID secondary to defects in these DNA repair genes is associated with increased cellular sensitivity to radiation and chemotherapy, which may lead to additional toxicity when conditioning regimens are used for HSCT. Schuetz and colleagues[16] compared the outcomes of HSCT for patients with Artemis mutations (radiation sensitive) versus patients with *RAG1* and *RAG2* mutations (normal radiation sensitivity). Survival after MSD HSCT was comparable in the two groups. However, patients with Artemis deficiency had an increased rate of late complications, including poor growth and requirement for nutritional support, autoimmune manifestations, growth hormone deficiency, hypothyroidism, and dental anomalies, emphasizing the increased susceptibility to toxicity for patients with SCID with DNA repair gene defects.

All patients born with SCID who undergo HSCT do remain at risk for complications of the organ toxicities that may occur before treatment (e.g., infections) and from the treatment, probably throughout their lives. A 2017 publication provides guidelines for screening and management of late effect in patients with SCID patients.[17]

Transplantation for Other Severe Primary Immune Deficiencies

A large number of other PIDs have been successfully treated with HSCT (Box 11.4). For several decades now, allogeneic HSCT has been considered first- or second-line therapy for such well-known disorders as CGD, WAS, and HLH and is often used for other severe immunodeficiencies, such as leukocyte adhesion deficiency (LAD), X-lymphoproliferative disorder, hyper-IgM syndrome, and others. Transplantation for PIDs other than SCID are almost always performed after conditioning, either fully myeloablative or of reduced intensity.

Transplantation for PIDs requires defining the optimal time and disease status to perform the HSCT. Results vary, in terms of overall survival and disease-free survival, based on the specific disorders, the type of donor and conditioning used, the disease status at transplant, and preexisting comorbidities, among other factors.

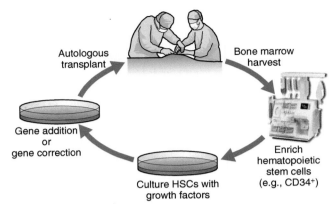

• **Fig. 11.2** Gene therapy using autologous hematopoietic stem cells *(HSCs)*. Bone marrow is harvested from the patient with primary immunodeficiency. In the laboratory, the HSCs are enriched by immune affinity with a monoclonal antibody to the CD34 antigen. The CD34-enriched cells are cultured with hematopoietic growth factors to activate the cells, and then gene addition or gene editing is performed. The HSCs are then transplanted by intravenous infusion back into the patient.

Transplantations for PIDs have improved to the present time, with many factors contributing, including higher stringency of HLA cross-matching, improved conditioning regimens tailored for each specific disorder that support engraftment with reduced toxicity, and better supportive care for infectious complications and organ toxicities from conditioning, and for some autoinflammatory disorders. Generally it is better to perform a transplantation in a patient with PID when the patient is in a good relative state of health and without active infections or inflammatory complications. Disease-specific steps to optimize the patient's medical condition at the time of transplantation have been important for reducing transplant-related morbidities. One such important measure is the use of immunosuppressive medications to "calm down" inflammatory complications before HSCT, such as sirolimus for X-linked immunodeficiency with polyendocrinopathy and enteropathy (IPEX), Campath for HLH, steroids for CGD, or JAK inhibitors for some autoinflammatory conditions (e.g., signal transducer and activator of transcription 3 *[STAT3]* gain of function).

More recently, HSCT is being applied to a variety of disorders characterized by immune dysregulation with complications being primarily inflammatory rather than infectious, recently termed *primary immune regulatory disorders* (PIRDs) (see Box 11.4). The PIRDs include disorders such as immune dysregulation, polyendocrinopathy, enteropathy, X-linked (IPEX) syndrome, *STAT1* gain of function, *STAT3* gain of function, interleukin-10R (IL-10R) deficiency, lipopolysaccharide-responsive and beige-like anchor protein (LRBA) deficiency, CTLA4 haploinsufficiency, DOCK8 deficiency, and so on.[18]

For each PIRD there may be specific levels of donor stem cell chimerism needed for disease response. In some, a relatively low level of donor stem cell chimerism (e.g., 5%–20%) can ameliorate the disease, such as in HLH and IPEX, in which a missing cell population is needed (cytotoxic T lymphocytes for HLH and regulatory T cells for IPEX). In other PIRDs, essentially 100%

donor chimerism, achieved using full-dose cytoablative conditioning, may be needed for disease remediation, such as *STAT1* and *STAT3* gain of function disorders, in which the constitutively active STAT-mediated signaling leads to overactive cell populations that can cause problems even at low frequencies. Treating these disorders is an emerging area of clinical research, and it is likely that indications and outcomes will continue to increase.

The posttransplant care of patients with PID after transplant entails continued protective isolation and antibiotic, antifungal, and antiviral prophylaxis, with immunoglobulin replacement therapy used when hypogammaglobulinemia or specific antibody deficiencies are present. These measures may be reduced and eliminated as immune recovery occurs.

The rare nature of the PIDs, the severe immunologic defects and abnormalities they entail, and the need to continually improve therapies mean there are usually some unknowns for each treatment. Transplantations still may be considered experimental in these cases and are best done in organized clinical trials, when available, or using standardized guidelines (e.g., from the European Society for Immunodeficiencies).

Gene Therapy

Gene Addition

Gene therapy is a means to use autologous HSCT to treat genetic blood cell diseases, such as the PIDs, by correcting the genetic defect in the patient's HSCs, which should allow each patient to be his or her own perfectly matched donor and avoid the risks of GvHD and the need for pretransplant and posttransplant immunosuppression (Fig. 11.2). The defective gene responsible for the cellular or humoral defect may be either augmented by adding a normal copy of the gene to replace its function or, in the near future, directly corrected by gene editing. The technical capacities to genetically correct primary HSC and re-engraft them in the patient have developed over the past three decades, borne out of the development of molecular biology techniques that allowed cloning of normal genes and construction of recombinant viral genomes that could serve as vectors to carry the human genes into patient cells with high efficiency.[19,20] Gene therapy took several decades to advance, from an early era (circa 1990–1999) when there was no significant clinical benefit conferred in initial trials (i.e., adenosine deaminase [ADA] deficiency, SCID, CGD, and LAD), which were all done without use of pretransplantation cytoreductive conditioning, through a middle period (circa 2000–2009) in which clear-cut immune reconstitution was achieved for multiple PIDs (i.e., X-linked SCID [XSCID], ADA SCID, CGD, and WAS), but the gamma-retroviral vectors used led to high frequencies of leukemic complications in a fraction of the patients, to the current time (2009–present) when lentiviral vectors are routinely conferring sustained restoration of immunity without vector-related complications.

Lentiviral vectors were primarily developed at the Salk Institute in the laboratories of Inder Verma, Didier Trono, led by then postdoctoral fellow Luigi Naldini.[21] They are derived from the human immunodeficiency virus-1 (HIV-1) because of the high efficiency with which this virus can transport its genetic information into the chromosomal DNA of target cells. All of the viral genes have been removed from the vectors, which carry only the human gene(s) of interest. The HIV proteins needed to produce a one-way delivery vector virus particle are provided *in trans* during packaging, but the gene encoding the HIV proteins are not transferred to the patient's cells, and, thus, no new virus can be made in transduced cells. There have been no instances of "live" virus somehow being created, spreading, and causing problems in now more than several hundred treated patients. The lentiviral vectors also have been engineered to remove the strong enhancer elements that were present in the earlier murine retroviral vectors and that were the cause of the leukemias seen as a result of *trans*-activation of cellular oncogenes when the retroviral vectors happened to insert near them during the stem cell modification process. Significant preclinical studies in murine and nonhuman primate gene therapy HSCT models indicated that the lentiviral vectors had undetectable risks for causing cellular transformation,[22] and this safety profile has been held up in the clinical trials performed to date.

For gene therapy, autologous HSCs are collected from the PID patient, either by bone marrow harvest or by mobilization into peripheral blood (e.g., with granulocyte colony-stimulating factor [G-CSF]) and leukapheresis. HSCs are partially enriched by immunoselection for the CD34 glycoprotein that is present on the surfaces of human hematopoietic stem and progenitor cells. These CD34-enriched cells are then cultured in an appropriate medium containing a mixture of recombinant hematopoietic growth factors (e.g., ckit ligand, flt-3 ligand, thrombopoietin) to activate the cells, followed by addition of the vector to the cells in culture. This process may take 1 to 3 days, after which the cells may be either prepared and administered to the patient directly or cryopreserved for later use. Use of cryopreserved cells allows complete characterization of the cell product before administration, to measure the percentage of cells that acquired the gene, the colony-forming activity of the modified stem cells, the functional activity of the new gene, and sterility and other purity properties. Additionally, frozen products allow the pretransplantation conditioning to be given over multiple days, with measurement of drug clearance and dose adjustment to achieve specific drug exposure targets, which generally was not possible within the shorter period between stem cell harvest and reinfusion, when producing and using cells freshly from culture.

Successful clinical trials have been reported using gene therapy with lentiviral vectors to treat WAS, ADA SCID, XSCID, and X-linked CGD (XCGD).[21,23] All have used partial or complete cytoreductive conditioning with busulfan, with trials for WAS also incorporating fludarabine (and rituximab in some trials) to ablate potentially autoreactive lymphocytes. Patients have appreciated protective immune recovery in a high percentage of the treatments, although platelet counts have been improved only moderately in many of the patients with WAS. There have been no vector-related complications, and these transplants are generally clinically mild, without GvHD complicating the posttreatment course. New clinical trials are in progress or under development for Artemis SCID, LAD, autosomal recessive forms of CGD, the perforin defect of HLH, and others.

One of the limitations of gene therapy is that each genotype (e.g., ADA SCID, XSCID, Artemis SCID, etc.) requires a gene-specific vector and package of preclinical studies and clinical trials, in contrast to allogeneic transplant that is more "one size fits all" diseases. Because of the high success rates with gene therapy, they are advancing to become licensed treatments. Currently, only ADA SCID has an approved gene therapy. Strimvelis was developed by the San Raffaele Telethon Institute For Gene Therapy (TIGET) in Milan, licensed to GSK, who achieved marketing approval in the European Union from the European Medicines Agency, and is now provided by Orchard Therapeutics. During the transition phase from academic investigations to regulatory approval, these proven beneficial therapies may become unavailable, which creates a dilemma for patients/parents and providers about waiting for an undetermined time for their approval or proceeding to allogeneic HSCT. Nonetheless, this progression from initial academic-based studies to commercialization of gene therapy is a sign of success for gene therapy after more than three decades of research.

Gene Editing

The new technology of in situ gene editing, augmented by site-specific endonucleases, such as zinc finger nucleases or the more recently identified CRISPR/Cas9 system, is an emerging approach to treating genetic diseases by directly correcting the defective gene in the patient's HSCs (Fig. 11.3). Gene editing would have advantages over vector-mediated gene addition in that the corrective gene would be in its normal chromosomal location, which may be essential for genes that need precise expression regulation (e.g., *BTK* for X-agammaglobulinemia) and would avoid the risks of random transgene insertion by vectors that imposes risks of leukemic transformation. The efficiency of gene editing in HSC is improving and soon may be able to produce sufficient frequencies of gene-corrected stem cells to treat the most favorable diseases with low thresholds of gene correction frequency for expected clinical benefit, such as genetic forms of SCID.

New Directions

As described here, there is exciting progress for both allogeneic and autologous/gene therapy transplants for PIDs and PIRDs. These advances are providing better outcomes in terms of survival and immune reconstitution, with reduced complications from conditioning and adverse immune responses, such as GvHD. An important goal is to develop methods to condition patients to accept transplants that do not use chemotherapy. Several monoclonal antibodies targeting stem cells are being assessed for use in conditioning, starting with applications to transplants for SCID.[24–26] Antibodies to ckit, a tyrosine kinase surface cytokine receptor on stem cells are being assessed in a clinical trial, with initial reports indicating some activity to facilitate engraftment. Other antibodies (e.g., anti-CD45, anti–IL-3 receptor alpha) are in development, either as unconjugated antibodies or as conjugates to toxins

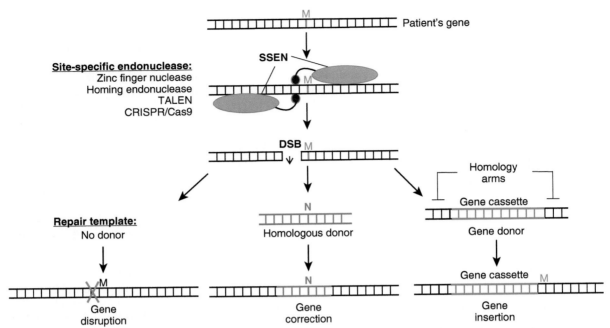

• **Fig. 11.3** Gene editing using site-specific endonucleases. For correcting a genetic mutation *(red M)*, site-specific endonucleases can be used to facilitate the repair process by producing a double-strand break (DSB) in the DNA near the mutation. The DSB may be resolved in several ways. If no donor is provided *(left)*, nonhomologous end joining may relink the cut ends of the DNA, but often creates base-pair insertions or deletions (indels), leading to gene disruption. If a homologous donor is introduced that contains the normal sequence *(green N; center)*, homology-driven repair may use the donor as a template to repair the DSB, copying the normal sequence into the genome for gene correction. If a donor is provided that contains the relevant complementary DNA (cDNA) with a polyadenylation signal flanked by homology arms to the sequence at the DSB *(right)*, the cDNA-polyA signal may be copied into the DSB, leading to gene insertion.

to increase target cell clearance. Effective condition methods that avoid the use of chemotherapy may greatly decrease the morbidity and mortality of transplantation.

In gene therapy, the design of lentiviral vectors is growing in sophistication, with lineage-specific expression being used to limit expression of the transgene to specific blood cell types produced from transduced HSC, such as a vector expressing *FOXP3* to treat IPEX using the endogenous expression regulatory elements of the *FOXP3* gene to restrict expression to regulatory T cells.[27] Gene editing methods continue to expand, as more CRISPR/Cas9-like proteins are studied that have broadened target specificities and with the production of fusions between the Cas9 protein and other enzymes to activate or repress expression of specific genes, edit specific bases in genes, and make other targeted gene modifications. Finally, gene therapy is advancing from an exploratory research basis to commercialization and licensure of gene therapy products. In the near future, it may be possible to obtain somatic cells from a patient (e.g., by skin biopsy), perform ex vivo gene addition or gene correction, dedifferentiate the cells to induced pluripotent stem cells (iPS), convert the iPS to transplantable HSCs, and perform an autologous transplant (Fig. 11.4). It is the goal of all of these activities to provide safer and more effective treatments for patients with severe PIDs.

The reference list can be found on the companion Expert Consult website at http://www.expertconsult.inkling.com.

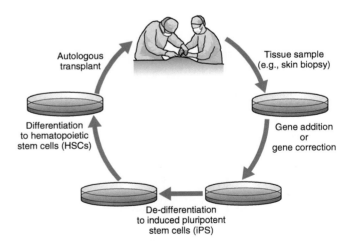

• **Fig. 11.4** Gene therapy using autologous hematopoietic stem cells *(HSCs)* made from induced pluripotent stem cells *(iPS)*. Somatic cells from a patient with primary immunodeficiency (PID), such as skin fibroblasts or keratinocytes, can be obtained from a skin biopsy. These cells can be cultured and genetically corrected by gene addition or gene correction methods. The cells can then be de-differentiated to produce iPS. The iPS can then be directed to differentiate to HSCs that can be used for transplantation. The gene correction of the cultured somatic cells can be analyzed and selected for clones with complete appropriate gene correction and safe gene integration sites for use in the production of HSCs.

12

Diagnosis of Human Allergic Disease

ROBERT G. HAMILTON

KEY POINTS

- Allergen-specific immunoglobulin E (IgE) antibody is a marker of allergic sensitization and a risk factor for allergic disease; however, alone it does not make the definitive diagnosis of allergic disease. Confirmation of allergic sensitization with a positive IgE antiallergen analysis increases the likelihood that the patient's symptoms may be a result of an immediate-type hypersensitivity response.
- Quantitative IgE antibody levels to selected foods (e.g., milk, egg, fish, and peanut), if above a predefined IgE antibody threshold, may eliminate the need for tedious and expensive double blinded placebo controlled food challenges (DBPCFC). However, caution needs to be exercised in consideration of the predictive threshold levels that vary across clinical studies

- because of the differences in study populations, protocols, and statistical analyses employed.
- Food antigen–specific IgG and IgG4 antibody levels are not diagnostically useful because they do not correlate with the results of oral food challenges.
- Clinically successful aeroallergen immunotherapy is almost always accompanied by high (microgram per milliliter) levels of allergen-specific IgG antibody in serum.
- Mast cell tryptase is a serine esterase used as a marker of mast cell activation during anaphylaxis. Immunoreactive tryptase levels in serum of healthy adults are typically less than 5 µg/L. Elevated mature tryptase levels (>10 µg/L) are detectable 1 to 4 hours after the onset of systemic anaphylaxis with hypotension.

Introduction

The diagnosis of human allergic disease begins and ends with the patient's clinical history and physical examination.[1] When the clinical history identifies allergic symptoms that are in temporal relationship to a definable and relevant allergen exposure, immunoglobulin E (IgE) antibody sensitization is then confirmed with in vivo skin tests (puncture/intradermal) or in vitro blood tests (allergen-specific IgE antibody serologic assays). If there is a mismatch between the patient's clinical history and the results of these primary diagnostic tests for sensitization, a secondary provocation test (open or placebo-controlled food challenge, nasal challenge, bronchial challenge) may adjudicate the veracity of the history-driven diagnosis.[2] This chapter discusses the contribution that in vivo and in vitro sensitization tests provide to the diagnostic algorithm and analytes that serve as diagnostic confirmatory tests when there is high suspicion of allergic disease based on a clinical history.

Immediate (Type 1) Hypersensitivity Response

Prausnitz and Kustner[3] first described the immediate-type hypersensitivity allergic reaction using an in vivo test in which serum

from Kustner, who was allergic to fish, was injected into the skin of Prausnitz. An immediate wheal and flare reaction in the skin was then induced when extracted fish antigen was subsequently injected into the same skin site. A serum factor or atopic reagin was later shown to be a novel IgE.[4,5]

Box 12.1 summarizes the immune system components that are involved in the induction of IgE antibody and elicitation of the effector mechanisms of type 1 hypersensitivity. Inhalation, skin, or parenteral exposure to allergens is the initiating event, during which these foreign molecules are presented to antigen-presenting cells on mucosal surfaces. Antigen-presenting cells process antigenic epitopes to T helper cells that secrete cytokines (interleukin-4 [IL-4], IL-10, IL-13), which induce B cell lymphocyte proliferation. As allergen-specific IgE antibody is produced, it circulates and binds onto FcεR1 receptors on mast cells and basophils. On re-exposure, allergen cross-links receptor-bound IgE, causing an influx in calcium, which triggers preformed mediator release (histamine, proteases) and newly synthesized mediators (leukotrienes, prostaglandins). The pharmacologic effects of these mediators on blood vessels and airways produce a spectrum of clinical symptoms, including hay fever, asthma, eczema, and anaphylaxis. Released cytokines (IL-4, IL-5, IL-6) from degranulating mast cells serve to enhance the inflammatory response and IgE production.

An investigation that employed engineered antibodies and allergens showed that four parameters of the immune response (concentration, specific activity [ratio of specific IgE to total IgE], affinity [tightness of binding], and clonality [epitope specificity] of the IgE antibody response) independently have an impact on effector cell activation.[6] The study concluded that higher levels of basophil activation occur with higher total serum IgE antibody concentrations, higher ratios of allergen-specific IgE to total IgE, broader clonality, and higher IgE antibody affinities. Future serologic assays for IgE antibody need to monitor more effectively these four important humoral immune response parameters.[7]

Allergens

Allergens are substances, usually glycoproteins, released from weeds, grasses, trees, animal danders, molds, house dust mites, parasites, insect venoms, occupational substances such as natural rubber latex, drugs, and foods. They are capable of inducing IgE antibody (sensitization) in atopic or genetically predisposed individuals. Each of these source materials may be extracted with a physiologic buffer to produce a final product (extract) that contains a complex mixture of allergenic and nonallergenic material. With the advent of molecular cloning techniques in the late 20th century, many clinically important allergenic components have been identified and purified out of these complex allergen extracts. A systematic allergen nomenclature for allergenic extracts and components has been adopted that involves the first three letters of the genus, the first letter of the species, and, for the allergen

component, a number. This scheme was established to identify each unique allergen extract and component specificity. For instance, Ara h 1 signifies the group 1 allergen in peanut *(Arachis hypogaea),* which is a carbohydrate-bearing 7S vicilin-like globulin.

Allergenic components are adopted into the World Health Organization/International Union of Immunological Societies (WHO/IUIS) Nomenclature Committee database once they have an established purity to homogeneity, physical-chemical characterization by molecular weight, isoelectric point and glycosylation pattern, nucleotide and/or amino acid sequence, and immunoreactivity to IgE antibody.[8] Allergenic molecules are further classified into protein families according to their structure and function. Different allergenic molecules often share common epitopes, which can result in immunologic cross-reactivity. Other allergenic molecules can serve as unique markers for a particular allergen specificity. Examination of the combined protein family (PFAM) database and structural database of allergenic proteins (SDAP) identified approximately 12,000 protein families, of which only approximately 2%, or 236 PFAMs, are known to contain allergenic proteins. Of these families, 31 protein families contain multiple allergenic proteins (homologs, orthologs). Thus, allergens account for a small fraction of the total number of protein families and they possess particular biologic structures and functions. They tend to be pervasive or abundant in nature and stable to processing (e.g., heat and digestion) as a result of multiple cysteine linkages. They tend to form aggregates or polymers, and many tend to be related to plant defense or involved in lipid transport. Importantly, not every member of a protein family is allergenic or cross-reactive. Box 12.2 lists the nine principal allergen families that manifest cross-reactivity because of structural similarity. In addition, it presents their principal biologic function in nature and illustrative members of these allergen families.

Since 1968, complex physiologic extracts of allergenic materials have been used as reagents in serologic assays for IgE antibody quantification in serum as they in theory contain all the principal allergenic components for that specificity. There has been increasing interest in the use of native and recombinant component allergens as serologic reagents because component-resolved diagnosis may better identify genuine sensitization from cross-reactivity in polysensitized patients. In food allergy, components have become particularly useful for certain foods, such as peanut and hazelnut, because they can facilitate the assessment of risk for a severe versus more mild allergic reaction and thus reduce the need for an oral food challenge. By identifying the specific components to which an individual is sensitized, more targeted immunotherapy also may be conducted. Thus, instead of measuring IgE antibody to crude cat dander extract, clinically used singleplex and multiplex microarray assays can measure IgE antibody specific to component allergens produced by cats, namely Fel d 1 (uteroglobin), Fel d 2 (cat albumin), Fel d 3 (cystatin), Fel d 4 (lipocalin), Fel d 5 (cat IgA), Fel d 6 (cat IgM), and Fel d 7 (cat IgG). Use of component allergens allows more effective dissection of the IgE antibody response into allergen families that share structural homologies and thus cross-react with each other.

Possibly the most well-studied family of cross-reactive allergens is the pathogenesis-related proteins (PR10 family), which are present in pollens, pomaceous and stone fruits, vegetables, and nuts. These 17-kd proteins function as ribonucleases and carriers of steroids. Most PR10 proteins are sensitive to heat and digestion. The group 1 allergen from birch tree pollen, Bet v1, has a number of homologs. These include allergenic proteins from alder tree pollen (Aln g 1), hazelnut pollen (Cor a 1), apple (Mal d 1), peach (Pru p 1),

• BOX 12.2 Principal Cross-Reactive Food-Aeroallergen Families

Profilin: An actin-binding protein in tree/grass/weed pollen and foods of plant origin that is involved in the dynamic turnover and restructuring of the actin cytoskeleton (12–15 kd); sensitive to heat and digestion

Birch *(Betula verrucosa)*	Bet v 2
Natural rubber latex *(Hevea brasiliensis)*	Hev b 8
Mercury *(Mercurialis annua)*	Mer a 1
Timothy grass *(Phleum pratense)*	Phl p 12

Serum albumin: Protein in milk, blood, and epithelia of animals that functions to transport hemin and fatty acids to muscle tissue and maintains oncotic pressure; sensitive to heat and digestion

Cow *(Bos domesticus)*	Bos d 6
Dog *(Canis familiaris)*	Can f 3
Horse *(Equus caballus)*	Equ c 3
Cat *(Felis domesticus)*	Fel d 2
Chicken *(Gallus domesticus)*	Gal d 5

Pathogenesis related proteins: PR10 family (Bet v 1 homologs)—present in pollens, pomaceous and stone fruits, vegetables, and nuts; function as ribonucleases and carriers of steroids (17 kd); most PR10 proteins are sensitive to heat and digestion

Birch *(Betula verrucosa)*	Bet v 1–
Hazel pollen *(Corylus avellana)*	Cor a 1.010–
Hazelnut *(Corylus avellana)*	Cor a 1.040
Apple *(Malus domesticus)*	Mal d 1
Peach *(Prunus persica)*	Pru p 1
Soybean *(Glycine max)*	Gly m 4
Peanut *(Arachis hypogaea)*	Ara h 8
Kiwi *(Actinidia deliciosa)*	Act d 8
Celery *(Apium graveolens)*	Api g 1

Procalcin: Present in weed/grass/tree pollens but not foods that function to bind calcium and regulate calcium levels; moderately stable

Birch *(Betula verrucosa)*	Bet v 4–
Timothy grass *(Phleum pratense)*	Phl p 7

Nonspecific lipid transfer proteins: Present in fruits, vegetables, nuts, and pollen; functions to shuttle phospholipids and other fatty acids between cell membranes; stable to heat and digestion (7–9 kd)

Peanut *(Arachis hypogaea)*	Ara h 9
Hazelnut *(Corylus avellana)*	Cor a 8
Walnut *(Juglans* spp.*)*	Jug r 3
Peach *(Prunus persica)*	Pru p 3
Mugwort *(Artemisia vulgaris)*	Art v 3
Olive pollen *(Olea europaea)*	Ole e 7
Plane tree *(Platanus acerifolia)*	Pla a 3

Lipocalin: Present in furry animals; functions to transport small hydrophobic molecules such as steroids, bilins, retinoids, and lipids; stable protein

Cat *(Felis domesticus)*	Fel d 4, 7
Dog *(Canis familiaris)*	Can f 1, 2, 4, 6

Parvalbumin: Present in fish and amphibians; binds calcium and is involved in calcium signaling in fast-contracting muscles; stable to heat and digestion

Cod fish *(Gadus morhua)*	Gad c 1
Shrimp *(Crangon crangon)*	Cra c 4, 6

Tropomyosin: Present in crustaceans, mites, cockroaches, and nematodes; functions as an actin-binding muscle protein that regulates actin mechanics in muscle contraction; stable to heat and digestion

Anisakis—herring worm *(Anisakis simplex)*	Ani s 3
German cockroach *(Blattella germanica)*	Bla g 7
Dust mite *(Dermatophagoides pteronyssinus)*	Der p 10
Shrimp *(Penaeus monodon)*	Pen m 1

Storage proteins: Present in seeds and nuts; function as nutrient storage (e.g., 2 S albumin) and are stable to heat and digestion

Peanut *(Arachis hypogaea)*	Ara h 1, 2, 3, 6
Hazelnut *(Corylus avellana)*	Cor a 9
Walnut *(Juglans* spp.*)*	Jug r 1, 2
Soybean *(Glycine max)*	Gly m 5, 6

soybean (Gly m 4), peanut (Ara h 8), celery (Apr g 1), carrot (Dau c 1), and kiwi (Act d 8). A primary sensitivity to Bet v 1 may result in oral allergy symptoms after exposure to any of these structurally similar allergenic molecules. The chip-based microarray system discussed later is a comprehensive research tool that uses allergen molecules for identifying IgE antibodies in a given patient's serum that cross-react with components from seemingly disparate allergen sources.

Diagnosis of Type 1 Hypersensitivity

The diagnostic algorithm for human allergic disease begins with a thorough clinical history and physical examination. A suggestive history is followed by in vivo skin testing, in vitro serologic assays, and, in select cases (e.g., food allergy), provocation challenge tests as confirmatory measures for detection of IgE antibodies (Box 12.3).

The interrelationship between each of these components of the diagnostic plan is illustrated in this chapter using natural rubber latex as a model allergen system.

Clinical History

Latex allergy diagnosis begins with a comprehensive clinical history.[9] A child may present with complaints of hives, rhinoconjunctivitis, asthma, or anaphylaxis that are temporally associated with exposure to a product that contains natural rubber. The allergist probes the child's general atopic and specific latex allergy history using questions designed to identify predisposing risk factors, such as an atopic state (seasonal rhinitis, early-onset asthma, eczema, food allergy); the frequency, consistency, and magnitude of latex exposure (e.g., multiple surgeries); the presence of concomitant food allergy; and hand dermatitis.[10,11] Exposure to

- Allergen-specific IgE antibody is a marker of allergic sensitization and a risk factor for allergic disease, but, alone, it does not make the diagnosis of allergic disease. It is performed as a confirmatory test in support of a clinical history that strongly suggests an allergic disorder.
- Allergen-specific IgE antibody is measured by nonisotopic autoanalyzers that employ a two-stage noncompetitive immunoassay format. In the assay, allergen-specific antibodies are bound to a solid phase allergosorbent and bound IgE antibodies are detected with labeled antihuman IgE. A heterologous total serum IgE calibration curve is used to interpolate response levels into quantitative estimates of allergen-specific IgE.
- Quantitative IgE antibody results are reported in kU_A/L, traceable to the World Health Organization IgE Reference Preparation (1 U = 2.4 nanograms of IgE).
- The multiallergen screen is a qualitative assay that measures allergen-specific IgE antibody to multiple aeroallergens and/or food allergens in a single test. The multiallergen screening assay produces qualitative (positive or negative) results that lead to subsequent investigation of the patient's serum or skin for IgE antibodies specific for individual clinically defined allergen specificities.
- A competitive inhibition format of IgE antibody assays is used to define the relative potency of allergen extracts used in skin testing to identify the extent of cross-reactivity of human IgE antibody for structurally similar allergens (e.g., vespid versus *Polistes* wasp venom allergens) and in *Hymenoptera* venom allergy to select appropriate venoms for immunotherapy.
- Quantitative IgE antibody levels to selected foods (milk, egg, fish, and peanut) if above a predefined IgE antibody threshold may eliminate the need for tedious and expensive double blinded placebo controlled food challenges (DBPCFC). Caution, however, needs to be exercised because the predictive threshold levels vary across clinical studies, because of differences in study populations, protocols, and statistical analyses employed.
- Allergenic components for peanut (Ara h 1, Ara h 2, Ara h 3, Ara h 8, and Ara h 8) and hazelnut (Cor a 1, Cor a 8, Cor a 9, and Cor a 14) provide clarity to the clinical diagnosis of peanut- and hazelnut-associated food allergy, and they have thus become routine tests in diagnostic allergy laboratories.
- Food antigen–specific IgG and IgG4 antibody levels are not diagnostically useful because they do not correlate with the results of oral food challenges.

rubber-containing products provides clues that strengthen the clinical suspicion of latex allergy. The rapid onset of allergic symptoms around toy balloons, dental dams, or other dipped rubber products (latex gloves, rubber toys) that contain high levels of allergen is supportive.[12] In contrast, respiratory or upper airway symptoms around latex paint that does not contain natural rubber diminish the likelihood of latex allergy. The type of exposure, time of onset, and duration and severity of the symptoms can help differentiate between an immediate type 1 (protein-allergen induced) and delayed type 4 (rubber-chemical induced) hypersensitivity. Finally, a genetic predisposition for atopic disease or parental history of allergy, chronic infectious or acute viral illness, relative contribution of Th1/Th2 cells to the immune response, and the nutritional status of the individual are other potential risk factors.

In Vivo Diagnostic Provocation Methods

As early as the 1900s, skin provocation testing has been used to detect atopic sensitization.[3] Nasal and bronchial provocation are rarely performed clinically, and in the case of food allergy in children, open and masked oral food challenges are performed in

select cases (see Chapter 41). Routine diagnostic skin tests are performed by prick/puncture and intradermal injection methods.[13] Skin prick testing allows the use of allergen extracts up to 1000-fold more concentrated than used for intradermal testing. The physiologic extract of a biologic material is applied on the skin, and a puncture introduces it into the dermis or it is injected intradermally. Positive (histamine) and negative (saline) controls are performed in parallel with the allergen to rule out dermagraphism or false positive irritant responses. Within 15 to 20 minutes, a measurement is performed on any visual wheal or erythema. A 3-mm wheal is generally considered a threshold for a positive puncture reaction. Wheal sizes up to 15 mm can be seen for highly sensitized individuals. The wheal diameter provides a relative indication of the degree of sensitization. For intradermal applications, a 5- to 10-mm wheal (+1 reaction) is usually considered evidence of sensitization to the allergen. More quantitative measures of sensitization can be obtained using an end-point titration method[14] in which serial 10-fold dilutions of allergen extract are applied. The end-point titer is defined as the greatest dilution producing a +1 intradermal reaction.

Diagnostic Laboratory Methods

Analytes that are measured in the clinical immunology laboratory to support the diagnosis and management of patients suspected of having allergic disease are summarized in Box 12.4. Historically, total serum IgE was used as a diagnostic marker for allergic disease.[15] However, the wide overlap in the total serum IgE levels between atopic and nonatopic populations[16] caused it to be superseded by allergen-specific IgE as the single most important laboratory analyte in the diagnostic workup for human allergic disease. Since 2003, one continuing application of total serum IgE involves anti-IgE therapy (omalizumab) in which the patient must first have a total IgE between 30 and 700 kilo–international units [kIU]/L of IgE, which is equivalent to approximately 2.4 nanograms of IgE) to be a candidate for treatment. The clinician uses the total serum IgE level to compute the starting omalizumab dose using package insert criteria.

The radioallergosorbent test (RAST), developed in 1968, was the first assay for the detection of allergen-specific IgE antibodies in human serum.[17] The RAST was a noncompetitive, heterogeneous (separation step included), solid phase immunoradiometric (radiolabeled antibody) assay in which allergen is covalently coupled to a solid phase (e.g., cellulose paper disc). In an initial incubation, human serum is added to the allergosorbent, during which time antibodies of all human isotypes, if present, bind to immobilized antigens. After a buffer wash, bound IgE is detected with iodine-125–labeled antihuman IgE Fc. After a second buffer wash to remove unbound radiolabeled antihuman IgE, bound radioactivity is measured in a gamma counter. The level of counts per minute associated with the solid phase is proportional to the amount of allergen-specific IgE in the initial serum specimen.

The basic RAST chemistry has remained essentially unchanged for more than 50 years. However, there have been major advances in assay automation and reagent quality. For instance, the number and quality of allergen extracts and especially component molecular allergens used in preparing allergosorbents have increased as a result of extensive research using new methods of extraction and quality control and the use of recombinant DNA techniques. The original paper disc solid phase that is still being used in one assay is being phased out of use. It is being replaced by newer matrix materials, such as the cellulose sponge (Phadia ImmunoCAP) and

• BOX 12.4 Analytes Measured in the Clinical Immunology Laboratory

Diagnosis
- Allergen-specific IgE
  - Multiallergen-specific IgE screen (adult and pediatric forms)
  - Individual allergen specificities (extracts and component allergens)
- Total serum IgE[1]
- Precipitating antibodies specific for proteins in organic dusts
- Tryptase (total and mature) (mast cell protease and used as a marker for mast cell–mediated anaphylaxis)
- Other tests: complete blood count (CBC), sputum examination for eosinophils and neutrophils

Management
- Allergen-specific IgG *(Hymenoptera)*
- Indoor aeroallergen quantitation in surface dust
  - Der p 1/Der f 1 (dust mite, *Dermatophagoides*)
  - Fel d 1 (cat, *Felis domesticus*)
  - Can f 1 (dog, *Canis familiaris*)
  - Bla g 1/Bla g 2 (cockroach, *Blattella germanica*)
  - Mus m 1 (mouse, *Mus musculus*)
  - Rat n 1 (rat, *Rattus norvegicus*)
- Cotinine (metabolite of nicotine measured in serum, urine, and sputum and used as a marker of smoke exposure)

Research Analytes
- IgE-specific autoantibodies
- Eosinophil cationic protein
- Mediators[2,3]
  - Preformed biogenic amine: histamine
  - Newly formed
  - Leukotriene C4 (LTC4)
  - Prostaglandin D2 (PGD2)
- Proteoglycans[2]
  - Heparin
  - Chondroitin sulfate E
- Proteases[2]
  - Mast cell chymase
  - Mast cell carboxypeptidase
  - Cathepsin G
- Fibroblast growth factor (bFGF)[2]
- Cytokines
  - Tumor necrosis factor (TNF)-alpha
  - Interleukins (ILs) 4, 5, 6, 13[3]

[1]Total serum IgE is the only one of these tests listed that is regulated under the CLIA 88.
[2]Primarily released from mast cells.
[3]Primarily released from basophils.

the use of biotinylated allergens (Siemens Immulite, Hycor Biomedical Noveos) that bind to immobilized avidin-coated beads. These advances have enhanced the binding capacity and reduced the nonspecific binding levels of allergosorbents. Various polyclonal and monoclonal anti-IgE detection antibody combinations ensure maximal assay sensitivity while maintaining their required specificity for human IgE. Microprocessor-driven automation has improved intraassay precision and interassay reproducibility. Nonisotopic labels have lengthened the shelf-life of immunochemical reagents and made the assays more user-friendly. The various assays now use a common calibration system in which a (heterologous[18]) total serum IgE curve using the third WHO IgE standard allows conversion of the allergen-specific IgE assay response data into quantitative dose estimates of IgE antibody in kilo units of allergen (kU$_A$)/L units. One kUa/L is equivalent to 2.4 ng/mL of IgE. These modifications have resulted in assays with superior analytical sensitivity and specificity. They are more quantitative, reproducible, and automated than their earlier counterparts. These improvements have made the serologic assay for IgE antibody diagnostically competitive with its in vivo puncture skin test counterpart. The intradermal skin test still appears to possess an inherent advantage in terms of analytical sensitivity and a major disadvantage involving the loss of diagnostic specificity.[1,19]

A consensus guideline (I/LA20-A3) established by the Clinical Laboratory Standards Institute on allergen-specific IgE assays has been prepared by an international body of scientists from academia, industry, and government regulatory agencies.[20] This effort has led to a more uniform strategy among the various assay manufacturers in reporting IgE antibody results using a common unit (kU$_A$/L) with a total serum IgE calibration system. In spite of the use of a common calibration scheme, the clinically used assays measure different populations of IgE antibody.[21,22] This observed interassay difference is thought to stem from the use of extracts containing different compositions of allergens and possibly different mathematical algorithms for interpolating specific antibody data from the heterologous total IgE calibration curve. The consequence is that published IgE antibody data generated with one assay cannot be directly extrapolated to published predictive outcomes that are based on IgE antibody levels from a second assay method. Specific IgE antibody levels measured in different commercial assays are currently not interchangeable or equivalent.[20]

Until recently, all allergen preparations used in clinical IgE antibody assays have been mixtures of proteins derived from biologic extracts of raw material that varies in its composition (i.e., molecular weight, charge [isoelectric point], relative content) and allergenic potency. The factors that contribute to allergen extract interlot variability include the season in which the raw material is collected, the degree of difficulty in identifying a pure source of raw material, the presence of morphologically similar raw materials that may cross-contaminate, and differences in the allergen extraction process used by various manufacturers. Once prepared, allergen extracts undergo extensive quality control involving total protein, isoelectrofocusing, sodium dodecyl sulfate–polyacrylamide gel electrophoresis, crossed immunoelectrophoresis, high-performance liquid chromatography tracings, and western immunoblotting. Issues of stability during storage, heterogeneity of the human IgE antibody–containing quality control sera, and different acceptance criteria for extract-based allergen-containing reagents also contribute to intermethod variability. Thus, allergosorbents from different manufacturers can be expected to bind different distributions of IgE antibodies for any given allergen specificity.

It is assumed that the physiologic extract of a biologic source material will contain all the principal allergenic molecules that are clinically relevant. Unfortunately, this is not always the case because some extracts contain labile molecules that are denatured or removed during the extract processing. This is why some allergen extracts used in IgE antibody assays are supplemented with recombinant allergens that are either low in quantity or missing in the extract. One successful supplementation involves the crude latex extract in which recombinant Hev b 5 has been added because it is labile and does not survive the extraction process from natural rubber products. The addition of recombinant Hev b 5 by one manufacturer to the latex reagent has increased the diagnostic sensitivity of their latex-specific IgE antibody assay by 10%, with no apparent loss of specificity.[23] However, a problem can occur when recombinant protein supplementation of an allergen extract is performed without the knowledge of the clinician who ultimately uses the IgE antibody results in patient management. When hazelnut extract that is used on an allergosorbent was supplemented with recombinant Cor a 1, it caused enhanced detection of IgE antibody to its structurally similar birch pollen homolog Bet v 1.[24] This led to exceptionally high levels of IgE antihazelnut being detected in patients with a concomitant birch pollen sensitivity because of the structural similarity and immunologic cross-reactivity of Car a 1 with Bet v 1 from birch pollen.

In 2002, microarray chip technology emerged.[25] Its commercialized version, the ImmunoCAP ISAC or immuno-solid phase allergen chip (Thermofisher Scientific/Phadia), has 112 native/recombinant component allergens that are spotted in triplicate onto glass slides. Thirty microliters of serum is pipetted onto the chip, and antibodies specific for the allergens attached to the chip bind during a 2-hour incubation period. After a buffer wash, bound IgE is detected with a fluorescence-labeled antihuman IgE conjugate. The chip is read in a fluorometer and fluorescence signal units are interpolated into Immuno-Solid Phase Allergy Chip (ISAC) units (ISU) as semiquantitative estimates of specific IgE antibody in the original serum. The analytical sensitivity of the ISAC varies as a function of the allergen specificity. It is generally less than the ImmunoCAP singleplex system when the same component allergen is coupled to the CAP sponge. The strength of the microarray system is its ability to identify cross-reactivity among structurally similar allergens from different biologic substances, as noted in Box 12.2. Knowledge of the extent of IgE cross-reactivity must be factored into the diagnostic process within the context of the patient's clinical history.

Performance of Immunoglobulin E Antibody Confirmatory Tests Using a Defined Positive Cut-Off Point

The practicing medical professional needs to know how well the available IgE antibody confirmatory assays perform analytically and diagnostically. The analytical performance of the available clinical immunoassays is readily defined because they are all calibrated using the same WHO total serum IgE reference preparation. In general, available clinically used assays detect allergen-specific IgE antibody down to 0.1 kU_A/L ($\approx$0.24 ng of IgE) and false positive nonspecific binding typically occurs only with extremely high total IgE levels (e.g., >20,000 IU/mL).[20] In terms of specificity, caution should be exercised with select IgE antibody assays that use a carbohydrate solid phase, with which the presence of IgE antibody in a patient's serum to cross-reactive carbohydrate determinants can produce elevated background responses up to 2 kUa/L that are not allergen-specific.[26] Otherwise, analytical specificity is a principal function of the quality of the allergen component and the specificity of the anti-IgE conjugate used in the assay.

The allergen-specific IgE antibody analysis is a test for allergic sensitization and not for making the definitive diagnosis of allergic disease. Confirmation of allergic sensitization with a positive IgE antiallergen analysis increases the likelihood that the patient's symptoms may be a result of an immediate-type hypersensitivity response. Thus, it is difficult to define the relative "diagnostic" sensitivity and specificity of IgE antibody assays because these parameters require, first, differentiating individuals who have allergic disease from those who do not have allergic disease. No perfect gold standard method exists for defining the presence of human allergic disease. The diagnostic algorithm indicates, however, that

the clinical history should be the primary decision criterion in making the final diagnosis of allergic disease. Unfortunately, a patient's history is not infallible.[27]

Gendo and Larson[28] have proposed three strategies for defining the presence of human allergic disease with the expressed purpose of judging the performance of confirmatory IgE antibody tests. The *clinical criteria gold standard* correlates the patient's symptoms and signs with clinical criteria that have been established by expert opinion. It is easy to use and applicable to most patients, but, unfortunately, it is prone to recall bias.[27] Box 12.5 lists the principal patient and medical care professional factors that can influence the accuracy of the clinical criteria based the gold standard approach. The *composite gold standard* combines the clinical history and physical examination information with one or more IgE antibody confirmatory test results (skin tests or serologic tests). This approach is generally more robust than using just the history alone; however, it tends to overestimate the index test's diagnostic sensitivity and specificity if the index test is a part of the composite gold standard. Box 12.5 also lists variables that influence the accuracy of skin test and serologic test results. The third and possibly most rigorous strategy for defining the presence of allergic disease is the *challenge gold standard*. Use of a challenge test to verify the presence of an allergic disease process on the surface sounds ideal. However, it too can be problematic because of differences in threshold of organ sensitivity, a lack of standardization of methods and outcome measures, and the use of a higher allergen dose than is found in nature to elicit a clinically measurable response. Skin and serologic tests and provocation testing are analytical methods, and thus they are inherently variable.[21,22,29] Therefore, the validity of their results must always be critiqued, especially if inconsistent with the history-based diagnosis.

A number of clinical studies have used one of these three gold standard approaches to define the presence of aeroallergen-related allergic disease.[19,29,30] With the cases defined, the investigators computed the diagnostic sensitivity and specificity of puncture skin tests and/or serologic tests for IgE antibody to a limited number of aeroallergen specificities. Because the patient population studied, positive cut-off criteria, reagent sources used, and statistical methods varied across the studies, generalized conclusions from the data in these studies are not possible. Within the limits of these studies, the performance of the puncture skin test ranged from 55% to 98% (diagnostic sensitivity) and 70% to 90% (diagnostic specificity) using the clinical or composite gold standard to identify allergic disease. In the same studies, the performance of the serologic tests for IgE antibody with the same allergen specificities ranged from 55% to 80% (diagnostic sensitivity) and 82% to 99% (diagnostic specificity) using the clinical or composite gold standard. Performance improved slightly for both the skin test and serology when a challenge-based gold standard was used to define the presence of clinical disease. In a 2014 comparative study,[30] substantial discordance was demonstrated between IgE antibody serology and skin testing results performed on the same individuals. The two methods of IgE antibody detection appeared to complement each other, and ideally they should not be interpreted interchangeably.[31] Importantly, using the IgE antibody results from either serology or skin testing alone can lead to a misdiagnosis of every fourth allergically sensitized patient as nonsensitized.

For food allergy diagnosis in which the skin testing food extracts are highly variable, serologic IgE antibody assays may be more reliable and reproducible. If the confirmatory test result is inconsistent with the history-based diagnosis, it should be repeated with the same or an alternative confirmatory test for verification. Both skin and serologic tests for IgE antibody are analytical methods with their inherent variability, and thus repetitive confirmation is often needed to minimize error associated with random or systematic bias.

Performance of Immunoglobulin E Antibody Confirmatory Tests Using a Probability of Clinical Disease

Current assay technology produces quantitative estimates of IgE antibody in serum as international units per milliliter that are traceable to the WHO International Reference Preparation for human IgE. Rather than examine the dichotomized IgE antibody data as a positive or negative result using a positive cut-off value, the alternative has been to examine the risk of clinical allergy associated with different quantitative IgE antibody levels as a series of probabilities. A 1997 study retrospectively investigated sera from 196 children and adolescents (mean age 5.2 years, 60% male) with atopic dermatitis who were evaluated for food allergy over a 10-year period.[32] Levels of IgE antibodies specific for cow's milk, chicken egg, peanut, wheat, soy, and fish were correlated with a diagnosis of food allergy as defined by positive double-blind, placebo-controlled food challenges or a convincing history of food-induced anaphylaxis. They were able to identify IgE antibody levels using the ImmunoCAP system that could predict clinical reactivity (positive food challenges) with more than 95% certainty for egg (6 kU_A/L), milk (32 kU_A/L), peanut (15 kU_A/L), and fish (20 kU_A/L). The significance of this report rests in its potential for identifying truly food-allergic individuals using the quantitative level of a positive IgE antibody serology and thus eliminating the need for a food challenge in children suspected of having IgE-mediated food allergy. In a 2001 report,[33] a prospective study was performed with sera from 100 children and adolescents (mean age: 3.8 years, 62% male) who had been referred for evaluation of food allergy. This prospective study verified the retrospective study based on 95% predictive decision points for egg, milk, peanut, and fish allergy. The study also confirmed that use of the positive criteria correctly diagnosed food allergy in more than 95% of children using the serum IgE antibody level. The study showed that quantitative food-specific IgE antibody measurements can be judiciously used to define the probability or risk of symptomatic allergies related to egg, milk, peanut, and fish in the pediatric population. The important conclusion of these studies is that careful use of quantitative serologic IgE antibody test results may eliminate the need for food challenges in some children. Equally important, however, is the fact that the 95% confidence limit (CL) decision thresholds do vary across different studies as a function of the subject population's disease state, the food specificity examined, and the mathematical algorithm used to compute the 95% CL decision threshold.[20]

For inhalant allergies, quantitative cat allergen-specific IgE antibody measurements have been shown to be equivalent to puncture skin tests and superior in performance to intradermal skin tests in the diagnosis of clinical reactivity to cat allergen.[19] Compared with a positive cat inhalation challenge outcome, IgE antibody levels by the ImmunoCAP system displayed a diagnostic sensitivity of 69%, specificity of 100%, positive predictive value of 100%, and negative predictive value of 73%. In the dust mite system, a significant correlation was observed between the concentration of dust mite–specific IgE and the concentration of sensitizing mite allergen in the individual's mattress dust ($P = .001$).[34] The authors reported a 77% probability of being exposed to high dust mite allergen (>10 μg/g of dust) when the serum IgE anti-mite levels were greater than 2 kU_A/L and vice versa. Finally, using specific IgE as a continuous variable, the risk of current wheeze and reduced lung function in children increases significantly with increasing summed measurements of IgE antibody specific for dust mite, cat, and dog.[35] These data indicate that quantitative estimates of serum IgE antibody can identify individuals who are not only sensitized but also who are in need of avoidance practices that they accomplish through environmental control measures. Other illustrations of the importance of quantitative allergen-specific IgE to respiratory allergy are reviewed elsewhere.[36] As a general rule for inhalant allergen specificities, the results of the skin test and quantitative IgE antibody immunoassay can be viewed as diagnostically interchangeable. One exception is in the monitoring of patients on immunotherapy, in which a decrease in the positivity of the puncture skin test titration alone has been shown to predict continued remission after cessation of allergen immunotherapy.[37]

Multiallergen IgE Antibody Screening Assays

When a patient provides an equivocal history for allergic disease, it can be difficult to pinpoint with reasonable certainty the appropriate IgE antibody specificities for further diagnostic investigation. A multiallergen screen is a single IgE antibody analysis that has the highest negative predictive value for atopic disease of any single laboratory test currently available. Multiple companies have multiallergen screens that cover a broad number of specificities (e.g., 10–15 common indoor and outdoor aeroallergens that induce most upper and lower airway–related allergic disease). Other multiallergen screens are specifically targeted at a limited number of specific allergens in a group such as foods (e.g., chicken egg, cow's milk, peanut, soybean, wheat, and fish/shellfish). A negative multiallergen screen reduces the likelihood that allergic disease is the cause of the individual's clinical problems. Multiallergen screen results are particularly useful in the diagnosis of pediatric allergic diseases, in which there is a need to detect allergen-specific IgE antibody in serum as a marker for sensitization. For this reason, the biomarkers committee of a workshop organized by the National Institutes of Health on asthma outcomes has recommended that the multiallergen screen be performed on all participants in asthma clinical trials to define their atopic status.[38]

In one illustrative study,[39] 143 children and adolescent patients were assigned an allergy status (103 positive, 40 negative) based on a combined history, skin prick test, and specific IgE antibody (ImmunoCAP) to seven common inhalants (mite, oak, ragweed, grass, dog, cat, and *Alternaria* spp.). The multiallergen screen (Phadiatop, Thermofisher Scientific/Phadia) that was run on these same sera correctly identified the allergy status of all subjects, verifying the diagnostic sensitivity and specificity of Phadiatop in differentiating sensitized individuals from those who are not sensitized to common inhalant allergens.

Mast Cell Tryptase

Serum levels of tryptase can be useful as a marker of mast cell activation in making the definitive diagnosis of anaphylaxis. Tryptase is a 134,000-Da serine esterase with four subunits, each containing an enzymatically active site.[40] When tryptase becomes dissociated from heparin, it spontaneously degrades into enzymatically inactive monomeric subunits. It is released from activated mast cells in parallel with previously stored histamine and other newly generated vasoactive mediators. The total protryptase concentration in blood is considered a measure of the mast cell number, and it is estimated by subtracting the mature tryptase from the total tryptase concentration. In contrast, mature tryptase levels in blood are considered a measure of mast cell activation.

An enzyme immunoassay is available to measure total tryptase levels in human serum. It uses a capture monoclonal antibody that binds both protryptase and mature tryptase.[41] Mature tryptase is measured with a solid phase noncompetitive immunoassay that uses a mature tryptase-specific capture monoclonal antibody. Before analysis, tryptase in the blood is converted into an enzymatically inactive form. Total serum tryptase concentrations in healthy (nondiseased) individuals range from 1 to 10 ng/mL (average 5 ng/mL). If baseline total serum tryptase levels exceed 20 ng/mL, systemic mastocytosis should be suspected. A mature

tryptase less than 1 ng/mL is observed in nondiseased individuals, and mature tryptase levels greater than 1 ng/mL indicate mast cell activation. For optimal results, blood samples should be collected from 0.5 to 4 hours after the initiation of a suspected mast cell–mediated systemic reaction.[42] A peak mature tryptase level greater than 10 ng/mL in a postmortem serum suggests systemic anaphylaxis as one probable cause of death. Systemic anaphylaxis induced by an insect sting can produce mature tryptase levels that peak at greater than 5 ng/mL by 30 to 60 minutes after the sting and then decline with a biologic half-life of ≈2 hours.[43]

Serum Markers of Hypersensitivity Pneumonitis

Extrinsic allergic alveolitis or hypersensitivity pneumonitis is an inflammatory reaction involving the lung interstitium and terminal bronchioles.[44] A heavy exposure to antigenic organic dusts (e.g., molds, bird droppings) can induce chills, fever, malaise, cough, and shortness of breath within hours of exposure. Although histologic examination of the lung lesions indicates that a cell-mediated pathologic factor is involved in hypersensitivity pneumonitis, most individuals have high levels of IgG antibody in their serum to the offending antigen that is used as a marker of the disease. Precipitating IgG antibody specific for antigens in organic dusts has been measured in human serum to support the differential diagnosis of this condition. The classic double diffusion (Ouchterlony) analysis is routinely performed to detect precipitating antibodies in the diagnosis of this disease. In this assay, crude antigen extract and antibody (control or patient's serum) are delivered into closely spaced wells in a porous agarose gel. Visible white precipitin lines confirmed by lines of identity with known human antibody controls are considered a positive test result. Precipitating antibodies, or precipitins, were detected in the serum of nearly all ill patients in one study, but also in the serum of 50% of asymptomatic individuals exposed to the relevant organic dusts.[44,45]

More recently, enzyme immunoassays for IgG antibody to selected organic dust antigens have been reported.[46,47] Unfortunately, the concentrations of serum IgG antibodies against the molds and mammal antigens measured by enzyme immunoassay methods does not differentiate between simple antigen exposure and the presence of hypersensitivity pneumonitis disease. These assays are too analytically sensitive and diagnostically nonspecific. Thus, the classic precipitin assays continue to be widely used for detecting IgG precipitins to antigens in pigeon serum, *Aureobasidium pullulans,* thermophilic actinomyces, *Aspergillus fumigatus,* and extractable proteins from fecal material produced by chickens, parakeets, and a variety of exotic household birds.

Management of Type 1 Hypersensitivity

The management of individuals with allergic disease involves the combined use of pharmacotherapy, immunotherapy, anti-IgE therapy, and avoidance therapy. A number of analytical measurements performed by the clinical immunology laboratory can aid the clinician in optimizing an immunotherapy regimen by monitoring the humoral (IgG antibody) immune responses in patients on venom immunotherapy (Box 12.6). Anti-IgE therapy begins with obtaining a total serum IgE level to determine proper dosing. Assays to monitor the level of free (non–anti-IgE bound) IgE in circulation of patients on omalizumab have remained research assays[48] because there is currently no documented clinical indication for their use. Finally, indoor aeroallergen levels may be measured in surface reservoir dust before remediation to document

- Clinically successful aeroallergen immunotherapy is almost always accompanied by high (microgram per milliliter) levels of allergen-specific IgG antibody in serum.
- Quantitative venom-specific IgG antibody levels can be useful in individualizing venom doses and injection frequencies for patients on maintenance venom immunotherapy for up to 4 years.
- Mast cell tryptase is a serine esterase that is used as a marker of mast cell activation during anaphylaxis. Immunoreactive tryptase levels in serum of healthy adults are typically less than 5 µg/L. Elevated levels (>10 µg/L) are detectable 1 to 4 hours after the onset of systemic anaphylaxis with hypotension.
- Indoor allergens from dust mites, animals (cat, dog, mouse, rat), cockroaches, and a limited number of molds are quantified in processed house dust to investigate individual risk for allergic symptoms or sensitization and to monitor effects of environmental control.

the need for and monitor the extent of allergen avoidance measures and after remediation to verify that the environment has been cleaned of allergen sources.

Optimizing Venom Immunotherapy

When considering the medically important *Hymenoptera*, cross-reactivity has been known to exist between the vespid venoms (yellow jacket, white-faced hornet, and yellow hornet) and *Polistes* wasp venom proteins. Results from a competitive inhibition format of the *Polistes* wasp venom–specific IgE antibody serology have allowed allergists to select the venom specificities more effectively and minimize the number of venoms that must be administered during immunotherapy.[49] This targeted venom therapy is especially important for children, in whom unnecessary administration of *Polistes* wasp venom may lead to de novo sensitization to *Polistes* allergens. More recently, component-resolved diagnosis using recombinant venom allergens (Api m1, Ves v 1, Ves v 5, and Pol d 5) permits more effective identification of cross-sensitization that results from dual sensitization to honeybee and vespid venoms. This allows venom immunotherapy to be performed with the relevant single venom rather than multiple venoms.[50,51]

Aeroallergen Measurements of Indoor Environments to Facilitate Avoidance Therapy

Dust mite *(Dermatophagoides pteronyssinus, Dermatophagoides farinae)*, cat epithelium/dander *(Felis domesticus)*, dog epithelium/dander *(Canis familiaris)*, German cockroach *(Blattella germanica)*, mouse *(Mus musculus)*, rat *(Rattus norvegicus)*, and molds are known sources of potent indoor aeroallergens.[52] Allergic proteins from each of these biosources are being used as "indicator" allergens for relative levels in surface reservoir dust in the home, workplace, and school (see Box 12.6).

A surface dust specimen is collected from air ducts, floors, or other horizontal surfaces (bed, upholstered furniture) using an inexpensive dust collector that is attached to a standard household vacuum cleaner. Crude dust is sent to a clinical immunology laboratory, where it is sieved, extracted, and quantified using a monoclonal antibody–based immunoenzymetric assay in plates (enzyme-linked immunosorbent assay [ELISA]) or on fluorescent beads (BioPlex). A high level of one or more indoor aeroallergens identifies an allergen source that can sensitize or induce an allergic reaction in a sensitized individual. Levels of Der p 1/f 1 allergen

greater than 2000 ng/g of fine dust have been associated with an increased risk of allergic symptoms in sensitized individuals. In contrast, cat allergen levels greater than 8000 ng/g of Fel d 1 in fine dust have been suggested as the threshold for sensitization. Comparable risk targets have been used for dog (Can f 1) allergen levels in indoor environments. For cockroach, mouse, and/or rat urinary allergen, any detectable allergen in the indoor environment places individuals allergic to cockroach, mouse, or rat allergens at risk for symptoms and further sensitization.[53]

Mold and Fungus Evaluation in Indoor Environments

Accurate quantitation of the mold content of an environment is a challenge. *Alternaria, Aspergillus, Cladosporium,* and *Penicillium* spp., account for the majority of indoor molds.[53] The total spore counts (nonviable and viable) can be determined by collecting particulate from an air impactor or suction device and then assessing the spore's morphology for the purpose of speciating the mold. Viable fungal spores that grow when environmental conditions are favorable are considered by some allergists as more clinically important because they can colonize indoor environments and, in some cases, the respiratory tract. In one clinical laboratory, a qualitative viable mold spore analysis is performed on 5 mg of fine dust that is distributed over a microbiologic culture plate containing Sabouraud's dextrose agar. Visual inspection of the plate at 24 and 48 hours allows the total number of mold colonies to be quantified. The colony count at 24 hours is an estimate of the mold burden of the environment. Repetitive subculturing and morphologic identification allows speciation of the predominant molds; however, this is infrequently performed. Rather, once a mold contamination has been identified, remediation by cleaning with bleach and reducing humidity is generally instituted.

There are no established mold spore contamination ranges that can be considered safe, partly because mold is ever present; different individuals have different relative sensitivities; and the target airborne mold allergens are difficult to sample and verify. Thus, it is not possible to identify an environment that will place a mold-allergic person at risk for symptoms. Multiple variables associated with mold spore heterogeneity, differential growth based on nutrients and environmental conditions, the degree of aerosolization, and variable specificity of the patient's IgE antibody complicate the interpretation of a mold spore measurement when attempting to predict a clinical outcome from any environmental exposure. Sometimes the indoor mold levels are compared with the outdoor mold levels collected at the same time to judge if airborne mold spores are significantly higher and thus playing a more significant role in the allergy and asthma symptoms experienced indoors. Mold spore levels greater than 25,000 colonies/g of fine dust have been identified in one study as a level that places a home in the 75th percentile for random homes monitored across the United States. When this proposed threshold level is exceeded, the allergic individual is encouraged to remediate the environment, which often involves replacing air duct filters, removing plants, decreasing indoor humidity, removing carpet from floors, and removing upholstered furniture, and stuffed toys.

Conclusions

The diagnostic allergy laboratory exists to provide serologic testing that supports the clinician in the diagnosis and management of patients suspected of type 1 hypersensitivity reactions. To this end, the most important analyte measured in the clinical laboratory is allergen-specific IgE antibody using allergen extracts and more recently allergenic components as allergosorbents. Selection of the laboratory and the IgE antibody assay methods and standards that it employs to ensure quality are the ultimate responsibility of the referring physician.[54] Performance on national diagnostic allergy proficiency surveys and successful inspections leading to federal licensure under the Clinical Laboratory Improvement Act of 1988 are benchmarks that can be used by the healthcare professional to ensure that the clinical laboratory provides quality diagnostic allergy testing.

The reference list can be found on the companion Expert Consult website at http://www.expertconsult.inkling.com.

13

Outdoor Allergens

RICHARD W. WEBER

KEY POINTS

- Sources of airborne allergens vary from microscopic to large fauna.
- Outdoor aeroallergenic particles include intact pollen grains or spores, cell fragments, and submicronic particles.
- Preferred samplers measure a calculable volume of air to determine the density of aeroallergens and have capture efficacy of particles down to 3 to 5 microns.

- Meteorologic parameters having the greatest impact on airborne pollen concentration are temperature and precipitation.
- Increased atmospheric temperature and carbon dioxide concentration increase allergenic plant biomass and pollen production.

Introduction

Aeroallergens may be on various-sized particles and dispersed from various sources (Table 13.1).[1] The airborne particle may be a cell, intact pollen grain, cytoplasmic component, fungal spore or mycelia, epidermal scale, dust particle, or protein dissolved in a water droplet. Outdoor sources are frequently of plant origin, animal allergens are more likely indoors, and fungal spores may be either. Practitioners involved with clinical patient care need to be aware of the local exposures facing their allergic patients to plan and initiate appropriate therapeutics. This requires a familiarity with the plant exposures specific to their locale. This is accomplished by personal observation and contact with municipal or academic experts. Key issues, or clinical pearls, are summarized in Box 13.1.

General Principles of Allergen Aerobiology

Pollen

Vascular plants propagate through extension, trunk or root shoots, rhizomes, and stolons, or by seed. Sexual reproduction is accomplished by transport of the pollen or spore. Dispersal is by the wind, anemophily, or a vector such as an insect, entomophily. Some amphiphilous plants use both mechanisms. Insect-pollinated plants are less frequently inducers of hay fever.

Fungi

Fungi have chitin-containing cell walls, a polysaccharide also present in insect exoskeletons. Fungi may be unicellular, syncytial, or multicellular. Life cycles may have multiple stages, with both sexual and asexual reproduction. Gene sequencing and mitochondrial analysis have verified the identity of such life stages belonging

to single organisms, making the taxon "fungi imperfecta," a paraphyletic group united only by asexual propagation, artificial and obsolete.[2]

Animals

Primarily indoors, animal sources also may be outdoor allergens. Heavy hatches of caddis flies or mayflies or miller moth infestations induce allergic symptoms, as do pine tree tussock moths for lumberjacks and sewer flies for municipal sanitation workers.[3,4] Horse dander allergen can be sampled downwind from stables.[5]

TABLE 13.1 Aeroallergen Sources and Types

Allergen Source	Particle Type
Bacteria	Cells, fragments, metabolites
Thermophilic actinomycetes	Spores, metabolites
Algae	Cells, fragments, metabolites
Protozoa	Metabolites
Fungi	Spores, mycelial fragments, metabolites
Ferns and mosses	Spores
Grasses, weeds, and trees	Pollens, cytoplasmic particles
Arthropods	Feces, saliva, body parts
Birds	Feces, serum proteins, epidermal debris
Mammals	Dander, saliva, urine

Modified from Burge HA. Monitoring for airborne allergens. Ann Allergy 1992;69:9–18.

Submicronic Allergenic Particles

Ragweed was the first pollen aeroallergen shown to be carried on submicronic particles.[6,7] Airborne birch antigenic activity can be found in particles smaller than 2.4 microns. Cytoplasmic starch granules are prominent in grass (Poaceae) and dock (*Rumex* spp., Polygonaceae) pollen, the former having heavy concentrations of groups 1, 5, and 13 allergens.[8–11] Although storm-driven raindrops may disrupt grass pollen grains and release respirable allergen-laden starch granules, Schäppi and colleagues[9] and Suphioglu and associates[12] demonstrated that a moisture-drying cycle releases starch granules through the grass pollen aperture.

Characteristics of Wind-Pollinated Plants

Wind pollination may appear a simpler process than vector-facilitated pollination, but it is a later evolutionary mechanism.[13] Characteristics are summarized in Box 13.2. Pollen grains tend to be small and dry, with reduced ornamentation to minimize turbulence and little resinous pollenkitt.

Erdtman[14] reported that a single birch catkin produced about 6 million pollen grains, an alder catkin 4.5 million, and an English oak catkin 1.25 million grains.[14] Tabulating the number of catkins on trees, Erdtman calculated the pollen produced in a single year. A birch tree released over 5.5 billion grains, an alder 7.2 billion, and an oak 0.6 billion. Cereal rye grass produced 4.25 million pollen grains per inflorescence.[14]

In 1930 August Thommen set out five principles necessary for a plant to be an important inducer of pollinosis (Box 13.3). With some caveats, Thommen's Postulates have remained correct.[15] Pollen must contain an excitant of hay fever: proteins or glycoproteins that are easily elutable or coat the surface of expelled respirable cytoplasmic particles. Although most pollinosis inducers are wind-pollinated, some primarily insect-pollinated plants may release sufficient airborne pollen to cause sensitization. Most pollen grains come to rest within meters of their source, although grains may be transported for hundreds of miles.[14]

Floristic Zones

The distribution of individual plant species depends on several factors: average high and low temperatures, ambient humidity, and average precipitation. Soil factors such as mineral content, pH, and density also have an impact on plant adaptation and selection.[16] Some plants are cosmopolitan, adapting to diverse circumstances; others are niche-limited, adapting to extremes of moisture or temperature. The range of indigenous species may be limited by niche selectivity. The extent an introduced plant will spread is determined by its adaptability, its aggressiveness, and the length of time from introduction.

The U.S. Department of Agriculture has defined "hardiness zones." The 10 climatic zones in the North American continent are based on the average annual minimum temperature. These isotherms define the northern limits of species, determined by winter cold survivability. Weber[16,17] presented floristic zones of North and Central America, modified from Takhtajan, listing 15 regions from the Arctic tundra to the tropics, with representative allergenic plants. A useful reference giving the distribution maps of many native allergenic plants is *Airborne and Allergenic Pollen of North America*.[18] However, numbers of introduced major allergenic plants do not have distribution maps.

Characterized Allergens

A list of fully sequenced allergens is maintained online (allergen.org) by the International Union of Immunological Societies.[19] Conventional allergen nomenclature is the first three letters of the genus, the first letter of the species, and a number; for instance, the major allergen of short ragweed is Amb a 1. Isoallergens are variations in the molecular weight or charge because of amino acid substitutions or glycosylation and are designated by a decimal point followed by four digits (e.g., Phl p 5.0102 and Phl p 5.0201).

Aeroallergen Sampling

Table 13.2 lists the types of samplers used in monitoring aeroallergens. Gravimetric samplers such as the Durham sampler and agar Petrie dishes are no longer adequate for meaningful study, although the latter has the advantage that the growth medium allows identification of viable spores through distinctive colony characteristics. Disadvantages of gravimetric samplers are that they are quantified in terms of surface area (square centimeters) and do not estimate particle burden in a volume of air. Capture is skewed to larger particles, because smaller mold spores may not have an impact.

Volumetric devices sample volumes of air over a given time interval and report in particles per cubic millimeter in 24 hours

TABLE 13.2	Types of Aeroallergen Samplers	
Type	Example	Comment
Gravimetric	Durham Petrie dish	Large particles overrepresented Particles per surface area (p/cm²)
Volumetric		Particles per air volume (p/m³)
Impaction		
Intermittent rotary	Rotorod	Easily overloaded
Suction drum	Burkard	Wind orientation necessary
Cascade	Anderson	Indoor or outdoor use
Filtration	Accu-Vol	Microscopic or immunoassay
Personal sampler		Clinically relevant exposure
Automatic counter	NTT-Shinyei KH300 BAA500 Plair PA-300	Misreading likely Lack of sensitivity Fully automated image recognition pollen monitoring systems

(see Table 13.2). The Rotorod seen in Fig. 13.1A is a rotary impaction device that spins two small plastic rods at fixed time intervals, usually for 1 minute in every 10. The silicone-greased leading side of the rod has a fixed surface area (length and width) that sweeps a given length of air (circumference of the circle) for a given length of time. It is not affected by wind direction. A disadvantage is lost capture efficiency as the surface becomes loaded with impacted particles, hence intermittent sampling. Suction devices move air through an aperture to impact on tape on a rotating drum (with the Burkard) or an advancing microscope slide (Kramer-Collins). The Burkard (see Fig. 13.1B) can be configured for a 24-hour or 7-day sample. Capture efficacy is best for particles down to 3 to 5 microns, when the aperture is facing into the wind and the wind velocity matches the intake flow. The Burkard has a large weather vane to orient the aperture into the wind. The Lanzoni is a similar device popular in Europe. The Andersen cascade impactor can segregate particles by size over several stages. Fig. 13.1C and D shows the Andersen intact and disassembled. Agar plates can be placed to identify fungi via culture characteristics. Personal-sized samplers are useful in indoor occupational risk assessment. High-volume suction devices with fiberglass filters can be scanned microscopically or eluted and stained with specific monoclonal antibodies. The subtleties of outdoor sampling and interpretation and the importance of pauci-micronic particles carrying allergen has been described.[20] Immunochemical techniques to measure outdoor allergen have come into vogue; however, the number of allergens contributing to the aeroallergen burden exceeds by several orders of magnitude the number of available monoclonal-specific allergen immunochemical assays.[21,22]

Outdoor aeroallergen sampling has been based on labor-intensive microscopic examination with morphologic pattern recognition identification.[23] Initial evaluation of an automated system by Delaunay and associates[24] showed drawbacks of misidentification and high detection threshold. More recent reports on computerized pattern recognition programs such as the BAA500 are encouraging.[25,26]

Representative Pollens

Grasses

Poaceae has several subfamilies and numerous tribes. The Pooideae subfamily is very important in pollinosis, with a wide range throughout the United States and Europe. Members include Kentucky bluegrass, timothy, and cereal rye (Fig. 13.2A) and have strongly cross-reactive major allergens.[27] Bermuda (*Cynodon dactylon*) is an important southern grass, as is Johnson grass (*Sorghum halepense*), extending from the Eastern Agricultural zone across the Arid Southwest.

Conifers

The most important member of the order Pinales is the cedar family (Cupressaceae), containing cedars, junipers, and cypresses (*Juniperus, Thuja*, and *Cupressus* spp.). In Texas and Oklahoma, mountain cedar (*Juniperus ashei*) counts may be greater than 20,000 grains/m³. A subfamily includes bald cypress, redwoods, sequoias, and the foremost producer of pollinosis in Japan, Japanese red cedar (*Cryptomeria japonica*). Members of this family are strongly cross-reactive.[27] Pinaceae contains pines (*Pinus* spp.), spruces (*Picea* spp.), hemlocks (*Tsuga* spp.), and firs (*Abies* spp., *Pseudotsuga* spp.). This family produces copious amounts of pollen, but induces little hay fever.

Other Trees

Deciduous trees are scattered throughout a great number of botanical orders and families, with little cross-reactivity between these diverse plants. Cottonwoods, aspens, poplars, and willows are within Salicaceae. Aspens are prevalent in the Rocky Mountains and the Canadian boreal forest; poplars and cottonwoods are common in the Great Plains and eastward. Birch (*Betula*) and alder (*Alnus*) are found throughout the Northern Forest, Northwest Coastal, California Lowlands, and Great Basin. Alder is especially prevalent in the Northern Forest and Vancouverian Pacific Maritime zones. Red and white oaks (*Quercus* spp.) have a wide range from the East Coast through the Central Plains. American elm (*Ulmus americana*) has been diminished by disease, with Siberian and Chinese elms (*Ulmus pumila* and *Ulmus parvifolia*) now more common. Numerous maples (*Acer* spp.) are found across the United States, with box elder (*Acer negundo*) having a wide range (see Fig. 13.2B). Box elder is an entirely wind-pollinated, prodigious pollen producer, whereas other maples are amphiphilous. Ash trees are widely found and have strong cross-reactivity with European olive. Linden, or basswood (*Tilia* spp.), is another amphiphilous tree that produces large amounts of airborne pollen, causing significant sensitization.

Weeds

Sorrel and dock pollination coincides with the grass pollen season. Sheep sorrel (*Rumex acetosella*) is a moderate hay fever inducer, whereas curly dock (*Rumex crispus*), is common, but a lower pollen producer. Nettle (*Urtica* spp.) is widespread, as is the related pellitory (*Parietaria* spp.). Under-appreciated as an aeroallergen, nettle produces large amounts of small, pale pollen. Pellitory is a major pollinosis inducer in the Mediterranean basin. Amaranthaceae members are major causes of hay fever in the later summer. Their pollen grains are similar and difficult to discriminate

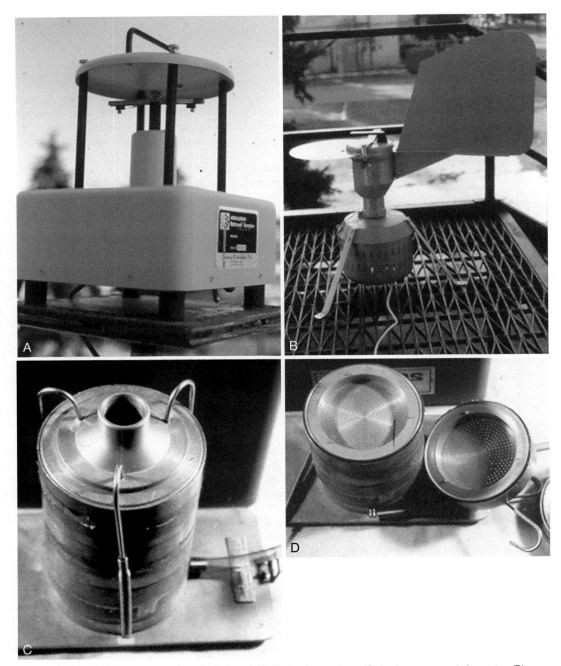

• **Fig. 13.1** Aeroallergen samplers. (A) Rotorod. (B) Burkard spore trap. (C) Andersen cascade impactor. (D) Andersen sampler showing inner layers.

by species. Pigweeds such as *Amaranthus retroflexus* are ubiquitous. The two major introduced tumbleweeds, Russian thistle *(Salsola kali)* and burning bush *(Bassia scoparia),* have expanded throughout the central states to the gulf and California coasts. Lamb's quarter *(Chenopodium album),* a modest pollen producer, has a worldwide distribution. Plantains *(Plantago* spp.) are moderate pollen producers, but pollinating from spring into fall.

Short *(Ambrosia artemisiifolia)* and giant *(Ambrosia trifida)* ragweed predominate in the eastern states and Central Plains, with false *(Ambrosia acanthicarpa)* and western *(Ambrosia psilostachya)* ragweed common in the western states (see Fig. 13.2C). These four major ragweed plants strongly cross-react.[27] Cocklebur *(Xanthium commune)* and the marshelders *(Iva* spp.) are related to

ragweed, but of lesser significance. Mugwort *(Artemisia vulgaris)* in the east and several western sages *(Artemisia* spp.) are important pollen producers in the late summer, rivaling the importance of ragweed in the western states.

Representative Fungi

Long and Kramer[28] demonstrated that some airborne fungal spora are facilitated by dry windy conditions and some by increased humidity or precipitation. In the Central Plains, fungi such as *Alternaria, Cladosporium,* and *Epicoccum* have spores released through wind turbulence and are present in greatest concentrations on dry windy afternoons (Fig. 13.3). Many Basidiomycetes and Ascomycetes have spore release dependent on humidity and are in greatest concentrations during or after rainfall and during damper hours of darkness.[28] Although *Alternaria* spp. are recovered on samplers in much fewer numbers than *Cladosporium* spp., it is a more potent allergenic source and has been incriminated in severe asthma and life-threatening events.[29,30] *Epicoccum* spp. and basidiospores also have been linked with decreases in pulmonary function and asthma admissions.[31,32]

Meteorologic Variables

Factors such as rain, humidity, wind speed and direction, temperature, and amount of sunshine have both immediate and cumulative effects on bioaerosols.[33] Precipitation and humidity decrease particle air burden acutely, and preseasonal moisture is necessary to ensure proper growth of flower buds on perennials and trees. Ambient temperature rise is necessary for pollen anthesis in many plants, and cumulative heat above a threshold value has been linked to onset and intensity of pollination in grasses, weeds, and trees. Thunderstorms may greatly increase aeroallergen burden because of outflows from storm cells resulting in pollen grain disruption with increased airborne submicronic particles.[34,35]

Dispersal of mold spores is intimately linked to precipitation and humidity. However, effects may be diametrically opposed, depending on the type of fungi. Certain ascospores and basidiospores require active rainfall for release of spores, whereas others will be suppressed by precipitation.

Impact of Climate Change on Aeroallergens

Pollen anthesis is a useful monitor of anthropogenic climate change. Over a 16-year period, oak pollen onset in Poland advanced by 9 days, correlating with temperature increase.[36] Increased ambient carbon dioxide and higher temperatures both result in short ragweed *(A. artemisiifolia)* biomass, and pollen production increases of 61% to 90%.[37–39] Because the content of Amb a 1 varies in ragweed plants from site to site and year to year, does increased pollen production necessarily imply an increase in airborne allergenic load?[40,41] Ziska and associates[42] collected ragweed pollen along an urban transect in Maryland, using the urban environment as a surrogate for climate change. The urban site averaged 2° C higher and the carbon dioxide level was 30% higher than in the rural site. The urban ragweed grew faster with greater above-ground biomass, flowered earlier, and produced more pollen than plants in the rural site. There was about a 2-fold greater concentration of Amb a 1 per microgram of protein in the rural versus the other sites. However, there was a more than 7-fold production of pollen from the urban sites compared with the rural site, documenting a greater airborne allergenic burden. The aggressive northern expansion of invasive ragweed in Europe has been linked to climate change.[43]

Climate change has an impact on numerous allergenic plants.[44,45] Increased carbon dioxide increases plant biomass and pollen production. It is conceivable that higher airborne pollen numbers will increase the efficiency of windborne pollination, thereby potentiating propagation. The outcome will be increasing amounts of robust allergenic plants and increasing aeroallergen burden for inhalant allergy sufferers. The rise of other pollutants in association with carbon dioxide may have a potentiating effect. Increased allergenicity of birch pollen has been linked with increased ozone levels.[46]

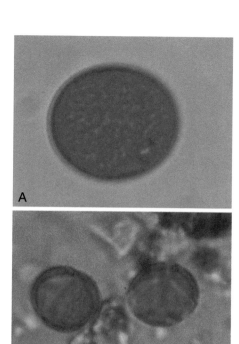
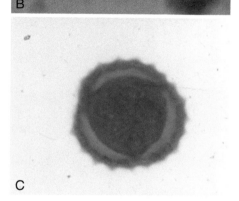

• **Fig. 13.2** Representative pollens. (A) Grass. (B) Maple. (C) Ragweed.

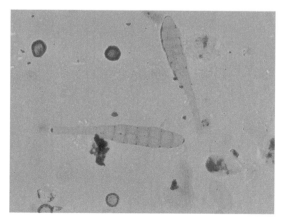

• **Fig. 13.3** *Alternaria.* Two club-shaped *Alternaria;* four clear cigar-shaped *Cladosporium* in lower right quadrant; two pairs of dark brown Basidiomycete smut spores in upper and lower left quadrants.

Conclusions

Airborne allergens are derived from a variety of sources ranging in size from microscopic to large fauna. These allergens may be transported on pauci-micronic particles such as cell fragments to intact pollen grains or fungal spores. It is clinically useful to assess the extent of allergen exposure. Volumetric samplers can determine the intensity or density of aeroallergens. Preferred samplers measure a calculable volume of air to determine the density of aeroallergens and have capture efficacy of particles down to 3 to 5 microns. Ideally, labor-intensive examination of microscope slides or tapes by individuals will soon be replaced by automated pattern recognition programs.

Local climate is defined by geographic and topographic characteristics and weather patterns. Meteorologic parameters having the greatest impact on airborne pollen concentration are temperature and precipitation. Climate change is driven by increasing concentration of greenhouse gases such as carbon dioxide and methane. Increased atmospheric temperature and carbon dioxide concentration increase allergenic plant biomass, pollen production, and timing of pollination.

The reference list can be found on the companion Expert Consult website at http://www.expertconsult.inkling.com.

14

Indoor Allergens

WILLIAM J. SHEEHAN, WANDA PHIPATANAKUL

KEY POINTS

- Studies in both inner city and suburban locations indicate that more than 80% of school-age children with asthma are sensitized to at least one indoor allergen.
- The level of early life environmental exposure to a specific indoor allergen influences the development of sensitization to that allergen and subsequent atopic conditions.
- Humidity levels greater than 50% promote house dust mite growth, and house dust mite allergy has been associated with asthma development, severity, and morbidity.

- Given the lack of scientific evidence, it is standard for current guidelines to state that hypoallergenic cats and dogs should not be recommended for individuals who are sensitized.
- In urban environments, several important studies have demonstrated the relationship between cockroach and/or mouse exposure and poor asthma outcomes in children.

Introduction

Over the past few decades, the investigation of the important role of indoor allergens in the pathogenesis of allergic disease has included the identification of the most important allergens, the evaluation of the effect of allergen exposure on allergic disease, and the development of techniques to accurately monitor allergen exposure. The primary indoor allergens include allergens from house dust mites, pets such as dogs and cats, molds, and pests such as cockroaches and rodents.[1] This chapter reviews the structure and biologic function of indoor allergens, the clinical significance of the primary indoor allergens, and the methods for assessing environmental exposure.

Allergen Structure and Function

Allergens are proteins or glycoproteins that are readily soluble and able to penetrate the nasal and respiratory mucosae. A systematic allergen nomenclature has been developed: the first three letters of the source genus followed by a single letter for the species and a number denoting the chronologic order of allergen identification. For example, the abbreviated nomenclature for the house dust mite allergen, *Dermatophagoides pteronyssinus* allergen 1, is Der p 1. Only a limited group of proteins (with certain structural features) have the potential to become allergens[2,3]; however, detailed structural analyses have not revealed any common features or motifs that are associated with the induction of immunoglobulin E (IgE) responses.

Allergens belong to protein families with diverse biologic functions, including enzymes, enzyme inhibitors, lipid-binding proteins, ligand-binding proteins, structural proteins, or regulatory proteins (Box 14.1).[4] Some dust mite allergens are digestive

enzymes excreted with the feces, such as Der p 1 (cysteine protease), Der p 3 (serine protease), and Der p 6 (chymotrypsin). Enzymatic activity of mite allergens promotes IgE synthesis and local inflammatory responses.[5–8] Most animal allergens are ligand-binding proteins (lipocalins) or albumins. In contrast, Fel d 1 (*Felis domesticus* 1) is a calcium-binding, steroid-inducible, uteroglobin-like molecule.[9] Fel d 1 has two amphipathic water-filled cavities that may bind biologically important ligands. Rat and mouse urinary allergens are pheromone- or odorant-binding proteins. The cockroach allergen Bla g 4 (*Blattella germanica* 4) is a lipocalin that is produced in utricles and conglobate glands of male cockroaches and may have a reproductive function. Other important cockroach allergens include Bla g 1, a gut-associated allergen; Bla g 2, an inactive aspartic proteinase; Bla g 5 (glutathione transferase family); and the group 7 tropomyosin allergens.[10]

> **• BOX 14.1 Clinical Pearls**
> *Indoor Allergens: Structure and Function*
>
> - Allergens are soluble proteins or glycoproteins of molecular weights of 10 to 50 kd.
> - Allergens have diverse biologic functions and may be enzymes, enzyme inhibitors, lipid-binding proteins, lipocalins, or regulatory or structural proteins.
> - Allergens promote T cells to differentiate along the Th2 pathway to produce interleukin-4 (IL-4) and IL-13 and initiate isotype switching to immunoglobulin E (IgE).
> - Biologic functions of allergens, such as proteolytic enzyme activity or other adjuvant-like effects, can enhance IgE responses, damage lung epithelium, and cause allergic inflammation.

Clinical Significance of Indoor Allergens

Exposure data collected in epidemiologic studies, population surveys, and birth cohort studies have investigated the association between indoor allergen exposure and the pathogenesis of allergic respiratory diseases, including asthma and allergic rhinitis. Childhood asthma is more closely linked to allergen exposure and allergic sensitization than adult asthma. Sensitization to indoor allergens likely occurs earliest in life, because young children have been shown to have higher rates of sensitization to indoor allergens compared with outdoor allergens.[11] Studies in both inner city and suburban children with asthma indicated that more than 80% of school age children with asthma are sensitized to at least one indoor allergen and that allergic sensitization is a strong predictor of disease persistence in later life.[12–15] The majority of patients with severe asthma are sensitized to multiple allergens, and the number of sensitivities correlates with asthma severity.[16,17] Epidemiologic studies have demonstrated risk of allergic sensitization to be attributable to certain levels of allergen exposure among different populations of atopic individuals. The relationship between early-life allergen exposure and the development of asthma is complex, with conflicting results that may depend on the specific allergen investigated or other nonallergen exposures such as the home microbiome.[13,14,18,19]

Dust Mites

The two principal mite species, Der p 1 and Der f 1, account for the majority of mite fauna in U.S. house dust samples. These house dust mites are found in dust and products with woven material or stuffing such as mattresses, pillows, stuffed animals, and bedding. Warm temperatures and high humidity are the major factors that promote dust mite growth. Rabito and colleagues[20] found that, in New Orleans, asthmatic children living indoors with average humidity greater than 50% were three times more likely to be exposed to elevated levels of house dust mites. In contrast, house dust mite levels are generally low or undetectable in areas of high altitude or low humidity. In fact, maintaining an indoor humidity below 50% is one of the recommended components of interventions to reduce dust mite exposure.[21]

More than half of children and adolescents with asthma are sensitized to house dust mites.[22] There is strong evidence for a dose-response relationship of exposure to house dust mites and sensitization in both cross-sectional[23–25] and prospective studies.[14,26–28] Persistent exposure of atopic individuals to approximately 2 µg/g of mite allergen is likely to result in sensitization in a majority of atopic individuals, increasing as mite allergen levels exceed 2 µg/g. A prospective study of German schoolchildren demonstrated a 7-fold increase in sensitization to dust mites for children exposed to the highest levels of dust mite allergen.[27] Exposure to dust mite allergen levels greater than 10 µg/g is considered high risk for sensitization, and findings from Arbes and colleagues[29] indicate that these levels are found in approximately 23% of U.S. homes.

Asthma development,[30–33] severity,[34] and morbidity[22,23] have been strongly associated with house dust mite allergy. Sporik and co-workers[14] demonstrated dust mite exposure to be associated with the development of childhood asthma, particularly if there was exposure to high levels in the first year of life. Tovey and colleagues[28] showed a nonlinear relationship between levels of dust mites in homes and the development of asthma at 5 years of age in a high-risk cohort of children. The trends showed increasing prevalence of sensitization and asthma correlating with dust mite exposure up to a critical point and then sharply dropping at the highest levels of exposure. The explanation of attenuated disease development with very high levels of dust mite exposure is unclear but may indicate that high concentrations of nonallergenic immune modifiers such as endotoxin are accompanying the house dust mites. Celedon and associates[26] found a dose-response relationship between levels of dust mite exposure in high-risk infants at age 2 to 3 months and asthma at school age. In this study, the high allergen threshold was 10 µg/g or greater, much lower than the critical threshold found in Tovey's evaluation. A survey of middle school children in Virginia showed that dust mite sensitization was independently associated with asthma (odds ratio 6.6, $P <$ .0001) and that dust from 81% of homes contained more than 2 µg/g mite group 1 allergen.[33] In addition to the implications for developing asthma, sensitization to dust mites predicts worse lung function compared with those not sensitized.[22]

Pets (Cat and Dog)

The major cat allergen, Fel d 1, is primarily found in cat skin and hair follicles and is produced in sebaceous, anal, and salivary glands. The major dog allergen, *Canis familiaris* 1 (Can f 1), is found in hair, dander, and saliva. What distinguishes pet allergen exposure from other indoor allergens is the wide range of exposure levels (from <0.5 to >3000 µg/g) and the ubiquitous allergen distribution. The small particles of cat and dog allergen can scatter easily in the air and adhere to clothing for further dispersal.[35,36] Therefore, these allergens are found in homes without pets, schools, daycare centers, and public places.[35,37–47]

Data on cat and dog allergen exposure in relation to sensitization are more difficult to interpret because there is a nonlinear relationship.[24] Exposure to Fel d 1 of less than 0.5 µg/g is considered to be low and is a low risk for sensitization.[25] Paradoxically, the prevalence of sensitization is also reduced among atopic individuals who are continuously exposed to high levels of Fel d 1 (>20 µg/g).[24,48,49] Studies have demonstrated that infants exposed to the highest levels of cat allergen had decreased cat-specific IgE levels and high allergen-specific IgG levels corresponding to a low-risk phenotype for atopy.[50,51] This may help explain why early exposure to cat has been found protective for asthma and other atopic conditions.[18,19,52,53] In countries such as New Zealand, where 78% of the population owns cats and high levels of allergen occur in houses, the prevalence of sensitization to cat is only 10%, and cat is not as important a cause of asthma as dust mites.[54] Most houses that contain cats or dogs have Fel d 1 or Can f 1 levels of greater than 10 µg/g, whereas homes that do not contain these pets usually have allergen levels of 1 to 10 µg/g, placing those inhabitants at the highest risk for sensitization.[37,38,41]

In addition to risk of sensitization, studies have demonstrated that certain levels of cat allergen exposure early in life are associated with the development of asthma.[32,55,56] In geographic areas where dust mite levels are low, dog and cat have been found to be the primary allergens associated with asthma.[41] Pet allergen exposure in sensitized individuals accounts for a high number of the asthma attacks and emergency visits for asthma annually in the United States.[57] Furthermore, Bertelsen and colleagues[58] reported that cat exposure led to an increased risk of asthma independent of cat sensitization. This result indicates a possible nonallergic mechanism. Additionally, an already sensitized child who lives in a home without a cat can become symptomatic by visiting homes or attending schools where cat allergen is present, even if those locations do not physically have any cats. Schools are the best example of this phenomenon. A Swedish study showed a 9-fold increased risk of asthma exacerbations at school among elementary schoolchildren who attended classes with other students from cat homes compared with children who attended classes with fewer than 18% cat owners.[59] Therefore, passive exposure of schoolchildren to animal allergens can exacerbate asthma, even among children who are purposely avoiding pets.

Similar to cat allergen, dog allergen has a nonlinear dose-response relationship between exposure and development of sensitization. A medium-dose exposure of Fel d 1 (1–8 μg/g) is most strongly associated with the development of sensitization. Dog exposure and the development of asthma is less studied. A meta-analysis noted a slightly increased, statistically significant relative risk of asthma in pet owners, not taking into account allergic sensitization.[53] Other birth cohort studies have not been suggestive of an association.[60]

More recently, issues regarding so-called "hypoallergenic" pets have arisen. There is no scientific evidence to support the existence of "hypoallergenic" pets.[61–63] In fact, Vredegoor and colleagues[63] actually found higher levels of Can f 1 in hair and fur samples of "hypoallergenic" dog breeds compared with nonhypoallergenic breeds. In the homes of these pets, the same study found that there were not any differences in Can f 1 levels in settled floor dust or air samples between the two groups. Currently, it is standard for guidelines to state that hypoallergenic cats and dogs should not be recommended for individuals who are sensitized.[62]

Cockroach

The German (*Blattella germanica*) and American (*Periplaneta americana*) cockroaches are the most common species to cause allergies. The major allergens, Bla g 1, Bla g 2, and Per a 1, are found in saliva, fecal material, secretions, cast skins, and debris. Urban environments, low socioeconomic status, multifamily homes, and old buildings are risk factors for cockroach infestation and higher levels of cockroach allergen.[1,64,65] The National Cooperative Inner-City Asthma Study found that 85% of collected dust samples had detectable levels of cockroach allergen.[66] In public housing residences of New York City, 77% were found to have evidence of cockroaches.[67] Cockroach allergen exposure is typically assessed by measuring Bla g 1 and Bla g 2, which cause sensitization in 30% and 60% of cockroach-allergic patients, respectively.[68] Most dust samples from cockroach-infested homes contain both allergens, and there is a modest, but significant, correlation between levels of the two allergens.[69]

Increased cockroach exposure leads to increased risk of sensitization. Although the highest levels of cockroach allergen are typically found in kitchens, Eggleston and associates[12] demonstrated that the bedroom concentration of cockroach allergen was most associated with cockroach sensitization.[12] Chew and colleagues[70] showed this relationship to be dose responsive between inner city home cockroach level and cockroach sensitization in children. Atopic individuals develop IgE-specific responses after exposure to 10-fold to 100-fold lower levels of cockroach allergen compared with dust mite or cat.[25]

Several important studies have demonstrated the relationship between cockroach exposure and poor asthma outcomes in children.[16,66,71] Most notably, Rosenstreich and colleagues[66] demonstrated that asthmatic children living in inner cities who were sensitized to cockroach and exposed to high levels of cockroach allergen had significantly more frequent hospitalizations, more

days with wheezing, more unscheduled medical visits for asthma, more missed school days, and more nights with lost sleep. In that inner city study, similar patterns were not seen for dust mites or cat. A follow-up study confirmed these findings, with cockroach allergen having a greater effect on asthma morbidity in the inner city compared with dust mite or pet allergens.[16] Although cockroach allergen exposure has been shown to increase the risk of development of childhood wheeze in certain studies,[72–74] a 2018 study demonstrated that higher cockroach exposure in early childhood was associated with a decreased risk of the development of childhood asthma, possibly related to concurrent exposure to higher levels of protective bacteria in the home microbiome.[19] These findings highlight the complex relationship between environmental exposures and the development of atopy in cases in which allergen exposure is only a part of the greater exposome, as seen in Fig. 14.1.[75]

Mouse

The major mouse allergens are *Mus musculus* 1 and 2 (Mus m 1 and Mus m 2). These allergens are found in mouse urine, dander, and hair.[76] Factors that increase mouse infestation are high population density, clutter, and integrity of the residence.[1] The presence of mouse allergen spans environments from inner city to suburban and rural areas, affecting both homes and schools.[42,44,47,77–81] Phipatanakul and co-workers found that 95% of inner city homes in multiple U.S. cities had detectable mouse allergen levels and the highest levels in those homes were found in the kitchens.[78] Similar high rates have been seen in a recent study from the National Health and Nutrition Examination Survey (NHANES). Exposure to mouse allergen is not limited to homes. Detectable mouse allergen has been discovered in urban schools, and the levels of mouse allergen found in those schools can be higher than the surrounding homes.[42,44,79]

Data from inner city studies have shown that subjects living in homes with higher mouse allergen concentrations had significantly higher rates of mouse sensitization.[82] In sensitized individuals, exposure to mouse allergen affects clinical asthma outcomes, leading to increased asthma morbidity.[83–85] Ahluwalia and associates[86] demonstrated that in a city with high levels of both mouse and cockroach allergens, mouse allergen was more strongly and consistently associated with worse asthma outcomes. Supporting these results, a different inner city study found that sensitization to mouse allergen, but not cockroach, was an independent risk factor for rhinitis in children with asthma.[87] Aside from those sensitized to mouse, exposure to mouse allergen may lead to current wheeze by acting as a direct irritant, as seen in laboratory workers.[88] Similarly, exposure to high levels of mouse allergen in urban schools was associated with increased asthma symptoms and decreased lung function among students with asthma independent of their sensitization status.[79] In contrast to exacerbating current disease, the relationship between exposure to mouse allergen and asthma development is less clear. Early-life mouse exposure has been shown to be associated with increased risk of wheezing in early life[89]; however, there are data to suggest that early-life mouse exposure may not predict or may even be protective for wheeze and asthma development later in life.[19,89]

Evaluation of Allergen Exposure

Allergens are typically measured in dust samples collected by either vacuuming settled dust or gathering airborne dust from

Interplay of exposures that may affect development of atopy

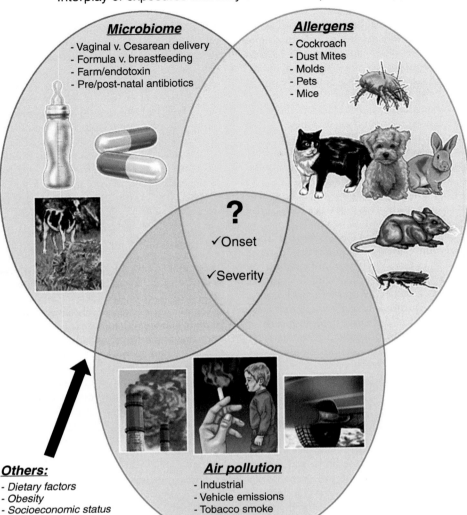

• **Fig. 14.1** Indoor allergens as a piece of several important exposures having an impact on the development of atopy in young children. Allergic disease development is influenced by many different factors. This figure notes that indoor allergen exposures are an important factor, but only one of several of the identified environmental triggers that increase susceptibility to allergic disease. (Modified from Burbank AJ, Sood AK, Kesic MJ, Peden DB, Hernandez ML. Environmental determinants of allergy and asthma in early life. J Allergy Clin Immunol 2017;140:1–12.)

filtered air within a room. Samples may be collected from multiple sites within a home or different rooms. Common sampling areas include mattresses, bedding, bedroom or living room carpet, soft furnishings such as sofas, or kitchen floors. After dust collection, fine dust can be filtered and extracted for further testing and analysis. For dust mite evaluation, collection of dust in bedding and mattresses has been the standard for investigating exposure[90]; however, Tovey and colleagues developed a novel method to measure an individual's dust mite exposure over 24 hours and found beds may not always be the main site of exposure. Cat and dog allergens are widely distributed throughout the house. Not surprisingly, the highest concentrations of cockroach and mouse allergens are usually

found in kitchens, although in heavily infested homes allergens accumulate throughout the home.

The decision to sample dust or air has to account for the aerodynamic properties of allergens.[38,91,92] Dust mite and cockroach allergens occur on large particles (10–40 µm in diameter) and cannot be detected in room air under undisturbed conditions. After a disturbance, such as using a vacuum cleaner without a filter, these particles remain airborne for only a short time of approximately 20 to 40 minutes. In contrast, cat and dog allergens can be carried on small airborne particles (1–20 µm in diameter), allowing for easier detection in air samples under undisturbed conditions and persistence in the air for several hours.[93] While airborne, pet allergens are easily able to adhere to clothing for further dispersal.

Monitoring Allergen Exposure as Part of Asthma Management

The most recent National Asthma Education and Prevention Program (NAEPP) Expert Panel Report 3 (EPR-3) significantly strengthened guidelines recommending allergen avoidance as an important goal of asthma management (Box 14.2).[94] Targeted interventions in the homes of allergic individuals can significantly improve health and should be part of the management of children with asthma. Studies of inner city asthma demonstrated that reduction of indoor allergen exposure leads to improvement of asthma symptoms, associated with a reduced use of medication and also a reduction in lost work or school time because of asthma.[95] Although patient use of home allergen monitoring devices may become more common in the future,[96] current guidelines recommend using patient histories and allergic sensitization as evidence of allergen exposure but do not include any formal allergen assessment.[94] Targeted indoor allergen avoidance strategies must account for geographic considerations and living conditions to attempt to identify the specific troublesome exposures for a specific patient.[1] Furthermore, given the ease of spread of many allergens, assessing true exposure may not always be as simple as asking families about obvious conditions in the home.[97] This is especially true of pet allergens.

Conclusions and Future Directions

Exposure to common indoor allergens has been associated with the development of atopic conditions and the worsening of already present allergic disease. The biologic function of these allergens may enhance IgE responses and play a direct role in causing allergic inflammation. The NAEPP-EPR 3 guidelines for the management of asthma recommend that for any patient with persistent asthma, the clinician should (1) use skin testing or in vitro testing to assess

---

• **BOX 14.2** **Practical Tips for the Office Setting**
Control of Indoor Allergens That Affect Asthma (NAEPP EPR-3)

- For patients who have persistent asthma, the clinician should evaluate the potential role of indoor allergens.
- Use the patient's medical history, skin testing, or in vitro testing to identify allergen exposures that may worsen the patient's asthma.
- Patients who have asthma at any level of severity should reduce, if possible, exposure to allergens to which the patient is sensitized and exposed.
- Know that effective allergen avoidance requires a multifaceted, comprehensive approach.
- Consider allergen immunotherapy when there is clear evidence of a relationship between symptoms and exposure to an allergen to which the patient is sensitive.

---

specific sensitivities to indoor allergens, (2) identify relevant allergen exposures, and (3) implement environmental controls to reduce exposure to relevant allergens. Avoidance procedures that can help reduce exposure to indoor allergens have been developed and can reduce symptoms and medication requirements. Future research will continue to focus on feasible strategies to reduce personal exposure to troublesome allergens. More development of practical methods for patients to monitor their home allergen exposures may provide additional assistance and encouragement in home allergen reduction. Finally, future research will likely focus on further investigating the relationship between home allergens and the home microbiome, as seen in Fig. 14.1.[75] It will be important to delineate the complex web among these multifactorial environmental exposures and intrinsic factors, such as genetics, within a specific patient.

The reference list can be found on the companion Expert Consult website at http://www.expertconsult.inkling.com.

15

Environmental Control

TORIE GRANT, ROBERT A. WOOD

KEY POINTS

- The major indoor allergens include dust mites, animal danders, cockroaches, rodents, and molds.
- Indoor allergen exposure and sensitivity should be considered for all patients with chronic allergic symptoms, including asthma, allergic rhinitis, and atopic dermatitis.

- Allergen avoidance should be considered the first line of therapy for patients with indoor allergen sensitivities.
- Allergen avoidance should be approached with a comprehensive specific environmental control strategy based on the patient's sensitivities and exposures.

Introduction

Aeroallergens play a major role in the pathogenesis of allergic disease, including asthma, allergic rhinitis, and atopic dermatitis. Among these, the indoor allergens, including house dust mites, domestic pets, molds, and pests such as cockroaches and rodents, are of particular importance. The relative importance of these different allergens varies in different environments depending on a variety of geographic, climatic, and socioeconomic factors. All studies agree, however, that children with asthma have a high likelihood of becoming sensitized to whichever of these allergens are prominent in their local environments. This chapter focuses on the possible role that allergen avoidance may play in the management of allergic disease.

As a general concept, it is important to recognize that allergen avoidance should be based on knowledge of the patient's specific allergic sensitivities and their environmental exposures. Based on this information, it is important to recommend a comprehensive strategy to reduce exposure to as many relevant allergens as possible. Although most of the studies in which environmental control has been proved effective used a multifaceted approach tailored to the patient's sensitivities and environment,[1–6] emerging evidence suggests that single allergen intervention could possibly be effective in reducing asthma morbidity.[7,8]

Dust Mites

Dust mites are arachnids that live in the dust that accumulates in most homes, particularly the dust contained within fabrics, such as carpets, upholstered furniture, mattresses, pillows and bedding materials, and stuffed toys. Their major food source is shed human skin scales, which are present in high numbers in most of these items. The major dust mite species known to be associated with allergic disease are *Dermatophagoides pteronyssinus* and *Dermatophagoides farinae*.[1,9–11] Dust mites grow optimally in warm and humid climates, and they grow very poorly when the relative humidity remains below 40%.[12]

Dust mite allergens settle quickly, and therefore, exposure is best sampled from settled dust rather than airborne sampling devices.[13] There is a general agreement that dust mite levels of greater than 2 μg of group 1 allergen per gram of dust should be considered a risk factor for sensitization and that levels greater than 10 μg/g of dust are a risk factor of increased asthma morbidity.[11,14–18]

The prevalence of dust mite sensitivity in patients with asthma or allergic rhinitis varies considerably from one geographic area to another, ranging from 5% in asthmatic children in Los Alamos, New Mexico; to 66% in Atlanta, Georgia; to 91% in Papua New Guinea,[19,20] and roughly correlates to mite exposure. Additionally, there is evidence that mite exposure contributes to the development of asthma.[1] In a prospective trial, Sporik and colleagues[17] demonstrated a significant increase in asthma and mite sensitivity in 11-year-old children who had experienced high mite exposure during infancy. Observational studies have also demonstrated a striking association between asthma development and mite sensitivity.[19,21–23] However, although these studies suggest mite avoidance early in life could potentially prevent development of asthma, studies of prevention have yielded inconsistent and mostly disappointing results.[24–31]

Extensive evidence also exists to support a relationship between ongoing mite exposure and disease activity.[1,32–35] With regard to chronic symptoms, mite exposure has been associated with medication requirements and asthma severity, as evidenced by bronchial hyperreactivity, peak expiratory flow rate variability, and forced expiratory volume in 1 second (FEV_1), in mite-sensitized adults with asthma.[32,34] Several studies have also demonstrated mite exposure to be a risk factor for acute asthma and emergency room visits.[18,35] Perhaps most compelling for the role of dust mites in asthma, classic mite avoidance studies from the 1980s demonstrated that through either mite control in the home or the removal of mite-allergic patients from their homes, patients experienced reduced asthma symptoms and wheezing, reduced medication requirements, and a reduction in bronchial reactivity.[36,37]

• BOX 15.1   Environmental Control of House Dust Mites

First Line (Necessary and Cost Effective)
- Encase mattresses and pillows
- Wash bed linens weekly, preferably in hot water
- Remove stuffed toys
- Regularly vacuum carpeted surfaces
- Regularly dust hard surfaces
- Reduce indoor relative humidity (dehumidify and do not add humidity)

Second Line (Helpful but More Expensive)
- Remove carpets, especially in the bedroom
- Remove upholstered furniture
- Avoid living in basements

Third Line (Limited or Unproven Benefit)
- Acaricides
- Tannic acid
- Air cleaners

Most subsequent trials of mite avoidance have yielded similar results.[38–42] In a 1-year trial, Ehnert and colleagues[40] placed 24 children with asthma and mite sensitivity into one of three treatment groups: (1) mattresses, pillows, and comforters covered with impermeable encasements; (2) mattresses and carpets treated with an acaricide (benzyl benzoate); and (3) mattresses and carpets treated with placebo. Only the group who received impermeable encasements had significant reductions in dust mite allergen levels and a highly significant reduction in bronchial hyperreactivity. In another study, Murray and colleagues[43] found children with impermeable encasements had a lower risk of hospitalization and emergency department visit requiring oral steroids versus placebo encasements; however, no effect was seen on the overall use of oral steroids, suggesting the encasements possibly affected the severity of the exacerbation, but not the overall risk of exacerbation.

However, it is important to recognize that there have been several important negative studies of mite avoidance, especially when using a single intervention such as bedding encasements,[44–46] and that meta-analyses on the efficacy of mite avoidance have yielded conflicting results.[47–52] For example, in one study of 1100 mite-sensitized adults with asthma, Tovey and colleagues[53] found that although impermeable covers resulted in significant decreases in mite allergen in mattress dust, asthma symptoms were not significantly reduced.

Dust Mite Control Measures

The exact approach to dust mite control remains controversial, because some environmental control measures have not been adequately studied; studies of their efficacy have yielded conflicting results; and, in many studies, a combination of environmental control measures was used, making it difficult to determine which measures actually led to the observed benefit. Specific environmental control measures will therefore be reviewed individually. They are summarized in Box 15.1.

It is very clear that mite-impermeable encasements for mattresses and pillows significantly reduce dust mite exposure.[1,40,51–53] In the study by Ehnert and colleagues,[40] polyurethane mattress encasements produced a 91% decrease in mite allergen by day 14 of treatment, which rose to 98% by month 12 of the study.

Encasements of the mattress, pillows, and box springs should therefore be recommended for all patients with mite sensitivity, and modern encasements made of tightly woven fabrics are more comfortable.[54]

Vacuum cleaning can reduce the allergen reservoir, but live mites are difficult to remove from carpeting, and vacuum cleaning in the absence of other measures will provide only limited benefit.[1] Patients should also be warned that vacuuming transiently increases airborne mite levels; therefore, vacuum cleaners equipped with high-efficiency particulate air (HEPA) filters may be recommended to help prevent this problem.[55] There is some evidence that wet vacuum cleaning or steam cleaning may provide additional benefit,[56,57] although one study showed that wet vacuum cleaning led to a subsequent increase in mite numbers.[58]

A variety of carpet treatments, including acaricides such as benzyl benzoate and denaturing agents such as tannic acid, also have been developed in an effort to control dust mite allergen exposure. At best, both approaches provide only modest, short-lived effects and should not be recommended for routine use.[1,39,59,60]

Because of the limitations of both vacuuming and chemically treating carpets, carpet removal is always best when feasible, especially from the bedroom of the allergic person. Additionally, excess pillows, linens, stuffed animals, and other soft furnishings are known mite reservoirs and should be removed whenever possible. Washing bedding and other soft materials in hot water (greater than 55° C) is ideal in that it both removes allergen and kills dust mites[61] but may not be achievable in many homes because of safety concerns. Washing in cooler water does not kill mites, but does remove most live mites and mite allergens very effectively. Dry cleaning also kills dust mites,[62,63] as does tumble drying at temperatures greater than 55° C for at least 20 minutes.[51]

Dust mites are susceptible to the effects of both low and high temperatures. Freezing in a typical household freezer for 24 hours will kill most dust mites, although the mite allergen in the object will not necessarily be reduced.[64] Exposing carpets to direct sunlight for several hours will also kill dust mites because of the high temperature, the low humidity, or both.[65] It also has been shown that electric blankets will reduce mite growth.[4,66] None of these methods has been established in clinical trials.

Because of the reliance of dust mites on humidity for growth, studies have shown that reducing indoor humidity below 7 g/kg by ventilation[67] or below 35% for at least 22 hours a day[68] can significantly reduce or prevent mite growth. Air conditioning and dehumidification also may help deter mite growth and should be used whenever possible; humidifiers should be avoided.[69]

Finally, air filtration devices are frequently purchased by patients for the control of their dust mite allergies; however, there is little evidence to support their use[70–73] because dust mite allergens do not remain airborne for extended periods.

In summary, effective dust mite control can be accomplished in most homes with a combination of mattress and pillow encasements; weekly hot washing of bed linens; removal of excess pillows, linens, stuffed animals, and other soft furnishings; and carpet removal.[1] Because of the convincing benefits provided through dust mite avoidance in mite-sensitive patients with asthma, these measures should be routinely recommended, and compliance with these recommendations should be reassessed at each subsequent visit.

Animal Allergens

Animal allergens are also potent causes of both acute and chronic asthma and allergy symptoms.[4,74] Cat and dog allergens are the most relevant in American homes, although significant exposure to a wide variety of other furred animals is not uncommon. Sensitivity to cat and dog allergens is very common in asthmatic children, and in some settings these are clearly the dominant indoor allergens.[20,75,76]

A number of studies have investigated the distribution of cat and dog allergens in the home and other environments.[4,20,76–79] Using settled dust analysis, cat and dog allergen levels are clearly highest in homes housing these animals; however, cat and dog allergens also have been documented in a variety of other settings, including homes without pets, office buildings, public transit, daycare facilities, and schools.[80–85] Whereas most of the environments with no animals have relatively low allergen levels compared with those with a cat or dog, it is not uncommon to find rather high levels in some of these homes. This widespread distribution is presumed to occur primarily through passive transfer of allergen from one environment to another. The particles carrying animal allergens appear to be very sticky, and, unlike dust mite allergens, can be found in high levels on walls and other surfaces within homes.[86]

The characteristics of airborne cat allergen also have been extensively studied. Cat allergen has been shown to be carried on particles that range from less than 1 μm to greater than 20 μm in mean aerodynamic diameter.[87,88] Although estimates have varied, studies agree that at least 15% of airborne cat allergen is carried on particles less than 5 μm. Dog allergen is distributed very much like cat allergen, with about 20% of airborne dog allergen being carried on particles less than 5 μm in diameter.[89] Because cat allergens are detected in cat-free homes, one study placed cat allergic participants in an experimental cat exposure facility to varying levels of cat allergen.[90] It was found that allergen levels of less than 100 ng/m^3 were capable of inducing upper and lower respiratory tract symptoms and significant pulmonary function changes. These levels are similar to those found in homes with cats and a subset of homes without cats, suggesting that even patients without known cat exposure may be exposed to clinically significant concentrations of airborne cat allergen on a regular basis.

Control of Animal Allergens

Less is known about the control of animal allergens than about the control of dust mite allergens,[91] and there are still very few studies on the clinical benefit of environmental control measures for animal allergens, although it is assumed that removing an animal from the home will lead to clinical improvement in patients. One prospective, nonrandomized study did evaluate 20 animal-sensitized asthmatic adults either who chose to find their pet a new home or keep their pet. After 1 year, there was a significant improvement in airway hyperresponsiveness and a reduction in inhaled corticosteroid use in the pet removal group compared with the pet keeping group.[92] Even fewer data are available regarding the potential benefits of methods that might be used in lieu of animal removal. The overall approach to the control of animal allergens is summarized in Box 15.2.

To begin, it should be stated that in any asthmatic patient who is known to be cat or dog sensitive and whose asthma is thought to be related to a significant degree to the pet, the most appropriate recommendation is to remove the pet from the home; however, a high proportion of patients are either reluctant or completely unwilling to remove a household pet. Once a cat has been removed from the home, it is important to recognize that

> ### • BOX 15.2   Environmental Control of Animal Allergens
>
> - Remove source (e.g., find a new home for the pet)
>   - Allergen levels fall slowly—benefit would not be expected for weeks to months.
>   - Follow by aggressive cleaning to remove reservoirs of allergen.
> - If the pet is not removed:
>   - Install high-efficiency particulate air (HEPA) filter air cleaners, especially in the bedroom.
>   - Remove carpeting, especially in the bedroom.
>   - Encase mattresses and pillows.
>   - Wash animals (not likely to help unless done at least twice a week).
>   - These measures may not reduce allergen levels enough to help highly allergic patients.

the clinical benefit may not be seen for a period of at least several months, because it can take 4 to 6 months for cat allergen levels to fall to those seen in homes without cats.[79] Levels may fall much more quickly with the removal of carpets, upholstered furniture, and other reservoirs from the home. This information points to the fact that thorough and repeated cleaning will be required once the animal has been removed. It also has been shown that cat allergen may persist in mattresses for years after a cat has been removed from a home,[93] so new bedding or impermeable encasements also should be recommended.

A number of studies have investigated other measures that might help reduce cat allergen exposure without removing the animal from the home. De Blay and colleagues[94] demonstrated significant reductions in airborne cat allergen (Fel d 1) with a combination of air filtration, cat washing, vacuum cleaning, and removal of furnishings, although these results were based on a small sample size and did not include any measure of clinical effect. Subsequent studies of pet washing have shown either no or only a transient reduction in pet allergen levels,[95–97] with the need to wash dogs at least twice a week.[97]

Information is very limited, and inconsistent clinical benefits have been seen in regard to these environmental control measures if one or more pets is allowed to remain in the home. Studies have evaluated different combinations of control measures, and although all have shown reductions in allergen levels, clinical effect was less consistent.[98–101] Two studies showed a clear benefit; one showed benefit only in the group in which environmental control was performed along with intranasal steroid treatment, and the fourth showed no clinical benefit whatsoever. It therefore still remains to be seen whether allergen exposure can be sufficiently reduced to produce a clinical effect in the absence of animal removal.

Although the notion of hypoallergenic cats and dogs is increasingly popular, there are no studies confirming that any specific breeds are predictably less allergenic.[102] Further, there is no evidence that the size, hair length, hair type, or degree of shedding have any effects on indoor allergen levels or allergenicity.[4,103] Finally, in one observational study of Swedish children,[104] children raised in homes with dogs classified as hypoallergenic were found to have a higher risk of allergy at age 6, but not asthma. However, it must be noted these hypoallergenic dogs were more commonly found in homes where parents reported having either allergies or asthma, and thus it is possible that there was residual confounding.

In families who insist on keeping their pets, the following should be recommended pending more definitive studies.[4] The animals should be restricted to one area of the home and certainly kept out of the patient's bedroom. HEPA or electrostatic air cleaners should be used, especially in the patient's bedroom. Carpets and other reservoirs for allergen collection should be removed whenever possible, again focusing on the patient's bedroom. Finally, mattress and pillow encasements should be routinely used. Although tannic acid has been shown to reduce cat allergen levels, the effects are modest and short-lived when a cat is present, so this treatment should not be routinely recommended. Similarly, cat and dog washing appears to be of such transient benefit that it is only likely to add significantly to the other avoidance measures if it is done at least twice a week.

Cockroach Allergen

The importance of cockroach allergen in asthma and allergy has been recognized for over 50 years.[105,106] Cockroach allergens play a major role in asthma, particularly in urban areas.[2,107] Significant cockroach exposure has been demonstrated in a number of cities and has been associated with high-density, urban living and low socioeconomic status.[108,109] The prevalence of cockroach sensitivity in urban patients with asthma has been shown to range from 23% to 60%,[18,108,109] with a prevalence of 21% in one suburban population.[110] In addition, cockroach exposure has been associated with higher rates of sensitization.[111] The combination of cockroach exposure and cockroach sensitization has been shown to be a risk factor for increased asthma morbidity and acute asthma exacerbations.[18,35,77]

In the first comprehensive study on the problem of asthma in inner city children, 1528 children with asthma from eight major inner city areas were extensively investigated with regard to the factors, both allergic and otherwise, that contributed to their disease.[77] Although sensitivity to cockroaches, dust mites, and cats were all common (36.8%, 36.9%, and 22.7%, respectively), exposure to cockroach allergen was much more common than exposure to either dust mite or cat (50.2%, 9.7% and 12.8%, respectively). The combination of cockroach sensitivity and high cockroach exposure was associated with significantly more hospitalizations, unscheduled medical visits for asthma, days of wheezing, missed days from school, and nights with sleep loss because of asthma. Such a correlation was not seen for dust mite or cat allergens. These data argue persuasively that cockroach allergen is a major factor, if not *the* major factor, in the high degree of morbidity seen in this patient population.

Two cockroach species, the German cockroach *(Blattella germanica)* and the American cockroach *(Periplaneta americana),* are the most common causes of both household infestation and allergic sensitization. Several allergens from each species have been identified and characterized,[112,113] with the most important among these being Bla g 1, Bla g 2, and Per a 1. There is significant cross-reactivity between *B. germanica* and *P. americana,* although most patients in the United States are primarily sensitized to *B. germanica.*

The highest cockroach allergen levels tend to be found in kitchens, although the allergen is widely distributed through the home, including the bedroom.[2,77,113] In fact, in the inner city asthma study noted previously, the 50.2% exposure rate was found in bedroom dust samples.[77] It has been suggested that cockroach allergen levels of greater than 2 U/g are associated with sensitization and levels greater than 8 U/g are associated with disease

---

• BOX 15.3 Environmental Control of Cockroach Allergen

- Regular and thorough extermination
- Thorough cleaning after extermination
- Extermination of neighboring dwellings
- Roach traps
- Repair leaky faucets and pipes
- Repair holes in walls and other entry points
- Behavioral changes to reduce food sources
- Clean immediately after cooking
- Clean dirty dishes immediately
- Avoid open food containers
- Avoid uncovered trash cans

---

activity.[77] Cockroach allergen also has been detected at significant concentrations in schools in urban Baltimore.[114] Finally, much like dust mite allergen, cockroach allergen has little or no measurable airborne allergen in the absence of significant disturbance.[107]

Cockroach Allergen Control

Chemicals for control of cockroach infestation include chlorpyrifos, diazinon, boric acid powder, and bait stations that contain hydramethylnon. These agents have been extensively studied, are readily available, and can reduce cockroach numbers by 90% or more, except boric acid, which reduces numbers by 40% to 50%. Several studies have shown that a combination of extermination and thorough cleaning can reduce cockroach allergen levels by 80% to 90%.[115–117] Although most studies to date have not convincingly demonstrated that cockroach eradication alone is capable of significantly reducing disease activity,[118–120] Rabito and colleagues[7] demonstrated fewer asthma symptoms and unscheduled healthcare utilization through the use of insecticidal bait.

In addition to these measures, integrated pest management also includes other strategies that help reduce cockroach infestation, including eliminating food sources and hiding and entry points (Box 15.3).[2,121] All foods should be stored in sealed containers, and the kitchen should be cleaned regularly. Finally, extensive cleaning should be performed after extermination to remove the cockroach debris as completely as possible. Even with the most aggressive measures, however, it may be difficult to reduce cockroach exposure adequately in some environments, such as older, multiple-dwelling units that house a preponderance of inner city residents. In a more encouraging study related to inner city pediatric asthma, a multifaceted, allergen-specific environmental control program[5] that included education, a HEPA-filtered vacuum cleaner, allergen-proof bedding encasings, and a bedroom HEPA filter, Bla g 1 in floor dust was reduced by 53% compared with 19% in the control group. More importantly, symptoms were also significantly reduced in the treated group. This trial supports the concept that integrated environmental avoidance strategies have the highest likelihood of producing beneficial clinical effects.

Rodent Allergens

Mice and rats produce allergens, primarily urinary proteins, that have been shown to cause sensitization and disease in both occupational and home environments.[3] Mouse allergens are measurable in nearly all inner city homes, as many as 75% of suburban homes, and have a significant impact on asthma morbidity,

---

• **BOX 15.4**   **Environmental Control of Rodent Allergens**

- Regular and thorough extermination
- Thorough cleaning after extermination
- Keep food and trash in covered containers
- Seal cracks in walls, door, and floors

• **BOX 15.5**   **Environmental Control of Mold Allergens**

- Identify sites/sources of mold growth
- Clean moldy areas with a fungicide
- If cleaning is not possible, discard moldy items (e.g., carpets, furniture)
- Dehumidify
- Repair leaks and maximize drainage
- Run vent in bathroom and kitchen
- Clean refrigerator, dehumidifier, and humidifier with fungicide

---

especially in urban populations.[122–131] Mouse allergen levels in inner city homes are 100-fold to 1000-fold higher compared to those in suburban homes.[132] Mouse exposure has been associated with increased sensitization, poorer asthma control, and increased healthcare utilization in pediatric and adult populations.[3,123–128,133] Like cat and dog allergens, mouse allergen is readily airborne.[129–131]

Reduction of mouse allergen and its clinical effects have been increasingly studied over the last 15 years, with Phipatanakul and colleagues[134] demonstrating a 75% or greater reduction in mouse allergen exposure using an integrated pest management strategy that included filling holes with copper mesh, vacuuming, cleaning, and baiting of traps with low-toxicity pesticides.[134] Another study in which integrated pest management intervention was performed by study participants, mouse allergen levels were only reduced by approximately 27%[135]; however, in a subset who achieved a 50% reduction in mouse allergen, there were fewer missed school days, reduced sleep disruption, and reduced caretaker burden. In 2017, Matsui and colleagues[8] reported that reduction of mouse allergen was associated with a reduction in asthma symptoms, emergency department and urgent visits for asthma, and rescue inhaler use.

Based on these studies and general information about pest management, recommendations for mouse allergen control include professional extermination, thorough cleaning after extermination, keeping food and trash in covered containers, cleaning food scraps from the floor and countertops, and sealing cracks in the walls, doors, and floors (Box 15.4).[3]

Mold Allergens

A wide variety of mold species can be present in both indoor and outdoor environments. *Aspergillus* and *Penicillium* spp. are generally regarded as the most numerous indoor molds, whereas *Alternaria* is important in both indoor and outdoor environments. Mold exposure has been associated with chronic asthma symptoms and asthma exacerbations.[136–138]

Molds tend to grow best in warm, moist environments, with basements, window sills, shower stalls, bathroom carpets, and air conditioners and humidifiers being common sources of significant mold exposure.[139,140] Airborne mold allergens have been shown to be carried on particles ranging in size from less than 2 μm to greater than 100 μm.[141]

The control of mold allergens requires a concerted approach combining fungicides, measures to reduce humidity, and the removal of mold-infested items whenever possible[136] (Box 15.5). With more severe infestation, such as after flooding has occurred, professional remediation may be required. A variety of fungicides are commercially available that are highly effective as long as the sites of mold growth are carefully investigated. Measures to reduce humidity should be recommended, including dehumidification, air conditioning, increased ventilation, and avoidance of humidifiers and vaporizers. Moldy items, such as a basement carpet that has suffered water damage, should be removed altogether.

Although no specific data are available, air filtration devices may also assist in reducing mold exposure; no clinical studies on the efficacy of mold avoidance measures have been undertaken.

Indoor Air Pollution

Although a detailed discussion of indoor air pollution is beyond the scope of this chapter, it should be emphasized that effective environmental control cannot be achieved without attention to a variety nonspecific irritants. The deleterious effects of passive cigarette smoke on pediatric asthma have been well documented,[142,143] and a variety of other indoor pollutants, such as nitrous oxide, have been documented to exacerbate pediatric asthma, especially in inner city environments.[144,145] Smoking cessation and passive smoke avoidance should be strongly recommended.

Outdoor Allergens

There is far less ability to control exposure to outdoor allergens than indoor allergens. Source control is rarely an option because the airborne pollens and molds travel so widely. Local mold control may be accomplished by ensuring good drainage, removing accumulated organic debris, and limiting the use of mulch. Exposure may be reduced by staying indoors when pollen and mold counts are high and keeping windows and doors closed. An air filter may help reduce exposure; some activities, such as lawn mowing or leaf raking, may need to be avoided altogether. After being outside, allergic individuals should wash their hands and faces immediately, wash their hair daily, and shower/bathe preferably at night.

Early-Life Allergen Exposure

Although repeated studies have shown that allergen exposure is associated with sensitization and subsequent allergic disease, more recent literature suggests that exposure to cat, cockroach, and mouse early in life can be protective against wheeze[146] and asthma.[147] More specifically, exposure to cat, cockroach, and mouse allergens in the first year of life was associated with a lower risk of recurrent wheeze at age 3 and exposure to cat, cockroach, and mouse allergens in the first 3 years of life was associated with a lower risk of asthma at age 7 in urban children at high risk for asthma. It is important to note that these were studies of early allergen exposure as primary prevention of allergic disease. Once allergic disease is diagnosed, these allergens switch to being associated with allergic morbidity and should be avoided.

Conclusions

Indoor allergens are of tremendous importance to pediatric allergic disease. Exposure is a risk factor for the development of

• BOX 15.6   Practical Tips for the Office Setting

- Perform skin testing or in vitro testing to assess specific sensitivities to indoor allergens.
- Identify exposures, keeping in mind exposure can occur in the home or school and in the absence of the known allergen (such as pet allergen in homes without pets).
- Create patient education material with practical environmental control recommendations and distribute to patients based on their sensitivities.

asthma and for more severe disease; however, evidence now suggests early-life exposure may be protective against atopic wheeze and asthma in high-risk populations. Integrated pest management can help reduce exposure to most allergens, significantly reducing symptoms and medication requirements. The guidelines for the management of asthma that were originally published in 1997 and most recently revised in 2007[148] have consistently stressed the importance of indoor allergens and environmental control, stating that for any patient with persistent asthma the clinician should (1) identify allergen exposures, (2) use skin testing or in vitro testing to assess specific sensitivities to indoor allergens, and (3) implement environmental controls to reduce exposure to relevant allergens. With all the time, effort, and money put forth for the use of medications and immunotherapy for asthma and allergic rhinitis, it is very important that we do not lose sight of this logical, feasible, and important recommendation. Box 15.6 Presents Practical Tips for the Office Setting in the management of allergies.

Helpful Websites

Allergy & Asthma Network Mothers of Asthmatics (www.aanma.org)

The American Academy of Allergy, Asthma & Immunology website (www.aaaai.org/)

American Lung Association (www.lung.org)

Association of Asthma Educators (www.asthmaeducators.org)

Asthma and Allergy Foundation of America (www.aafa.org)

Centers for Disease Control and Prevention (www.cdc.gov)

National Heart, Lung, and Blood Institute Information Center (www.nhlbi.nih.gov)

National Institute of Allergy and Infectious Diseases (www.niaid.nih.gov)

U.S. Environmental Protection Agency National Center for Environmental Publications (www.airnow.gov)

The reference list can be found on the companion Expert Consult website at http://www.expertconsult.inkling.com.

16

Immunotherapy for Allergic Disease

POOJA VARSHNEY, ELIZABETH C. MATSUI

KEY POINTS

- Immunotherapy is the only disease-modifying treatment for certain allergic diseases.
- Subcutaneous immunotherapy is an effective treatment for selected pediatric patients with allergic rhinitis with or without allergic conjunctivitis, allergic asthma, and stinging insect hypersensitivity.
- Sublingual immunotherapy is an approved and effective treatment for children with seasonal allergic rhinitis because of grass pollen allergy.

- There is a small but real risk of systemic allergic reactions with immunotherapy, and the risk associated with subcutaneous immunotherapy appears to be greater than that for sublingual immunotherapy.
- Immunotherapy is associated with changes in humoral and cellular immune responses and effector cell responsiveness.
- Various forms of immunotherapy are being actively investigated as treatments for food allergy.

Introduction

In 1911 Noon[1] found that by administering increasing doses of grass pollen extract he could induce a marked decrease in conjunctival sensitivity to grass pollen. It was this observation that eventually led to the widespread use of immunotherapy for the treatment of allergic disease.[1] *Allergen immunotherapy* is the term used to describe a prolonged process of repeated administration of allergen extracts to reduce symptoms in patients with allergic disease and confirmed relevant allergic sensitization. It is also termed *desensitization,* referring to the process of attenuating the allergic response over time. Immunotherapy is a disease-modifying treatment and is a key therapeutic option for several allergic diseases, along with allergen avoidance and symptomatic drug therapy.

Principles of Immunotherapy

In allergic rhinitis, the effectiveness of immunotherapy has been demonstrated in many carefully conducted placebo-controlled trials. The results of a typical clinical trial are shown in Fig. 16.1.[2] Three groups of patients matched on the basis of their allergic sensitivity to ragweed allergen were treated with injections of whole ragweed pollen extracts, purified antigen E (Amb a 1), or placebo. Although everyone became symptomatic during the ragweed pollen season, those receiving placebo injections were more symptomatic than those receiving pollen extracts. These trials have been reviewed in detail elsewhere[3] and are addressed here only to review the principles learned for the safe and effective use of immunotherapy.

The first principle is that clinical effectiveness is antigen-specific and dose-dependent, A patient's response to treatment depends on proper identification of relevant allergens based on history, exposure, and presence of specific immunoglobulin E (IgE). A certain minimal dose of allergen extract must be administered to produce effective symptomatic control or reduced risk of systemic allergic reaction, in the case of venom hypersensitivity.[4,5] These extracts are prepared by suspending source material (pollen, fungal cultures, dust mites, animal pelts, venoms, or fire ant whole body extracts) in buffers to extract the water-soluble components into the buffer, and they are available commercially under license by the U.S. Food and Drug Administration (FDA). Extracts are complex mixtures of dozens of proteins, of which only a few are major allergens. Clinical trials that compare treatment with purified allergens or with partially purified extracts containing high concentrations of allergens with treatment with currently available crude extracts have shown them to be equally effective. For instance, symptoms are reduced to a similar extent with immunotherapy with purified ragweed allergen Amb a 1 and with whole ragweed extract in the study, as illustrated in Fig. 16.1. Another lesson from these studies is that therapeutic effectiveness of conventional immunotherapy increases with time. Significant improvement is generally seen soon after attaining maintenance dosing.[6] It is not clear why such a long time is needed, but in part it reflects the time required to increase the injected dose from the very small dose that can be tolerated initially to the 10,000-fold higher dose that produces immunologic and clinical effects. It is also apparent that immunologic effects

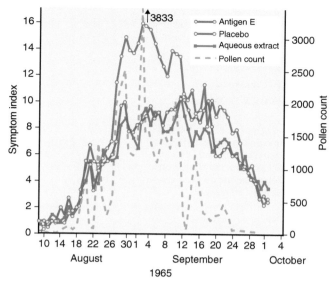

• **Fig. 16.1** Typical result of an immunotherapy trial in patients allergic to ragweed pollen. (From Norman PS, Winkenwerder WL, Lichtenstein LM. Immunotherapy of hay fever with ragweed antigen E: comparisons with whole pollen extract and placebos. J Allergy 1968;42(2):93–108.)

must be taking place very early in this process to allow the patient to tolerate increasing doses without anaphylaxis. Clinical benefit increases for several years after the maximal doses of antigens are achieved. It is important to note, however, that single-dose sublingual immunotherapy, which has been approved for pediatric use in the United States for grass allergy, has a more rapid onset of action, likely because no build-up phase is required, and is efficacious when given only part of the year, before and during the relevant pollen season.

In clinical trials when symptom scores are compared with those in untreated patients, a placebo effect is consistently seen. The placebo effect is especially easy to see in the asthma trials, in which most placebo-treated patients improve and 25% to 30% improve significantly.[7] This tenet was also notoriously illustrated by the field's decades-long practice of using whole-body immunotherapy for treatment of insect hypersensitivity until the publication of the key controlled trial of venom immunotherapy (VIT).[6] For clinical investigators, these lessons have underscored the vital importance of including a placebo group in any immunotherapy trial. For clinicians, it is important to recognize that there is a significant and powerful placebo effect associated with the repeated injections and frequent visits with sympathetic physicians and nurses. Only by administering concentrated antigen preparations to carefully selected patients are the benefits greater than those seen with sympathetic support.

The concepts of desensitization and sustained unresponsiveness, borne out of work developing food immunotherapy, are fundamental when considering the goals of immunotherapy. *Desensitization* refers to a diminished state of clinical reactivity dependent on continued allergen exposure. Although the term *tolerance* has been used to refer to the more enduring hyporesponsive clinical and immunologic state induced by treatment, *sustained unresponsiveness* may be a more accurate term, in that the duration of this state is largely unknown and may vary according to allergen, disease state, and host. For example, the

current understanding of food immunotherapy supports the need for ongoing treatment to maintain a desensitized state and potentially decrease the risk of a severe reaction (see Chapter 37). Additionally, investigating the attainment or duration of sustained unresponsiveness is challenging, in part the result of lack of long-term follow-up data and the unpredictable nature of allergic reactions. Consequently, in insect allergy, immunotherapy is continued indefinitely in patients with certain risk factors (see Chapter 43).

Mechanisms of Action

Many observations about patients' immunologic and cellular responses to immunotherapy have been made, but the precise mechanism of action of immunotherapy remains unknown. Fig. 16.2 depicts much of what is known about the immunologic changes seen during immunotherapy.[8] Suppression of mast cell and basophil activity is seen early in treatment, followed by the appearance of regulatory T and B cells and suppression of T_H1 and T_H2 responses. Specific IgE levels initially increase and gradually decrease late in treatment in some patients. Allergen-specific IgG and IgG4 levels increase early in treatment and continue to rise throughout treatment. Late changes include decreased number of tissue mast cells and eosinophils, reflected in decreased skin test reactivity.[8–11]

Antibody Response and Immunotherapy

Studies have consistently demonstrated an early and prolonged increase in allergen-specific IgE, with a slow decline months to years after starting immunotherapy. In contrast, allergen-specific IgG levels increase within months of starting immunotherapy and remain elevated, with allergen-specific IgG4 becoming more prominent than other isotypes. One trial of ragweed immunotherapy in adults that examined allergen-specific antibody responses can be seen in Fig. 16.3. Subjects demonstrated significant dose-dependent increases in ragweed-specific IgG long before symptom relief was seen. Ragweed-specific IgE initially increased and did not decrease until years into therapy.[9] Similar observations have been made by other investigators for both VIT and inhalant allergen immunotherapy, and it is noted that clinical response does not depend on reduction in IgE levels.

Allergen immunotherapy induces a shift toward a regulatory B cell phenotype, resulting in suppression of proinflammatory cytokines via production of interleukin-10 (IL-10) and induction of IgG4 production.[8] It has been suggested that allergen-specific IgG acts as a blocking antibody by either blocking antigen binding by IgE or preventing aggregation of the high-affinity IgE receptor (FcεRI) at the cell surface. Although allergen-specific IgG levels do not correlate with clinical efficacy, the functional blocking activity of allergen-specific IgG does appear to correlate with clinical efficacy, and the absence of allergen-specific IgG is associated with lack of clinical response.[10]

Effects on T Cells

Because a T_H2 phenotype has been associated with allergic disease and a T_H1 phenotype with protection against allergic disease, it has been hypothesized that immunotherapy exerts

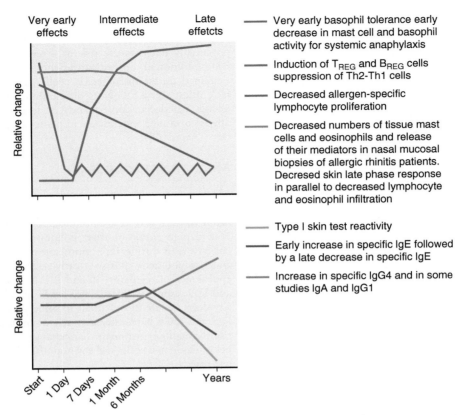

• **Fig. 16.2** Immunologic changes during the course of immunotherapy. A similar profile is seen regardless of route of administration. B_{REG}, Regulatory B lymphocytes; *Ig*, immunoglobulin; T_{REG}, regulatory T lymphocytes. (From Akdis M, Akdis CA. Mechanisms of allergen-specific immunotherapy: multiple suppressor factors at work in immune tolerance to allergens. J Allergy Clin Immunol 2014;133(3):621–631.)

its effects through modulation of the T helper phenotype. CD4+CD25+ regulatory T cells play a central role in this process and increase early in immunotherapy treatment, with associated increase in inhibitory cytokines IL-10 and/or transforming growth factor-beta (TGF-β).[8] IL-10 results in decreased B cell IgE production, increased IgG4 production, and decreased production of proinflammatory cytokines by effector cells.[8] There is the suggestion that regulatory T cells suppress both T_H1 and T_H2 responses early in immunotherapy, with a subsequent waning of this response and a shift from T_H2 to T_H1 responses[8] later in therapy.

Effects on Inflammatory Cells

There also is evidence that immunotherapy affects mast cells, basophils, and eosinophils. In the first few weeks of immunotherapy, the in vitro basophil response to allergen decreases sharply, just as it does during rapid desensitization regimens for patients with drug allergy.[8] One study demonstrated a significant decrease in metachromatic cells (mast cells and basophils) in nasal scrapings after dust mite immunotherapy.[11] Allergen-specific immunotherapy has also been demonstrated to decrease peripheral blood basophil histamine release.[12] In addition, successful immunotherapy has been associated with a decrease in the numbers of eosinophils from nasal and bronchial specimens.[13–15]

Specific Disease Indications

Allergic Rhinitis

Subcutaneous immunotherapy has been demonstrated to be quite effective in both seasonal and perennial allergic rhinitis. Many well-designed studies have examined the efficacy of immunotherapy for pollen-allergic patients with seasonal allergic rhinitis.[10,16,17] These randomized, controlled trials have been the subject of a meta-analysis that demonstrated significant symptom relief and reduction of medication requirements.[18] Immunotherapy also has been shown to be effective for mite-induced perennial allergic rhinitis[19] and also may be effective in mold-induced rhinitis.[20]

Sublingual immunotherapy tablets have been approved for treatment of allergic rhinitis with or without allergic conjunctivitis in pediatric patients with allergy to northern pasture grasses. A 2009 pediatric trial demonstrated improved allergic rhinoconjunctivitis and asthma symptoms with treatment initiated 8 to 23 weeks before the start of grass season and continued through the season.[21] A meta-analysis showed a small decrease in symptoms and need for rescue medications in patients receiving grass pollen sublingual tablets.[22]

Asthma

Many studies in the past decade have examined the efficacy of immunotherapy for allergic asthma.[23–27] Certainly, allergic

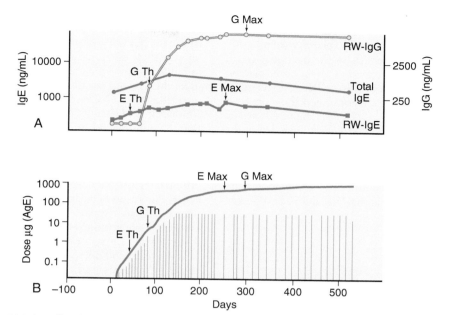

• **Fig. 16.3** A profile of a typical patient receiving ragweed immunotherapy. (A) Ragweed-specific immunoglobulin E (IgE) *(RW-IgE)*, IgG *(RW-IgG)*, and total IgE responses during ragweed immunotherapy plotted against time expressed in days. *E Max,* Maximum ragweed-specific IgE; *E Th,* threshold dose for ragweed-specific IgE response; *G Max,* maximum ragweed-specific IgE; *G Th,* threshold dose for ragweed-specific IgG response. (B) Cumulative dose *(curve)* and single doses *(lines)* plotted against time expressed in days. (From Creticos PS, Van Metre TE, Mardiney MR, Rosenberg GL, Norman PS, Adkinson NF, Jr. Dose response of IgE and IgG antibodies during ragweed immunotherapy. J Allergy Clin Immunol 1984;73(1 Pt 1):94–104.)

sensitization and subsequent allergen exposure contribute significantly to asthma morbidity in children, making immunotherapy an appealing option for children with allergic asthma. However, IgE-mediated mechanisms are only part of the underlying pathophysiology of asthma, making the rationale for immunotherapy as a treatment option in allergic asthma less straightforward. Still, the body of evidence supports the use of immunotherapy in allergic asthma, and the current asthma guidelines recommend consideration of subcutaneous immunotherapy in patients with confirmed aeroallergy who require controller therapy and demonstrate a clear link between symptoms and allergen exposure.[28]

Results of clinical trials examining the efficacy of immunotherapy in allergic asthma have been conflicting. To complicate matters further, many studies have not included placebo arms, making it difficult to draw any conclusions about efficacy from those studies. Abramson and colleagues[29] conducted a meta-analysis of randomized, controlled trials for immunotherapy in asthma. Eighty-eight trials met inclusion criteria of being double blind, randomized, and placebo-controlled. After analysis of the combined results from these trials, immunotherapy was found to reduce bronchial hyperreactivity and medication use and to improve asthma symptoms. There was no clear effect of immunotherapy on pulmonary function.

A comprehensive review also concluded that immunotherapy is effective in the treatment of asthma but in carefully selected circumstances.[30] The authors concluded that immunotherapy is effective in grass pollen asthma but that results from studies for ragweed asthma were inconclusive. In addition, mite immunotherapy with standardized extracts was effective in reducing symptoms and increasing the threshold dose of mite extract needed to induce bronchial obstruction in bronchial challenges. The authors also make the point that children receiving mite immunotherapy benefited to a greater extent

than adults, and a 2010 study demonstrated that mite immunotherapy had a steroid-sparing effect in children with asthma.[31]

Immunotherapy for animal-induced asthma has been more controversial. Some proponents of immunotherapy think there is a role for animal immunotherapy in the treatment of asthmatic patients who live with pets, but consensus statements from respected international organizations maintain that allergen avoidance is first-line therapy for these patients.[6] Carefully conducted placebo-controlled trials have demonstrated the efficacy of specific immunotherapy for cat asthma.[26,32] Studies have demonstrated a decrease in the quantitative airway responsiveness to cat allergen and decreased skin test reactivity in those treated with cat immunotherapy, but studies examining improvement in clinical symptoms have been inconclusive.

Clinical trials evaluating mold immunotherapy for asthma have been published for *Alternaria* and *Cladosporium* spp. One of the *Cladosporium* trials was conducted in children and demonstrated a decrease in allergen sensitivity on inhalation challenge but did not provide good evidence of a decrease in symptoms or medication use.[20] Some studies evaluating *Alternaria* immunotherapy have demonstrated an improvement in asthma symptoms and a decrease in medication use.[33] Although there is evidence to support the addition of certain mold extracts to an immunotherapy prescription, more data are needed before any firm conclusions can be made about immunotherapy in mold asthma.

Although many studies support a role for immunotherapy in the treatment of allergic asthma, some studies have not demonstrated the efficacy of immunotherapy for asthma. One of these was a well-conducted, placebo-controlled trial of immunotherapy for children with allergic asthma, and the investigators found little evidence to support the efficacy of polyvalent (i.e., a mixture of extracts of various allergens) immunotherapy.[23] Both the active treatment and placebo groups had a reduction in medication use and improvement in the provocative concentration of methacholine that causes a 20% drop in forced expiratory volume in 1 second (PD_{20} FEV_1), and the outcomes in the treatment group were not statistically significantly better than those in the placebo group. Despite the negative results of this well-conducted study, many other published studies have demonstrated the efficacy of immunotherapy for allergic asthma. One of the major differences in this trial is that multiple allergen extracts were included in the injections. Although this is the usual approach to immunotherapy for allergic asthma in the United States, European standards require therapy with a single allergen extract (e.g., dust mite, cat, *Alternaria* spp.), and this trial is the only one dealing with polyvalent immunotherapy. It is possible that this approach differs in some important way from immunotherapy with single-allergen extracts.

Stinging Insect

Immunotherapy for venom allergy is highly efficacious, affording protection for more than 95% of individuals undergoing treatment.[4] Although VIT is indicated in adults with evidence of IgE to Hymenoptera venom and a history of a systemic reaction to Hymenoptera, the indications in children are somewhat different. Studies of the natural history of venom allergy in children indicate that the risk of a serious reaction from a subsequent sting for a child with a history of a cutaneous systemic reaction is small. There is an approximately 10% incidence of subsequent systemic reactions in this patient population and a 0.4% incidence of more severe reactions involving the respiratory and cardiovascular systems.[34] In light of these findings, VIT has been reserved for those children who have had symptoms beyond systemic cutaneous reactions to Hymenoptera and evidence of IgE to Hymenoptera venom (see also Chapter 43), though it may be considered if requested by the child's parents or if frequent stings are anticipated.[35] Immunotherapy also can be considered in children with generalized cutaneous reactions to fire ant stings because less is known about the natural history of fire ant allergy and risk of re-exposure is generally high in endemic areas.[35]

Food

Although immunotherapy is not currently an approved treatment for food allergy, it is an area of active investigation, with evidence suggesting that first-generation treatments may be available for clinical use in the near future (see Chapter 37). Subcutaneous immunotherapy for foods has proved too risky to pursue as a treatment option. Recent studies have focused on oral, sublingual, and epicutaneous routes, with oral immunotherapy showing the greatest treatment response but a less favorable safety profile than the latter two routes.[36] Large phase 3 studies of oral[37] and epicutaneous[38] immunotherapy for peanut allergy have demonstrated desensitization in approximately 67% and 35% of subjects, respectively. These studies and others indicate immunotherapy shows promise, though several important questions remain, including optimal dose, frequency, and length of treatment.[36] It is likely that continued dosing is required to maintain the desensitized state, though further study will elucidate whether sustained tolerance is an achievable and realistic goal.

Reactions with treatment are common and unpredictable, particularly with oral immunotherapy.[39] Adverse events were reported by more than 95% of subjects in both the active and placebo groups, including events treated with self-injectable epinephrine, administered by 14% of subjects receiving active treatment and 6.5% of those receiving placebo.[37] Chronic gastrointestinal side effects are another well-known complication of oral immunotherapy. Epicutaneous immunotherapy generally results in local cutaneous reactions, with rare anaphylaxis or gastrointestinal side effects.[38] Clearly, safety will be an important factor to consider if food allergy treatment is implemented in a clinical setting, because the risk-to-benefit ratio would differ according to patient and family preferences. Although great strides have been made in developing potential food allergy treatments, one could argue that a state of equipoise still exists. A 2019 meta-analysis explored the risks and benefits of oral immunotherapy versus allergen avoidance and concluded that treatment does in fact increase the risk of allergic reactions, anaphylaxis, and epinephrine use over avoidance while inducing a modest degree of desensitization.[40] The researchers propose use of patient-centered outcomes, such as real-world food allergen exposures instead of supervised food challenge to measure efficacy in future trials. A more detailed discussion of immunotherapeutic treatments for food allergy can be found in Chapter 37.

Practical Considerations

Patient Selection

Given the generally long-term commitment required for successful treatment with immunotherapy, patient selection must take into account several different variables, including medical criteria, patient/family preference, adherence, medication requirement and response, adverse effects of medications versus immunotherapy, and desire to reduce need for medications.[6]

It is important to detail response rate and timeline to response, namely the delayed effect of immunotherapy, so patients have realistic expectations. Although immunotherapy is highly effective with careful patient selection, for most patients symptomatic improvement is partial and immunotherapy serves to decrease the severity of symptoms without totally eliminating them. In addition, a significant number of allergic patients, perhaps as many as 25%, do not benefit from immunotherapy regardless of the potency of the antigen or the length of therapy. The reasons why certain patients are "nonresponders" are unclear, but the point is an important one to bear in mind when discussing immunotherapy with patients.

Allergic Rhinitis

Immunotherapy should be considered for patients with clear evidence of IgE-mediated symptoms who have not been adequately controlled with first-line medical therapy, including antihistamines, nasal corticosteroids, and ocular antihistamines or anti-inflammatory medications. Other aspects of the patient's history should be taken into consideration. For example, successful immunotherapy requires that a patient be able to visit a physician's office weekly and spend a minimum of 30 minutes there. Certain medications, such as β-blockers and angiotensin-converting enzyme inhibitors, put a patient at higher risk for systemic reactions to immunotherapy.

Asthma

Although some of the same principles of patient selection apply, immunotherapy for asthma deserves separate commentary. As in allergic rhinitis, patients must have demonstrable IgE to allergens

TABLE 16.1	**Major Allergen Content of Extracts**						
Source	**Label**	**Allergen**	**N**	**Mean (μg)**	**Maximum (μg)**	**Minimum (μg)**
Orchard grass	100,000 BAU/mL	Dac g 5	14	918	2414	294
Short ragweed	1:10 wt/v	Amb a 1	13	268	458	87
Dermatophagoides farinae?	10,000 AU/mL	Der f 1	18	44	72	30
Cat hair	10,000 BAU/mL	Fel d 1	12	40	52	26
Dog hair	1:10 wt/v	Can f 1	4	5.4	7.2	2.7

AUs, Allergen units; *BAUs,* Bioequivalent allergen units; *wt/v,* weight to volume.

Modified from Nelson HS. The use of standardized extracts in allergen immunotherapy. J Allergy Clin Immunol 2000;106(1 Pt 1):41–5.

to which they are exposed and a clinical history of exacerbation of asthma symptoms with exposure to the allergens. A patient's ability to visit a medical facility weekly and his or her medications and age should be taken into consideration. Immunotherapy may be appropriate for treating asthma that has been difficult to control and is recommended as add-on therapy in the current asthma guidelines,[6] but it should not be prescribed for patients with unstable asthma and an FEV_1 less than 70% of predicted because of safety concerns. Additionally, screening questions assessing asthma control and β-agonist use proximate to the day immunotherapy is administered is recommended.

Allergen Extracts

Allergen Extracts for Immunotherapy

Allergen extracts are prepared by extracting bulk source materials (e.g., pollens, mite cultures, fungal cultures) in aqueous buffers; typically the potency of these extracts is expressed in a ratio of the weight of source material extracted to the extraction volume, such as 1:10 weight to volume (wt/v). Variations in the bulk sources and in the manufacturing process have led to vast differences in the quantity of active allergens in these extracts.[41] A second approach to labeling is based on the total protein content of the extract and is expressed in protein nitrogen units (PNUs); this method has little relationship to allergenic potency but is still commonly used in the United States. Efforts to standardize extracts in Europe and the United States have produced fundamentally different approaches. One approach measures the content of the major allergen or allergens in the mixture using crossed immunoelectrophoresis, immunodiffusion, radioallergosorbent test (RAST) inhibition or enzyme-linked immunosorbent assay (ELISA). Another approach compares the biologic activity of the material with the diameter of a control intradermal injection of histamine and expresses this as a biologic unit (BU). The FDA uses a slightly different approach to establish a BU, in which the flare diameter of reference extract in a select group of allergic volunteers is compared with a reference extract and expresses the result in allergen units (AU) or bioequivalent allergen units (BAUs). The results are somewhat confusing, and most commercially available extracts are labeled with more than one method to try to simplify administration of the materials. Studies that have established guidelines for effective maintenance doses for particular allergens report these doses in micrograms of major allergen, but translating wt/v, PNU, BU, AU, or BAU into microgram doses can be difficult. Fortunately, some products have also been standardized by the major

allergen concentration expressed as micrograms per milliliter (μg/mL). There are also some data translating allergen content into micrograms of major allergen; this information may be helpful in guiding dosing decisions. Table 16.1 is adapted from a comparison of labeling methods.[42] Where they are available, standardized extracts always should be used for therapy.

Storage

Some loss of potency is usual over time; therefore, manufactured extracts are supplied with expiration dates. These expiration dates are based on the assumption that the extracts will be refrigerated because loss of activity is more rapid at temperatures above 5° C. Loss of potency is faster in more dilute solutions, but it can be decreased by the addition of 50% glycerol or 0.03% human serum albumin. Because glycerol is irritating, most allergen solutions are diluted in albumin-containing buffers. Fungal, cockroach, and, to a lesser extent, dust mite extracts have been found to have significant protease activity[43] and therefore may accelerate the deterioration of allergen solutions. Some experts recommend that when mixing immunotherapy solutions, cockroach and fungal extracts should be placed in vials separate from other allergen extracts that do not contain protease activity. Dust mite extracts can be mixed with pollens and cat allergens.

Injection Regimens

A prescription for immunotherapy should reflect the patient's demonstrated specific IgE-mediated sensitization, clinical history of symptoms on exposure, and history of other medical illnesses. The decision is a complex one and should be made by a trained allergist rather than a manufacturer or testing service. Typically, a prescription is written for a treatment set, with one vial containing a 1:1 dilution of concentrated extract from a manufacturer and three or four other vials containing 10-fold dilutions (i.e., 1:10, 1:100, 1:1000, etc.). Each vial of the set should be clearly labeled with the patient's name, the allergens contained in the vial, the dilution, and an expiration date.

Administration and Dosing

Dosing instructions are shown in Table 16.2, modified from Cox[6]. There are two phases of immunotherapy: build-up and maintenance. The immunotherapy prescription is written for components of the concentrate vial; 10-fold dilutions are made to obtain the starting vial, typically a 1000-fold or 10,000-fold dilution of the maintenance vial. Various schedules are used for the build-up phase, most commonly increasing doses 1 to 3 times

TABLE 16.2 Allergen Extract Prescription[6]

The immunotherapy prescription is written for the concentrate vial (1:1). 10-fold dilutions are made to 1:1000 or 1:10,000 dilutions. Begin with the most dilute vial and administer injections subcutaneously 1–3 times/week until the maintenance dose is achieved, 0.5 mL of the 1:1 vial for aeroallergens or 100 µg of each venom. Intervals can then be spaced according to various schedules to once every 2–4 weeks for aeroallergens and once every 4–8 weeks for venoms.

The patient should remain for observation for 30 minutes after each injection. Dose adjustments should be made for lapses in treatment, large local reactions, and systemic reactions.[6]

1:1,000	1:100	1:10	1:1
0.05 mL	0.05 mL	0.05 mL	0.05 mL
0.1 mL	0.1 mL	0.07 mL	0.07 mL
0.2 mL	0.2 mL	0.1 mL	0.1 mL
0.4 mL	0.3 mL	0.15 mL	0.15 mL
	0.4 mL	0.25 mL	0.2 mL
	0.5 mL	0.35 mL	0.25 mL
		0.4 mL	0.3 mL
		0.45 mL	0.35 mL
		0.5 mL	0.4 mL
			0.45 mL
			0.5 mL

Modified from Cox L, Nelson H, Lockey R, et al. Allergen immunotherapy: a practice parameter third update. J Allergy Clin Immunol 2011;127(1 Suppl):S1–55.

• BOX 16.1 Minimum Resuscitation Equipment for Administering Immunotherapy

- Stethoscope
- Sphygmomanometer
- Tourniquet
- Syringes and needles (some 14 gauge)
- Equipment for administering oxygen by mask
- Oral airway
- Equipment for administering intravenous fluids
- Aqueous epinephrine 1:1000
- Parenteral and oral diphenhydramine
- Parental and oral corticosteroids
- Injectable vasopressor
- Glucagon kit for patients receiving β-blockers

per week. Generally, it takes 6 months to reach maintenance dosing, depending on the schedule, compliance with visits, and reactions. Alternative dosing schedules have been proposed in which the build-up doses are administered every 20 to 30 minutes (rush immunotherapy) or 2 or 3 times a week (cluster immunotherapy). These regimens allow a patient to reach the maintenance dose in a shorter time, but each has a greater risk of allergic reactions to the injections and are often not practical for children.

Duration of Immunotherapy

Once attained, maintenance doses are generally continued for 3 years or longer. If a patient is able to tolerate two sequential pollen seasons with minimal symptoms or none at all, they are able to stop immunotherapy without a relapse for up to 3 years. Although this has been shown in adult clinical trials,[10] it is likely to be true for children as well. Duration of treatment for asthma is less clear. Maintenance VIT is recommended for 3 to 5 years and may be continued indefinitely in certain cases, including in those with a history of near-fatal reaction, systemic reaction during VIT, honeybee allergy, increased baseline serum tryptase, or mast cell disorders.[35]

Reactions to Immunotherapy

The risks of immunotherapy are not trivial. The American Academy of Asthma, Allergy and Immunology and the American College of Asthma, Allergy, and Immunology initiated a surveillance

program of immunotherapy reactions in 2008, and the most recent results indicate a rate of 1 in 1 million injections for near-fatal reactions and 1 in 1000 injections for systemic reactions.[44] Such reactions are not surprising because patients are selected who are clearly allergic on the basis of skin tests and/or specific IgE tests and history of severe symptoms on allergen exposure. Reactions may be limited to urticaria, but 40% to 73% include respiratory reactions and almost 10% include hypotension; fatal reactions occur in 1 per 2 to 3 million injections.[45] From 70% to 90% of reactions begin within the first 30 minutes of an injection. The risk of reactions is greater during the build-up phase, but about half of the reactions occur during maintenance therapy. Reactions are more common in adolescents and young adults and possibly during pollen or mold seasons. Other risk factors for serious systemic reactions include severe asthma, age younger than 5 years, and use of a β-blocker.[46] For these reasons, injections should be given in a medical facility and by personnel who know how to recognize and treat a local and systemic reaction to allergenic extract and who are trained in basic cardiopulmonary resuscitation. Resuscitation equipment should be available (minimal equipment is summarized in Box 16.1). Patients should remain in the facility for 30 minutes after an injection and should report immediately if a reaction begins. Injections should not be administered at home.

Future Directions

Research in immunotherapy continues in several directions. Standardization of allergen extracts to make available products with consistent potency has dramatically increased the reliability of commercially available extracts. Studies have demonstrated the safety and efficacy of shortening the dose escalation phase with cluster, rush, and ultra-rush immunotherapy schedules. Investigators have been studying adjuvants to improve efficacy of immunotherapy and modified allergens to reduce the risk of serious reactions to immunotherapy. Other routes of administering allergen extracts are also being studied, as is the use of immunotherapy for other allergic diseases such as atopic dermatitis[47] and food allergy.[39] Finally, immunomodulatory therapies are currently in clinical trials; these include agents such as anti-IgE and anticytokine therapies.

Allergoids and Adjuvants

Allergoids are produced by chemically modifying or denaturing native allergens. The goal is to retain the ability of the allergen to elicit an immunologic response (specifically a T cell response) while decreasing the risk of anaphylaxis (the IgE-mediated response). Various chemical agents have been used, including urea, glutaraldehyde, and polyethylene glycol. Although some of these agents have appeared promising, the inability to standardize the process of chemical modification has made this approach impractical. Adjuvants are used with the allergen extract to boost immunologic response to immunotherapy in hopes of increasing its efficacy. Substances such as alum, tyrosine adsorbate, and Freund's adjuvant have been used with the rationale that they have the ability to boost T_H1-type immune responses, and more recently there has been interest in using innate immune stimulants such as TLR2, TLR4, and TLR9 ligands as adjuvants.

Peptides and Recombinant Allergens

As more is discovered about T cell epitopes, peptides of major allergens can be produced and used as a means of decreasing the risk of IgE-mediated reactions while retaining immunologic potency. In fact, fragments of both the dust mite allergens Der p 1 and Der f 1 and the cat allergen Fel d 1 were found to contain epitopes that were capable of inducing tolerance in mice.[48] This led to clinical trials that showed that injections of mixtures of small synthetic peptides containing the Fel d 1 epitope modified T cell responsiveness in allergic patients and decreased symptoms on exposure to cats.[49] The effects were modest, but other groups have improved on some of the immunologic and technical limitations of this prototype peptide vaccine and have begun to study the effect of the new formulation on cat allergy.[50]

Immune Modulators

Many immune modulators are being actively investigated as therapeutic strategies for allergic disease; these include treatment strategies aimed at IgE and those aimed at cytokines or their receptors. Several such therapies that have been approved for use in pediatric patients: anti-IgE humanized monoclonal antibody, a humanized monoclonal antibody to the IL-4 receptor α, and a humanized antibody to the IL-5 receptor α. Anti-IgE was evaluated as a treatment for allergic asthma and allergic rhinitis starting in the 1990s. Milgrom and colleagues[51] conducted a randomized, placebo-controlled trial of anti-IgE in adolescent and adult patients with moderate to severe allergic asthma. Symptom scores in the active treatment groups were improved compared with the placebo arm, but perhaps the most striking result was the steroid-sparing effect of anti-IgE. Anti-IgE also has been shown to be effective in reducing the symptoms of seasonal allergic rhinitis in adolescents and adults with ragweed allergy.[52] One randomized, double-blinded study in children and adolescents examined its therapeutic value in seasonal allergic rhinitis when added to immunotherapy. Those subjects receiving anti-IgE in addition to specific immunotherapy had significant reduction in symptoms compared with those receiving immunotherapy alone.[53] The currently available anti-IgE medication, omalizumab, is approved for use in patients 12 years and older with sensitization to a perennial aeroallergen and moderate to severe persistent asthma.

Monoclonal anti–IL-4Rα has been demonstrated to significantly reduce rates of severe asthma exacerbation and improve lung function.[54] It is also being studied for treatment of refractory atopic dermatitis in children, having recently gained approval for use in adults. Anti–IL-5Rα has been shown to reduce the annual asthma exacerbation rate and improve symptoms and lung function.[55] Antagonists to IL-4, IL-13, thymic stromal lymphopoietin

(TSLP), tumor necrosis factor-alpha (TNF-α), and IL-17 are also in various stages of development.[56,57]

Alternative Routes of Administration

Interest in sublingual swallow immunotherapy (SLIT) began in Europe as a method to reduce the risk of serious allergic reactions to therapy. Since then, many clinical trials have examined efficacy and safety, and the results of these trials have been examined in recent meta-analyses. In adults with allergic rhinitis, 49 high-quality randomized clinical trials were identified and demonstrated a significant reduction in symptoms ($P < .0001$) and medication requirements ($P = .0001$).[58] In children with asthma, nine high-quality trials were examined and the reduction in symptoms and medication requirements was significant, although less consistent than that seen in adults.[59,60] Dose requirements of relevant aeroallergens are now better defined and an order of magnitude larger than those used for injection immunotherapy. Successful studies using these doses produce symptomatic changes and immunologic changes similar to those seen with injection immunotherapy. However, the increasingly common off-label use of multiallergen sublingual drops made from commercial allergen extracts has not been endorsed by professional societies because of the lack of placebo-controlled studies and paucity of data regarding effective dose ranges.[61]

Systemic reactions to SLIT are uncommon, but local (oral and gastrointestinal) reactions are common. SLIT for grass pollen and ragweed for patients with allergic rhinitis has been approved by the FDA for use in the United States, and data on perennial allergen SLIT are emerging. The ragweed formulation is only approved for adults, and the two grass pollen formulations are approved down to ages 5 and 10 years, respectively. SLIT products generally contain either a single dose of allergen or two doses of allergen, so there is little to no build-up phase, and they can be used before and during the relevant pollen season. Contraindications include severe, unstable or uncontrolled asthma; eosinophilic esophagitis; a history of a severe allergic reaction or any severe local reaction to sublingual allergen immunotherapy; and hypersensitivity to any of the inactive ingredients. Patients should take the first dose in a medical setting and be observed for 30 minutes and have auto-injectable epinephrine available for subsequent home doses. Other routes under study include intralymphatic and epicutaneous immunotherapy.

Immunotherapy as Prevention

Immunotherapy has traditionally been used as a therapeutic intervention rather than a preventive one. However, some evidence suggests that specific immunotherapy may have a future role in the secondary prevention of allergic diseases. The Preventative Allergy Treatment Study is a European multicenter, randomized trial of specific immunotherapy for seasonal allergic rhinitis. Among the children without asthma, those who had received 3 years of immunotherapy had significantly fewer asthma symptoms than those in the open control group.[62] The children who had received immunotherapy continued to be at lower risk for asthma 10 years after initiation of treatment.[63] In addition, a study evaluating dust mite immunotherapy in monosensitized children demonstrated a decreased risk of the development of additional sensitizations in the active treatment group compared with the control group.[64] The evidence is preliminary, but there is a suggestion that immunologic intervention at an early stage of immune development may alter the natural progression of the allergic phenotype.

Conclusions

Immunotherapy is an effective treatment option for selected pediatric patients with allergic rhinitis with or without allergic conjunctivitis, asthma, and stinging insect hypersensitivity (Box 16.2). There is a small but definite risk of systemic allergic reactions; therefore, facilities administering immunotherapy should be adequately prepared to handle such an event, and patient safeguards must be in place (Box 16.3).

Immunotherapy may act to suppress allergic symptoms through modification of antibody responses, lymphocyte responses, or target cell responses to allergen. Studies are under way to determine whether modifications of immunotherapy reagents or dosing route will improve its efficacy or reduce side effects. Immunotherapy is also being pursued as a treatment option for food allergy. Additionally, immunotherapy is unique in its potential to be a disease-modifying treatment; there is some evidence to suggest that immunotherapy may alter the natural progression of allergic disease, either alone or in combination with newer biologic therapies. In both its current forms and in future applications, immunotherapy will likely remain a key therapeutic modality.

 The reference list can be found on the companion Expert Consult website at http://www.expertconsult.inkling.com.

• BOX 16.2   Key Concepts
Principles of Immunotherapy

- Efficacy is antigen-specific and dose-dependent.
- Clinical effectiveness occurs after maintenance doses are reached.
- There is a significant placebo effect.
- Approximately 75% of patients respond.
- A major risk is systemic reaction.

• BOX 16.3   Therapeutic Principles of Allergen Immunotherapy

- Immunotherapy is effective only in immunoglobulin E (IgE)-mediated diseases such as allergic rhinitis and asthma and stinging insect anaphylaxis.
- Patient selection should be based on demonstrated specific IgE relevant to clinical symptoms.
- Successful therapy requires that maximal tolerated doses of allergen extracts be given and requires months to years to reach maximal benefit.
- Because of the risk of anaphylaxis during therapy, injections should be administered in a physician's office or other medical facility that can support cardiorespiratory resuscitation. Patients should be observed for 30 minutes after an injection is administered.

17

Allergic Rhinitis

THOMAS EIWEGGER, MICHAEL B. SOYKA

KEY POINTS

- Allergic rhinitis (AR) represents 50% of all cases of rhinitis in childhood and adolescence.
- Based on the time of clinical symptom presentation, AR is classified as seasonal, perennial, or mixed (perennial with seasonal exacerbation).
- A detailed history and physical examination in conjunction with a confirmation of allergic sensitization are the hallmarks of AR.
- Diagnostic tests for AR include skin prick testing and specific

immunoglobulin E (IgE) measurements.
- Nasal allergen provocation and/or measurement of allergen-specific IgE in nasal secretions are tests of choice in complex cases.
- The treatment of AR consists of topical corticosteroids, topical antihistamines, oral nonsedating histamine 1 antihistamines, reduction of allergen exposure, and allergen-specific immunotherapy.

Introduction

Rhinitis is defined as inflammation of the membranes lining the nose and is characterized by one or more of the following nasal symptoms: sneezing, itching, rhinorrhea, and nasal congestion. Rhinitis is frequently accompanied by symptoms that involve the eyes, ears, and throat.[1,2] Approximately 50% of all cases of rhinitis are caused by allergy. In allergic rhinitis (AR), symptoms arise as a result of inflammation induced by an immunoglobulin E (IgE)-mediated immune response to specific allergens that involves the release of inflammatory mediators and the activation and recruitment of cells to the nasal mucosa.[1,2] A careful history and physical examination are the most effective tools for diagnosing AR, and specific diagnostic testing should be pursued when indicated. Management options for AR include treatment with pharmacologic agents and measures such as reduction of allergen exposure and allergen immunotherapy (AIT).[3]

Epidemiology

There are several limitations regarding epidemiologic studies of AR. First, most data regarding the true prevalence of AR are difficult to interpret, because the majority of studies use either a physician diagnosis of disease or results from patient-administered surveys and/or phone interviews. Results of both types of studies are likely to underreport the actual prevalence of AR.[2–7] In particular, perennial AR is more difficult to identify because its symptom complex often overlaps with those of chronic rhinosinusitis, adenoid hypertrophy, recurrent upper respiratory tract infections, and nonallergic rhinitis. Seasonal AR is easier to identify because of a timely association of symptoms with pollen exposure.

The prevalence of AR has been reported in up to 42% of children. In 2013 AR was reported to affect about 60 million people in the United States, with about 40% of those affected being children. The Allergies, Immunotherapy, and RhinoconjunctivitiS (AIRS) surveys reported seasonal symptoms in 78% of subjects, with the most common triggers being pollen (53%), dust (26%), and grass (26%) and nasal congestion being the most bothersome symptom.[1,4] The frequency of AR in the general population has risen in parallel with that of all IgE-mediated diseases during the past decade. The International Study of Asthma and Allergies in Childhood (ISAAC) showed that the prevalence of AR in U.S. children rose from 13.4% in 1994 to 19.1% in 2003.[5] More recent unselected cohort data at the age of 10 years from the Isle of Wright in 1999 to 2000 and the Food Allergy and Intolerance Research (FAIR) in 2011 to 2012 reported an increase of prevalence of rhinitis by 5.5% within 12 years to 28.1%.[6] Comparable trends have been reported for an adult Danish population.[7] At ages 6 to 7, boys with AR outnumber girls; however, at ages 13 to 14, girls outnumber boys[8] or show a comparable prevalence.[6,9]

Symptoms of AR develop before the age of 20 years in approximately 80% of cases. Children in families with a bilateral family history of allergy generally have symptoms before puberty; those with a unilateral family history tend to have symptoms later in life or not at all.[10–12]

Risk Factors

The exact cause of AR is not understood. The environment, in particular during the perinatal phase, plays a decisive role in the development of AR.[13] A 2018 systematic review on the role of siblingship and twin pregnancies suggests a relevant role of genetic factors on the development of AR. In the CHILD cohort study, atopic dermatitis and allergic sensitization at the age of 12 months were associated with an adjusted risk ratio of 4.44 and 4.85 to develop AR at the age of 3 years, with a relative risk of interaction of 2.65.[14] In a Mongolian population family history, adverse food and drug reactions, age, increased family income, and male gender were associated with an enhanced risk of developing AR.[15] These results match studies suggesting the prevalence is higher in more affluent socioeconomic classes, minorities, areas with heavy outdoor air pollution, individuals with a family history of allergy, firstborn children, and individuals born during pollen season.[16] Childhood studies provided evidence that the disease risk is increased in those with early introduction of food or formula, maternal tobacco smoking, indoor allergen exposure, elevated serum IgE levels, positive allergy skin test results, and parental allergic disorders. Studies published in 2018 and 2019 demonstrated associations between obesity,[17] nutrition,[18] perinatal stress stress/anxiety,[19] and poor housing and allergic predisposition. Currently there is little to no evidence for a protective effect of vitamin D,[20] probiotics,[21] and n-6 or n-3 polyunsaturated fatty acids (PUFAs) early in life.[22]

Socioeconomic Impact

Because of the high prevalence of AR, impaired quality of life, costs of treatment, and the presence of comorbidities such as asthma, rhinosinusitis, and otitis media, it has a tremendous impact on society. The severity of AR ranges from mild to seriously debilitating. The cost of treating AR and indirect costs related to loss of workplace productivity resulting from the disease are significant and substantial. AR was noted as the illness that caused the greatest loss of productivity in the workplace. The estimated costs of AR, based on direct and indirect costs, were approximately $11 billion for 2005, exclusive of costs for associated medical problems such as sinusitis and asthma.[23] In Europe, because of indirect costs, including work absenteeism, up to €110 billion was discussed for the year 2011 (Global Atlas of Allergic Rhinitis and Chronic Rhinosinusitis, EAACI 2015). In children with AR, the quality of life of both the parents and the child, including the ability to learn, may be affected.

Pathophysiology

Under normal conditions, the nasal mucosa efficiently humidifies and cleans inspired air. This is the result of orchestrated interactions of local and humoral mediators of defense and mucociliary clearance. In AR, these mechanisms do not function appropriately and contribute to signs and symptoms of the disorder.[13]

Components of the Allergic Response

Exposure to allergens in a type 2–favoring environment by antigen-presenting cells to CD4+ T lymphocytes results in the education of naïve allergen-specific T cells to develop to memory T cells, which then release interleukins (ILs), such as IL-4, IL-5, IL-9, and IL-13 (Fig. 17.1).[13,24–26] In particular, IL-4 is instrumental in IgE production against these allergens by favoring the isotype switch to IgE. Local IgE production by plasma cells and the mucosal infiltration and actions of mast cells, basophils, and eosinophils are key events in response to the allergen on exposure in sensitized individuals. Allergens cross-link membrane-bound IgE with immediate mediator release and the induction of mediator

synthesis in basophils, mast cells, and eosinophils. Moreover, local allergen-specific T cells are recruited and activated. In addition, allergen-related factors or inherent activities affect epithelial barrier function and facilitate the release of epithelial alarmins such as IL-25, IL-33, and thymic stromal lymphopoietin (TSLP),[27,28] which affect antigen-presentation and polarization of antigen-presenting cells and alter the threshold of key effector cells such as mast cells, eosinophils, and basophils, which trigger a cascade of events that result in the symptoms of AR (see Fig. 17.1). The manifestation of AR is facilitated by a lack or suboptimal functionality of regulatory B and T cell subsets.[27,29,30] The immunologic response in AR can be divided into two phases: the early-phase response and the late-phase response.

Early Phase

On exposure to allergens and cross-linking of membrane-bound IgE, degranulation and release of preformed mediators takes place. Products of this process include preformed mediators such as histamine, tryptase (mast cell–specific marker), chymase (connective tissue mast cells only), kininogenase (generates bradykinin), heparin, and other enzymes. In addition, mast cells secrete several inflammatory mediators after de novo synthesis, including prostaglandin D_2 and sulfidopeptidyl leukotrienes C_4, D_4, and E_4. These mediators cause blood vessels to leak and produce the mucosal edema and watery rhinorrhea characteristic of AR. Glands secrete mucoglycoconjugates and antimicrobial compounds and dilate blood vessels to cause sinusoidal filling and consequently occlusion and congestion of nasal air passages. In addition, sensory nerves that convey the sensation of nasal itch and congestion and recruit systemic reflexes such as sneezing are stimulated. These responses develop within minutes of allergen exposure and thus constitute the early-phase allergic response.[20] Sneezing, itching, and copious, clear rhinorrhea are characteristic symptoms during early-phase allergic responses, although some degree of nasal congestion also can occur.

Late Phase

The mast cell–derived mediators released during early-phase responses are hypothesized to act on postcapillary endothelial cells to promote the expression of vascular adhesion molecule and E-selectin, which facilitate the adhesion of circulating leukocytes to the endothelial cells. Chemoattractant cytokines such as IL-5 promote the infiltration of the mucosa with eosinophils, neutrophils, basophils, T lymphocytes, and macrophages.[31] During the 4- to 8-hour period after allergen exposure, these cells become activated and release inflammatory mediators, which in turn reactivate many of the proinflammatory reactions of the immediate response. This cellular-driven, late inflammatory reaction is the late-phase response. This reaction may be clinically indistinguishable from the early phase, but congestion tends to predominate. Eosinophil-derived mediators such as major basic protein, eosinophil cationic protein, and leukotrienes have been shown to damage the epithelium, ultimately leading to the clinical and histologic pictures of chronic allergic disease. In addition to mast cells and eosinophils, basophils also play a role in this process. Basophils and mast cells are potent sources of type 2 cytokines and chemokines, apart from the previously mentioned preformed and newly synthesized mediators.

Subsets of the T helper lymphocytes are the likely orchestrators of the chronic inflammatory response to allergens. T helper type 2 (T_H2) cells promote the allergic response by releasing mediators such as IL-4, IL-5, IL9, IL13, thymus- and activation-regulated

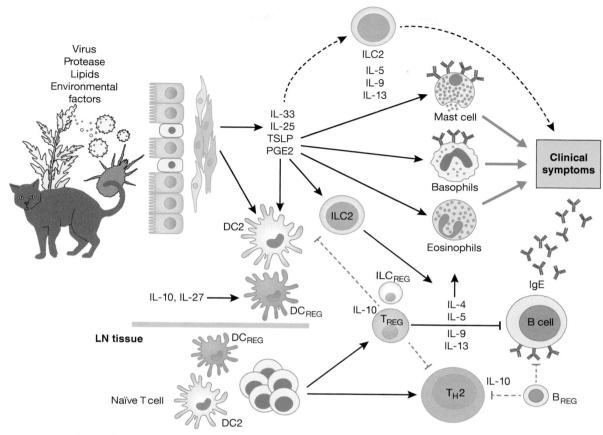

• **Fig. 17.1** Pathomechanisms of allergic rhinitis. *B*REG, Regulatory B lymphocyte; *DC2*, dendritic cell type 2; *D*REG, regulatory dendritic cells; *IgE*, immunoglobulin E; *IL*, interleukin; *ILC2*, type 2 innate lymphoid cell; *LN*, lymph node; *PGE2*, prostaglandin E2.

chemokine (TARC), and many more that promote IgE production, eosinophil chemoattraction, and survival in tissues and mast cell recruitment and activation.[31] T_H17 cells contribute to immune responses in AR by increasing the production of proinflammatory cytokines in the epithelium on IL-17A release.[32,33] T_H17 cells in concert with type 2 inflammation elevate the sensitivity to allergens on recurrent exposure. This process is called *priming* and is hypothesized to be a result of the influx of inflammatory cells that occurs during late-phase allergic responses. The exposure to one relevant allergen may promote an exaggerated response to other allergens to which the individual is susceptible.[32] The priming phenomenon, together with the well-established linkage of epitope spreading and disease severity, emphasizes the need to intervene in the allergic cascade at an early point by the prompt initiation of preseasonal, prophylactic antiinflammatory therapy or even primary and secondary preventive strategies.[34–36]

Inflammatory cytokine responses cause barrier function impairment, induction of epithelial inflammation, up-regulation of adhesion molecules, release of alarmins, and ultimately reshaping of the mucosal structure. Furthermore, pollen and environmental allergens seem to cause epithelial barrier dysfunction, alarmin release, and leakiness through protease activity.[37–42]

Classification

AR can be classified depending on the time and type of exposure in a seasonal and perennial form. In general, seasonal AR is usually caused by outdoor allergens such as pollen and mold, whereas perennial AR most frequently is due to indoor allergens such as house dust mite and animal dander. The 2001 ARIA guidelines introduced the new terms of *intermittent* and *persistent* AR, which are not widely used in clinics and research.[43] Most of the cases are either perennial or mixed with seasonal exacerbations; only about 20% are strictly seasonal.

Seasonal Allergic Rhinitis

The seasonal form of AR is commonly caused by outdoor allergens, including pollen and mold spores. In these cases, symptoms occur in a locally defined time span or season according to the geographic location and pollinating season of trees, grasses, and weeds of the respective area. Mold spores can occur the whole year through, and certain outdoor molds show seasonal variations and higher spore levels in summer and fall.[13,44] It is of utmost importance to know the local pollen calendar and to match it with a thorough clinical history of a patient to judge the relevance of a positive allergy test in the context patient complaints. It is a common mistake not to discern between irrelevant sensitizations and truly allergic symptoms. Most patients will report classic rhinitis symptoms, including watery rhinorrhea, nasal congestion, itching, and sneezing, along with ocular symptoms in those who have allergic conjunctivitis. Unspecific nasal hyperresponsiveness to temperature changes and exogenous triggers, including perfumes and smoke exposure, may persist even longer than the actual pollen season.[45]

Perennial Allergic Rhinitis

The definition of persistent AR in patients with perennial symptoms, according to the ARIA guidelines, includes the presence of symptoms on more than 4 days per week and a duration of more than 4 weeks. The severity of symptoms may be further divided into mild (no impairment of daily activities) and moderate to severe (with abnormal sleep or impairment in daytime activities). In contrast to seasonal AR, nasal congestion and mucus production, including postnasal drip, are predominantly present and sneezing, itching, and watery rhinorrhea might be less pronounced.[46] In perennial AR the triggering factor may be more difficult to be elucidated, and situational changes such as alleviation of symptoms during high-altitude stays might be important hints for specific factors such as mite allergies. Overlaps between forms can occur, depending on the extent of sensitizations to different allergens.

Differential Diagnosis

Other conditions may mimic symptoms of AR, and in children infectious rhinitis and adenoid hypertrophy are the most common. Box 17.1 summarizes the broad spectrum of differential diagnoses and groups of diseases. Differential diagnoses in AR pose a diagnostic challenge because many conditions share the same symptoms, and nasal hyperreactivity is found in allergic and nonallergic rhinitis forms.[47] In patients with short duration of symptoms (2–4 weeks or less) a watchful waiting strategy is justified.

In persistent unilateral (fetid) rhinorrhea, a foreign body should be suspected and thorough nasal examination, including bilateral nasal endoscopy, is warranted to exclude other nasal lesions or a

---

• BOX 17.1   Causes of Rhinitis

Allergic Rhinitis
- Seasonal
- Perennial
- Perennial with seasonal exacerbation
- Local allergic rhinitis

Nonallergic Rhinitis
- Infectious
- Idiopathic
- Nonallergic rhinitis with eosinophilia
- Drug-induced
- Hormonal
- Atrophic
- Gustatory
- Toxic/occupational
- Autoimmune
  - Granulomatosis with polyangiitis
  - Eosinophilic granulomatosis with polyangiitis
  - Sarcoid

Anatomic
- Adenoid hypertrophy
- Foreign body
- Choanal atresia
  - Tumors
  - Cerebrospinal fluid leaks

Rhinosinusitis
- Chronic with and without nasal polyps
  - Cystic fibrosis
  - Primary ciliary dyskinesia
  - Fungal/allergic fungal

---

contralateral foreign body. Bloody discharge, unilateral breathing impairment, and pain pose alarm signs that should lead to specialist ear, nose, and throat examination.

In the absence of a good correlation between clinical symptoms and allergy test results (refer to "Diagnostic Tests" section), other tests, including bacteriologic examinations, cytologic studies, a sweat test, nasal nitric oxide measurement, and ciliary microscopy, may help exclude other diagnoses such as cystic fibrosis and primary ciliary dyskinesia. Blood sampling may help identify patients with immunodeficiencies or autoimmune disease, and computed tomography can rule out chronic rhinosinusitis or sinonasal tumors. Even in cases without trauma history, β-trace or β-transferrin tests are indicated when a cerebrospinal fluid leak is suspected in watery (unilateral) discharge; glucose testing of secretions is not recommended because of its lack of sensitivity and specificity. No conventional radiographs should be obtained in sinonasal disorders.

Evaluation and Management

History and Physical Examination

Obtaining a thorough history and performing a careful physical examination are most effective in diagnosing AR.[1] This will not only allow discrimination between relevant and irrelevant type 1 sensitizations but will also help identify the trigger factor. AR diagnosis is often delayed because of misdiagnosis of recurrent colds in children. It is of utmost importance to also focus on potential comorbidities such as asthma, atopic dermatitis/eczema, and otitis media and to perform the respective diagnostic tests with a very low threshold.[48] Family history of allergic disease, atopic dermatitis, and asthma may be helpful in finding the correct diagnosis. Asthma occurs in approximately 20% of AR cases.

The typical signs and symptoms are summarized in Box 17.2. Most patients will present with a stuffy nose and rhinorrhea, and sneezing and itching are frequently reported as well. Some patients might report specific factors triggering symptoms but also alleviating them, providing good hints for potential causes. In children with oral allergy syndrome, also called pollen-food allergy syndrome; allergic reactions; and intolerances to specific food should be investigated.[49] Component testing may be helpful (see discussion of specific IgE [sIgE] testing). Nasal obstruction can lead to xerostomia, especially at nighttime, and sometimes snoring. This may cause sleep disturbances and daytime sleepiness or difficulties in concentration at school and work. Even depressive mood has been reported in children with AR.[50] Similarly to patients with adenoid facies, patients with

---

• BOX 17.2   Signs and Symptoms of Allergic Rhinitis

- Clear, watery rhinorrhea (bilateral)
- Itching of nose, eyes, ears, palate, and throat
- Sneezing, often repetitive
- Nasal congestion
- Trouble with middle ear ventilation
- Mouth breathing
- Postnasal drip
- Chronic, nonproductive cough
- Frequent throat clearing
- Sleep disturbance
- Daytime fatigue

AR and chronic mouth-breathing may develop a specific facial appearance that many experienced clinicians think is typical for AR. A typical but nonspecific appearance of patients with AR includes the allergic crease, a horizontal wrinkle in the supratip-region of the nose that is caused by repetitive upward rubbing of the outer nose with the palm of the hand. This is often also referred to as the "allergic salute."[51] Some authors think that darkening of the skin beneath the eyes, so called shiners, are more often observed in patients with AR.

A nasal voice, snorting, sniffing, and repetitive clearing of the throat are more often observed in older children and adults. Frequent nose blowing and picking of the nose may lead to epistaxis. Hyposmia or anosmia is reported by children, especially of younger age, and should prompt the treating physician to perform or indicate nasal endoscopy to rule out olfactory cleft disease.[52]

There is no specific endonasal finding in AR. Inferior turbinates may appear swollen, bluish, and hyperemic. The mucosa is boggy, and clear secretions are found throughout the nasal cavity. Swollen mucosa in the middle meatus points toward involvement of the sinuses. The nares often form fissures and redness of the skin as a result of chronic irritation by nasal discharge and frequent cleaning.

Extranasal findings include conjunctival edema and redness and watery eyes. The absence of eardrum movement on Valsalva or Toynbee maneuver points toward eustachian tube dysfunction. In very severe cases, serous otitis media may be observed. Cough and wheezing will point the clinician toward the presence of concomitant asthma. All findings are aggravated in the peak pollen seasons.

Evaluation and Management

Diagnostic Tests

Confirmation of sensitization to specific allergens such as dust mites, pollen, and animal dander is helpful in establishing a specific allergic diagnosis. Consequently, it is imperative for physicians to remember that positive test results for allergen sIgE are not by themselves sufficient for a diagnosis of allergic disease. A decision about whether the sIgE antibodies are responsible for clinically apparent disease must be based on the physician's assessment of the entire clinical picture. The current standard for the diagnosis of allergic disease remains the combination of (1) positive history, (2) the presence of sIgE antibodies, and (3) demonstration that the symptoms are the result of IgE-mediated inflammation (i.e., treatment response, potentially local provocation). Testing should be closely oriented to the history, seasonal and perineal reaction patterns, and geographic location to avoid unnecessary testing and unintended avoidance behavior.

The skin prick test (SPT) assesses the relevance of mast cell–bound IgE in the skin. It is easy to perform, is inexpensive, and can be done in a child of any age. Sensitization to inhalant allergens increases over time, and it is less likely to show positive results in very young children. However, this should not prevent the clinician considering environmental allergies as a cause of chronic rhinitis in very young children. Physicians should be selective in the use of allergens for skin testing, focus on common allergens of potential clinical importance, and have cross-reactivities in mind. The geographic location is very important for pollen allergy, and so are the living conditions of the family and the associated likelihood of exposure to allergenic sources. Therefore, allergens used for skin testing must be individualized and should be selected on the basis of prevalence in the patient's geographic area and home and school environments.

The most important allergens for testing in a child with perennial inhalant allergy are dust mite, animal dander, and molds and fungi. Allergens that are important in the diagnosis of seasonal AR are weed, grass, and tree pollen, and some molds such as *Alternaria alternata* can have a very strong seasonal character.

sIgE to allergen extracts and specific allergens (often referred to as *components*) can be measured in serum and on a research basis in nasal lavage. Serum IgE measurements have advantages and disadvantages over the SPT [39] (Table 17.1). Over the last decade component-specific testing, which focuses on allergen sIgE versus extract sIgE has been established. It is considered to be of a higher specificity because allergens belonging to protein families, which show a high degree of conservation over time, can be omitted or tested for specifically. These cross-reactive allergens may significantly confound clinical interpretation of the test results with extracts. In addition to single tests for specific components, microarrayed, recombinant, or purified allergens have been established. These assays allow for the assessment of sensitization to an array of allergens. Although these methods are available in some areas in Europe, there is very little availability in North America. These array technologies are likely to change the future diagnostic landscape for AR. The major advantage of microarray testing lies in the potential to incorporate hundreds of allergens that could be assayed in parallel with a very small amount of serum. Additionally, potential exists for a greater resolution between clinical reactivity and asymptomatic sensitization with this platform. It requires a basic understanding of allergen protein families and cross-reactivity (see Molecular Allergology User's guide, EAACI 2016).

The array design implies that lower amounts of allergen are available for binding, which results in a higher rate of competition with other allergen-specific antibody isotypes (e.g., IgG). This in turn may cause a lower sensitivity compared with single-allergen solutions such as the most commonly applied ImmunoCAP system. Therefore, direct comparison between arrays and the ImmunoCAP system is possible only to a certain extent.

Specific Nasal Testing

Local IgE may be more specific in predicting clinical reactivity. In cases in which SPT or serologic IgE diagnosis is in doubt, the nose poses an almost perfect organ to directly test for an allergic response. Sometimes it is necessary to evaluate whether a positive SPT result is of real relevance for a patient, before desensitization.[53] Furthermore, in some patients with high suspicion of allergy with negative SPT or IgE test results, local AR (local sensitization in the absence of a systemic response) must be ruled out.[54] In these cases, nasal provocation and measurement of sIgE in nasal secretions are tests of choice and may be safely performed in children.[55] These procedures are reserved to a few centers, and local IgE measurements lack standardization.

Sensitization testing is very important and should be performed in the context of clinical and diagnostic consequences for the patient. Panel testing, in particular to extracts, should be avoided. Given the importance of specific recommendations for immunotherapeutic interventions, the relative contribution of individual sensitizations may be assessed. Evidence-based treatment

TABLE 17.1   Immunoassays to Assess Allergic Sensitization

Skin Prick Test	Specific IgE Extracts	Specific IgE Allergen/Component
Extract based/cross-reactivity	Extract-based/cross-reactivity	Complementary to extract testing Specific allergens within an allergen extract
Less expensive	Expensive	Expensive
General availability	Broad availability	Not generally available in every country
Results available immediately	Often batchwise testing/days	Often batchwise testing/days
Depends on a number of medications (antihistamines, immunosuppressants, leukotriene receptor antagonists, antiepileptic drugs)	Not suppressed by antihistamines	Not suppressed by antihistamines
Quantification is limited	Results are quantitative	Results are quantitative
Unspecific reactions as a result of local irritation	Preferable to skin testing in: Dermatographism Widespread dermatitis Uncooperative children	Risk assessment pollen-fruit syndromes versus "true" food allergy
Minimal chance of a systemic reaction	No patient risk	No patient risk
High sensitivity	High sensitivity	Lower sensitivity

preparations for subcutaneous or sublingual immunotherapy (i.e., products that have been tested in placebo-controlled trials) should be favored over nontested mixtures.

Guidelines for Diagnosis and Management

Strategies for the evaluation and management of AR are summarized in an algorithm compiled by the Joint Task Force on Practice Parameters in Allergy, Asthma and Immunology[2] (Fig. 17.2). A similar approach has been emphasized in the MACVIA clinical decision algorithm (Fig. 17.3).[56] As outlined, the initial evaluation of a patient with rhinitis symptoms (e.g., rhinorrhea, nasal congestion, sneezing, nasal pruritus, postnasal drainage, and conjunctivitis) should be performed by a primary care physician. The primary care physician should institute an appropriate therapeutic trial. On follow-up, the primary care physician should determine whether the patient has responded to treatment and/or meets the criteria for consultation with an allergist, as summarized in Box 17.3. One of the primary purposes of a consultation with an allergist is the differential diagnosis of AR based on the combined results of a detailed medical history, physical examination of the airway, and ancillary tests, particularly skin tests.

Effective management of AR may require a combination of aggressive avoidance measures including education regarding allergen avoidance and the administration of pharmacologic therapy, AIT, management of co-existing conditions, and adjustments in pharmacologic therapy. Co-operative follow-up is an essential part of the successful management of AR and ideally includes the patient, the family, and all healthcare providers. With the common goal of reducing symptoms and improving functional ability, all involved would cooperatively manage exacerbations and complications through the optimal use of environmental avoidance measures, medications, and immunotherapy in appropriately selected patients. Periodic assessments and continued patient education should be included in the follow-up protocol.

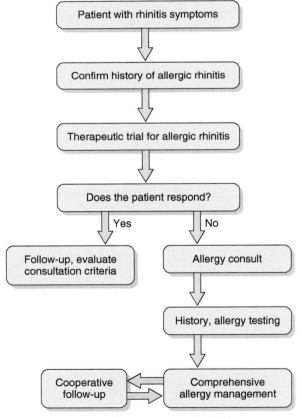

• **Fig. 17.2** Diagnosis of allergic rhinitis.

Management

Specific treatment options include environmental controls for allergen avoidance, pharmacotherapy, and immunotherapy. In all cases, the primary goal of treatment is to control the symptoms

Assessment of Control in **Untreated** Symptomatic Patient

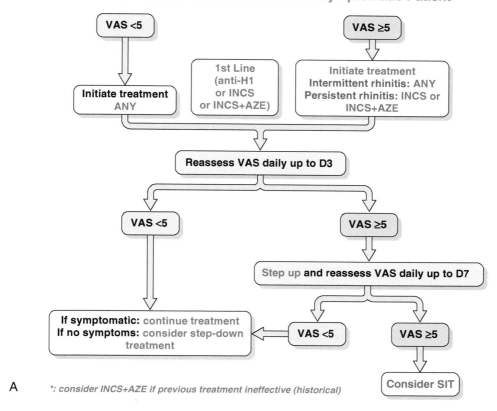

A   *: consider INCS+AZE if previous treatment ineffective (historical)

Assessment of control in **treated** symptomatic patient

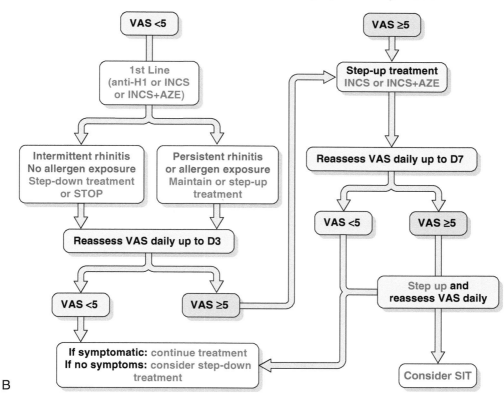

B

• **Fig. 17.3** Step-up algorithm in untreated (A) and treated (B) patients using Visual Analogue Scale (adolescents). If ocular symptoms remain once treatment has been initiated, add intraocular treatment. VAS levels are shown in ratios. *AZE,* Azelastine; *D3,* day 3; *D7,* day 7; *INCS,* intranasal corticosteroid spray; *SIT,* specific immunotherapy. (With permission from Bousquet J, Schünemann HJ, Togias A, et al. Next-generation Allergic Rhinitis and Its Impact on Asthma (ARIA) guidelines for allergic rhinitis based on Grading of Recommendations Assessment, Development and Evaluation (GRADE) and real-world evidence. J Allergy Clin Immunol 2020;145(1):70–80.)

TABLE 17.2   Environmental Control of Allergen Exposure

Allergens	Control Measures
Dust mites	Encase bedding in mite-proof covers Wash bedding in water at temperatures >130° F Remove wall-to-wall carpeting Remove upholstered furniture Daily vacuum-cleaning in bedrooms Remove stuffed animals from bed Consider air-cleaner
Animal dander	Avoid furred pets Keep animals out of patient's bedroom
Cockroaches	Control available food supply Keep kitchen/bathroom surfaces dry and free of standing water Professionally exterminate
Mold	Destroy moisture-prone areas Avoid high humidity in patient's bedroom Repair water leaks Check basements, attics, and crawl spaces for standing water and mold
Pollen	Keep automobile and house windows closed Control timing of outdoor exposure Restrict camping, hiking, and raking leaves Drive in air-conditioned automobile Air-condition the home Install portable, high-efficiency particulate air filters Wash hair regularly before bedtime

and improve the quality of life without altering the patient's ability to function. A second but equally important goal is to prevent the development of sequelae of AR such as asthma exacerbations.[2,57]

The Joint Task Force on Practice Parameters in Allergy, Asthma and Immunology previously published guidelines on the diagnosis and management of AR, and in 2019 the next Generation Allergic Rhinitis and its Impact on Asthma Guidelines (ARIA) were published, including real-world data generated by mobile technologies and provocation chamber data.[58a] It clearly highlighted the disconnection between recommendation and actual adherence, emphasizing the importance of communication and shared decision making.

Environmental Control for Allergen Avoidance

Educating families about avoiding exposure to allergens is an essential part of the treatment of AR (Table 17.2). Unfortunately, the specific measures are often highly impractical; moreover, they may have negative psychosocial ramifications for children that should not be ignored. Avoiding outdoor sports in the springtime and banishing furred pets from the home, for example, may have adverse effects on children that range beyond allergen control. Nevertheless, families should be taught about the importance of environmental control measures and advised to adhere to them to the extent possible.[2]

Antihistamines

Oral antihistamines are available as first-generation (sedating) antihistamines and so-called nonsedating or second-generation antihistamines (Table 17.3). Sedating antihistamines are not recommended for the treatment of AR because of their side effect profile (binding to the H1 receptors in the central nervous system [CNS]); antiserotonergic, anticholinergic, α-adrenergic blocking activities; and sedative and performance-impairing effects.[58b]

Antihistamines are available in both oral and nasal formulations. The practical decision in choosing between an oral or nasal formulation is often driven by a variety of factors, including insurance coverage, side effects, and patient preference. Nasal antihistamines relieve sneezing, nasal itching, congestion, and postnasal drip. Additionally, they have some efficacy against nasal and ostial congestion. Onset of action is within minutes, and these are often administered on an as-needed basis. Side effects of these products include a bitter taste, drowsiness, and fatigue.[59] Oral antihistamines achieve comparable results but are less effective regarding nasal congestion, and, consequently, combinations

with topical corticosteroids or short-term decongestants may be indicated.

Decongestants

Decongestants produce vasoconstriction within the nasal mucosa through α-adrenergic receptor activation and therefore are effective in relieving the symptoms of nasal obstruction. However, these agents have no effect on other symptoms such as rhinorrhea, pruritus, or sneezing and may be most effective when used in combination with other agents, such as antihistamines. The most commonly used decongestant is pseudoephedrine. The most common side effects of oral decongestants are CNS (i.e., nervousness, insomnia, irritability, headache) and cardiovascular (i.e., palpitations, tachycardia) effects.

Topical intranasal decongestants are sometimes used by patients with AR. However, when these agents are used for longer than 3 to 5 days, many patients experience rebound congestion after withdrawal of the drug. If patients continue to use these medications over several weeks, a form of rhinitis, rhinitis medicamentosa, will develop that can be difficult to treat effectively.[59–61]

Intranasal Corticosteroids

Topical intranasal corticosteroids (INCSs) represent the most efficacious agents for the treatment of AR, are considered superior to H1 antihistamine therapy, and are useful in relieving symptoms of nasal pruritus, rhinorrhea, sneezing, and congestion. These drugs exert their effects through multiple mechanisms, including vasoconstriction and reduction of edema, suppression of cytokine production, and inhibition of inflammatory cell influx. These

TABLE 17.3 Nonsedating Antihistamines

Medication	Formulations	Recommended Dosage
Azelastine	Nasal spray	≥12 yr: 2 sprays per nostril bid
		5–11 yr: 1 spray per nostril bid
Cetirizine	Tablets 5, 10 mg	≥12 yr: 10 mg/day
	Syrup 5 mg/5 mL	6–11 yr: 5–10 mg/day
		6 mo–5 yr: 5 mg/day
Desloratadine	Tablets 5 mg	≥12 yr: 5 mg/day
	Syrup 2.5 mg/5 mL	6–11 yr: 2.5 mg/day
		1–5 yr: 1.25 mg/day
		6–11 mo: 1 mg/day
Fexofenadine	Capsules/tablets 30, 60, 180 mg	≥12 yr: 60 mg bid or 180 mg/day
	Syrup 30 mg/5 mL	2–11 yr: 30 mg bid
Rupatadine	Syrup	2–11 yr, 10–25 kg: 2.5 mg/day
		2–11 yr, >25 kg: 5 mg/day
	Tablets 10 mg	≥12 yr: 10 mg/day
Levocetirizine	Tablets 5 mg	≥12 yr: 5 mg/day
	Syrup 2.5 mg/5 mL	6–11 yr: 2.5 mg/day
Loratadine	Tablets 10 mg	≥12 yr: 10 mg/day
	Syrup 5 mg/5 mL	6–11 yr: 5–10 mg/day
		2–5 yr: 5 mg/day
Olopatadine	Nasal spray	≥12 yr: 2 sprays per nostril bid
Bilastine	Tablet	≥12 yr: 20 mg/day

TABLE 17.4 Intranasal Corticosteroid Sprays

Corticosteroid	Dose per Actuation (mcg)	Recommended Dosage
Beclomethasone	42	≥6 yr: 168–336 mcg/day bid
Budesonide	32	≥12 yr: 64–256 mcg/day
		6–11 yr: 64–128 mcg/day
Ciclesonide	50	≥6 yr: 200 mcg/day
Flunisolide	25	≥14 yr: 200–400 mcg/day bid
		6–14 yr: 100–200 mcg/day bid
Fluticasone furoate	27.5	>12 yr: 110 mcg/day
		2–11 yr: 55 mcg/day
Fluticasone propionate	50	≥4 yr: 100–200 mcg/day
Mometasone furoate	50	≥12 yr: 100–200 mcg/day
		2–11 yr: 100 mcg/day
Triamcinolone acetonide	55	≥12 yr: 110–220 mcg/day
		6–11 yr: 110 mcg/day

agents work best when taken regularly on a daily basis or prophylactically in anticipation of an imminent pollen season. A number of glucocorticoid compounds are available for intranasal use in both aerosol and aqueous formulations (Table 17.4). Clinical trials have been unable to demonstrate significant differences in efficacy.[43,59–61]

The most important pharmacologic characteristic differentiating these agents is systemic bioavailability. After intranasal administration, the majority of the dose is swallowed. Most of the available compounds, including beclomethasone dipropionate, budesonide, flunisolide, and triamcinolone acetonide, are absorbed readily from the gastrointestinal (GI) tract into the systemic circulation and subsequently undergo significant first-pass hepatic metabolism. The resulting bioavailabilies can be as high as 50%. However, fluticasone propionate, fluticasone furoate, and mometasone furoate are not well absorbed through the GI tract, and the small amount of drug that reaches the portal circulation is rapidly and thoroughly metabolized. The newest agent, ciclesonide, is administered as a prodrug and metabolized to a bioactive metabolite by esterases in the nasal mucosa. Ciclesonide has low oral bioavailability because of low GI absorption and high first-pass metabolism. The lower systemic availabilities of these newer agents may be most important in growing children and in

patients who are already using INCSs for asthma. Nevertheless, no studies exist at this time to document the comparative effects of nasal corticosteroids on growth and development.[62–64]

INCSs may cause dryness and irritation of the nasal mucous membranes in 5% to 10% of mild cases and mild epistaxis in approximately 5%. For mild adverse events, the dose of INCS may be reduced if tolerated, and/or saline nasal spray should be instilled before the drug is sprayed. Correct application of the spray will reduce side effects and increase efficacy (Fig. 17.4).

Combination Nasal Products

In the classic step-up approach in patients not responding to monotherapy with H1 antihistamines or topical corticosteroids, the combination product containing azelastine and fluticasone has shown superiority in a pediatric population and can be used in children older than 6 years or 12 years (depending on the country of application).[65,66] It has the advantage of delivering both an antihistamine and a nasal corticosteroid in one product and may subsequently improve compliance (Table 17.5). This combination nasal product has been shown to improve symptoms of nasal congestion, rhinorrhea, itchy nose, and sneezing compared with treatment with placebo or treatment with either an antihistamine or a nasal corticosteroid. Adverse effects are similar to those listed for the individual drug components. In addition to the azelastine-fluticasone product, several other combination products are currently under development.

Mast Cell Stabilizers

Mast cell stabilizers, such as cromolyn sodium, can be useful in relieving nasal pruritus, rhinorrhea, and sneezing; however, they have minimal effects on congestion. Cromolyn sodium is generally well tolerated and is most efficacious when taken prophylactically,

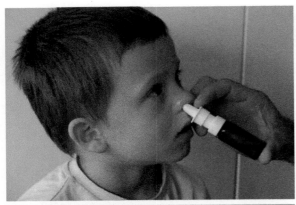

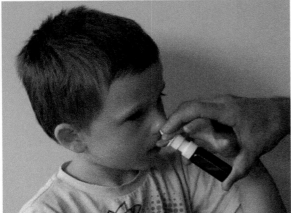

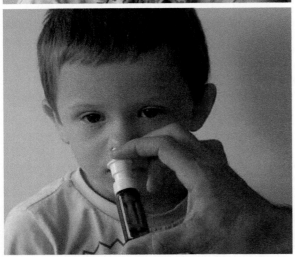

• **Fig. 17.4** The application of a nasal spray needs to be explained thoroughly to both the patient and parents. Incorrect use of topical corticosteroids may not only lead to injuries, epistaxis, and thus maladherence but may also have an impact on the effectiveness of the spray. In older children the spray may be applied by the child with or without the help of a parent. The nozzle should always point away from the nasal septum. The head is slightly inclined. A technique using the left hand for the right nostril, and vice versa, may aid in using the device correctly. In younger children the spray must be applied by an adult, again pointing toward the lateral nasal wall rather than the septum. No deep breath or sniffing should be performed while applying the spray, because it will lead to particle deposition in the pharynx rather than the nose. Other techniques might be necessary for corticosteroid drops.

TABLE 17.5	Intranasal Corticosteroid-Antihistamine Combination Spray		
Corticosteroid		Dose per Actuation (mcg)	Recommended Dosage
Azelastine hydrochloride and fluticasone propionate		137 mcg 50 mcg	≥12 yr: 274/100 mcg/ day

Adapted from Tran NP, Vickery J, Blaiss MS. Management of rhinitis: allergic and nonallergic. Allergy Asthma Immunol Res 2011;3:148–156.

well in advance of allergen exposure. In addition, because of its short duration of action, it should be taken four times per day; as a result, compliance is difficult for many patients.

Leukotriene Receptor Antagonists

Leukotriene receptor antagonists are effective in the treatment of seasonal and perennial AR compared with placebo and in combination with antihistamines over monotherapy.[67–70] Because AR often co-exists with asthma, and montelukast is approved for both of these diagnoses, montelukast may be considered in such patients. It also should be considered in patients who are unresponsive or noncompliant with INCSs. Montelukast has an excellent safety profile, is approved down to 6 months of age, and is available in generic formulations. An attractive attribute of this drug is that it is available as a once-daily oral formulation. Dosing is one 10-mg tablet daily for patients 14 years and older, one 5-mg chewable tablet daily for patients aged 6 to 13 years, and 4 mg daily (chewable tablet or granules) for children of 6 months to 5 years of age. Adverse effects are rare, with the most common being headache or stomachache shortly after dosing.

Saline

Saline is not part of the guidelines but can be of benefit in reducing symptoms and improving quality of life in some patients with AR. A 2012 study demonstrated that hypertonic saline was more effective than isotonic saline in improving outcomes.[71] Various mechanisms of action, including improvement in mucociliary clearance, removal of allergen and inflammatory mediators, and a protective effect on nasal mucosa, have been proposed but not confirmed. Side effects are minimal and include local burning and irritation and nausea. Optimal delivery techniques, volumes, concentrations, and dose frequency have not been established in AR. For patients with concomitant chronic rhinosinusitis, high-volume, low-pressure rinses with salt formulations with a high pH that are rich in calcium and magnesium and have lower levels of sodium chloride should be preferred to increase ciliary beat frequency and wound healing.[72]

Allergen Immunotherapy

AIT is a useful and important treatment for many patients with AR.[57,58] Although AIT was initially administered by the subcutaneous route, sublingual immunotherapy has proved to be efficacious and direct comparisons suggest comparable reductions in symptom scores and drug reductions. In pediatric populations, in particular, the less invasive sublingual treatment is widely applied. The mode of therapy to be applied underlies a classic joint decision-making process between the patient and the caregivers. Positive and potentially negative effects of regular office

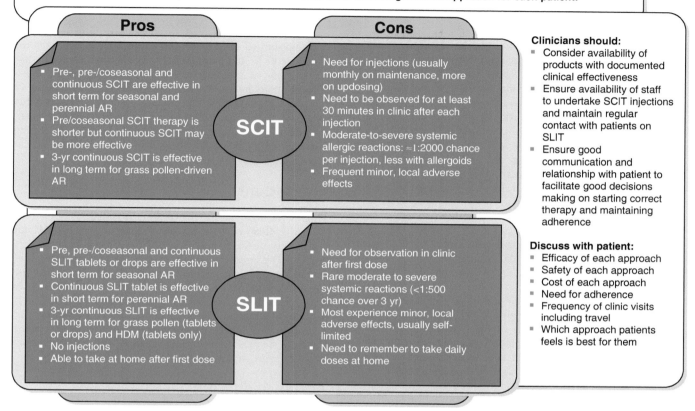

AIT should be considered if all are present:
- Moderate-to-severe symptoms of allergic rhinitis, +/– conjunctivitis, on exposure to clinically relevant allergen(s)
- Confirmation of IgE sensitisation clinically relevant allergen(s)
- Inadequate control of symptoms despite antihistamines and/or topical corticosteroids and allergen avoidance measures and/or unacceptable side-effects of medication

Pros and cons of the various options need to be considered when choosing the best approach for each patient:

Pros

Cons

SCIT
- Pre-, pre-/coseasonal and continuous SCIT are effective in short term for seasonal and perennial AR
- Pre/coseasonal SCIT therapy is shorter but continuous SCIT may be more effective
- 3-yr continuous SCIT is effective in long term for grass pollen-driven AR

- Need for injections (usually monthly on maintenance, more on updosing)
- Need to be observed for at least 30 minutes in clinic after each injection
- Moderate-to-severe systemic allergic reactions: ≈1:2000 chance per injection, less with allergoids
- Frequent minor, local adverse effects

SLIT
- Pre, pre-/coseasonal and continuous SLIT tablets or drops are effective in short term for seasonal AR
- Continuous SLIT tablet is effective in short term for perennial AR
- 3-yr continuous SLIT is effective in long term for grass pollen (tablets or drops) and HDM (tablets only)
- No injections
- Able to take at home after first dose

- Need for observation in clinic after first dose
- Rare moderate to severe systemic reactions (<1:500 chance over 3 yr)
- Most experience minor, local adverse effects, usually self-limited
- Need to remember to take daily doses at home

Clinicians should:
- Consider availability of products with documented clinical effectiveness
- Ensure availability of staff to undertake SCIT injections and maintain regular contact with patients on SLIT
- Ensure good communication and relationship with patient to facilitate good decisions making on starting correct therapy and maintaining adherence

Discuss with patient:
- Efficacy of each approach
- Safety of each approach
- Cost of each approach
- Need for adherence
- Frequency of clinic visits including travel
- Which approach patients feels is best for them

• **Fig. 17.5** Approach to decide on allergen immunotherapy. (With permission from Roberts G, Pfaar O, Akdis CA, et al. EAACI guidelines on allergen immunotherapy: allergic rhinoconjunctivitis. Allergy 2018;73:765–798)

• BOX 17.4 Key Concepts
Allergic Rhinitis

- Allergic rhinitis is one of the most common chronic disorders of childhood.
- Allergic rhinitis in children is an inflammatory airway disease.
- The distinction between allergic and nonallergic forms of rhinitis is important in children.
- Treatment should be individualized, aggressive, and targeted toward decreasing inflammation.
- Attention should be given to decreasing environmental exposures (e.g., allergens, tobacco smoke) and the use of intranasal corticosteroids and nonsedating antihistamines.
- Intranasal steroids constitute very effective therapy for allergic rhinitis and are safe despite a potential small drug-specific effect on growth rates.
- Allergic rhinitis in children may predispose to the development of otitis media, sinusitis, and asthma.

visits for the administration of injections have to be considered to optimize patient compliance. Subcutaneous immunotherapy must be administered by a physician who is experienced in its use, and there is a small risk of systemic reactions. Therefore, the office needs to be set up to deal with the management of adverse allergic reactions, including anaphylaxis.

Sublingual formulations for the treatment of grass, house dust mite, and ragweed pollen allergy have received U.S. Food and Drug Administration approval, but not all of them have been approved for children and adolescents yet.[59–61] Other sublingual formulations are under development (cat), under review (tree pollen), or approved outside of the United States. This route of delivery appears to be safer, with side effects usually restricted to the upper airways and GI tract. Safety data on patients with a history of anaphylaxis, eosinophilic esophagitis, or uncontrolled asthma is still scarce. When prescribing sublingual immunotherapy, the first dose must be administered in an allergy specialist's office. In

North America the patient must be instructed on the signs and symptoms of anaphylaxis and the use of an epinephrine autoinjector and must be discharged with an anaphylaxis action plan. In other settings the prescription of an epinephrine autoinjector for immunotherapy is not standard of care.

Patients with a narrow sensitization spectrum and clear exposure-related symptoms have better treatment responses. If necessary, several AIT courses to multiple allergenic sources can be applied. In general, one immunotherapy approach is conducted after the other. Whereas preformulated immunotherapy predominates in Europe, formulations by the physician still represent a frequent approach in North America. This is limited by the lack of standardization and available Phase III studies confirming the efficacy over placebo that could be as high as 60%. The time of application varies by the individual product. Both preseasonal and co-seasonal protocols are used. Moreover, continuous application for 3 to 4 years is also possible. The standard duration of AIT is 3 years. The improvement in rhinitis symptoms persists for several years after the treatment is discontinued.[3,73] The overall improvement in symptom scores over placebo is in the range of 15% to 30%. This is reflected in a significant reduction in symptoms on exposure and reduction in medication scores.

AIT is a human model of desensitization and to a certain extent tolerance induction. Research highlighted the parallel mechanisms that come into action during AIT compared with natural tolerance development.

The sequence of immunologic events is characterized by a typical sequence of events. Initially desensitization takes place. Moreover, a transient expansion of the type 2 responses kicks in that is paralleled by the generation of allergen-specific regulatory T cells, the exhaustion of effector cells and the generation of blocking antibodies of an IgA, IgG, and specifically IgG4 type. At a later stage, allergen sIgE tends to decline. The induced reduction in mediator release and tissue inflammation is reflected in clinical improvement.[63] AIT should be considered in patients with AR who (1) may need an additional option when they do not respond to a combination of environmental control measures and medications, (2) have a confirmed IgE sensitization of clinical relevance to environmental allergens, or (3) experience substantial side effects with symptomatic medications (Fig. 17.5).[3]

Biologic Agents in Allergic Rhinitis Treatment

Recent developments in AR treatment include the use of novel drugs with specific targets and combinations of established treatments.[13] Biologic agents are increasingly becoming a more mainstream approach.[74] Despite the advances in various fields of medicine with these drugs, there is very limited evidence for their use in AR alone, especially in children. In principle, omalizumab, a monoclonal anti-IgE antibody, could represent a valid option in AR that has demonstrated clinical efficacy.[75] Because of its high cost and limited long-term experience, there is not yet sufficient evidence for its standard use in this indication alone. In cases of severe atopic manifestations such as uncontrolled asthma or in chronic spontaneous urticaria, its use may be considered. Other biologic agents targeting the IL-4/IL-13 axis, such as dupilumab, which has been approved for chronic rhinosinusitis with nasal polyps and atopic dermatitis, are currently being investigated regarding their ability to modify allergen-specific responses and change disease progression in the context of AIT.

Conclusions

Despite the high prevalence of AR in the pediatric population, this disease is often overlooked or undertreated. Untreated AR impairs the quality of life of the child and his or her parents. Accurate and timely diagnosis of AR in children relies on awareness of the symptoms and signs of the disease and its comorbidities, including asthma, rhinosinusitis, and otitis media. Clinicians should understand the differential diagnosis of AR in children and pursue specific diagnostic testing when indicated. Treatment options include environmental controls and the use of INCSs, nonsedating antihistamines, and immunotherapy. The key concepts of AR in children are summarized in Box 17.4.

Acknowledgment

This chapter is based on the chapter in the third edition, which was written by Deborah A. Gentile, Nicole Pleskovic, Ashton Bartholow, and David P. Skoner.

18

Sinusitis

KENNY H. CHAN, MARK J. ABZUG, ANDREW H. LIU

KEY POINTS

- Sinusitis is diagnostically challenging because symptoms (i.e., nasal discharge, congestion, and cough), signs, and radiographic findings are similar to those in other common upper respiratory tract infections. Coronal sinus computed tomography scans may be helpful in chronic, recurrent, or complicated sinusitis.
- Respiratory infections (viruses, bacteria), bacterial biofilms, and microbiome disruption have pathogenic roles. The most common causes of bacterial sinusitis are *Streptococcus pneumoniae* (20%–30%), *Haemophilus influenzae* (20%–30%), and *Moraxella catarrhalis* (10%–20%); 30% to 35% of sinus aspirates are sterile.
- Antibiotic resistance is common with *S. pneumoniae* (15%–50% penicillin resistant), *H. influenzae* (25%–80% β-lactamase positive), and *M. catarrhalis* (90%–100% β-lactamase positive). Antral irrigation can provide sinus specimens for bacterial culture and

targeted antimicrobial therapy in patients with chronic, refractory, and complicated disease.
- Young children with chronic sinusitis have mucosal pathologic findings and inflammation that typically differ from those in from adults. In adults, chronic sinusitis is characterized by mucosal thickening, goblet cell hyperplasia, subepithelial fibrosis, and persistent Type 2 eosinophilic inflammation. In young children, panimmune inflammation (CD8+ T lymphocytes, B lymphocytes, neutrophils), with reduced basement membrane thickness, fewer mucous glands, and less epithelial injury, is common.
- Management of uncomplicated, acute sinusitis consists of antimicrobial treatment aiming for symptom relief and prevention of complications and recurrence. Severe intraorbital and intracranial complications require aggressive medical and surgical intervention.

Introduction

This chapter on sinusitis in children will provide an overview of the pathogenesis and management of acute and chronic sinus disease. Although acute sinusitis has been substantially investigated, relatively little is known about chronic sinusitis in children.

Sinus Development in Childhood

The four pairs of paranasal sinuses in humans are maxillary, ethmoid, frontal, and sphenoid. The maxillary and ethmoid sinuses are present at birth and become radiographically visible in the first 1 to 2 years of life (Fig. 18.1). In comparison, frontal and sphenoid sinuses begin to develop in the first few years of life and gradually become radiographically visible between 7 and 15 years of age. The maxillary anterior ethmoid and frontal sinus ostia enter the nasal cavity through the middle meatus, under the middle turbinate (i.e., ostiomeatal complex; see Fig. 18.1). The sphenoid and posterior ethmoid ostia join the nasal cavity through the superior meatus above the middle turbinate.

Clinical Definitions of Sinusitis

Several descriptive modifiers for sinusitis are commonly used. In terms of sinusitis duration, (1) *acute* sinusitis refers to sinus symptoms of 10 to 30 days, with complete resolution of symptoms[1]; (2) *subacute* sinusitis refers to symptoms that last 30 to 90 to 120

days; and (3) *chronic* sinusitis is used for symptoms that last more than 90 to 120 days. *Recurrent* sinusitis occurs in patients who improve with sinus therapy but experience multiple episodes. *Refractory* sinusitis refers to patients who do not respond to conventional therapy for sinusitis.

The uses of the terms *sinusitis* and *rhinosinusitis* have been debated; *sinusitis* implies that the disease is the manifestation of an infectious process of the sinuses.[2] In comparison, the term *rhinosinusitis* implies that the nasal and sinus mucosae are involved in similar and concurrent pathogenic (e.g., inflammatory) processes.[1] In this chapter the two terms will be used interchangeably.

Epidemiology and Health Burden

Sinusitis is a common problem in childhood. Studies have found incidence rates of acute sinusitis in children between 4% to 8%.[3] In a prospective study, sinusitis was diagnosed in 9% of upper respiratory tract illnesses.[4] In a large birth cohort study, the main risk factors for sinusitis were current allergic rhinitis and grass pollen hypersensitivity.[5]

The U.S. National Center for Health Statistics reported that from 1980 to 1992 sinusitis was the fifth leading diagnosis for which antibiotics were prescribed.[6] The annual outpatient visit rates for sinusitis increased about 3-fold over this period, and the use of amoxicillin and cephalosporin antibiotics for sinusitis also increased significantly. Antibiotic resistance of bacterial pathogens

147

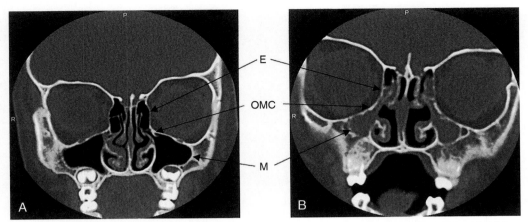

• **Fig. 18.1** Computed tomography scans of the paranasal sinuses. Coronal views of a 4-year-old child with (A) normal maxillary and ethmoid sinuses and patent ostiomeatal complex and (B) opacified maxillary and ethmoid sinuses consistent with sinusitis. *E,* Ethmoid sinus; *M,* maxillary sinus; *OMC,* ostiomeatal complex.

from the sinuses of children with acute[7] and chronic sinusitis[8] is common. Severe alterations in quality of life can result from chronic recurrent sinusitis in children. Using a standardized child health questionnaire, children with chronic sinusitis and their parents reported more bodily pain and greater limitation in their physical activity than were typically reported by children with asthma or juvenile rheumatoid arthritis.[9] Complications of sinusitis, such as intracranial or intraorbital extension of bacterial infection from the sinuses, are life-threatening medical emergencies. Neuropsychiatric disturbances associated with sinusitis also have been described.[10]

Etiology

A combination of anatomic, mucosal, microbial, and immune pathogenic processes is believed to underlie sinusitis in children. Children with congenital mucosal diseases (e.g., cystic fibrosis [CF], ciliary dyskinesias) and lymphocyte immunodeficiencies (congenital and acquired) typically have chronic recurrent sinus disease. In addition, allergic airway diseases in children have both epidemiologic and pathogenic links to sinusitis.

Anatomic Pathogenesis

Anatomic obstructions of the sinus ostia in the nasopharynx have long been suspected causes of sinusitis. The pathophysiologic process of ostiomeatal obstruction leading to sinusitis is thought to be similar to that of otitis media.[11] For the middle ear space, animal model studies reveal that a lack of ventilation (i.e., oxygenation) of the middle ear results in negative pressure in the closed space, leading to mucosal vascular leakage, edema, inflammation, and middle ear fluid accumulation.[12,13] Both anatomic obstructive lesions and mucosal disorders such as mucosal injury from viral upper respiratory tract infections (URTIs), inhalant allergies, cystic fibrosis, and ciliary dyskinesias may begin this cascade of pathogenic events. Anatomic variations associated with sinusitis in children in uncontrolled studies include concha bullosa (10%), paradoxical turbinates (4%–8%), lateralized uncinate process with hypoplastic maxillary sinus (7%–17%), Haller cells (5%–10%), and septal deviation (10%).[14,15] Importantly, these anatomic abnormalities are common in asymptomatic patients.[16] Recent studies have failed to establish a relationship between anatomic variations

and the severity and extent of chronic sinusitis in children.[17,18] Adenoid hypertrophy also has been implicated as a possible predisposing factor to sinusitis, especially in younger children, by serving as a mechanical obstruction to nasal drainage and/or as a focus of bacterial biofilm colonization; however, an etiologic role has not been established.[16,19,20] Therefore, it is not prudent to base surgical intervention on anatomic variations alone.

Microbial Pathogenesis

Both viral and bacterial infections have integral roles in the pathogenesis of sinusitis. Viral URTIs commonly cause sinus mucosal injury and swelling, resulting in ostiomeatal obstruction, loss of ciliary activity, and mucus hypersecretion. Indeed, radiologic sinus imaging studies of adults and children with common colds revealed that sinus mucosal abnormalities are the norm, and even air-fluid levels in the maxillary sinuses and opacification of the maxillary sinuses are common.[21,22] Specifically, coronal sinus computed tomography (CT) scans of adults with URTIs revealed that 87% had abnormalities of one or both maxillary sinuses, 77% had obstruction of the ethmoid infundibulum, 65% had abnormal ethmoid sinuses, 32% had abnormal frontal sinuses, and 39% had abnormal sphenoid sinuses.[22]

Sneezing and nose blowing are thought to introduce nasal flora into the sinuses. Chronically infected adenoids, which may be colonized by bacterial biofilms, and intracellular bacteria (in particular, *Staphylococcus aureus*) in the nasopharynx have been proposed as nasopharyngeal reservoirs of pathogens that may be introduced into the sinuses.[20,23] Normal nasopharyngeal flora such as alpha streptococci and anaerobes may elaborate bacteriocins and other inhibitory compounds that interfere with colonization and infection by pathogenic bacteria.[24] Bacterial growth conditions are favorable in obstructed sinuses, reflected by bacterial concentrations of up to 10^7 bacterial colony-forming units (cfu)/mL in sinus aspirates. Additionally, bacterial biofilms have been demonstrated in sinus mucosal specimens obtained from 45% to 80% of children and adults with chronic sinusitis.[25,26] White blood cell counts in excess of 10,000 cells/mL in sinus aspirates are evidence of a robust inflammatory response to infection. The combination of infection, biofilm formation, and inflammation can result in intense epithelial damage and transmucosal injury.[27,28]

TABLE 18.1 Microbiology of Acute, Subacute, and Chronic Sinusitis

Microorganism	FREQUENCY		
	Common	Occasional	Uncommon
Streptococcus pneumoniae	A, C		
Haemophilus influenzae, nontypeable	A, C		
Moraxella catarrhalis	A, C		
Streptococcus pyogenes		A, C	
Other streptococcal species (including *Streptococcus milleri*)		A, C	
Staphylococcus aureus (including methicillin-resistant *S. aureus*)		C	A
Diphtheroids		C	
Coagulase-negative staphylococci		C	
Other gram-negatives, *Moraxella*, *Neisseria*		C	A
Anaerobes		C	A
Respiratory viruses		A, C	
Fungi (*Aspergillus*, *Alternaria*, other dematiaceous fungi, zygomycetes)*		C	A
Acanthamoeba†			A

*Primarily in immunocompromised hosts or associated with allergic fungal sinusitis.
†Primarily in immunocompromised hosts.
A, Acute and subacute sinusitis; C, Chronic sinusitis.

Microbiology of Acute and Subacute Sinusitis

The gold standard for microbiologic diagnosis of bacterial sinusitis has been the recovery of 10^4 cfu/mL or greater of pathogenic bacteria from a sinus aspirate.[1,29] Studies employing sinus aspirates indicate that the pathogens responsible for acute and subacute sinusitis are similar to each other and mirror those responsible for acute otitis media[29–34] (Table 18.1). *S. pneumoniae* is recovered in 20% to 30% of cases, nontypeable *H. influenzae* in 20% to 30%, and *M. catarrhalis* in 10% to 20%. Similar to observations for acute otitis media, a modest reduction in the proportion caused by *S. pneumoniae* and a corresponding increase in the proportion caused by *H. influenzae* is suggested in populations with routine pneumococcal conjugate vaccination of young children.[24] Before availability of the 13-valent pneumococcal conjugate vaccine, a significant proportion of *S. pneumoniae* isolates have intermediate- or high-level resistance to penicillin because of alterations in penicillin-binding proteins

(15%–50%); rates of penicillin-resistance among *S. pneumoniae* isolates have fallen significantly with use of this vaccine.[35] *H. influenzae* and *M. catarrhalis* isolates are frequently positive for β-lactamase (25%–80% and 90%–100%, respectively), and a minority of *H. influenzae* are ampicillin resistant because of altered penicillin-binding proteins and/or an efflux pump.[24,36] Actual resistance rates vary with time period, geographic region, and the prevalence of risk factors for resistance (e.g., age younger than 2 years, daycare attendance, recent antibiotic exposure). *Streptococcus pyogenes* and other streptococcal species are generally recovered in only a small number of cases, although several series have highlighted a frequent association between recovery of *Streptococcus anginosus* group with acute sinusitis leading to intraorbital and/or intracranial complications in children and adults.[37–39] *S. aureus* and anaerobes are uncommon causes of acute and subacute pediatric sinusitis; however, they are more frequently identified in severe, complicated disease or, in the case of anaerobes, associated with dental disease.[40] Less commonly recovered bacteria include gram-negative organisms such as *Eikenella corrodens* and other *Moraxella* and *Neisseria* spp. Fungi are uncommonly recovered in acute sinusitis except in immunocompromised patients.[30] The protozoan *Acanthamoeba* has also been identified as a rare cause of sinusitis in severely immunosuppressed hosts.[41,42] Sinus aspirates are sterile in 30% to 35% of children with clinically and/or radiographically diagnosed sinusitis.[1,29,33,43] Acute sinusitis in children has been associated with rhinovirus URTIs.[44]

Microbiology of Chronic Sinusitis

Infection is a key component in pediatric chronic sinusitis, although concomitant factors may be an important contributor to the chronic inflammatory process.[45] In numerous studies, 65% to 100% of children with chronic sinusitis have positive cultures of sinus aspirates.[8,46–50] Rates of recovery of specific organisms vary among studies; this variability is likely to be explained by differences in patient populations, sinuses evaluated, specimen collection methods, and microbiologic culture techniques. Despite these differences, certain general observations can be made. *S. pneumoniae*, *H. influenzae*, and *M. catarrhalis* are frequently isolated from children with chronic sinusitis, mirroring acute and subacute sinusitis[8,47,51] (see Table 18.1). With increasing chronicity, other organisms also may be recovered, including *S. aureus*, *S. pyogenes*, alpha streptococci (including the *Streptococcus anginosus* group), group D streptococci, diphtheroids, coagulase-negative staphylococci, *Neisseria* spp., gram-negative aerobic rods (including *Pseudomonas aeruginosa*), and anaerobes; infection is frequently polymicrobial.[46,48–50] *S. anginosus*, *S. aureus*, and anaerobes tend to be disproportionately associated with protracted, severe, or complicated disease.[52–57] In concert with the overall increase in community-acquired methicillin-resistant *S. aureus* (MRSA) infections, an increased frequency of MRSA-associated sinus infections has been observed.[58] Recovery of anaerobes (e.g., *Peptococcus*, *Peptostreptococcus*, *Propionibacterium acnes*, *Prevotella*, *Veillonella*, *Fusobacterium*, *Bacteroides*, and *Actinomyces* spp.) has varied widely from less than 5% to more than 90%, depending on the populations and sinuses evaluated and microbiologic methods employed.[46–50,59,60] Many anaerobic isolates produce β-lactamase.[40,61]

Antibiotic resistance is an important factor in the microbiology of chronic sinusitis. For example, in a 4-year retrospective review of maxillary sinus aspirates from children with sinusitis for more than 8 weeks (before pneumococcal conjugate vaccination), rates

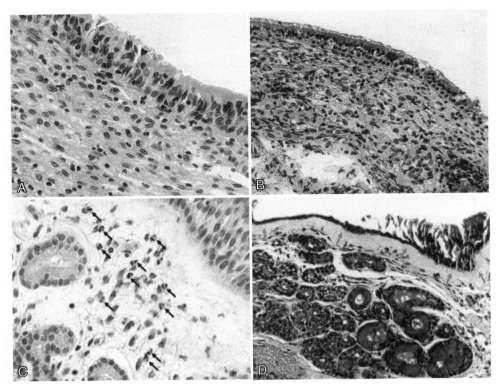

• **Fig. 18.2** Chronic sinusitis: sinus mucosal biopsies from children (A and B) and adults (C and D). (A) and (C), Hematoxylin and eosin–stained (original magnification 400×). *Arrows* on the adult photo (C) point to some of the eosinophils in this image. There is a relative abundance of lymphocytes and scarcity of eosinophils in the pediatric specimen (A) compared with adult tissue (C). (B) and (D), Pentachrome stained (original magnification 200×). *Arrows* on the adult photo (D) point to thickened basement membrane. Basement membrane thickening, mucous gland hyperplasia, and hypertrophy, and loss of columnar epithelium in the adult sample (D) are not seen in the pediatric sample (B).

of nonsusceptibility of *S. pneumoniae* (recovered in 19% of cultures) were 64% for penicillin, 40% for cefotaxime, and 18% for clindamycin.[8] Of *H. influenzae* isolates (recovered in 24%), 44% were nonsusceptible to ampicillin, and all *M. catarrhalis* isolates (recovered in 17%) were positive for β-lactamase.

Studies using modern profiling techniques to determine the sinus microbiome in chronic rhinosinusitis have demonstrated great diversity of the sinus microbiome.[62] In one study, an abundance of a single fastidious species, *Corynebacterium tuberculostearicum,* and depletion of *Lactobacillus sakei* were identified compared with healthy controls.[63] In a mouse model, *C. tuberculostearicum* was demonstrated to be a sinus pathogen after pretreatment with amoxicillin-clavulanic acid, and protection against this organism was conferred by pretreatment with *L. sakei.*

Fungi, including *Aspergillus, Alternaria,* and other dematiaceous species (e.g., *Bipolaris* and *Curvularia*) and zygomycetes are occasionally isolated, although invasive disease is uncommon except in immunocompromised children.[49] Respiratory viruses are occasionally identified in sinus mucosal or lavage specimens.[64,65] Interestingly, bilateral cultures of the sinuses are often discordant.[8,50]

Chronic rhinosinusitis (CRS) also has been associated with nasal respiratory viruses. Comparing nasal lavage from participants with CRS with non-CRS controls: nasal respiratory virus detection (50% versus 26%), especially rhinovirus (26% versus 10%), parainfluenza virus (23% versus 8%), influenza virus (13% versus 4%), respiratory syncytial virus (11% versus 2%),

and multiple respiratory viruses (24% versus 4%, respectively).[66] Respiratory viruses have been recovered from approximately 10% of sinus aspirates, although sinus aspirates and biopsy investigations with more sensitive modern viral detection methods may provide additional insights.[29] Whether respiratory viruses have a direct pathogenic role in sinusitis is poorly understood, but it is clear that viral rhinosinusitis and bacterial sinusitis may have overlapping clinical and radiographic features that make clinical diagnosis of the latter entity challenging.[36]

Immune Pathogenesis

There are few studies in the literature on the immunopathology of sinusitis in children. Most of our knowledge is derived from studies conducted on adults with chronic hyperplastic sinusitis and nasal polyposis (CHS/NP). In adults, chronic sinusitis is characterized by mucosal thickening, goblet cell hyperplasia, subepithelial fibrosis, and persistent inflammation[67] (Fig. 18.2). These fibrotic changes are thought to be driven by activated eosinophils and their products, including the profibrotic transforming growth factor-β,[68] granulocyte-macrophage colony-stimulating factor (GM-CSF),[69,70] and interleukin (IL)-11.[71] Tissue fibroblasts are stimulated to increase the synthesis and deposition of collagen and matrix products, resulting in thickening of the sub-basement membrane layer.

Current views associate sensitivity to aeroallergens as a primary pathologic mechanism in the development of chronic sinusitis in both adults[72,73] and children.[74] Many studies have shown that the composition of the inflammatory substrate in chronic sinusitis is similar to that seen in allergic rhinitis and the late phase response to antigen challenge.[72,75]

T_H2-Mediated Eosinophilic Inflammation

Although many immune cell types are involved in the pathogenesis of chronic sinusitis, a specific subclass of T lymphocytes (i.e., T helper cell type 2 [T_H2] lymphocytes) and eosinophils appear to have a central role. The orchestration of cellular recruitment and activation of the inflammatory infiltrate in CHS/NP has been largely attributed to the T_H2 cells and their cytokines (i.e., IL-3, IL-4, IL-5, IL-9, IL-13, GM-CSF). Among immune cell types, eosinophils are the most characteristic and are found in 80% to 90% of nasal polyps.[76] A histopathologic study has investigated the inflammatory cells in pediatric chronic sinusitis and reported similar findings: the numbers of eosinophils, and to a much lesser extent mast cells and T lymphocytes, are significantly increased in children with chronic sinusitis compared to control subjects[77] (see Fig. 18.2). The degree of tissue eosinophilia was not affected by the allergic status of patients. This is in agreement with published studies on chronic sinusitis in the adult population, in whom the level of eosinophilic infiltration was found to be similar between allergic and nonallergic patients with either chronic sinusitis without nasal polyps[78,79] or CHS/NP.[80,81] Levels of neutrophils are also increased in the sinus lavage fluid of adults with chronic sinusitis, particularly in nonallergic patients.[82]

Allergic fungal sinusitis (AFS), an uncommon condition resulting from an intense and chronic allergic reaction to fungi growing in allergic mucin within the sinus cavities, is thought to be pathogenically similar to allergic bronchopulmonary mycoses.[83,84] *Aspergillus* spp. and dematiaceous fungi (e.g., *Alternaria, Curvularia, Bipolaris* spp.) have been cultured from affected sinuses. Nasal polyposis, facial deformity, bony erosion of the sinuses, proptosis, and fungal hyphae in allergic mucin filling the sinuses are common in children with AFS.[85–87] Because of its destructive nature, AFS is managed aggressively, with topical and oral corticosteroids after surgical debridement.[83,87] Antifungal therapy (e.g., itraconazole, voriconazole) has been associated with clinical improvement, oral steroid reduction, and resolution of disease in some series.[88,89]

Chronic rhinosinusitis in young children differs from the common phenotype in older children and adults. Sinus mucosal biopsies from younger children (median age 3.9 years; range 1.4–8.2) with chronic rhinosinusitis (i.e., despite at least two courses of antibiotics, one with a second-line agent), when compared with adult sinusitis controls, had significantly fewer eosinophils, less basement membrane thickness, fewer submucosal mucous glands, and less epithelial injury (see Fig. 18.2).[90] These young children had more CD8+ (cytotoxic T lymphocytes), CD20+ (B lymphocytes), myeloperoxidase-positive (neutrophils), and CD68+ (monocytes, macrophages) cells in sinus epithelium and/or submucosal tissues.[91] Those whose sinus cultures grew a bacterial pathogen (55%) had significantly more submucosal neutrophils. This pan-immune histopathologic finding might indicate inadequate and/or dysregulated immune responses to bacterial biofilms, pathogenic microbiomes, and/or common respiratory viruses.

Asthma and Allergy Risk Factors

Along with histologic evidence that the immune pathologic processes of chronic sinusitis and asthma can be similar, epidemiologic, radiographic, and clinical studies also link sinusitis with asthma. In a large European survey study, a strong association of asthma with chronic rhinosinusitis (adjusted odds ratio [aOR] 3.47) was observed at all ages, and was stronger in those also reporting allergic rhinitis (aOR 11.85).[92] Using plain radiography of the sinuses, the prevalence of radiographic sinus abnormalities was significantly higher in children with asthma (31%) than nonasthmatic controls (0%).[93] In children with asthma who were hospitalized for an acute exacerbation, significant radiographic abnormalities of the sinuses were revealed in 87%.[94] A study of patients undergoing surgery for chronic sinusitis found that sinus CT evidence of extensive disease was associated with asthma, allergen sensitization, and peripheral blood eosinophilia.[95] Of those with eosinophilia, 87% had extensive sinus disease.

Allergic rhinitis and inhalant allergen sensitization also have been associated with sinusitis in children. In a large birth cohort study, both allergic rhinitis and grass pollen sensitization were significant and independent risk factors for sinusitis in childhood (i.e., age 8 years).[5] Experimentally, in subjects with allergic rhinitis, nasal provocation with allergen-induced sinus radiographic changes (i.e., mucosal thickening, sinus opacification) and symptoms of headache and pressure in the maxillary sinuses.[96]

Genetic Risk Factors

Association studies between chronic sinusitis and a few candidate gene markers have been reported. In children, chronic rhinosinusitis and sometimes nasal polyposis are hallmark features of CF and primary ciliary dyskinesia, two autosomal recessive inherited disorders. A small proportion of patients with chronic sinusitis without CF are carriers of mutations in the CF transmembrane regulator *(CFTR)* gene, especially in association with the M470V polymorphism[97,98]; however, siblings of patients with CF, who are all *CFTR* mutation carriers, do not have an increased prevalence of rhinosinusitis.[99] Modest linkages of single-nucleotide polymorphisms (SNPs) in other CRS candidate genes include tumor necrosis factor-alpha (TNF-α) (CHS/NP),[100] LTC4 synthase,[101] transforming growth factor-beta 1 (TGF-β1),[102] TNF-β2 (chronic sinusitis),[103] and the major histocompatibility B54 haplotype.[104] A replication study of 53 CRS-associated SNPs replicated significance for SNPs in seven good gene candidates, especially prolyl-tRNA synthetase 2 (OR 0.77), TGF-β1 (OR 0.81), and nitric oxide synthase 1 (OR 0.84).[105]

Other Risk Factors

Medical conditions that render children susceptible to acute and chronic sinus disease include immunodeficiencies (especially patients with T and B lymphocyte defects or acquired immunodeficiency syndrome [AIDS] and those receiving immunosuppressive medications), CF, and primary ciliary dyskinesias. Low immunoglobulin G (IgG) subclass levels and/or specific antibody responses have been implicated in some children with recurrent and/or chronic sinusitis, as have possible defects in local innate immunity and mucociliary clearance.[16,106] The association of gastroesophageal reflux disease (GERD) with chronic sinusitis has also received attention. GERD, diagnosed by pH-monitored nasopharyngeal acid reflux[107] or esophageal biopsy,[108] was associated with rhinosinusitis in children in some studies, but there is lack of consensus regarding the contribution of GERD to chronic sinusitis.[3,109] Phipps and colleagues[110] also reported significantly increased nasopharyngeal reflux in children with chronic sinusitis when compared with a historical control group. Antireflux treatment of their GERD-positive cohort resulted in a 79% improvement in chronic sinusitis symptoms.

• BOX 18.1   Differential Diagnosis and Risk Factors for Acute and Chronic Sinusitis in Children

Acute Sinusitis
- Prolonged viral upper respiratory tract infection
- Foreign body in the nose
- Acute exacerbation of inhalant allergies
- Acute adenoiditis or adenotonsillitis

Chronic Sinusitis
- Rhinitis, allergic and nonallergic
- Anatomic causes of nasopharyngeal obstruction
  - Turbinate hypertrophy
  - Adenoid hypertrophy
  - Nasal polyps
  - Severe septal deviation
  - Choanal atresia
  - Asthma
- Neoplasms of the nose and nasopharynx
  - Juvenile angiofibroma
  - Rhabdomyosarcoma
  - Lymphoma
  - Dermoid cyst
- Cystic fibrosis
- Lymphocyte immune deficiencies
  - B lymphocytes—antibody deficiencies
  - T lymphocyte deficiencies—congenital and acquired
- Primary ciliary dyskinesias
- Wegener's granulomatosis
- Churg-Strauss vasculitis
- Dental caries/abscess
- Gastroesophageal reflux disease with nasopharyngeal reflux

Sinusitis Management

Overview

Medical histories and physical examinations can help distinguish sinusitis in children from URTIs and other masqueraders and identify complications from sinusitis and underlying risk factors for chronic recurrent disease. Radiographic imaging studies are particularly helpful in evaluating children with chronic, recurrent, or complicated sinusitis. Sinus washings for bacterial culture and targeted antimicrobial therapy, although ideal, are surgical procedures (e.g., antral irrigation) that require general anesthesia in children. Therefore, their use is generally reserved for (1) children with chronic sinusitis that does not adequately improve with multiple courses of antibiotics, (2) children with sinusitis with complications, and (3) sinusitis in immunocompromised hosts. Differential diagnostic considerations are provided in Box 18.1.

Consensus-based guidelines on the management of sinusitis in children have been published,[111] including guidelines from the American Academy of Pediatrics (AAP),[1] the Infectious Diseases Society of America (IDSA),[112] the American Academy of Allergy, Asthma and Immunology,[113] and the American Academy of Otolaryngology–Head and Neck Surgery[109,114] and in the International Consensus Statement on Allergy and Rhinology: Rhinosinusitis.[3] These consensus guidelines, along with randomized controlled trials, systematic reviews, and meta-analyses of specific management topics, have been considered in the following discussion.

History and Physical Examination

Acute Sinusitis

Persisting, nonimproving symptoms, such as nasal discharge (76%) and cough (80%), lasting longer than 10 to 14 days are the most common presentation of acute sinusitis in children.[1,29,112] Nasal discharge can be of any quality, and cough can be daytime, nighttime, or both. Fever may accompany the illness. Less common presentations include severe symptoms such as high fever, purulent nasal discharge, or facial pain for 3 to 4 days or longer at the start of illness or worsening symptoms after 5 to 6 days of a viral URTI that had been improving.[1,112]

Although headaches and sinus tenderness are generally thought to be the hallmarks of sinusitis, a study of 200 patients with sinusitis did not find a significant correlation of facial pain or headache with abnormal findings on sinus CT.[111] Additionally, the reported regions of facial pain did not correlate with radiographically identified sinus abnormalities. The nasal cavity is usually filled with discharge, and the nasal mucosa and turbinates are generally edematous. After decongestion of the nasal cavity, purulent drainage coming from the middle meatus can sometimes be observed in older children. Tenderness over the frontal sinus in older children may indicate frontal sinus disease, but tenderness in general is uncommon in children with acute disease. Transillumination, considered by some to be a useful tool in adults, is unreliable in children. Nasal endoscopy may be helpful in diagnosing invasive fungal sinusitis in immunocompromised children.[115]

Chronic Sinusitis

The most common symptoms associated with chronic sinusitis in children are nasal discharge (59%), facial pain/discomfort (33%), nasal congestion (30%), cough (19%), and wheezing (19%).[114] Nasal discharge can be of any quality, but purulent discharge is the most common. Daytime mouth-breathing and snoring are common complaints. Examination of the nasal cavity may or may not reveal nasal discharge. The nasal turbinates are generally enlarged and can be edematous or erythematous. Although facial pain or discomfort may be a common complaint, tenderness over the sinuses is an uncommon finding in children.

Radiographic Imaging

A consensus report provided by the American College of Radiology[116] provided appropriateness criteria of different radiographic imaging modalities in assessing pediatric sinus disease. Currently, coronal CT is the recommended examination for imaging potential complications or persistent or chronic sinusitis in patients of any age. Plain sinus radiographs (Waters and Caldwell projections), although widely available, can both underdiagnose and overdiagnose sinus soft tissue changes. Magnetic resonance imaging provides superior soft tissue delineation; however, it is expensive, has limited availability, and does not provide bony details of the ostiomeatal complex. Conventional tomography, nuclear medicine studies, and ultrasound have significant limitations for imaging the sinuses.

It is tempting to consider sinus mucosal abnormalities and associated anatomic variations seen in imaging studies in symptomatic patients as clear indications for sinusitis therapy (e.g., antimicrobial therapy and sinus surgery). However, the clinical importance of such findings is challenged by studies that have revealed a high prevalence of such soft tissue findings in people without sinusitis symptoms or with URTIs.[21,22] In these studies,

TABLE 18.2 Sinusitis Complications (by Sinus Involvement)	Maxillary Sinus	Ethmoid Sinus	Frontal Sinus	Sphenoid Sinus
Complication				
Osteomyelitis	+		+ +	
Mucocele	+ +	+ +	+ +	+
Preseptal cellulitis		+ + +		
Orbital cellulitis		+ + +	+	
Subperiosteal abscess		+ + +		
Orbital abscess		+		
Meningitis			+ +	
Epidural abscess			+ +	
Subdural abscess			+	
Brain abscess			+	

+, Least frequent; ++, less frequent; +++, frequent.

URTI symptoms and associated radiographic sinus abnormalities have improved without specific sinusitis therapy (i.e., no antibiotics or surgery for sinusitis).

The American College of Radiology consensus report has the following recommendations: (1) the diagnoses of acute and chronic sinusitis should be made clinically and not on the basis of imaging findings alone; (2) no imaging studies are indicated for acute sinusitis except for cases in which complications are suspected or cases that are not responding to therapy; and (3) if imaging information in patients with chronic sinusitis is desired, coronal sinus CT is recommended. The use of plain radiographs of the sinuses (i.e., Waters and Caldwell views) is generally discouraged in this report, except in children younger than 4 years of age. The use of Waters view radiographs in children is supported by a study in which the sensitivity and specificity of a Waters view radiograph to diagnose chronic sinusitis in children were 76% and 81%, respectively.[117] In the same study, limited coronal CT scans were better than sinus x-rays and nearly as good as full sinus CT evaluations. CT angiography or magnetic resonance angiography are used for evaluation of possible venous thrombosis.[118]

Sinusitis Complications

Complications of sinusitis include orbital and intracranial extension and frontal bone osteomyelitis (Pott's puffy tumor) (Table 18.2). These complications are generally thought to be acute events that result from a combination of outflow obstruction and spread of pathogenic bacteria from the sinuses. Intracranial extension of infection is by direct erosion, thrombophlebitis, or extension through preformed pathways (e.g., fracture lines). The incidence of intracranial complications in children hospitalized for sinusitis was 3%.[119]

Orbital complications from sinusitis are primarily the result of acute ethmoid disease but could occasionally be extensions of

frontal disease.[120] A classic description of the progression of sinusitis to orbital complications is as follows: inflammatory edema, orbital cellulitis, subperiosteal abscess, orbital abscess, and cavernous sinus thrombosis.[121] The most common presentations of orbital complications include eyelid edema, orbital pain, diplopia, painful extraocular movements, proptosis, and chemosis, fever, nasal discharge, and headache.[122] In a cohort of hospitalized children with orbital complications from sinusitis, 72% had a history of a URTI and 24% had received oral antibiotic therapy before their presentation with orbital complications.[122] It can be difficult to differentiate between preseptal cellulitis and orbital cellulitis on clinical parameters alone (i.e., based on lid edema and pain) without an imaging study. In orbital cellulitis, proptosis progresses and chemosis, ophthalmoplegia, and reduced visual acuity may ensue. Orbital abscesses and cavernous sinus thrombosis caused by bacterial sinusitis are uncommon and can result in loss of vision.[123]

Intracranial complications from sinusitis primarily result from frontal or sphenoid sinus disease and include meningitis, epidural and subdural abscess, and brain abscess.[119] There are many similarities between the pathogenesis of intracranial extension of sinusitis and that of otitis media. Intracranial extension of infection is by direct erosion, thrombophlebitis, or extension through preformed pathways (e.g., fracture lines). In children, intracranial complications occur most frequently in adolescent males.[124] The incidence of intracranial complications in children hospitalized for sinusitis in one series was 3%.[120] Current mortality rates for these complications are between 3% and 20%. Cavernous sinus thrombosis is a unique intracranial complication of ethmoid and sphenoid sinusitis by direct extension or venous communication. This complication is characterized by a toxic-appearing patient with infectious/inflammatory involvement of cranial nerves III, IV, and VI, resulting in ophthalmoplegia. Progressive disease within the cavernous sinus can lead to carotid artery thrombosis and mycotic aneurysm formation, resulting in neurologic sequelae and death.

Complications of maxillary sinusitis are rare. Mucoceles in the maxillary sinus are occasionally encountered in children with CF. Osteomyelitis of the maxillary sinus, more prevalent in the preantibiotic era and in adults with dental disease, is rare today.

Sinusitis Treatment

Antimicrobial Therapy

Acute and Subacute Sinusitis

The goals of therapy for acute and subacute sinusitis are to hasten clinical improvement, prevent intracranial and orbital complications, and prevent mucosal damage that may predispose to chronic sinus disease[30,31] (Box 18.2). The actual benefit of antibiotics in achieving these goals has not been conclusively proven. A pivotal randomized trial showed that antibiotic therapy (amoxicillin or amoxicillin-clavulanic acid) for acute sinusitis, defined by clinical and plain radiograph criteria, was associated with symptom resolution in 66% of children at 10 days, significantly greater than the 43% rate of resolution among placebo-treated subjects.[125] Two subsequent randomized trials call into question the benefit of antibiotic treatment. One compared amoxicillin, amoxicillin-clavulanate, and placebo in children with clinically diagnosed acute sinusitis and found no differences in symptom improvement at 14 days (79%–81%) or relapse or recurrence rates.[126] The other compared cefuroxime and placebo in children with nonimproving respiratory symptoms and abnormal maxillary sinus ultrasonography; no difference in rates of improvement or cure at 14 days

(84%–91%) was observed.[127] A fourth trial randomized children with acute sinusitis to receive amoxicillin-clavulanate or placebo. Antibiotic treatment was associated with a superior cure rate (50% versus 14%) and less treatment failure (14% versus 68%).[128] An additional randomized study of amoxicillin and nasal saline irrigation versus placebo and intranasal saline did not show a difference

in clinical cure between groups.[129] In the IDSA guidelines, a meta-analysis of antibiotic randomized controlled trials of children with acute sinusitis concluded modest benefit with approximately five children requiring therapy for one additional child with cure or improvement.[112] Meta-analyses of studies in adults with acute sinusitis suggest similar modest benefit of antibiotic therapy, in part because approximately two-thirds of adults with acute sinusitis improve without antibiotic treatment.[112,130–134]

Despite lack of definitive proof of efficacy, antibiotic treatment is recommended for most children with acute and subacute sinusitis because bacterial pathogens are recoverable from the majority of affected sinuses,[1,20] antibiotic treatment may be associated with greater rates of clinical improvement, and preventing sinusitis complications is a major concern.[1,112] Several days of watchful waiting for spontaneous clinical improvement before initiating antibiotic treatment is an alternative for persistent, nonsevere symptoms.[1] There is a paucity of trial data in children to indicate which antibiotics may be superior, although studies performed in adults suggest comparable clinical efficacy of commonly used agents.[24] Antibiotic selection is frequently directed by typical susceptibility profiles of frequently isolated bacteria and pharmacokinetic properties of candidate antibiotics[30,31] (Table 18.3). Because their microbiology is similar, the approach to antibiotic selection for acute and subacute sinusitis is similar. Amoxicillin is commonly recommended for previously untreated, mild, and uncomplicated acute sinusitis based on its excellent tolerability, low cost, narrow spectrum, and track record for both sinusitis and otitis media; this option is preferred in the AAP guidelines for uncomplicated, mild to moderate disease in children lacking risk factors for antibiotic resistance.[1,135,136] This parallels recommendations for adults, in whom meta-analyses

---

> • BOX 18.2 **Key Concepts**
> *Use of Antimicrobials in Sinusitis*

- For acute and subacute sinusitis, target therapy toward the same pathogens responsible for acute otitis media: *Streptococcus pneumoniae, Haemophilus influenzae,* and *Moraxella catarrhalis.*
- Broad-spectrum antibiotics targeting β-lactamase–producing organisms and resistant *S. pneumoniae* should be used when there is:
  - Poor response to first-line antibiotics
  - Moderate to severe chronic or recurrent disease
  - Complicated or potentially complicated disease (including frontal or sphenoidal involvement)
  - High risk for first-line antibiotic-resistant organisms: antibiotic therapy within the preceding 30 to 90 days, daycare attendance, age younger than 2 years, high endemic rates of resistant pathogens
- Treat acute sinusitis for at least 10 to 14 days and until asymptomatic plus an additional 7 days.
- Consider sinus aspiration for microbiologic identification and targeted antimicrobial therapy if disease is:
  - Severe
  - Associated with orbital or intracranial complications
  - Unresponsive to multiple antibiotic courses
  - In immunocompromised patients

TABLE 18.3 Selected Antibiotics for Acute, Subacute, and Chronic Sinusitis

Antibiotic	Comments
Penicillins Amoxicillin Amoxicillin-clavulanate	Untreated, mild, uncomplicated disease; high dose targets resistant *Streptococcus pneumoniae* Poor response to amoxicillin; moderate to severe, complicated or protracted disease; or high risk for antibiotic resistance High dose of amoxicillin component targets resistant *S. pneumoniae*
Cephalosporins Cefuroxime Cefpodoxime Cefprozil Cefdinir Cefixime Cefotaxime Ceftriaxone	Poor response to amoxicillin or amoxicillin-clavulanate; moderate to severe, complicated or protracted disease; penicillin allergy; or high risk of antibiotic resistance. May be combined with clindamycin for additional gram-positive (*S. pneumoniae, Staphylococcus aureus,* streptococci) coverage. Intravenous agents (cefotaxime, ceftriaxone) for severe or complicated disease or disease unresponsive to oral antibiotics
Macrolides Clarithromycin Azithromycin	Recommended only if significant β-lactam allergy limits other options; increasing resistance of *S. pneumoniae* and *Haemophilus influenzae*
Trimethoprim-sulfamethoxazole	Recommended only if significant β-lactam allergy limits other options or if known methicillin-resistant *S. aureus;* increasing resistance of *S. pneumoniae* and *H. influenzae*
Clindamycin	Activity against gram-positive aerobes (including many *S. pneumoniae,* many methicillin-susceptible and methicillin-resistant *S. aureus,* and streptococci) and anaerobes; can be combined with cephalosporin to provide broad coverage; option if significant β-lactam allergy or poor response to β-lactam antibiotics
Levofloxacin	Fluoroquinolone antibiotic; option if severe penicillin allergy or poor response to β-lactam antibiotics
Vancomycin	Intravenous; severe or complicated disease or disease unresponsive to oral antibiotics

of randomized trials support the efficacy of amoxicillin (and penicillin) for acute sinusitis.[130,137,138] However, a 5% to 20% failure rate can be expected with amoxicillin because of resistant *S. pneumoniae, H. influenzae,* and *M. catarrhalis.*[1,34] High-dose amoxicillin (80–90 mg/kg/day) can be used to improve eradication of potentially nonsusceptible *S. pneumoniae* in children with risk factors for antibiotic resistance (e.g., antibiotic therapy within the preceding 30–90 days, daycare attendance, age younger than 2 years, and/or high local rate of penicillin-nonsusceptible *S. pneumoniae*).[1,30,112] Initial therapy with a broader antibiotic targeting β-lactamase–producing organisms and resistant *S. pneumoniae* should be considered in the following circumstances: a history of poor response to amoxicillin; moderate to severe, complicated, or potentially complicated disease (including frontal or sphenoidal involvement); protracted or recurrent disease; and high risk for antibiotic resistance (age younger than 2 years, daycare, recent antibiotic use).[1,34,112,136] Amoxicillin-clavulanic acid (80–90 mg/kg/day of amoxicillin component) is generally recommended in these situations and, in the ISDA guidelines, is the preferred first-line therapy.[1,112] Alternatives include cephalosporins (e.g., cefuroxime, cefpodoxime, cefprozil, cefdinir, cefixime), combination cephalosporin with clindamycin to provide extended gram-positive (e.g., *S. pneumoniae,* methicillin-susceptible and methicillin-resistant *S. aureus*) and anaerobic coverage, or the fluoroquinolone levofloxacin.[1,112] Of note, improved outcomes with broad-spectrum antibiotics have not been demonstrated.[139] Macrolides (e.g., azithromycin) are generally not recommended because of increasing resistance of *S. pneumoniae* and *H. influenzae* unless other options are limited by allergies.[1,30,112,136] The role of trimethoprim-sulfamethoxazole (TMP-SMX) has similarly been reduced by increasing resistance of both *S. pneumoniae* and *H. influenzae;* it remains an option in patients with β-lactam allergy or known infection with MRSA.[1,30,31,112,136]

If amoxicillin is chosen for initial therapy, lack of clinical response within 48 to 72 hours should prompt a change to a broader agent (e.g., amoxicillin-clavulanate).[1,31,34] If amoxicillin-clavulanate is used initially without clinical response, options include either a combination of cephalosporin with clindamycin, or levofloxacin.[1,112] If the disease becomes severe, protracted, associated with orbital or intracranial complications, or unresponsive to multiple antibiotic trials, sinus lavage for microbiologic diagnosis can be considered. Intravenous antibiotic therapy, including staphylococcal and anaerobic coverage, is indicated if severe or complicated disease is present (e.g., combinations among cefotaxime or ceftriaxone, vancomycin, and clindamycin or metronidazole).[1,22,118,136] In immunocompromised hosts, sinus lavage should be considered earlier because of their increased risk for atypical and resistant organisms and their impaired immune response to them.[34,136]

There has been no systematic evaluation of the optimal duration of antibiotic therapy for acute sinusitis in children. Data obtained in adults suggest that treatment for 10 days affords microbiologic cure rates in excess of 90%, whereas 7-day courses are associated with microbiologic failure in 20%. However, treatment courses as short as 1 to 5 days in children have had encouraging clinical results in a limited number of trials.[140–142] In general, a 10- to 14-day treatment course is recommended for the majority of children, tailored to a patient's response (e.g., treat until asymptomatic plus an additional 7 days).[1,34,112,136,143] Longer courses (e.g., 3–4 weeks) should be considered for severe disease or if resolution is unusually slow.[30,36,136,143]

Chronic Sinusitis

Few studies of the efficacy of antibiotics in hastening clinical improvement from and preventing complications of chronic sinusitis have been reported; furthermore, their findings are inconsistent. In atopic children with chronic sinusitis, amoxicillin and TMP-SMX were associated with higher response rates than either erythromycin or an oral antihistamine/decongestant without antibiotic.[144] However, in other studies of subacute or chronic sinusitis, response rates with antibiotic therapy plus decongestant were not greater than those with decongestant plus nasal saline[145] or with placebo or drainage procedures.[51] A Cochrane review found little evidence that systemic antibiotics are effective in adults or children with chronic sinusitis.[146]

Despite lack of firm evidence of efficacy, antibiotics are generally prescribed for chronic sinusitis because pathogenic bacteria in the sinuses have been well documented. Broad-spectrum antibiotics are chosen for empirical therapy, with the choice dependent on previous treatments and anticipated resistance patterns of pathogens such as *S. pneumoniae, H. influenzae, M. catarrhalis,* and *S. aureus* (see Table 18.3). Favorable options include amoxicillin-clavulanic acid, cefuroxime, and third-generation cephalosporins such as cefpodoxime and cefdinir. If these agents are unsuccessful, a trial of clindamycin to target β-lactam–resistant *S. pneumoniae,* methicillin-susceptible and methicillin-resistant *S. aureus,* and anaerobes is reasonable.[30,147,148] TMP-SMX may be helpful for a patient with known infection with MRSA resistant to clindamycin.[149] The roles of oxazolidinones (e.g., linezolid) and newer fluoroquinolones such as levofloxacin for pediatric chronic sinusitis are yet to be determined. After multiple failed antibiotic courses, concern for resistant organisms increases, and sinus lavage for culture and susceptibilities should be considered to facilitate targeted antibiotic treatment.[8,34,47,136,150] Nasal swabs have insufficient positive predictive value to accurately guide antibiotic therapy.[1,43,50,64,112,151] Middle meatus swabs may have better, although still imperfect, correlation with sinus cultures.[1,43,50,64,112,151] Patients with very resistant isolates and/or extremely refractory disease may benefit from intravenous therapy with agents such as cefotaxime, ceftriaxone, cefuroxime, ampicillin-sulbactam, piperacillin-tazobactam, vancomycin, or clindamycin.[47,136,150,153] For invasive fungal sinusitis, surgical debridement, and systemic antifungal therapy are indicated.[154]

The optimal duration of therapy is unknown. A minimum of 14 days is generally recommended if there is a prompt response. Longer courses (e.g., 3–6 weeks) can be considered for slower responses, and treatment for 7 days beyond the patient becoming symptom-free has been suggested.[36,136,143] It also has been suggested that prolonged courses of intravenous antibiotics may be effective for treating bacteria in sinus-containing biofilms; however, this concept remains to be proved.[20]

Antibiotic prophylaxis with agents such as amoxicillin or sulfonamides was previously used for children with recurrent sinusitis by analogy with recurrent otitis media; benefit of prophylactic azithromycin also has been suggested.[34,114,155] An alternative approach was short-term, preemptive prophylaxis with the onset of URTIs in children who have frequently recurrent sinusitis triggered by URTIs, a strategy that was beneficial for recurrent otitis media.[156] However, increasing rates of antibiotic resistance and the resulting impetus to reduce antibiotic exposure have restricted prophylactic antibiotic strategies.[36,157]

Sinus Surgery

Acute Sinusitis

The indications to perform sinus surgery on a child with acute and uncomplicated sinusitis are limited. Acute sinusitis symptoms are generally relieved by medical therapy consisting of antibiotics and adjunctive medical therapy. However, acute frontal or sphenoidal sinusitis in an adolescent may benefit from emergent surgical drainage for pain relief. In immunocompromised hosts, sinus irrigations to obtain specimens for microbial staining and culturing may be needed to identify potentially unusual, opportunistic pathogens.

Chronic Sinusitis

Endoscopic sinus surgery (ESS) was popularized after sinus surgery using endoscopes was imported from Europe by American surgeons in the 1980s. The safety and efficacy of this procedure in pediatric sinusitis cases have been reported, based primarily on satisfaction questionnaires.[158–160] A meta-analysis using data from 13 studies on the outcomes of pediatric ESS concluded that ESS is a safe and effective treatment for chronic sinusitis in children.[161] However, it is important to note that the studies included in this analysis lack an untreated control group, and most of the data sources were retrospective chart reviews.

Others have reported symptomatic and clinical improvements after ESS in special populations such as children and adults with asthma[162,163] and CF,[164] although polyp recurrence in cystic fibrosis exceeds 50%.[161] Opposing this trend have been sporadic commentaries challenging the impression that pediatric sinusitis is a surgical disease.[157,165] Indeed, in a cohort of children who underwent ESS at an early age, a markedly higher rate of revision surgeries (50%) was required (e.g., for postsurgical ostiomeatal scarring), in comparison with a control group of young patients with chronic sinusitis who had not had prior sinus surgery (9%).[166]

Despite its unproved clinical efficacy and uncertain indications, ESS has safety attributes that surpass those of its predecessors. ESS with pediatric instrumentation can provide sinus drainage and sinus ablation. Specifically, the ostium of the maxillary sinuses can be widened by endoscopic antrostomy. By performing endoscopic ethmoidectomy, the ethmoid cells and polypoid tissue can be removed, frontal duct drainage can be enhanced, and the sphenoid sinus can be entered and drained. A technologic advance in ESS—balloon sinuplasty—uses angioplasty balloon technology to expand the sinus ostium to increase sinus aeration and/or establish drainage. The therapeutic benefit of balloon sinuplasty has not yet been determined,[109,167] but case series suggest benefit.[168,169] The light angioplasty guide wire can be used to enter the frontal sinus for bacteriologic sampling and irrigation.

Surgery for Sinusitis Complications

The type of sinusitis complication dictates whether an otolaryngologist will need the additional expertise of an ophthalmologist or a neurosurgeon. Generally, the participation of a pediatrician or an infectious disease consultant in the care of a child with sinusitis complications is beneficial.

Subperiosteal and orbital abscesses can be drained through either an external or endoscopic approach. Small intraorbital or epidural abscesses may be treated medically. Other intracranial abscesses are usually drained by a neurosurgeon, often in association with ESS.[170] Complicated frontal sinusitis (e.g., mucocele, osteomyelitis of the frontal bone) is treated through an external approach, with the intent to achieve drainage and debridement.

Severe cases in which long-term antimicrobial therapy has failed may need sinus obliteration, cranialization, and/or other reconstructive procedures. Mucoceles of the ethmoid and sphenoid sinuses can be drained endoscopically. Children with toxic shock syndrome from sinusitis should undergo sinus irrigation for culture and drainage. Neurosurgical drainage is sometimes indicated.

Adjunctive Surgical Procedures

Adenoid hypertrophy is a cause of chronic sinusitis, and the benefits of adenoidectomy for chronic sinusitis have been suggested by earlier uncontrolled studies.[171,172] A meta-analysis of 10 trials (six cohort and four case series) showed significant reduction of postoperative sinusitis symptoms.[173] The basis for improvement by adenoidectomy is unknown. No correlation between maxillary sinus and adenoid cultures in patients with chronic rhinosinusitis was found.[19] An abundance of bacterial biofilm coating the surface of adenoid surgical specimens in patients with chronic rhinosinusitis versus obstructive sleep apnea was observed.[174] Patients with chronic sinusitis with nasal obstruction from adenoid hypertrophy are likely to have some symptomatic benefit from an adenoidectomy regardless of effects on the sinuses.

Some children with chronic sinusitis have inferior turbinate hypertrophy causing nasal obstruction. There are no published reports on the efficacy of inferior turbinate cauterization or reduction in the treatment of chronic sinusitis. In subjects in whom intranasal corticosteroid therapy for nasal obstructive symptoms associated with inferior turbinate hypertrophy has failed, a turbinate reduction procedure for symptomatic relief may be considered.

Adjunctive Medical Therapy

Clinicians have used an assortment of agents in conjunction with oral antibiotics for the treatment of both acute and chronic sinusitis in children, including nasal saline washes (isotonic and hypertonic), topical and oral decongestants and antihistamines, topical anticholinergics, leukotriene receptor antagonists, topical antiinfectives, and corticosteroids (intranasal and oral). The use of these agents is largely based on their theoretical benefits of improving associated rhinitis and rhinorrhea by decreasing mucosal inflammation, edema, and mucous production and increasing mucociliary transport, thereby improving nasal patency and presumably ostial drainage. Data are limited, and use of these agents is generally discouraged in treating acute sinusitis in children.[1,113,175] In particular, there is limited support for intranasal corticosteroids as monotherapy or in combination with oral antibiotics for acute sinusitis.[10,16,176]

Cochrane reviews addressing the efficacy of intranasal saline washes[177] and intranasal corticosteroids[168,178] for rhinosinusitis (primarily in adults) identified improvement in chronic sinusitis symptoms with saline washes and intranasal corticosteroids. Additionally, in adults with chronic rhinosinusitis with nasal polyposis, intranasal corticosteroids improved polyp scores and symptoms and reduced postoperative polyp recurrence.[35] Consistent with these observations, intranasal saline irrigation and intranasal corticosteroids are generally recommended for children with chronic sinusitis.[3,109] Very limited data also suggest possible benefit of short-course oral corticosteroids for chronic sinusitis.[3,16,179] Studies to support use of nasal decongestants and antihistamines for pediatric chronic sinusitis are lacking.[3] Topical antibiotic and antifungal therapies have been purported to benefit patients with chronic rhinosinusitis, but data indicating benefit of these treatments are also lacking.[3,39,109]

For the treatment of chronic rhinosinusitis with nasal polyposis in adults (18 years of age and older), dupilumab is a new anti–IL-4/IL-13 "biologic" therapy that has recently been approved by the U.S. Food and Drug Administration (FDA)-approved as 300 mg by subcutaneous injection every 2 weeks.[180] Current interventions for this chronic sinusitis phenotype are limited and include intranasal and systemic corticosteroids and nasal polypectomies. Because the pathologic hallmark of this phenotype is T_H2-type eosinophilic inflammation with sinus mucosal hypertrophy and polyp formation (see Immune Pathogenesis section and Fig. 18.2, earlier), monoclonal antibody therapies developed to block key mediators in this inflammatory pathway are therapeutic considerations. Dupilumab is a human monoclonal antibody targeting IL-4 receptor-α to inhibit the actions of both T_H2 cytokines IL-4 and IL-13. Dupilumab was approved by the FDA for use in adults and adolescents ages 12 years and older for moderate to severe asthma and atopic dermatitis, and for adults with chronic rhinosinusitis with nasal polyposis. For rhinosinusitis with nasal polyposis, three randomized controlled trials (including two FDA Phase III trials) demonstrated significant and substantial improvements in nasal polyp size and burdens assessed endoscopically, sinus opacification assessed radiographically, symptom scores, nasal obstruction/congestion severity, sense of smell, systemic corticosteroid/nasal polyp surgery use, quality of life, and sick leave days.[181–183] The most common adverse effects reported in the clinical trials were injection site reactions, conjunctivitis, arthralgia, and gastritis. Other biologic therapies directed against T_H2-type inflammation currently under investigation for treatment of this chronic sinusitis phenotype include omalizumab (anti-IgE), mepolizumab (anti-IL5), and benralizumab (anti-IL5 receptor).[184]

Conclusions

Sinusitis in children is a common problem. Diagnosis is challenging because of the overlap of symptoms, physical findings, and radiographic findings with those of common URTIs. Sinusitis rarely leads to severe, life-threatening complications as a result of direct extension of bacterial infection from the sinuses. Management of uncomplicated, acute sinusitis consists of antimicrobial treatment aiming for symptom relief and prevention of complications and recurrence. Radiographic imaging studies (e.g., coronal sinus CT scans) may be helpful in chronic, recurrent, or complicated sinusitis. Antral irrigation can provide sinus specimens for bacterial culture and targeted antimicrobial therapy in patients with chronic, refractory, and complicated disease. Sinus surgery in uncomplicated sinusitis, especially in young children, should generally be avoided. Great reductions in mortality caused by sinusitis complications coincide with advances in antimicrobial and surgical therapies.

The reference list can be found on the companion Expert Consult website at http://www.expertconsult.inkling.com.

19

Chronic Cough

JULIE M. MARCHANT, SUSANNE G. LAU, ANNE B. CHANG

KEY POINTS

- Chronic cough (>4 weeks duration) causes impaired quality of life in the child and parents and should be systematically assessed.
- Daily chronic wet or productive cough should never be ignored.
- The causes of chronic cough in children are different from those in adults, although still depending on age and setting.

- Treatment for chronic cough in children should be based on cause and medications for upper airways, gastroesophageal reflux, and asthma and should not be used when there are no other supportive symptoms or signs.
- The most common cause of chronic wet cough in children in some settings is protracted bacterial bronchitis, an infection of the lower airways.

Chronic Cough in Children

Chronic cough in children is one of the most frequent reasons for medical review and a common reason for referral for specialist consultation.[1] The burden of chronic cough has been well documented with impaired quality of life, use of medications, and multiple visits to doctors for parents and children.[2,3] An approach to the diagnosis and management of this common symptom is presented here. Although this chapter is included in the "Upper Airways" section, cough is a symptom of the lower airways.

Definition

Most guidelines around the world define chronic cough in children as a daily cough lasting for more than 4 weeks.[4] However, in the absence of data that have specifically examined whether cough management or testing algorithms should differ depending on the duration of chronic cough, this is primarily based on expert opinion and is now incorporated into American College of Chest Physicians (ACCP) guidelines.[5–7] It is based on evidence that cough related to acute upper respiratory tract infection will have resolved in the majority (>90%) of children within this time frame.[8] Importantly, in these studies, children with persistent cough were not evaluated. In addition, in children the definition of chronic cough of more than 4 weeks allows for the identification of potentially serious and life-threatening conditions that may otherwise be left untreated.[2] A prospective multicenter study that used a cough algorithm documented a serious potentially progressive underlying respiratory illness (bronchiectasis, aspiration lung disease, or cystic fibrosis [CF]) in 18% of children newly referred to pediatric pulmonologists.[2] Further published studies that systematically assessed outcomes of individual children with

acute cough (at a children's specialist hospital) that persisted for longer than 4 weeks found a new and serious chronic lung disease (e.g., chronic pneumonia, bronchiectasis) in up to 30.8% children.[9,10] However, the prevalence of these illnesses would likely be lower in primary care.

Chronic cough can be categorized into *specific cough* and *nonspecific cough*. Specific cough is cough that is caused by an identifiable underlying abnormality or cause. Initial clinical evaluation will usually highlight signs and symptoms that suggest the specific cause of the cough (see Box 19.2, later in chapter). These specific cough markers can be used to identify a likely underlying cause for the cough.[5] Each of these markers has its own varying specificity and sensitivity and associated likelihood ratios.[11] Importantly, an absence of all of these markers makes a specific cause for the cough very unlikely.[11]

Nonspecific cough is a dry chronic cough in which a thorough history, examination, chest radiography, and spirometry do not reveal any specific cough markers, and no identifiable cause can be found. Therefore, this type of cough will usually resolve without therapy, but review and re-evaluation for the development of a wet cough or other specific cough markers is necessary until the cough resolves.

One of the most important markers in the approach to chronic cough in a child is the nature of the cough—wet/productive or dry.[11] It has been shown that compared with assessment by clinicians, parental assessment of wet cough holds good clinical validity in young children.[12] In older children, who are able to expectorate, the term *productive cough* is used. The presence of a daily wet or productive cough for longer than 4 weeks indicates the presence of increased airway secretions[12] and a specific cause for the cough.[11] Thus, when discussing the differential diagnoses of chronic childhood cough in this chapter, the causes will be addressed in this framework.

Pathophysiology

Cough Reflex in Health

Cough is a protective reflex, with both voluntary and involuntary elements of control, that functions to clear the airways of inhaled particulate material and airway mucus and is essential for respiratory health. It is a complex reflex that responds to chemical and mechanical stimuli via sensory vagal nerve fibers in pulmonary and extrapulmonary sites (afferent limb). These fibers feed into the brainstem, whereby further modulation can occur (central limb). Output occurs by phrenic, intercostal, laryngeal, and abdominal motor neurons to the muscles involved (efferent limb).[13]

The afferent limb of the cough reflex is primarily mediated via chemosensitive and mechanosensitive vagal fibers. The chemosensitive bronchopulmonary C-fibers are sensitive to inflammatory mediators, such as bradykinin, and irritants, such as capsaicin, and account for the majority of bronchopulmonary afferent nerves. Numerous animal studies have concluded that they are primarily responsible for cough reflex initiation.[13,14] The second afferent limb is myelinated vagal nerves described first by Widdicombe as "cough receptors."[15–18] These mechanosensitive and acid-sensitive nerves, although not truly receptors, play a central role in cough. They do not respond to capsaicin but to punctate mechanical stimulation and are found only in the extrapulmonary airways (i.e., larynx, trachea, and main bronchi).[19]

After cough initiation, the afferent limb nerves converge at the brainstem, particularly the nucleus of the solitary tract. A synergistic interaction of C-fibers and cough receptors can occur at this level, to enhance or inhibit cough (discussed further later). The central limb of cough then involves the brainstem respiratory network. This extensive network, including the ventrolateral medulla, raphe nuclei, and pons, controls phases of cough. Finally, higher brain processing (cortical and subcortical) is involved in the consciousness, perception, and emotional elements of cough, such as voluntary suppression of cough.

The efferent motor limb involves the laryngeal and spinal motor neurons (to phrenic, intercostal, and abdominal muscles) controlling all three phases of cough: inspiratory, compressive, and expiratory.

Mechanically, an effective cough involves three phases: inspiratory, compressive, and expiratory[20] (Fig. 19.1). The inspiratory phase of cough involves the inhalation of gas. Inhaling to higher volumes assists the expiratory muscles to lengthen and optimize positive intrathoracic pressures. The compressive phase follows, which involves glottic closure. Glottic closure increases intraabdominal and intrathoracic pressures and further improves the force-length relationship for the expiratory muscles.[20] Once the glottis is open, the expiratory phase of cough begins with high expiratory flow rates. Hence an optimal cough involves high intrathoracic pressures to generate optimal airflow velocities, maximal expiratory pressures, and dynamic airway compression for airway clearance.

After the previously described mechanical phases, an effective cough will clear the airway of mucus and particulate matter through several mechanisms. The increased velocity of the airflow will promote the dispersion of mucus into the airstream for removal, termed "misty flow."[20] Second, these high airflow velocities can promote waves of mucus to be cleared during cough.

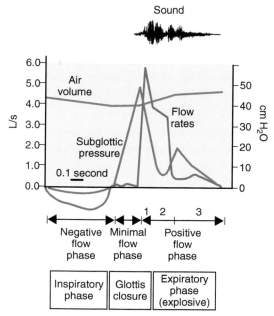

• **Fig. 19.1** Changes in flow and subglottic pressure during cough. (From Bianco S, Robuschi M. Mechanics of cough. In: Braga PC, Allegra L, editors. Cough. New York: Raven; 1989).

Finally, the higher pressure can cause the airways to vibrate and compress, loosening mucus to help its clearance. These processes, combined with mucociliary apparatus, can lead to clearing of mucus from as distally as the 7th to 12th (out of total of 23) airway generations.[21]

Cough Reflex in Pediatric Chronic Cough

Like almost everything in health, there is a maturation aspect to cough. In neonates the predominant reflexes are laryngeal chemoreflexes, including swallowing, apnea, and laryngeal closure, and the cough reflex is underdeveloped, which is particularly important in premature infants.[22] With maturation, these protective reflexes decrease and the coughing reflex becomes more pronounced. The age at which the coughing reflex is fully mature is not known, but these maturational effects can have clinical implications[13]; for instance, inhaled foreign bodies are more common in young children.

"Cough receptor" sensitivity in postpubertal adolescents and adults depends on gender and increases in clinical situation such as chronic dry cough. In children, unlike in adults, age but not gender influences cough receptor sensitivity measurements.[23] An increase in cough sensitivity can be seen during coughing illness, such as in a respiratory tract infection, and is thought to be due to increased inflammatory mediators and neuromodulation.[24] Although cough sensitivity remains increased when children are actively coughing, this is thought to return to normal levels when the coughing resolves.[25]

An impaired cough reflex can have significant consequences for respiratory health, such as in bronchial obstruction and children with neuromuscular disorders. Children with neurologic disorders may have a compromised cough reflex with an abnormal afferent limb leading to an increased predisposition to chest infections through aspiration, further highlighting the importance of this protective reflex. Although both the inspiratory phase and compressive phase of coughing are not essential for cough, glottic closure enhances cough, leading to a more effective cough. In patients with neuromuscular weakness, minor increases in intrathoracic pressure may be enough to generate an effective cough, but as disease progresses and respiratory muscle weakness increases, cough will become ineffective because of limited inhalation in the first phase, followed by impaired intrathoracic rise in the second and third phases of cough.[20] An assessment of cough effectiveness is an important element of diagnostic evaluation in children with chronic cough and neurodevelopmental or neuromuscular disorders.

Differential Diagnosis

Our differential diagnosis framework is based on one of the most important markers in the approach to chronic cough in a child—the nature of the cough as wet/productive or dry.[11] Although it has been shown that reporting of wet cough by parents holds good clinical validity,[12] it should be remembered that when the cough is mixed (i.e., reported as sometimes wet and sometimes dry), it should be classified as wet cough. Whereas the presence of a daily wet/productive cough indicates the presence of airway secretions,[12] the absence of wet cough does not exclude the possibility of a small amount of airway secretions. Therefore, children who present initially with a dry cough may have airway secretions, or cough may become wet/productive subsequently, and they should be reviewed and reassessed for symptom change.

Dry Cough

Nonspecific Cough

Dry cough with no other specific cough markers on history, examination, chest radiography, and spirometry is by definition *nonspecific* cough and will usually resolve without therapy. Management should involve a "watchful waiting" approach, with regular re-evaluation for the development of a wet cough or other specific cough markers until the chronic cough resolves.[11] Preceding respiratory viruses are the most likely common cause of nonspecific cough.[10]

Other infections, specifically *Mycoplasma pneumoniae* and *Chlamydia pneumoniae,* can cause a nonproductive chronic cough. The initial infections may vary from a mild respiratory tract infection through to a pneumonic process. Laboratory diagnosis is difficult and can only rarely be made with serology, polymerase chain reaction (PCR), or antigen detection.[26] Only patients with pneumonic processes should be treated empirically. In otherwise well patients with chronic cough the cough resolves with time, and treatment with antibiotics is not recommended.

Other respiratory organisms can lead to a persistence of cough beyond the acute illness; adenovirus, *Haemophilus influenzae,* and *Moraxella catarrhalis* have been implicated in the literature, but more often are associated with a wet cough and protracted bacterial bronchitis (PBB) (discussed later).[27–29] There are other specific causes of cough, which can present with dry cough, but in which other cough markers in history or examination are evident. These are presented in the following section.

Bordetella Pertussis Infection

Bordetella pertussis or *Bordetella parapertussis* infection can manifest as chronic nonproductive cough, with or without

the typical paroxysmal whoop. The classic disease pattern is modified by vaccination, and readers are referred to recent reviews.[30,31] With over 16 million cases diagnosed worldwide, this is particularly important in low-income countries, which account for 95% of cases.[32] Classic pertussis has three stages: catarrhal, paroxysmal, and convalescent. The first catarrhal stage is similar to a viral upper respiratory tract infection. The second paroxysmal phase sees the development of coughing spells, prolonged bursts of coughing with little inspiratory effort, and typical whoop.[31] The whoop is noise made by forced inspiratory effort and typically follows a coughing attack. Although the acute paroxysmal phase peaks early in the illness, it can persist for months in some cases.[33] In one prospective study, 20% of children with chronic cough had evidence of recent pertussis infection, most of whom had been immunized. Therefore, the diagnosis should be considered even in those fully immunized.[34]

Advances in diagnostic methods such as PCR and antibody detection in serum and oral fluid against pertussis toxin (PT) have occurred.[35] In the setting of chronic cough in older children, laboratory investigation (where available) should include immunoglobin G (IgG) to PT because a diagnosis is important for disease control measures and to avoid ongoing investigations for other causes of chronic cough, although no treatment is recommended.[31,32] In infants, PCR and culture are recommended and antimicrobial therapy may be recommended in the first 6 weeks of illness.[31]

Asthma

Although children with asthma can present with chronic cough, isolated chronic dry cough in the absence of other suggestive symptoms or signs is rarely asthma.[36] Symptoms and signs suggestive of asthma include exertional dyspnea, bilateral recurrent wheeze, and personal or family history of atopy. Investigation with spirometry (performed in children older than 6 years) that demonstrates a reversible obstructive pattern and chest radiograph that shows bilateral hyperinflation, and in some instances right middle lobe changes, would support the diagnosis of asthma in a child with a chronic cough. An absence of these symptoms and investigation results has been termed *cough-variant asthma,* but the term *cough-dominant asthma* is arguably a better term. Nevertheless, it manifests comparable to a nonspecific cough, but studies have suggested this is an uncommon cause of cough in children.[37,38] Despite this, in certain children a trial of asthma therapies is appropriate to consider because parental reporting of wheeze is not reliable.[39] If a trial of asthma medications is warranted, bronchodilators and low-dose inhaled corticosteroids are recommended for a defined period (usually 2 to 4 weeks) before re-evaluation for response. It must be remembered that cough therapies demonstrate a significant placebo effect and nonspecific cough will spontaneously resolve, so these asthma medications should be continued only if a definitive diagnosis is made. Furthermore, failure to respond to the medication trial makes the diagnosis unlikely (please refer to Section E for more extensive asthma specific information).

In some instances, children with diagnosed asthma have a chronic wet cough, and in these situations co-existing PBB (see later discussion) should be considered and treated appropriately because the two conditions can co-exist.

Allergy and Cough

Although some argue that "allergic cough" exists, there is little substantive evidence. One study involving 202 children found that atopy (defined on skin prick tests) had no significant influence on any of the cough outcomes (cough counts, cough score, or cough sensitivity to capsaicin).[40] The link between cough and allergy is likely through other conditions associated with chronic cough, such as asthma. Readers are referred to the chapters on allergic rhinitis and asthma. In contrast to adults, in whom eosinophilic bronchitis is a well-recognized cause of adult chronic cough, it is not yet defined as a distinct diagnosis in children.

Pediatric studies that have reported "upper airways cough syndrome" were not randomized controlled trials (RCTs), and most subjects in these studies were treated with antibiotics. Indeed, there are no RCTs on therapies for upper airway disorders in younger children with nonspecific cough. Finally, postnasal drip is not thought to be a common cause of chronic cough in children because a postnasal drip will end up in the gastrointestinal passages not in the airways.[41]

Data on fractional exhaled nitric oxide (FeNO) levels in children with cough presumed related to "upper airway cough syndrome" is conflicting. One study[42] reported elevated FeNO levels, and another[43] reported no elevation in levels. Thus, using FeNO levels alone for diagnosing and managing children with chronic cough without other cough markers is yet to be clearly defined.

Gastroesophageal Reflux Disease

Whether gastroesophageal reflux disease (GERD) causes chronic cough in pediatric individuals remains controversial, although in adult cough GERD is thought to be an important cause.[44] However, it has been suggested by experts that it is an uncommon cause except when associated with aspiration.[1,45] A 2017 systematic review of causes of chronic cough in children found GERD described as a common cause in only 2 of 10 prospective studies.[1] In addition, the causative role of GERD in chronic cough in children has been difficult to prove.[46] When acid reflux is measured with pH manometry and compared objectively with a cough-meter, more than 80% of coughs were not associated with a reflux event.[47] Furthermore, gold standard diagnosis of GERD in children is not well defined.[48]

A recent systematic review of GERD and cough in children has suggested children with chronic cough and no symptoms of GERD should not treated with anti-GERD management for their cough.[45] In children with chronic cough and with symptoms, signs, or positive investigations, treatment should be in accordance with the current evidence-based GERD-specific guidelines.[45,48] These guidelines suggest a trial of medications depending on child's age and of 4 to 8 weeks duration before review. Investigations should follow GERD-specific guidelines that are also specific to the child's age but in general recommend endoscopy before pH manometry.[48] Importantly, a trial of acid-suppressive therapy for cough symptomatology alone is not recommended, because meta-analysis data have found proton-pump inhibitors have not reduced cough in infants[49] and have serious adverse side effects.

Tic Cough (Habit Cough) or Somatic Cough Disorder (Psychogenic Cough or Dysfunctional Respiratory Symptoms)

A functional cough (tic or somatic cough disorder) is a persistent dry cough without a pathologic cause. A tic cough (previously

---

• BOX 19.1 Suggestion Therapy for Tic (Habit) Cough

- Instill confidence in the patient that the cough will stop.
- Explain the vicious cycle of irritation that may have caused the cough.
- Instruct the patient to concentrate only on holding back the urge to cough, sipping warm water if necessary.
- Repeat confidence in the patient's efforts to suppress the cough, use nodding of head.
- After 10 minutes during which the patient has suppressed the cough, ask "you're beginning to feel able to resist the urge to cough aren't you?"
- End the session with "do you feel you can resist the cough on your own now?"
- Explain "autosuggestion" for the patient to continue to suppress the cough at home.

Weinberger M, Lockshin B. When is cough functional, and how should it be treated? Breathe (Sheff) 2017;13(1):22–30.

---

known as *habit cough*) is a repetitive dry cough with the features of suppressibility, distractibility, and suggestibility.[50] It is characterized by a frequent loud and repetitive dry cough, often with characteristic honking or barking.[51] *A significant differentiating feature is the absence of cough in sleep.* It is often associated with secondary gains such as school absence and sometimes high-performance pressure, such as in competitive sports; it affects males and females equally. Typical age is school-age children and adolescence ages from 4 to 18 years, with a median age of 10 years.[52,53] The majority of children present to specialists having received multiple trials (median of three) of medications with no resolution of the cough.[53] Often antiasthma therapy has been prescribed without success.[54] These children have a normal examination and normal investigation findings, such as with spirometry, chest radiograph, and allergy tests. The treatment of tic cough is suggestion therapy, which involves reassurance and suggestion that the cough can be stopped (Box 19.1). This treatment can see cessation of cough within 15 minutes of initial therapy in 95% of patients when done by experienced pediatric respiratory physicians.[51,55]

Somatic cough disorder (previously known as psychogenic cough) presents with a similar repetitive dry cough, and the children fulfill criteria for somatic disorder, including the presence of one or more somatic symptoms as per the *Diagnostic and Statistical Manual of Mental Disorders,* 5th edition (DSM-5).[50] These somatic symptoms may include disproportionate thoughts about the seriousness of the cough, anxiety about the cough beyond expected levels, or excessive time devoted to the cough. They may respond to suggestion therapy, as outlined earlier, and if unsuccessful require referral to a psychologist or psychiatrist for further evaluation. Occasionally, these children who present with repetitive tic cough may have Tourette's syndrome, which involves motor and vocal tics, and need referral for further evaluation and management.[50]

Other Rarer Causes Chronic Dry Cough

Interstitial Lung Disease

Interstitial lung disease (ILD), more recently known as *diffuse lung disease,* represents a diffuse group of disorders in which there are changes to the alveolar and airway architecture that interfere with gas exchange.[56] The causes are broad and include primary genetic abnormalities, autoimmune disease, postinfection bronchiolitis obliterans, postradiation effects, or drug side effects. Typical presentation involves persistent tachypnea, dry cough, fine crackles on auscultation, digital clubbing, and failure to thrive. Other features may include feeding difficulties, hemoptysis, and fevers, and late diagnosis may have features of pulmonary hypertension. Exposure to birds is an important historical factor for hypersensitivity pneumonitis. A chest radiograph is usually abnormal but not usually specific, with bilateral pulmonary infiltrates being most common. Spirometry may show a restrictive pattern. Further investigation will include a high-resolution computed tomography (HRCT), which may be specific for some ILDs, but further investigation with bronchoscopy and bronchoalveolar lavage (BAL), genetic testing, and lung biopsy is often necessary.

Space-Occupying Lesions

A mediastinal mass, resulting from a malignancy, is a rare cause of chronic cough and will usually be evident on chest radiography during investigation. Further investigation with HRCT and referral to an oncologist is necessary.

Cardiac Disease

Underlying cardiac disease can cause chronic cough as a result of pulmonary hypertension or pulmonary edema. Pulmonary hypertension can be idiopathic or secondary to congenital heart disease, human immunodeficiency virus (HIV) infection, or connective tissue disorders. Cardiogenic pulmonary edema is most often due to left-sided congenital heart disease. Specific examination findings may include abnormalities in heart sounds or pulses or peripheral edema of extremities. A chest radiograph will often be abnormal and may show a large or abnormally shaped heart. Referral to a pediatric cardiologist, electrocardiogram, and echocardiogram is recommended.

Otogenic Cough

In a small number of people the external ear is innervated by a branch of the vagal nerve.[57] In these individuals, irritation to the ear canal (i.e., with cerumen) can cause chronic dry cough via the otogenic reflex. Removal of the irritants can relieve symptoms.

Wet Cough

Chronic Endobronchial Infection

As mentioned earlier, a daily wet/productive cough indicates the presence of airway secretions and holds good clinical validity.[12] Chronic wet cough in children most commonly represents chronic endobronchial infection. This includes a spectrum of disease from isolated PBB, recurrent PBB, chronic suppurative lung disease, and bronchiectasis.

It has been suggested that all three diseases represent a spectrum of disease with PBB at one end and irreversible bronchiectasis at the other (Fig. 19.2).[58] The three conditions share pathobiologic similarities with neutrophilic airway infection with typical organisms (*H. influenzae, M. catarrhalis,* and *S. pneumoniae*) and associated airway inflammation, with increased matrix metallopeptidase 9 (MMP-9), interleukin-1 beta (IL-1β), and interleukin 8 (IL-8).[59] A prospective longitudinal study found that 8% of 106 children with PBB progressed to

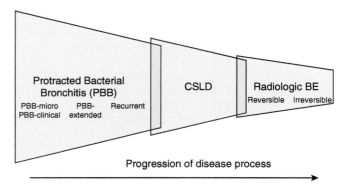

• **Fig. 19.2** Spectrum of chronic suppurative lung disease. (Courtesy Chang AB, Upham JW, Masters IB, et al. Protracted bacterial bronchitis: the last decade and the road ahead. Pediatr Pulmonol 2016;51(3):225–42.)

bronchiectasis over the 2-year study, with recurrent episodes of PBB and nontypeable *H. influenza* infection being significant risk factors.[60]

Protracted Bacterial Bronchitis

PBB is one of the most common causes of chronic cough in affluent countries, accounting for up to 40% of chronic wet cough presentations to tertiary clinics.[2,38] The diagnosis is based on clinical criteria, including (1) chronic daily wet cough (> 4 weeks duration), (2) absence of other specific cough markers, (3) resolution of cough with 2 weeks of appropriate antibiotic therapy (typically amoxicillin–clavulanic acid).[59]

Initially described in 2006 as part of a large cohort study, the diagnosis has now been incorporated into most international pediatric cough guidelines, including in the United States, Australia, and the United Kingdom.[5,61,62] The original description involved the presence of lower airway infection with airway neutrophilic inflammation with 10^4 colony-forming units (CFUs)/mL or more organisms collected by bronchoscopy and bronchoalveolar lavage (BAL). The organisms identified were typically common respiratory pathogens *H. influenzae, M. catarrhalis,* and *S. pneumoniae*.[38] Because the typical patient is preschool aged (younger than 5 years of age) and otherwise well, the requirement for lower airway fluid sampling by bronchoscopy and BAL has since been removed from the clinical definition.[59] Recommended treatment is 2 weeks of antibiotic therapy aimed at these typical organisms, based on systematic review of available RCTs.[63,64] The most commonly used antibiotic for PBB is amoxicillin–clavulanic acid because it is active against the β-lactamase–producing strains of *H. influenzae*. In cases of penicillin allergy, trimethoprim-sulfamethoxazole is an alternative. Macrolide antibiotics are not recommended because of concerns with increasing resistance of *H. influenzae* and *S. pneumoniae*.[65] In some children with more severe disease the cough may not resolve within 2 weeks and a further 2 weeks of antibiotics is required and a diagnosis of "PBB-extended" is used.[59]

The characteristics of these patients have now been well described,[66,67] and the natural history of this condition has been examined in longitudinal studies.[60] Typically, children with PBB are young (median age 1.8–4.8 years), although it also occurs in older children (older than 12 years) with a male predominance.[59] These children with PBB are not exposed to tobacco smoke more than are control groups. Atopic features, clinical history (e.g., eczema, rhinitis, etc.), elevated total IgE, positive test for specific serum IgE, or positive skin prick test for aeroallergens are similar in children with PBB and control groups.[68] On examination, these children are otherwise very well with normal growth and development. They may have or describe a "rattle" on chest auscultation, thought to be secretions moving in the large airways. A chest radiograph will be normal or show nonspecific changes of peribronchial thickening. Spirometry, if performed, is typically normal.[59] A significant proportion (44%) will have recurrent PBB, and 8% were diagnosed with bronchiectasis in the first 2 years after diagnosis.[57] Other studies have confirmed the recurrent nature in some children, and parents should be counseled about this risk and appropriate follow-up.[59,69]

For patients with recurrent PBB (>3 episodes/year) or wet cough that does not respond to 4 weeks of appropriate antibiotic therapy, it is recommended the children undergo further investigation and referral to a pediatric pulmonologist. This is because studies have shown (1) a wet cough that does not respond to an initial 4 weeks of antibiotic therapy increases the likelihood of underlying bronchiectasis at presentation (adjusted odds ratio [aOR] 20.9; 95% confidence interval [CI] 5.4–81.8)[70] and (2) recurrent PBB (defined as >3 episodes in 1 year) has been shown to be a significant risk factor for the development of bronchiectasis (aOR 11.5; 95% CI 2.3–56.5).[60] Significant other diagnoses may manifest in the same way (e.g., retained airway foreign body, H-type tracheoesophageal fistula, or bronchiectasis). These investigations include flexible bronchoscopy and BAL, HRCT chest scan, or lung magnetic resonance imaging (MRI), which has improved as a diagnostic tool, especially for inhomogeneity of ventilation and bronchiectasis, sweat test, immune evaluation, and other investigations for causes of bronchiectasis as considered necessary in the context of the clinical symptoms and signs (i.e., ciliary biopsy for suspected primary ciliary dyskinesia (PCD); see "Bronchiectasis" section).

Chronic Suppurative Lung Disease

Chronic suppurative lung disease (CSLD) is used to describe the clinical entity in which patients have a chronic wet cough that does not resolve with 4 weeks of appropriate oral antibiotic therapy, yet the patients do not have bronchiectasis on HRCT chest scan[71] or lung MRI. This diagnosis is thought to lie between PBB and bronchiectasis within the spectrum of chronic endobronchial infections (see Fig. 19.2).[58] Treatment is similar to that for bronchiectasis (described in the next section), with intravenous antibiotic therapy and airway clearance techniques often necessary for cough resolution.[71]

Bronchiectasis

Pediatric bronchiectasis is diagnosed in children with chronic wet cough and with a radiologic diagnosis on HRCT chest scan of airway dilation, confirmed with a bronchoarterial ratio greater than 0.8.[72] Other radiologic features include signet ring appearance, bronchial wall thickening, and failure of bronchial structure to taper toward lung periphery.[73] Historically it has been thought that the diagnosis was irreversible, but when diagnosed early with prompt and intensive treatment it has been postulated that it can be reversed in some cases.[74] Clinical history may include recurrent episodes of wet cough unresponsive to oral antibiotics, recurrent pneumonia, exertional dyspnea, feeding difficulties, coarse crackles on chest auscultation, and digital clubbing.

There are many underlying causes that vary in low- and high-income countries and include postinfectious (including posttuberculosis or bronchiolitis obliterans), CF, PCD, aspiration lung disease, foreign body inhalation, tracheomalacia, and immunodeficiency. Investigations after HRCT chest scan to define the cause of bronchiectasis are necessary, when available. These include, but are not limited to, the sweat chloride test; complete blood count; immunoglobulins; vaccine responses; and, when clinically indicated, tests for cilial motility, extended immune testing, bronchoscopy and BAL, and tuberculosis (TB) and HIV testing depending on the setting and clinical history. In some settings lung MRI is used, especially in clinical follow-up of CF,[75-77] but chest CT scan remains the gold standard for diagnosing bronchiectasis.[72]

Management involves treatment of airway infection and inflammation to prevent further air lung damage with targeted antibiotic therapy and airway clearance techniques, with airway clearance therapies, and is ideally carried out in a multidisciplinary clinic with children managed by a pediatric pulmonologist. Initial oral antibiotic therapy should be aimed at specific pathogens when known: amoxicillin–clavulanic acid for common respiratory pathogens, flucloxacillin for *Staphylococcus aureus*, and ciprofloxacin (plus addition inhaled antibiotics) for *Pseudomonas aeruginosa*.[72] Intravenous antibiotics are necessary when exacerbations are severe, or there is no cough resolution on oral treatment.

Tracheomalacia

Several studies have reported that children with tracheomalacia and other airway abnormalities, such as vascular rings and airway compression, have a chronic cough. Despite this finding of chronic cough in children with tracheomalacia determining causality is difficult. First, in cohort studies of patients with tracheomalacia, cough is reported in approximately 70% of children and not all cases.[78,79] Second, it has been shown that when underlying infection is treated the cough resolves.[38] Third, airway lesions can be found in asymptomatic children. Nonetheless, it is common for children with chronic endobronchial infection to have an airway lesion as a comorbidity. Tracheomalacia is found in approximately two-thirds of children with PBB[38,80] and reported as a comorbidity in 11% of children with bronchiectasis.[81] In addition, tracheomalacia is known to have a negative impact on airway clearance, and children have an increased frequency of airway infection and longer duration of symptoms.[82]

Chronic Lung Infections and Pneumonia

Chronic pneumonia and infections can manifest with chronic cough. Depending on the geographic area and the age of the child, infections with *Legionella* spp., *Chlamydia pneumoniae*, *Chlamydia trachomatis*, parasites, fungi, and mycobacteria should be considered in cases of chronic lung infections or pneumonia. Immunocompromised children are more at risk. Investigations include flexible bronchoscopy and BAL and HRCT chest scan. Specific investigations beyond this are guided by clinical suspicion.

Of particular importance remains the incidence of *Mycobacterium tuberculosis* (TB) because it remains endemic in many areas, such as India, some Asia-Pacific countries, and Africa (often because of acquired immunodeficiency by HIV infection). Cough, fever, and weight loss are frequent symptoms, especially in adults with postprimary TB or children with miliary TB, but many patients may have vague nonspecific symptoms, and so TB should always be considered in countries where the disease is prevalent or in individuals who have traveled to these countries or have known infected disease contacts.[83] Specific investigations include tuberculin skin test, interferon-gamma release assay (IGRA), or microbiologic tests on sputum samples (e.g., GeneXpert test for DNA to *M. tuberculosis*). GeneXpert for DNA in sputum is currently recommended as the first diagnostic test, particularly in countries with limited resources, because it offers a sensitivity of 89% and specificity of 99%.[83]

Inhaled Airway Foreign Body

A retained airway foreign body always should be considered in young children presenting with a chronic cough. Typically the cough is wet, but it may occasionally be dry. A history of onset after a choking episode or while eating or playing are specifically important historical questions. Even in the absence of this history, it always should be considered in children younger than 5 years of age. Chest examination may be normal or may present with signs of asymmetric breath sounds and focal sounds, most commonly a monophonic and unilateral low-pitched wheeze. Chest radiograph may show unilateral lung hyperinflation consistent with bronchial obstruction, which becomes more apparent on an expiratory film. Immediate urgent referral to specialist care for bronchoscopy and removal if found is appropriate management.

Aspiration Lung Disease

Primary, as a result of swallowing dysfunction, or secondary, related to gastroesophageal reflux, aspiration lung disease can be a cause of chronic cough. Primary aspiration should be particularly considered in children with a history of coughing with feeds and neurologic, neuromuscular, and developmental disorders. Airway disorders such as tracheoesophageal fistula or laryngeal cleft also can cause aspiration lung disease. Investigation when suspected may include videofluoroscopic swallow assessment, bronchoscopy and BAL, and/or esophageal pH monitoring.

Eosinophilic Lung Disease

Eosinophilic lung disease should be considered in children with elevated eosinophils in peripheral blood. The diagnosis can be confirmed only with bronchoscopy and BAL, which shows elevated eosinophils in airway fluid. An eosinophilic pneumonia is characterized by pulmonary infiltrates, which can be seen on chest radiograph. Eosinophilic disorders can be primary or secondary. In secondary cases, infection with parasites (e.g., *Ascaris lumbricoides*) or fungus (e.g., allergic bronchopulmonary aspergillosis) and serologic investigation for secondary causes should be considered.[84]

Upper Airway Pathology

In adults, upper airway cough syndrome, or postnasal drip, is thought to be a common cause of cough; however, in children it remains a controversial cause. A 2016 systematic review of causes in children with chronic cough has found upper airway cough syndrome was common in only 2 of 10 prospective studies (both from same country).[4] Chronic rhinitis or sinusitis should be treated, regardless of the presence of chronic cough, and have been discussed in detail in the preceding two chapters. Given the pathologic process of PBB with neutrophilic airway infection and the continuity of the airways from nose to bronchus, a response

---

• BOX 19.2   Specific Cough Markers

History
- Chronic wet/productive cough
- Hemoptysis
- Wheeze
- Dyspnea
- Recurrent pneumonia
- Symptoms from neonatal period
- Onset after choking episode
- Cough worsens when child is anxious; improves with distraction; can be voluntarily suppressed; does not occur during sleep
- Child has thoughts disproportionate to symptoms
- Cardiac disease
- Developmental/neurologic abnormalities
- Swallowing difficulties
- Failure to thrive
- Exposure to tuberculosis or pertussis; travel history
- Immunodeficiency or history of deep infections
- Autoimmune disease
- Angiotensin-converting enzyme inhibitor use
- Chronic fever

Examination
- Wet or productive cough
- Classically recognizable cough sounds*
- Digital clubbing
- Chest wall deformity
- Auscultatory findings (wheeze, crepitation, differential breath sounds)
- Hypoxia
- Cardiac abnormalities (including murmurs)

Investigations
- Abnormal chest radiograph
- Abnormal spirometry

*Refer to Table 19.1
From Chang AB, Glomb WB. Guidelines for evaluating chronic cough in pediatrics: ACCP evidence-based clinical practice guidelines. Chest 2006;129(1 Suppl):260S–83S.

---

to oral antibiotics with resolution of cough when antibiotic treatment for upper airways is prescribed may simply indicate the patients had PBB in addition to rhinosinusitis.

Diagnostic and Therapeutic Recommendations

When assessing a child with chronic cough, one should initially undertake a detailed history and physical examination, followed by chest radiograph and spirometry (where able). The history should be targeted at symptoms and signs to suggest specific cough markers (Box 19.2).

These specific cough markers can be used to identify a likely underlying cause for the cough.[5] The cough will then be able to be categorized into specific cough or nonspecific cough. One of the most important markers in the approach to chronic cough in a child is the nature of the cough, particularly wet or dry, as discussed.[11] In addition to the nature of cough, classically recognizable cough sounds should be considered (Table 19.1). These can lead to a specific cough diagnosis as a possible underlying cause.

Many pulmonology societies (e.g., British Thoracic Society and those based in the United States, Australia, and New Zealand) have developed guidelines for managing chronic cough in

TABLE 19.1	Classically Recognizable Cough Sounds
Cough Type	**Suggested Possible Diagnoses**
Barking or brassy	Tracheomalacia, tic (habit) cough
Honking	Tic (habit), somatic cough disorder (psychogenic), tracheomalacia
Paroxysmal (+/− inspiratory whoop)	*Bordetella pertussis, Bordetella parapertussis* infection
Staccato	*Chlamydia* spp. infection (infants)
Wet or productive cough	Chronic endobronchial secretions
Wet cough in mornings only	Suppurative lung disease (e.g., bronchiectasis)
Cough productive of casts	Plastic bronchitis, mucus plugs

Adapted from Weinberger M, Lockshin B. When is cough functional, and how should it be treated? Breathe (Sheff) 2017;13(1):22–30.

children.[5,6,61,62] The U.S. guideline suggests a pediatric-specific algorithmic management pathway; a version is presented in Fig. 19.3.[5] These algorithms have been evaluated in studies worldwide, and a systematic review has shown there is high level evidence to support the use in cough management algorithms.[4] This evidence has demonstrated that use of a child-specific cough algorithm can lead to earlier diagnosis of children, thus determining which require further investigations.[4] The only RCT that has assessed the algorithm found at study conclusion that a significantly higher percentage of children were cough free, with a significantly improved quality of life and a shorter cough duration in the early-intervention group compared with the delayed-intervention control group. In addition, irrespective of timing, the cough algorithm showed reliability and was advantageous at whatever timing in which it was used.[85] Nine studies were included in the systematic review, and all have agreed with these findings that a management pathway improves outcomes.[4] Thus, it is now recommended that all children be evaluated using a pediatric-specific cough management pathway.[6] In contrast to management in adults, empirical treatment for common causes is not routinely recommended in children.[6]

The algorithmic approach begins with assessment of cough markers (see Box 19.2), classic cough characteristics (see Table 19.1), and chest radiograph and spirometry. An illustration of initial diagnoses that may be reached with the algorithm include the following:

- *Asthma:* A provisional diagnosis of asthma should at this stage be evident, with history suggested by a chronic dry cough, recurrent wheeze, exertional dyspnea, and/or family or personal history of atopy. Importantly, no other significant cough markers will be present. A chest radiograph may show bilateral hyperinflation or right middle lobe change or may be normal. Spirometry may show a reversible obstructive pattern or may be normal.
- *Inhaled foreign body:* A provisional diagnosis of an inhaled foreign body always should be considered in young children with a history of choking or sudden onset of cough after eating. Examination may show focal signs; a monophonic, low-pitched, unilateral wheeze is pathognomonic. Chest radiograph

may show unilateral lung hyperinflation consistent with bronchial obstruction, which becomes more apparent on an expiratory film.

- *Tic (habit) or somatic cough disorder (dysfunctional respiratory symptom/psychogenic) cough:* A characteristic cough (see Table 19.1) will suggest this diagnosis. Confirmation is made by suppressibility, as shown in Box 19.1.
- *Bordetella pertussis infection:* A diagnosis should be suspected if characteristic paroxysmal coughing and/or inspiratory whoop is present.
- *Protracted bacterial bronchitis:* A wet cough in the absence of any other specific cough markers in an otherwise well child suggests PBB as a diagnosis.
- *Nonspecific cough:* A chronic dry cough and thorough history, examination, chest radiography, and spirometry that do not reveal any specific cough markers is likely to be a nonspecific cough.
- *Other specific types of cough:* In the presence of other specific cough markers, further investigation and management with tests specific to each diagnosis (as per earlier discussion) is recommended.

Specific management should be targeted to the confirmed cause as outlined in this chapter, where appropriate. Importantly, re-evaluation and review are necessary at regular intervals for development of new symptoms, signs, and markers to the cause of cough after an initial diagnosis. Treatment trials should be re-evaluated after an appropriate time (2–4 weeks, depending on therapy), and if the treatment cannot be proved effective, it should be stopped. Cough has a significant placebo effect and known "period" effect (i.e., resolution with time), and thus, if the cough resolves, a trial of ceasing the medication and watching for cough recurrence is necessary to confirm the diagnosis. Importantly, before cough resolution, parents should be advised against using cough suppressants, because there is no role for them in childhood cough, and they can have serious adverse effects.[5,61]

Finally, irrespective of the cause of chronic cough, exacerbating factors always need evaluation. Environmental exposures from indoor or outdoor air pollution contribute to poor respiratory health, particularly in low-income areas and developing countries. Air pollutants include tobacco smoke, heating (gas or wood), and dust mite, molds, and pets. Identification and discussion around avoidance is vital in cough management because exposure can contribute to persistence of symptoms in any cause of chronic cough. Of special mention is counseling of parents about cessation of smoking.

Parental expectations and the burden of chronic cough for the family is another factor that needs to be explored when seeing a child with chronic cough. The high burden has been documented for parents and children, with increased levels of stress in parents that resolves with cough resolution.[3] Clinicians need to be cognizant of this increased stress and emotional distress of parents and counsel them appropriately about the natural history of childhood cough and the expected time for resolution in each child.

Conclusions

Chronic cough is common and reasons for its cause vary widely, encompassing many organs and anatomic sites, for example, tracheomalacia, chronic infections such as PBB or others, asthma and bronchial hyperresponsiveness, foreign body aspiration, cardiac

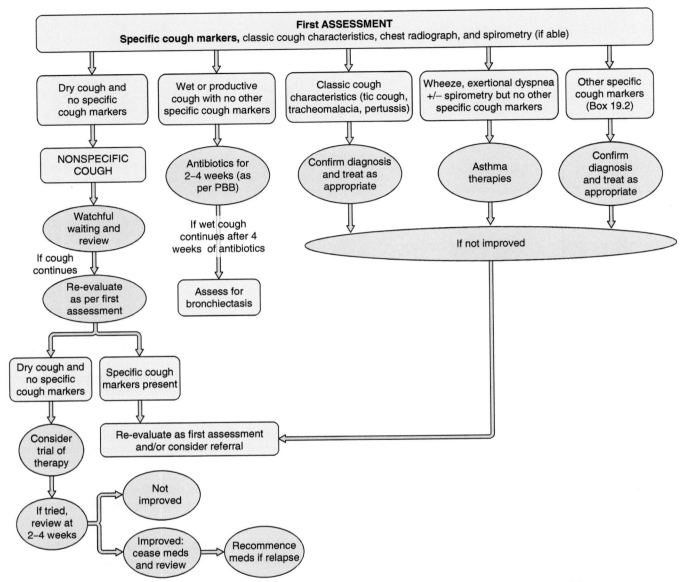

First ASSESSMENT
Specific cough markers, classic cough characteristics, chest radiograph, and spirometry (if able)

Dry cough and no specific cough markers	Wet or productive cough with no other specific cough markers	Classic cough characteristics (tic cough, tracheomalacia, pertussis)	Wheeze, exertional dyspnea +/− spirometry but no other specific cough markers	Other specific cough markers (Box 19.2)

NONSPECIFIC COUGH

Antibiotics for 2–4 weeks (as per PBB)

Confirm diagnosis and treat as appropriate

Asthma therapies

Confirm diagnosis and treat as appropriate

Watchful waiting and review

If wet cough continues after 4 weeks of antibiotics

If not improved

If cough continues

Re-evaluate as per first assessment

Assess for bronchiectasis

Dry cough and no specific cough markers

Specific cough markers present

Consider trial of therapy

Re-evaluate as first assessment and/or consider referral

If tried, review at 2–4 weeks

Not improved

Improved: cease meds and review

Recommence meds if relapse

• **Fig. 19.3** Algorithmic management pathway for chronic cough. *Dx,* Diagnosis. (Courtesy Marchant JM, Chang AB. Causes of chronic cough in children. In: Mallory GB, Hoppin, AG, editors. Waltham, MA: UpToDate; 2019.)

• BOX 19.3   Practical Tips for the Office Setting

- Children with wet cough without any other specific cough markers should receive 2 weeks of antibiotics (typically amoxicillin–clavulanic acid recommended).
- Children with wet cough without any other specific cough markers who are still coughing after 4 weeks of antibiotic therapy should be investigated further and/or referred to a pediatric pulmonologist.
- A chronic cough with a history of onset after a choking episode or after eating should alert the clinician to the possibility of a foreign body and be referred for evaluation.
- Children with nonspecific cough without any specific cough markers can be watched because there is a high chance the cough will resolve spontaneously. They should be re-evaluated for any new symptoms or signs at periodic intervals.
- Exacerbating factors, such as exposure to tobacco smoke or other allergens, always should be addressed.

diseases, and rarely also ILD (Box 19.3). This chapter presents an overview of the differential diagnoses of specific and nonspecific cough and dry and wet cough and suggests specific cough markers to help determine the correct diagnosis (see Box 19.2). Using a systematic approach to rule out underlying diseases, such as CF, or a deficiency in mucociliary clearance, such as PCD, are pivotal for the prevention of lung damage at an early stage. Furthermore, consideration of dysfunctional psychologic causes helps avoid unnecessary medication and provide adequate behavioral therapy. Allergy, although a common condition in children and adolescents, is less frequently the reason for chronic cough than expected but should be taken into consideration.

The reference list can be found on the companion Expert Consult website at http://www.expertconsult.inkling.com.

20

Immunology of the Asthmatic Response

OSCAR PALOMARES, CEZMI A. AKDIS

KEY POINTS

- Asthma is a complex syndrome encompassing different pheno-types and endotypes. Type 2 and non–type 2 asthma pheno-types are defined according to underlying molecular mecha-nisms. Type 2 asthma includes allergic asthma and eosinophilic asthma, representing the most common and severe asthma phenotypes.
- Allergen-specific T helper cell type 2 cells and immunoglobulin E are key components of allergic asthma, but Type 2 innate lym-phoid cells and other innate immune cells emerged as important players in type 2 asthma. Bronchial epithelial barrier disruption and production of alarmins after epithelial cell activation essential-ly contribute to inflammatory burden and asthma development.
- Airway remodeling is associated with asthma severity and chronicity and includes smooth muscle hypertrophy, goblet cell hyperplasia and mucus hypersecretion, basal membrane thickening, subepithelial fibrosis, epithelial destruction, and angiogenesis.

- Respiratory syncytial virus and rhinovirus infections are associ-ated with severe recurrent wheezing or asthma development and exacerbations.
- The reduction of environmental biodiversity accounts for the exponential growth of chronic inflammatory disorders, includ-ing asthma. Exposure to endotoxin, farm environment, and microbial diversity impairs inflammation and asthma develop-ment.
- Biologics significantly contribute to improving the quality of life of patients with asthma and to enhancing the knowledge of underlying immunologic mechanisms.
- Immune tolerance to allergens with the induction of T and B regulatory cells represents the major mechanisms of action of allergen immunotherapy for asthma treatment.
- A precision medicine approach in patients with asthma accord-ing to endotype-based stratification will contribute significantly to the development of better prevention strategies and novel therapeutic options.

Introduction

Asthma is one of the most common chronic inflammatory disor-ders of the airways. It is characterized by variable and recurring symptoms (cough, dyspnea, wheezing, or chest tightness), revers-ible airflow obstruction, bronchial hyperresponsiveness (BHR), and underlying inflammation.[1–3] Asthma is a complex syndrome encompassing several phenotypes with different pathophysiologic mechanisms that develops after environmental exposures, such as to innocuous allergens, infectious agents, and air pollutants, in genetically susceptible individuals. The label *asthma* includes a large number of heterogeneous patients in terms of sever-ity, lung function, comorbidities, natural history, and treatment response.[2,4–6] Patients can be stratified into type 2 and non–type 2 asthma according to the expression levels of type 2 biomark-ers, such as blood and/or sputum eosinophils, exhaled nitric oxide (FeNO), serum periostin, or bronchial epithelial cell (EC) gene signature after interleukin 13 (IL-13) in vitro stimulation.[6] The

combination of such biomarkers and clinical features further stratifies patients into type 2 asthma phenotypes (allergic asthma, late-onset eosinophilic asthma, or aspirin-exacerbated respira-tory disease) and non–type 2 asthma phenotypes (very-late-onset asthma, neutrophilic asthma, exercise-induced asthma, or pauci-granulocytic asthma).[6] Recent advances in multiple omics tech-nologies applied to precision medicine have started to delineate that these phenotypes might encompass different endotypes (sub-types characterized by specific pathophysiologic mechanisms).[1,7–9] Allergic asthma endotype is one of the best characterized.[10,11] It is associated with specific immunoglobulin E (IgE) sensitization to indoor and outdoor allergens[3,12] and with sometimes elevated total serum IgE levels, which represent major risk factors for asthma development and persistent wheezing in children.[13] Aller-gic asthma is characterized by a type 2 inflammatory immune response that involves increased circulating numbers and bron-chial submucosal infiltration of T helper cell type 2 (T_H2) lympho-cytes, type 2 innate lymphoid cells (ILC2s), eosinophils, B cells,

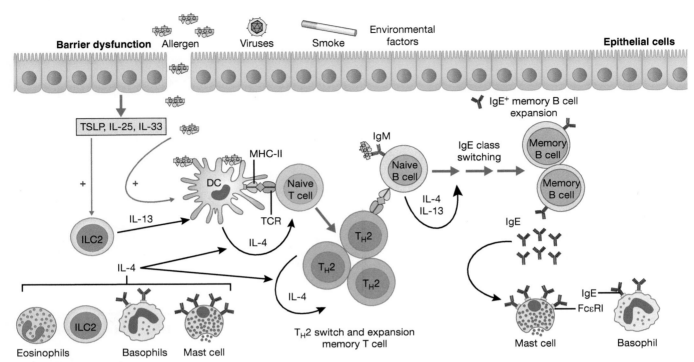

- **Fig. 20.1** Allergic sensitization in asthma. After encounter with allergens and other environmental factors, epithelial cell–derived alarmins such as thymic stromal lymphopoietin *(TSLP)*, interleukin-25 (IL-25) and IL-33 activate ILC2 and condition dendritic cells *(DCs)* to polarize allergen-specific T helper cell type 2 *(T_H2)* responses by mechanisms depending on IL-4. ILC2-derived IL-13 favors DCs migration to lymph nodes. Eosinophils, ILC2, basophils, and mast cells are also sources of IL-4 during T_H2 priming. IL-4 and IL-13 are essential for immunoglobulin E *(IgE)* class switching on B cells. IgE binds to high-affinity immunoglobulin E receptor *(FcεRI)* on effector cells, leading to the allergic sensitization.

basophils, epithelium, and smooth muscle cells leading to mucus production, edema, BHR, airway obstruction, and remodeling.

Mechanisms of Allergic Inflammatory Response

Allergic asthma consists of two different phases: (1) sensitization and memory and (2) effector phases—immediate phase response (IPR) and late phase response (LPR).[11] During sensitization, airway dendritic cells (DCs) uptake encountered allergens and transport them to the draining lymph node, where processed allergen peptides are presented in a major histocompatibility complex II (MHC-II) context to naïve CD4+ T cells that differentiate into allergen-specific CD4+ T_H2 cells by mechanisms depending on IL-4 and signal transducer and activator of transcription 6 (STAT6) signaling. The clonal expansion of such allergen-specific CD4+ T_H2 cells producing IL-4 and IL-13 is essential to induce IgE class-switching and clonal expansion of memory B cells, differentiation to plasma cells, and production of allergen-specific IgE antibodies. IgE binds to the high-affinity immunoglobulin E receptor (FcεRI) on the surface of mast cells and basophils, thus leading to the patient's sensitization (Fig. 20.1). A memory pool of allergen-specific T and B cells is also generated, which are essential in the subsequent phases. Bronchial ECs also contribute to allergic sensitization. On contact with allergens, pathogens, pollutants, and other substances, the integrity of the bronchial epithelium is altered as a result disruption of tight junction (TJ) proteins, favoring the accumulation of allergens and inflammatory substances in the submucosa and contributing to allergen polysensitization.[14] In addition, in response to environmental insults, bronchial ECs

produce large amounts of alarmins (i.e., thymic stromal lympho-poietin [TSLP], IL-33, and IL-25), which act on DCs, ILC2s, T cells, natural killer T (NKT) cells, basophils, and mast cells, leading to their activation and cytokine production, which also enhances allergen sensitization (see Fig. 20.1).[15] After new encounters with the causative allergens, IPR occurs. Allergens induce the cross-linking of the IgE-FcεRI complexes on sensitized mast cells and basophils, leading to the immediate release of preformed (e.g., histamine, proteases, heparin) and de novo synthesized (e.g., prostaglandins, leukotrienes, cytokines, chemokines) anaphylactogenic mediators responsible for wheezing, increased vascular permeability, fluid extravasation into the bronchial tissues, and BHR (Fig. 20.2).[3,4,16] If these mediators accumulate in the airways as a result of persistent local allergen contact, the LPR occurs 6 to 12 hours later. Memory allergen-specific T_H2 cells activated by mechanisms depending on IgE-facilitated presentation by antigen-presenting cells produce large amounts of IL-4, IL-5, IL-9, and IL-13, which contribute to the activation of effector cells, sustained local production of IgE, recruitment of eosinophils and other inflammatory cells into the airways, goblet cell hyperplasia, and contraction of smooth muscles, leading to strong inflammation, mucus production, and BHR, the cardinal features of reduced lung function in asthma (see Fig. 20.2).[12] Alarmin-activated ILC2s producing large amounts of IL-13, IL-5, and probably IL-4 also contribute to such effects in some patients with asthma.[15,17,18] The perpetuation of this type 2–mediated inflammatory response might contribute to airway remodeling, which is associated with the most severe manifestations of asthma, including exacerbations and chronicity. In some patients with allergy, other non–type 2 immune mechanisms led by T_H1, T_H17, or T_H9/T_H22 cells might be predominant under certain circumstances (see Fig. 20.2).[12]

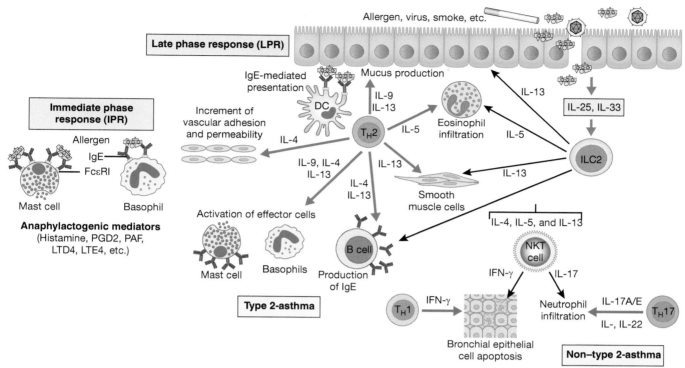

• **Fig. 20.2** Immediate phase response (IPR) and late phase response (LPR) in type 2 and non–type 2 asthma. Immunoglobulin E *(IgE)*-mediated high-affinity immunoglobulin E receptor *(FcεRI)* cross-linking in effector cells induces the activation and degranulation of anaphylactogenic mediators. LPR memory T helper type 2 (T$_H$2) cells are activated by antigen-presenting cells by IgE-facilitated presentation. Activated T$_H$2 cells produce type 2 cytokines that contribute to the different effects shown (i.e., eosinophilia, bronchial hyperresponsiveness [BHR], local IgE and mucus production, activation of effector cells, vascular permeability). ILC2s also significantly contribute to these processes, as shown in type 2–mediated asthma. Other cells participate in non–type 2 asthma: interferon-gamma *(IFN-γ)*-producing natural killer T *(NKT)* cells and T$_H$1 cells promote epithelial apoptosis and shedding; interleukin-17 *(IL-17)*-producing NKT and T$_H$17 cells contribute to neutrophilic inflammation. *LTD4,* Leukotriene D4; *PAF,* platelet activating factor; *PGD2,* prostaglandin D2.

Orchestration of Type 2 Immune Responses

Under normal conditions, type 2 immune responses are essential in the defense against parasites, venoms, and toxins.[19,20] Dysregulation of type 2 immune responses leads to the development of asthma and other allergic diseases, including rhinitis, atopic dermatitis, and food allergy.[11] Historically, allergic asthma has been considered a T$_H$2 cell–mediated disease, but ILC2s and other innate immune and effector cells also appear to contribute.[21,22] Therefore, the term *type 2 immune-mediated disease* is more adequate. The initiation and maintenance of type 2 immune responses require the coordination of proper innate and adaptive immune responses in a tightly regulated manner.[21] Different cell subsets directly contribute to these responses both locally and systemically (Fig. 20.3).

Dendritic Cells: The Link Between Innate and Adaptive Immune Responses

The best-characterized professional antigen-presenting cells are macrophages, B cells, and DCs.[23] Other type 2 innate immune cells such as basophils, masts cells, eosinophils, and ILC2s also could act as antigen-presenting cells under certain circumstances.[23]

A large number of alveolar macrophages in the lungs eliminate allergens in the airways and differentiate into alternatively activated M2 macrophages. They prime FOXP3+ regulatory T (T$_{REG}$) cells by a mechanism depending on IL-10.[24,25] B cells induce T$_H$2 responses in vitro, but their role in the induction of primary T cell responses in vivo is still controversial. House dust mite models of allergic asthma showed that B cells might contribute to the generation of follicular T helper cells (T$_{FH}$).[26]

DCs are the professional antigen-presenting cells linking innate and adaptive immune responses. Because of their migratory capacity, expression of costimulatory molecules and polarizing cytokines, DCs lining the bronchial epithelium and airway submucosa represent the most potent stimulators of naïve T cells, thus being indispensable for the initiation and maintenance of type 2 immune responses.[11,27,28] In humans, blood DCs are classified into myeloid dendritic cells (mDCs) and plasmacytoid dendritic cells (pDCs).[29] Two types of mDCs can be distinguished: type 1 mDCs and type 2 mDCs, which correspond to their mouse counterparts IRF8-expressing cDC1 and IRF4-expressing cDC2, respectively.[29] Type 2 mDCs, in both humans and mice, are the main DC subset involved in the induction and expansion of allergen-specific T$_H$2 cells in the airways. Immature DCs mainly promote tolerance through the generation of T$_{REG}$ cells, whereas fully mature DCs induce effector immune responses.[30,31] Fully mature DCs also can be involved in the generation of T$_{REG}$ cells.[32] Mature tonsil pDCs generate tolerogenic functional allergen-specific T$_{REG}$ cells in humans,[33] which could be disrupted by proinflammatory cytokines and specific Toll-like receptor (TLR)-ligands.[34] Other studies in humans and mice also suggest pDCs as a specific DC subset with intrinsic tolerogenic capacity contributing to the control and prevention of allergic asthma.[33,35–37]

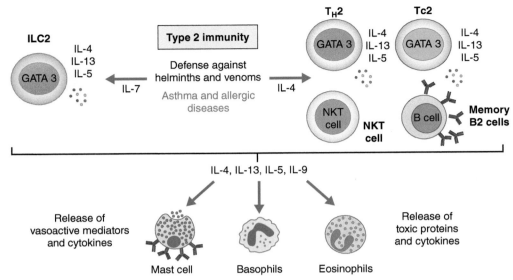

• **Fig. 20.3** Cells involved in type 2 immune responses. Under normal conditions, type 2 immunity is orchestrated against helminths, venoms, and other parasites and toxins. T helper cell type 2 *(TH2)* cells, type 2 CD8+ T (TC2) cells, natural killer T (NKT) cells, B cells, and ILC2 produce type 2 cytokines that exert different physiologic effects and contribute to the recruitment and activation of mast cells, basophils, and eosinophils. After activation, effector cells release anaphylactogenic substances, toxic proteins, and cytokines. Alterations in type 2 immune responses lead to asthma and other allergic diseases.

Adaptive Immune Responses: T Helper Cell Type 2 Cells and Cytokines

The clonal expansion of allergen-specific CD4+ T_H2 cells producing large amounts of type 2 cytokines is essential in the initiation and further development of allergic asthma. Activated T_H2 cells are found in large quantities in blood, lung biopsy samples, and bronchoalveolar lavage (BAL) fluid of patients with allergic asthma.[38–40] Allergen-specific T_H2 cells are also key in the development of allergen-specific IgE antibodies and allergic asthma during childhood. In mice, initial experiments demonstrated that depletion of CD4+ T_H2 cells or their corresponding T_H2 cytokines prevented asthma development,[41–43] whereas the transfer of allergen-specific T_H2 cells in naïve recipient mice could reproduce all allergic asthma features on allergen challenge.[44] In contrast, IL-12 administration generated interferon-gamma (INF-γ)-producing T_H1 cells able to suppress all typical features of allergic asthma.[45,46] Genetic and epigenetic studies confirmed that type 2 cytokine production by T_H2 cells is regulated by specific epigenetic inscriptions in corresponding gene locus, which is associated with asthma and atopy development.[47,48] Many patients with allergic asthma treated with omalizumab, a humanized monoclonal antibody (mAb) targeting free IgE, reported significant clinical improvement (Fig. 20.4A).[3,4,49,50] Omalizumab impairs IgE-binding to FcεRI on effector cells and DCs, thus avoiding mast cell and basophil degranulation and IgE-mediated allergen activation of T_H2 cells and subsequent type 2 cytokine production.[51,52]

Development of T Helper Type 2 Responses

Allergens and other stimuli, directly or after inducing the release of alarmins by ECs, condition the capacity of DCs to generate T_H2 responses.[15,23] DCs express OX40-L and Notch receptor ligands, which in the presence of IL-4 favor the generation of T_H2 cells. ILC2, basophils, and eosinophils, which can be found in the T cell areas of lymph nodes, have been proposed as potential initial sources of IL-4 during T_H2 generation. IL-4 binds to

two receptors (type I and type II IL-4R), which share the IL-4Rα chain.[53,54] Type I IL-4R, expressed by naïve and memory T cells, consists of IL-4Rα and the γ-common chain, which is also shared by IL-2, IL-7, IL-9, IL-15, and IL-21 receptors. Type II IL-4R consists of the IL-4Rα chain and the IL-13Rα1 chain and binds both IL-4 and IL-13.[53,54] Triggering of type I IL-4R activates signal transduction and STAT-6, which translocate to the nucleus and cooperate with GATA binding protein 3 (GATA-3), the master transcription factor for T_H2 cell differentiation and type 2 cytokine expression. STAT-6 and GATA-3 expression levels are significantly increased in the lung of patients with asthma.[55,56] Hypomethylation of GATA3 promoter at birth is associated with later asthma development.[57]

Effector T Helper Type 2 Cytokines as Targets in Asthma

IL-4 and IL-13 play a major role in allergic asthma.[54,58] Mice deficient in IL-4 and IL-13 reveal the important role of these cytokines for T_H2 differentiation, IgG1 and IgE production, goblet cell hyperplasia, and mucus production.[42,59] IL-13 overexpression in the lung reproduces classic asthma features.[60] IL-13 polymorphisms in humans are associated with enhanced asthma exacerbations in childhood, total IgE, and blood eosinophilia.[61] Both cytokines are produced by T_H2 cells, basophils, mast cells, NKT cells, and ILC2s. Although they are structurally and functionally similar cytokines sharing the IL-4Rα chain, they also perform nonredundant specific functions. T cells do not express the IL-13 receptor, and therefore IL-13 does not contribute to T_H2 cell priming. IL-4 with tumor necrosis factor-alpha (TNF-α) increase vascular permeability by inducing vascular cell adhesion molecule-1 (VCAM-1) expression on vascular endothelial cells.[54,58] IL-13 and transforming growth factor-β (TGF-β) contribute to tissue remodeling and fibrosis. IL-4 and IL-13 promote the activation of mast cells and increase the production of cysteinyl leukotrienes after IgE-mediated activation.[62] IL-13 activates eosinophils and favors their recruitment to tissues, prolonging their survival.

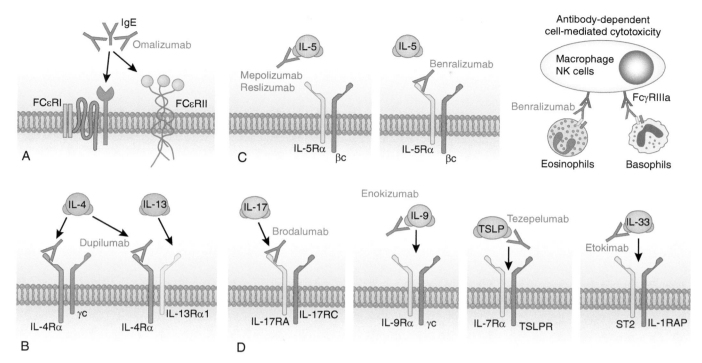

• **Fig. 20.4** Biologics approved and under development in asthma. (A) Omalizumab is a clinically used antiimmunoglobulin E *(IgE)* monoclonal antibody (mAb) blocking free IgE and avoiding binding to high-affinity immunoglobulin E receptor *(FcɛRI)* and low-affinity *(FcɛRII)* IgE receptors. (B) Clinically used anti–interleukin-5 (IL-5) signaling pathway mAbs. Mepolizumab and reslizumab bind IL-5 and prevent the binding to the receptor. Benralizumab binds to IL-5Rα chain, thus inducing antibody-dependent cell-mediated cytotoxicity. (C) Dupilumab is a clinically used mAb targeting IL-4Rα chain, thus inhibiting signaling mediated by both IL-4 and IL-13. (D) Several mAbs at different stages of development and their way of action are displayed. Brodalumab (mAb targeting IL-17RA), enokizumab (mAb targeting IL-9), tezepelumab (mAb targeting thymic stromal lymphopoietin [TSLP]), and etokimab (mAb targeting IL-33).

Dupilumab, a human mAb targeting the IL-4Rα chain that simultaneously blocks effects mediated by IL-4 and IL-13 has been approved for asthma (see Fig. 20.4B). Dupilumab reduces exacerbations and oral corticosteroid usage in patients with severe asthma, which is accompanied by significant improvements in lung function, clinical symptoms, and quality of life.[63,64] Other strategies using mAbs exclusively targeting IL-13, such as lebrikizumab, did not show clinical efficacy in Phase III studies,[65] suggesting that simultaneous blocking of IL-4 and IL-13 is required, likely because of the nonredundant effects of these two cytokines in the pathophysiologic processes of asthma.

IL-5 is another key type 2 cytokine in asthma mainly produced by T_H2 cells under the control of GATA-3 but also by ILC2s, mast cells, NKT cells, basophils, and eosinophils.[54,58] The IL-5 receptor consists of the IL-5R-α chain, to which IL-5 binds, and the β-common chain that is shared by IL-3 and granulocyte-macrophage colony-stimulating factor (GM-CSF) receptors. IL-5R is expressed on progenitors and mature eosinophils, basophils, and probably some B cells and ILC2s subsets. IL-5, in cooperation with IL-3 and GM-CSF, induces maturation, activation, and recruitment of eosinophils to the nose and lung. IL-5 and eosinophil levels are increased in BAL fluid, lung biopsies, and sputum of patients with asthma and the level of blood eosinophils correlates with the severity of the disease.[66–68] Biologics targeting IL-5 (mepolizumab and reslizumab) and IL-5R-α (benralizumab) are approved for severe eosinophilic asthma (see Fig. 20.4C).[69] Initial clinical trials with anti–IL-5 treatments did not show clinical efficacy when unselected patients with asthma were included.[70,71] However, subsequent studies in well-selected

refractory eosinophilic and steroid-dependent patients with asthma demonstrated clinical efficacy.[72,73] Mepolizumab[74–76] and reslizumab[77,78] reduced eosinophil counts, exacerbations, and oral corticosteroid use, showing lung function improvement in some cases. Benralizumab targets IL-5Rα and induces an antibody-dependent cell-mediated cytotoxicity, leading to the complete depletion of eosinophils and probably other target cells expressing the receptor (see Fig. 20.4C). Benralizumab depletes eosinophils and reduces basophil counts, exacerbations, and oral corticosteroid use and improves lung function.[79–81]

Beyond the T Helper Type 2 Paradigm in Allergies and Asthma

After the discovery of T_H1 and T_H2 cells in 1986,[82] it was accepted for a long time that T_H2 response was mainly involved in the development of allergic diseases, whereas INF-γ–producing T_H1 cells generated by IL-12 after induction of the master switch transcription factor T-bet mainly predominated in infections and autoimmunity. Infants with higher levels of cord blood IFN-γ are less likely to develop atopy,[83] and patients with asthma express lower levels of T-bet, IL-12R, and IL-12 in the airways.[84,85] The T_H2 paradigm explains many features of asthma, but it does not explain several other observations. In the airways of some patients with asthma and severe corticosteroid resistance, T_H1 cells able to induce bronchial epithelial apoptosis or T_H17 cells involved in neutrophil recruitment can be detected (see Fig. 20.2).[86–89] T_H9 and T_H22 cells also might play an important role in some patients with asthma.[90–92] T_{REG} and regulatory B (B_{REG}) cells suppress excessive immune response in the lung, play a role in development and maintenance of immune tolerance to allergens, and appear to be essential in healthy immune response to allergens in cases of high-dose allergen exposure.[11,93]

Other T Cell Subsets Involved in Asthma

T_H17 Cells

T_H17 cells, together with T cytotoxic (c)17 and ILC3, orchestrate type 3 immune responses against extracellular bacteria and fungi.[21,94,95] T_H17 cell differentiation and expansion is driven by TGF-β, IL-6, IL-1β, IL-21, and IL-23 under the control of the retinoic acid receptor–related orphan receptor γt/C2 (RORγt/RORC2), in mice and humans, respectively.[96–99] The main effector cytokine of T_H17 cells is IL-17A, but they also produce IL-17F, IL-22, and IL-26.[54,100] Aberrant T_H17 responses are associated with the development of different autoimmune diseases and psoriasis.[99] Mouse models and human data suggest a pathogenic role for T_H17 cells in the development of allergic diseases and asthma, but there is still controversy, with some reports indicating a potential protective role.[89,101,102] T_H17 cells have been associated with neutrophilic and macrophage influx in acute allergic airway inflammation, BHR, and steroid-resistant asthma.[88,89,103,104] IL-17 production is not always detected in the human airways despite their presence in blood.[22,105] Airway T_H17 cell numbers and IL-17 levels vary in a dynamic way according to recent exacerbations, periods of clinical stability, and the presence of neutrophils in tissues.[22] Genetic polymorphisms demonstrated an association of IL-17 and asthma, and T_H17 cells were shown to promote smooth muscle cell migration in allergic airways.[54,89] Brodalumab, an anti–IL-17A receptor mAb (see Fig. 20.4D), did not show global clinical efficacy in patients with asthma[106]; however, a possibility still exists for the existence of an endotype with high numbers of sputum neutrophils that could benefit from anti–IL-17 treatments.[106,107]

T_H9 and T_H22 Cells

IL-9–producing T_H9 cells are generated by TGF-β in the presence of IL-4.[90] IL-9 is also produced by ILC2s, T_H2 cells, and granulocytes, including mast cells, eosinophils, basophils, and probably neutrophils. The IL-9 receptor consists of the IL-9Rα chain and the common-γ chain and is expressed on mast cells, T cells, B cells, and ECs.[54] IL-9 contributes to the development of allergic asthma by promoting mast cell survival, eosinophilic inflammation, BHR, elevated IgE levels, increased mucus secretion, and airway remodeling.[54,108–111] The expression of IL-9 and IL-9R is increased in bronchial tissue of subjects with atopia and asthma.[112] Until the present, human clinical trials with the anti–IL-9 mAb enokizumab (see Fig. 20.4D) did not report clinical efficacy.[113] Mouse models showed that anti–IL-9 in combination with allergen-specific immunotherapy (AIT) might be a suitable strategy to treat patients with allergic asthma, but more studies are required.[114]

There is some evidence that IL-22–producing T_H22 cells also might be involved in asthma.[54,89] IL-22 is also produced by T_H1, T_H2, T_H17, natural killer (NK) cells, and ILCs.[115] IL-22 displays proinflammatory properties in the chronic phases of allergic skin diseases, especially in some atopic dermatitis endotypes.[116] In contrast, the role of IL-22 in asthma is still controversial.[115] Some studies suggest a more proinflammatory activity for IL-22, which in cooperation with IL-17 might enhance migration of airway smooth muscle cells.[89,117] Other studies have shown that

IL-22 inhibits the production of IL-25 by ECs and contributes to the modulation of DC function, thus impairing allergic airway inflammation and effector phases.[118] More research is required to delineate the specific contribution of T_H22 cells and IL-22 in different asthma endotypes.

Regulatory T and B Cells and Immune Tolerance

The generation and expansion of functional T_{REG} and B_{REG} cells is the hallmark of allergen-specific immune tolerance induction.[11,32,93,119] T_{REG} and B_{REG} cells exert their immunosuppressive properties by different mechanisms using a plethora of soluble and surface-bound molecules, such as IL-10, TGF-β, IL-35, granzymes, cyclic adenosine monophosphate (cAMP), adenosine, CD25, PD1, CD39, CD73, cytotoxic T lymphocyte–associated protein 4 (CTLA-4), lymphocyte-activation gene 3 (LAG-3), and histamine receptor 2 (HR2) (Fig. 20.5).[119,120]

Regulatory T Cells

T_{REG} cells are a heterologous T cell population able to suppress immune responses that are classified as the thymus-derived naturally occurring CD4+ CD25+ FOXP3+ T_{REG} (nT_{REG}) cells and the inducible T_{REG} (iT_{REG}) cells.[11,119,121] nT_{REG} cells constitutively express high levels of the IL-2Rα chain (CD25) and the suppressor costimulatory molecules CTLA4 and PD1.[122–124] In humans, FOXP3 mutations underlie the X-linked immunodeficiency with polyendocrinopathy and enteropathy (IPEX) or the X-linked autoimmune and allergic dysregulation syndrome (XLAAD).[125,126] In the periphery, IL-10–producing type 1 regulatory (T_R1) cells are essential to keep tolerance by inhibiting priming of naïve CD4+ T cells and development of memory T_H1, T_H17, and T_H2 cells (see Fig. 20.5).[127–129] During natural high exposure to venom allergens, venom-specific IL-10–Tr1 cells are clonally differentiated from allergen-specific T_H1 and T_H2 cells by mechanisms depending on HR2.[127–133] High-dose exposure to cat allergen significantly enhances the levels of allergen-specific IgG4.[130]

B Regulatory Cells

IL-10–secreting B_{REG} cells cooperate with T_{REG} cells in the generation of tolerance to allergens (see Fig. 20.5).[11,93] Phospholipase A–specific B cells from nonallergic beekeepers produced large amounts of IL-10 and IgG4 and suppressed T cell proliferation.[131,132] Human B cells that overexpressed IL-10 acquired a prominent immunoregulatory profile and mimicked the function of B_{REG} cells.[133] High-dose venom exposure induces similar IL-10–producing B_{REG} cells in healthy beekeepers and patients with allergy.[134] Der p 1–specific B cells in patients responding to 2 years of AIT are characterized by increased numbers of IgA- and IgG4-expressing Der p 1–specific B cells, plasmablasts, and IL-10+ B_{REG} cells.[132] Human CD40L+ ILC3s promote the generation of IL-10–producing B_{REG} cells in human tonsils by mechanisms depending on CD40, B cell activating factor (BAFF), and IL-15.[135]

Asthma Treatment and Induction of Immune Tolerance for a Protective Immunity

Current guidelines for asthma treatment are based on a stepwise approach that increases broad-spectrum medication (corticosteroids and bronchodilators) to achieve asthma control and minimize the risk of future exacerbations.[3,4] This approach is effective for many patients but not for all patients with asthma. The better

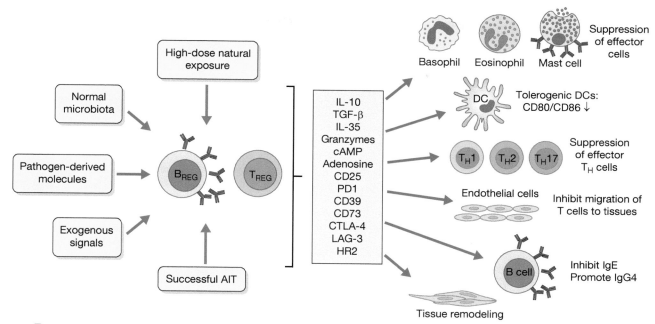

• **Fig. 20.5** The generation and maintenance of functional regulatory T (T_{REG}) and B (B_{REG}) cells is essential in suppressing inflammation in asthma, maintaining tissue homeostasis. Functional T_{REG} and B_{REG} cells are generated after natural high-dose exposure to allergens, successful allergen immunotherapy (AIT), normal microbiota, specific pathogen-derived molecules, and other exogenous signals. Functional T_{REG} and B_{REG} cells produce a large number of soluble and surface molecules with suppressive properties. They suppress the activation of effector cells such as mast cells, basophils, and eosinophils and different effector T_H subsets. They also promote the generation of tolerogenic dendritic cells (DCs) able to induce regulatory responses and favor the inhibition of immunoglobulin E (IgE)-producing B cells and the induction of functional blocking allergen-specific IgG4 antibodies. T_{REG} and B_{REG} are able to act on endothelial cells inhibiting the migration of inflammatory cells to the lung, contributing to tissue homeostasis and avoiding airway remodeling. cAMP, Cyclic adenosine monophosphate; CTLA-4, cytotoxic T lymphocyte-associated protein 4; HR2, histamine receptor 2; IL, interleukin; LAG-3, lymphocyte-activation gene 3; TGF-β, transforming growth factor-beta.

endotype-based diagnosis by omics technology would contribute to patient stratification and personalize medicine.[1,136,137] Most available asthma treatments are effective at controlling symptoms and reducing exacerbations, but, until the present, the only treatment for allergic asthma that showed a potential to modify the course of the disease is AIT.

AIT consists of the administration of high doses of the causative allergen to induce a state of permanent tolerance.[120,138] Systematic analysis has led to the recommendation of subcutaneous immunotherapy (SCIT) and sublingual swallow immunotherapy (SLIT) for both children and adults with controlled allergic asthma.[139,140] The generation of improved AIT vaccines could significantly pave the way toward AIT as an immune-modifying treatment with the potential to prevent and cure allergic asthma in many patients. Different immunostimulatory or vehicle adjuvants such as TLR ligands (TLR-Ls) or nanoparticles have been assayed to improve AIT vaccines with different rates of success.[141–143] In this regard, allergoids conjugated to mannan-targeting DCs and inducing functional T_{REG} cells represent promising next-generation vaccines for AIT.[143–145]

Innate Inflammatory Mechanisms in Asthma

Impairment of Epithelial Barrier Function in Asthma

Lung ECs were initially considered a mere physical barrier protecting the host against external aggression. However, bronchial ECs also orchestrate immune responses and inflammation by producing a large number of cytokines/alarmins, chemokines, growth factors, nitric oxide, and other mediators.[1,15,22] Defective

function of the epithelial barrier is reported not only in bronchial ECs in patients with asthma but also in sinus ECs of patients with chronic rhinosinusitis and keratinocytes in the skin of patients with atopic dermatitis.[146–150] Protease-containing allergens, pathogens, pollutants, toxins, and type 2 cytokines alter bronchial ECs by disrupting the integrity of TJ proteins. TJs are disrupted in airways of patients with asthma as assessed by biopsies and air-liquid interface cultures from the asthmatic bronchi.[151] Very high dilutions of laundry detergents and rinsing residues also disrupt human bronchial ECs, without affecting epigenome and TJ gene expression.[152] Pollutants such as ozone disrupt barrier integrity and induce IL-33 release, which precedes inflammatory injury induced by myeloid cells.[153] In contrast, bacterial CpG motifs enhance the integrity of TJ proteins and bronchial EC barrier.[154] Interestingly, IL-4 and IL-13 produced by activated T_H2 cells and ILC2s are driving bronchial TJ barrier leakiness, which contributes significantly to asthma pathogenesis.[155–157] Peptidase allergens down-regulate claudin-18 by mechanisms depending on IL-13.[158] Oncostatin M levels are increased in the BAL fluid and sputum of patients with allergic asthma after allergen challenge, which is associated with barrier dysfunction.[159] Opening of TJs is also important to drain inflammatory cells to the lumen, thus contributing to resolution of pathologic processes. Therefore, TJs could contribute to both aggravation of inflammation related to tissue damage and resolution of inflammation by drainage.

The Role of Epithelial Cell–Derived Alarmins in Asthma

TSLP is a member of the IL-2 cytokine family that play a key role in the regulation of type 2 immune responses.[15,54] It is mainly produced by human lung, gut, and skin ECs, but also by DCs, basophils, and mast cells. The functional receptor is a dimer of TSLP-R and IL-7Rα chains, which is expressed in ECs and sensory neurons and in many hematopoietic cells, such as DCs, ILC2s, T cells, NKT cells, mast cells, basophils, eosinophils, monocytes, and macrophages. TSLP instructs DCs to polarize T_H2 responses by mechanisms depending on OX40-L.[160] TSLP also directly acts on naïve T cells, promoting the generation of type 2–producing T_H2 cells in the absence of IL-4[161] and regulates IL-13–producing ILC2s during viral infections and asthma exacerbations.[162] TSLP expression is significantly increased in the asthmatic airways and in the skin of patients with atopic dermatitis and correlates with type 2 immunity and disease severity.[163,164] Tezepelumab is a mAb targeting TSLP that has shown promising results in Phase II clinical trials for asthma treatment by reducing exacerbations and improving lung function regardless eosinophil counts (see Fig. 20.4).[165]

IL-33 is a member of the IL-1 cytokine family that also plays a very important role in the regulation of type 2 immune responses in the airways.[15,54,166] IL-33 is produced by bronchial ECs, endothelial and stromal cells, myeloid cells, mast cells, platelets, and megakaryocytes. The IL-33 receptor consists of ST2 and IL-1 receptor accessory protein (IL-1RAP), which is mainly expressed on ECs and neurons, DCs, ILC2s, macrophages, B and T cells, mast cells, basophils, eosinophils, neutrophils, and NK and NKT cells.[15,54,167,168] IL-33 plays a pivotal role in allergic sensitization and asthma development, being loci susceptible to IL-33 and ST2 for asthma development.[169–171] IL-33 potently activates human eosinophils and mediates direct degranulation of mast cells in the absence of allergen. IL-33 affects all stages of allergy and type 2 inflammation, including the establishment of the immune environment in the perinatal lungs.[172,173] In mice, IL-33 generates airway inflammation through T_H2 cells and ILC2,[174,175] in addition to BHR and goblet cell hyperplasia by lymphocyte-independent mechanisms.[166] Etokimab is a mAb targeting IL-33 that showed efficacy for severe eosinophilic asthma in Phase II clinical trials (see Fig. 20.4).[15,69] Other mAbs targeting IL-33 and ST2 are under development for asthma treatment at different stages.[15,69]

IL-25, also known as IL-17E, belongs to the IL-17 cytokine family and plays a very important role in the initiation and amplification of type 2 immune responses.[15,176] IL-25 is secreted mainly by ECs, macrophages, basophils, mast cells, eosinophils, and T_H2 cells. IL-25 receptor, a heterodimer of IL-17RA and IL-17RB, is expressed on ECs, stroma cells, ILC2s, CD4+ T cells, DCs, invariant NKT (iNKT) cells, and myeloid cells.[15,54] IL-25 levels are increased in the lungs and skin of patients with asthma and atopic dermatitis.[177] In mice the expression of IL-25 in the lung and gut is mainly confined to tuft cells, a rare type of chemosensory ECs.[178] In asthma, IL-25 induces the production of T_H2 cytokines, enhances IgE synthesis, goblet cell hyperplasia, mucus production, and blood eosinophilia.[179] IL-25 drives the airway remodeling induced by house dust mite allergen.[180] IL-25 also contributes to the maintenance of the memory pool of T_H2 cells in cooperation with TSLP-activated DCs.[181] In allergic sensitized mice, the expression of IL-25 on antigen challenge is sufficient to induce airway inflammation and blocking of IL-25 restores homeostasis.[182]

Mast Cells, Basophils, and Neutrophils

After activation by IgE-dependent or IgE-independent mechanisms, sensitized mast cells and basophils produce large amounts of anaphylactogenic substances and type 2 cytokines during the IPR.[16] The frequency of activated airway mast cells is significantly higher in patients with asthma compared with healthy individuals, significantly contributing to BHR.[183] During LPR, basophils, neutrophils, eosinophils, and activated T cells infiltrate the exposition areas, trigger potent inflammatory responses, and contribute to BHR, mucus production, and chronicity. In vivo studies demonstrated that basophils and probably mast cells can acquire MHC-II molecules from DCs by trogocytosis.[184,185] Basophils contribute to the amplification of allergen-specific T_H2 and mast cells to the activation and expansion of memory and tissue resident T_H2 cells and T_{REG} cells.[23,27,186] In some patients, airway neutrophilia drives chronic severe asthma. The mechanisms by which neutrophils infiltrate the airways are not fully understood. Mechanisms dependent on IL-17–mediated production of IL-8 and other recruiting factors by ECs have been described and correlated with disease severity.[187] Neutrophil cytoplasts containing extruded DNA in the form of neutrophil extracellular traps have been shown to instruct DCs to polarize T_H17 responses, and in patients with asthma they correlate with IL-17 levels.[107]

Natural Killer T Cells, Natural Killer Cells, and Other Cells

NKT cells recognize lipids and glycolipids via their unique invariant T cell receptor after CD1d-mediated presentation. Activated NKT cells rapidly produce different types of cytokines that amplify adaptive immune responses. Different types of NKT cells contributing to BHR and asthma development according to their cytokine signature (*NKT1, NKT2,* or *NKT17*) have been described in asthma models. In allergic asthma, NKT2 cells producing IL-4 and IL-13 are required,[188] whereas in an ozone asthma model, IL-17–producing NKT17 cells drive neutrophil infiltration in the airways.[189] In these models, T_H2 cells and adaptive immunity have been dispensable for NKT cells to promote BHR, which might help explain some asthma endotypes. Recently the epigenetic repressor Ezh2 has been shown to perform an essential role in the capacity of NKT cells to induce asthma.[190] In humans, there is controversy on the frequency of NKT cells found in asthmatic lungs. The correlations are better found in BAL fluid and sputum but not in blood, which appears to be highly variable depending on asthma severity and symptom control.[190,191]

NK cells perform essential roles in killing tumor and virus-infected cells and in controlling microbial infections. Activated CD56bright CD16dull NK subset cells produce large amounts of both proinflammatory and antiinflammatory cytokines, and they might display a dual role in asthma. They contribute to exacerbation of airway inflammation, increase T_H2 cytokines and eosinophilia,[192] and suppress asthma development by producing high levels of IFN-γ after TLR9-L stimulation.[193] Activated NK cells also produced IL-22, which induces antimicrobial peptide production and enhances EC integrity.[89] In humans, a tiny subset of NK cells mainly producing T_H2 cytokines but not IFN-γ contribute to IgE production.[194] NK cells can also contribute to resolve inflammation in severe asthma by inducing eosinophil apoptosis.[195] In addition, an IL-10 producing regulatory NK-cell subset has been proposed that may suppress type 1 and type 2 immune responses.[196–198]

Other cell types such as γδ T cells or different types of CD8+ T cells (IFN-γ–producing T_C1 and IL-4– and IL-5–producing T_C2) might also play important roles in the orchestration of inflammation in different asthma endotypes.[1,199–202] Some reports showed increased γδ T cell numbers in BAL fluid from patients with asthma,[203] whereas others showed decreased numbers of peripheral blood γδ T cells.[204] T_C2 cells may contribute to asthma pathogenesis,[200] and T_C1 cells might have a dual role enhancing asthma symptoms in some endotypes[202] or displaying a protecting role in others by eliminating allergen-specific T_H2 cells.

Type 2 Innate Lymphoid Cells

ILC2s are present in human lungs and mucosa and require the transcription factors RORα and GATA3 for their development.[205] The alarmin IL-33–activated ILC2s produce large quantities of IL-5, IL-9, and IL-13 and significantly contribute to virus-induced BHR and allergic asthma.[168,206] After influenza virus infection, IL-33–activated ILC2s by alveolar macrophages contribute significantly to BHR.[168,207] Different mice models have shown the role of ILC2s in the pathophysiologic processes of asthma and allergic inflammation.[168,208] The number of ILC2s producing IL-5 and IL-13 is significantly increased in sputum from patients with severe eosinophilic asthma and after allergen challenge.[209,210] In patients with severe corticosteroid-resistant eosinophilic asthma, ILC2s contribute to local eosinophilopoiesis by mechanisms depending on large amounts of production of IL-5 and IL-13.[209] In children with severe therapy-resistant asthma, the levels of ILC2 were higher in BAL fluid.[18] Other studies have confirmed these observations supporting that virus- and allergen-induced BHR and asthma share these pathways to generate type 2 immune responses.[205]

Airway Remodeling in Asthma

Airway remodeling refers to the abnormal structural changes altering the physiologic function of the airways in patients with asthma.[211] These structural changes include smooth muscle hypertrophy, goblet cell hyperplasia and mucus hypersecretion, changes in extracellular matrix composition leading to basal membrane thickening and subepithelial fibrosis, epithelium destruction, and angiogenesis. These features correlate with an overall thickening of the airway wall and narrowing of the airway lumen and are frequently associated with the most severe manifestations of asthma and chronicity.

The epithelial-mesenchymal unit coordinates the regeneration and proper responses to tissue damage.[212] Different cytokines and growth factors play a key role in these processes. The conversion of mesenchymal cells into myofibroblasts producing large amounts of interstitial collagens leads to fibrosis and thickening of the subepithelial basement membrane.[213] Stromal cell–derived TGF-β induces the synthesis of collagen-I and inhibits collagenase production in an autocrine manner, thus contributing to fibrosis and airway remodeling in asthma.[206,212,214] In contrast, T_{REG} cell–derived TGF-β impairs airway inflammation.[119] Chronic inflammation has been linked to airway remodeling through mechanisms involving ECs, goblet cells, smooth muscle cells, and blood vessel cells. Various cytokines, chemokines, adhesion molecules, and matrix metalloproteinases cooperate during the complex and redundant process of cell trafficking to the lung in asthma. Other studies based on structural changes observed in children with asthma in the absence of classic inflammation suggest that airway remodeling might precede airway inflammation.[211,215] Supporting this concept, the airways are more prone to damage during embryonic and fetal development in the absence of inflammation and bronchoconstriction leads to compressive mechanical forces

that may also induce remodeling without inflammation. Another important factor contributing to airway remodeling is the higher frequency of exacerbations in patients with severe asthma that are normally associated with strong airway inflammation.[4,12,211] Both inflammation-dependent and inflammation-independent mechanisms might cooperate in airway remodeling. Genetic polymorphisms for asthma susceptibility have been described for several remodeling-related genes such as *ADAM33* and filaggrin *(FLG)*.[213,216]

The Role of Respiratory Viruses in Asthma Development and Exacerbations

Viral respiratory tract infections might be associated with asthma exacerbations in older children and adults and with asthma development early in life.[217,218] Respiratory syncytial virus (RSV) is the most common causative agent of bronchiolitis during the first year of life, followed by rhinovirus, which starts to predominate after the first year. Other less common viruses associated with asthma include the more recently identified bocaviruses and pneumoviruses, along with coronaviruses, parainfluenza viruses, and adenoviruses.[217,219] The persistence of respiratory viruses, virus load, and virus coinfections, probably as a result of impaired innate immune responses and predisposition to mount strong type 2 immune responses, correlate with the most severe respiratory illnesses. A high rate of respiratory bacterial infections also has been associated with asthma exacerbations, suggesting that, in general, respiratory infections may exacerbate rather than prevent the development of asthma. In contrast, other studies suggest that respiratory infections might have a preventive role for asthma development or contribute to the reduction of asthma symptoms.

Rhinovirus

Rhinovirus, the common cold virus, is the most frequent viral infection associated with asthma exacerbations.[220,221] In susceptible children, rhinovirus infections lead to asthma-like airway inflammation and severe wheezing. High-risk birth cohort studies have demonstrated that young children with rhinovirus-induced wheezing episodes are at high risk of school-age asthma development, with this risk higher in allergic sensitized children before 2 years of age.[222–224]

Rhinovirus-infected bronchial ECs and endothelial cells produce a large amount of proinflammatory mediators that contribute to the worsening of asthma episodes.[217,218] Human rhinovirus promotes type 2 immune responses and inhibits T_H1 or IL-10–producing T_{REG} cells, which together with impaired capacity to mount innate immune responses could justify rhinovirus infection and asthma exacerbations.[225–227] Rhinovirus is also able to enter and form viral replication centers in B lymphocytes inducing their proliferation.[219,228] IgE-mediated FcεRI cross-linking in human pDCs impairs IFN-α production, which favors viral replication and asthma exacerbations.[220,229] CDHR3, a receptor for rhinovirus C to enter the body, is a susceptible locus for early childhood asthma with severe exacerbations.[169] Several strategies to prevent the attachment of rhinovirus to host cells have been tried, but clinical translation is questioned because of safety issues and drug resistances. Accordingly, oral corticosteroid treatment for rhinovirus infection has demonstrated efficacy in suppressing lung inflammation and delaying the appearance of new episodes and asthma development, suggesting that early systemic antiinflammatory treatments might affect the natural course of asthma.[230]

Respiratory Syncytial Virus

RSV is the most common viral infection during the first year of life, leading to acute viral bronchiolitis associated with increased risk of severe recurrent wheezing and mildly increased risk of asthma.[224] Allergic asthma increases the risk of RSV infection, leading to severe lower airway illness and hospitalization.[231] In contrast, 2014 findings suggest that RSV infection is not causal to asthma and atopy development.[230] In very young infants, RSV infection is a strong inducer of EC-derived TSLP, IL-25, and IL-33, which subsequently boost the activation of IL-5–producing and IL-13–producing ILC2s and T_H2 cells, leading to eosinophil recruitment and mucus production. Because of the impaired T_H1 responses in neonates, RSV also promotes the generation of IL-17–producing T_H17 cells that contribute to a more severe disease state.[232] RSV also impairs the generation of functional T_{REG} cells.[11,233] B cell responses are not fully developed in very young children, and therefore babies born from mothers with high levels of neutralizing antibodies are better protected from RSV-induced severe disease.[217] The antiviral ribavirin treatment of children hospitalized with RSV bronchiolitis has been demonstrated to decrease the risk of subsequent allergic sensitization and asthma development, but toxicity still remains a concern.[217,234] Treatment of premature infants with palivizumab, an mAb preventing RSV infection, also reduced subsequent recurrent wheezing but not asthma.[235,236] Novel vaccines and molecules to prevent and treat RSV infection are currently under development.[217]

The Hygiene Hypothesis

The original hygiene hypothesis postulated that excessive hygiene measures, antibiotics, and vaccines decreased microbial burden exposure and infectious diseases, which results in a significantly lower activation of immune system cells and reduced numbers of functional T_{REG} cells. This would result in a significant increase of T_H2 and T_H1 cells accounting for the observed increment of prevalence for allergic diseases and autoimmunity.[32,119] More recent findings extended these observations to reduction in biodiversity of the environment and microbiota of the body and proposed that rapid urbanization, sedentary lifestyle, pollution, and climate change also contribute to the rapid observed increment in prevalence of different types of chronic noncommunicable diseases.[237]

Role of Endotoxins and Other Bacterial Products

In contrast to respiratory viral infection, early exposure to different microorganisms or their derived products might well contribute to preventing airway inflammation and asthma development. For example, gram-positive commensal bacteria (*Bifidobacterium* and *Lactobacillus* strains), *Helicobacter pylori* infection, histamine-producing bacteria, fiber-rich diets promoting short-chain fatty acids, flagellin B, vitamin A, and components excreted by helminths impair ECs inflammatory responses and promote tolerogenic DCs that polarize T_{REG} and T_H1 responses, which protect against the asthma development and allergic diseases.[11,32,238–241] Epidemiologic and mechanistic studies on farm environments showed that high bacterial lipopolysaccharide exposure confers protection against allergic sensitization and asthma development.[242,243]

Conclusions

Asthma is a very complex syndrome encompassing different subgroups with specific immune pathologic mechanisms termed *endotypes*. Our knowledge about the different clinical asthma entities and their specific molecular mechanisms significantly improved over recent years. Although allergen-specific T_H2 cells and IgE play a central role in the pathophysiologic processes of allergic asthma, findings have delineated that the integration of a much more complex network of cells and molecules such as ILC2s and other innate immune cells and their cytokines also significantly contribute to the initiation and severity of the disease that also represent molecular targets for the treatment. Viral infections have been associated with severe recurrent wheezing, asthma development, and exacerbations. The hygiene hypothesis has been reformulated, and the significant reduction of environmental biodiversity appear to account for the exponential growth of chronic inflammatory disorders, including asthma, that we have witnessed over the last century (Fig. 20.6). High-level exposure to endotoxin, farm environment, and diversity in microbial colonization impairs excessive

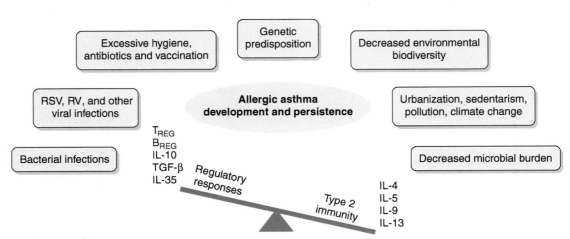

• **Fig. 20.6** Development and persistence of allergic asthma. Genetic predisposition and environmental factors contribute to immunologic alterations that promote type 2 immunity versus regulatory responses that lead to the exponential increase in the development and persistence of allergic asthma observed over recent decades. B_{REG}, Regulatory B cell; *IL*, interleukin; *RSV*, respiratory syncytial virus; *RV*, rhinovirus; *TGF-β*, transforming growth factor-beta; T_{REG}, regulatory T cell.

inflammation and asthma development. The establishment of functional allergen-specific T_{REG} and B_{REG} cells is a key event for long-term healthy immune responses to allergens. Tolerogenic DCs producing high levels of IL-10 and/or TGF-β are essential for immune tolerance to allergens, and strategies targeting these cells represent promising approaches to restore proper immune responses and homeostasis. Initial asthma therapies were based on relieving airway obstruction and inflammation using broad-spectrum drugs, but current biologic treatments move forward to more specific approaches targeting molecular pathways. Similarly, AIT emerged as a suitable strategy to restore the course of the disease in patients with controlled allergic asthma. Biotechnology and omics platforms offer promising approaches to better stratify patients in an endotype-based manner according to underlying mechanisms, which might well help the development of better prevention strategies and alternative therapeutic options in carefully selected asthma patients.

The reference list can be found on the companion Expert Consult website at http://www.expertconsult.inkling.com.

21

Lung Function Testing in Children

KAREN M. MCDOWELL, THERESA W. GUILBERT

KEY POINTS

- Objective measures of lung function are important in the diagnosis and management of asthma.
- Spirometry is the mainstay of pulmonary function testing in asthma.
- Methacholine challenge testing is helpful in identifying or excluding bronchial hyperresponsiveness in children with atypical history, persistent symptoms with normal lung function, abnormal examination or persistent symptoms, and/or airway obstruction despite appropriate asthma treatment.
- Impulse oscillometry (IOS), which is performed during tidal breathing, is a method for obtaining lung function measures in children too young or unable to perform spirometry.

- IOS can be useful in determining baseline lung function, demonstrating response to bronchodilator or bronchoprovocation, and predicting asthma exacerbations and loss of disease control.
- Fractional exhaled nitric oxide levels reflect eosinophilic inflammation and predict responsiveness to corticosteroids.
- Exhaled breath condensate includes volatile organic compounds and markers of inflammation that are elevated in asthma.

Introduction

Objective measures of lung function are important in the diagnosis and management of asthma. Spirometry is the pulmonary function test most widely used in asthma; however, multiple other pulmonary function tests are useful in assessment and monitoring of asthma. Spirometry requires respiratory maneuvers that may be difficult for young children. Impulse oscillometry (IOS) is a noninvasive method of measuring lung function during tidal breathing and thus is an ideal test for use in patients unable to perform spirometry. IOS has been shown to be more sensitive than spirometry in detecting peripheral airway obstruction, asthma exacerbations, and loss of control. Fractional exhaled nitric oxide (FeNO) levels correspond to eosinophilic inflammation and predict responsiveness to corticosteroids. Although FeNO has been used to discriminate among wheezing phenotypes, its role in preschool wheezing is less clear. Exhaled breath condensate (EBC) contains volatile organic compounds and biomarkers of inflammation that are elevated in asthma. EBC is appealing as an easily obtained, noninvasive test for asthma, yet more standardization is needed before widespread adoption for clinical use.

Spirometry is an important tool in the management of asthma and is recommended for the diagnosis and monitoring of asthma in both U.S. and European guidelines.[1,2] Although spirometry is the most commonly used method for objective assessment of lung function, multiple other pulmonary function tests are useful in the management of children with asthma. This chapter will review the role of lung function testing in asthma and summarize tests that are available for objective measurement of lung function in children.

Spirometry

Spirometry is the most widely used test for evaluation of children with asthma or suspected asthma. The role of spirometry is to evaluate for the presence or absence of airway obstruction. To establish an asthma diagnosis, reversibility of airway obstruction must be demonstrated. Importantly, most children with asthma, even those with severe disease, have normal spirometry when well[3,4]; thus, it may be necessary to perform spirometry when the child is symptomatic to document airway obstruction. Objective measurement of lung function is especially important in children because their perception of asthma symptoms and airflow obstruction is variable. Spirometry may reveal more severe obstruction than that estimated from the history and physical examination and can result in the child being placed in a more severe asthma category than using symptom frequency alone.[5]

To perform spirometry successfully, a child must be able to follow directions and execute full inspiration from functional residual capacity (FRC), the end of a tidal breath exhalation, to total lung capacity (TLC) followed by forced exhalation to residual volume (RV), ideally over a minimum of 6 seconds. An exhalation of 3 seconds or greater is acceptable for children younger than

10 years of age. In addition, the child must be able to provide reproducible efforts. The maximal respiratory maneuvers required for spirometry may be difficult for children under the age of 5 years, although with appropriate coaching, children as young as 3 years of age can learn to perform spirometry appropriately[6] (Box 21.1). The technical aspects of spirometry in children are outlined elsewhere,[7] but it is important to note that successful pulmonary function testing in children requires a child-friendly environment and technicians who are specifically trained in pediatric spirometry and able to help children feel at ease. Visual demonstration of maneuvers and simple but encouraging coaching directions are also crucial (Fig. 21.1).

Spirometry measures forced vital capacity (FVC), forced expiratory volume in 1 second (FEV_1), and forced expiratory flow (FEF) at 25%, 50%, 75% of FVC and flow between 25% and 75% of FVC (FEF_{25}, FEF_{50}, FEF_{75}, and FEF_{25-75}, respectively). Reference equations for spirometry are derived from several variables, including age, race, sex, height, and weight. Values within the 95% confidence interval of the calculated reference are considered normal.[8] Airway obstruction is defined by FEV_1/FVC that is lower than the 5th percentile of the predicted value. As disease progresses, the FEV_1 will become reduced as well.[8] The severity of obstruction is determined by the FEV_1 percent predicted. An abnormal (low) FEV_1 that is greater than 70% predicted is considered mild obstruction. FEV_1 of 60% to 69% of predicted reveals moderate obstruction, 50% to 59% predicted is moderately severe obstruction, and 35% to 49% of predicted indicates severe obstruction. FEV_1 percent of predicted that is less than 35% is evidence of very severe obstruction.[8] Reversibility of airflow obstruction is determined by measuring spirometry before and after bronchodilator. In adults, an improvement of 12% and 200 mL in FVC or FEV_1 after administration of a bronchodilator is considered to be clinically significant; however, in children an increase of 8% may be accepted as evidence of bronchodilator response.[9] Just as most children have normal spirometry when well, similarly they may not demonstrate a bronchodilator response at baseline or unless they are ill.

In addition to utility in establishing an asthma diagnosis, spirometry is valuable in monitoring of asthma and risk assessment. Decrease in FEV_1 is associated with future exacerbations

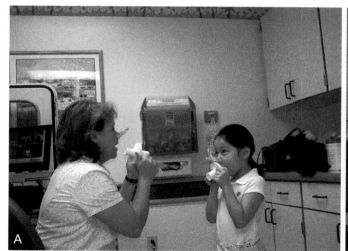
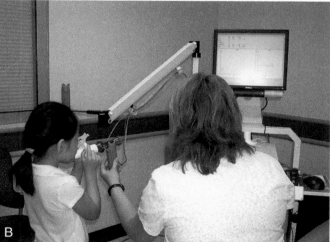

• **Fig. 21.1** Six-year-old girl performing spirometry in a pulmonary function laboratory. (A) The respiratory therapist prepares the child for the test by practicing with the nose clips and mouthpiece. (B) The child performs spirometry while the respiratory therapist observes flow-volume loops on the computer to ensure the test is technically adequate.

of asthma and healthcare usage for children who have mild to moderate asthma.[10] FEV_1/FVC is the most sensitive indicator of obstruction in children[11] and declines with increased asthma severity.[10,12] In children with asthma, lung function should be measured at the time of diagnosis and a minimum of annually thereafter.[1,2] International guidelines also recommend obtaining lung function values 3 to 6 months after initiation of treatment.[2]

A spirometry report includes a display of the flow-volume loop as performed by the child along with measured values, reference values, confidence interval, and percent of predicted reference value for each parameter. Many reports will also present a volume-time curve. The flow-volume loop demonstrates airflow on both inspiration and expiration. Analysis of the shape of the flow-volume allows detection of other patterns of airflow obstruction. Extrathoracic obstruction affects the inspiratory limb of the flow-volume loop, whereas intrathoracic obstruction generally affects the expiratory portion of the loop. The intrathoracic airway obstruction in asthma causes an abnormality in the expiratory curve, giving it a "scooped" appearance. Fixed airway obstruction, such as that caused by a large mediastinal mass compressing the trachea, will result in blunting of both inspiratory and expiratory limbs. Inducible laryngeal obstruction (previously known as vocal cord dysfunction) is a form of variable extrathoracic obstruction and produces flattening of the inspiratory portion of the flow-volume loop (Fig. 21.2). Examination of the shape of the flow-volume curve is important in the diagnosis of static and dynamic large airway obstruction and in the diagnosis of diffuse airways obstruction in asthma.[4,11]

Plethysmography

Plethysmography allows the measurement of lung volumes and airway resistance. Conductance (the inverse of resistance) and specific conductance (conductance corrected for the lung volume at which it is measured) also can be measured by plethysmography. The airway narrowing seen in asthma results in an increased airway resistance and decreased conductance; therefore, measurement of resistance and conductance offer additional methods of assessing airway obstruction. Specific airway conductance is a sensitive measure of mild airway obstruction even in younger children.[7] Lung volumes that are useful in assessment of asthma include TLC, thoracic gas volume (TGV), RV, and RV/TLC. Hyperinflation as a result of severe airway obstruction in asthma manifests as elevated TLC or TGV. Airway narrowing results in decreased exhaled volume, which in turn results in increased RV. Elevated RV/TLC is a measure of gas trapping, which is a sensitive measurement of pulmonary dysfunction in children with asthma.[4]

Bronchial Provocation

Bronchial provocation testing may be helpful in establishing the diagnosis of asthma by providing evidence of airway hyperreactivity (AHR). It is especially useful if any of the following are present: atypical history, persistent symptoms with normal lung function, abnormal examination findings or persistent symptoms, and/or airway obstruction despite appropriate asthma treatment. There are several methods of performing bronchial provocation testing, differing mostly by the stimulus used to elicit AHR. The most frequently used approaches are methacholine challenge and exercise challenge testing, although cold air, mannitol, histamine, and adenosine 5′-monophosphate also have been used.[4]

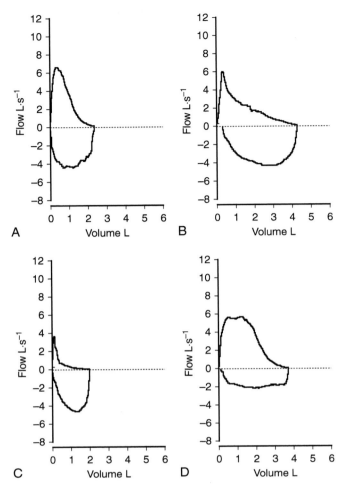

• **Fig. 21.2** Flow-volume loop patterns. (A) Normal flow-volume loop. (B) Moderate obstruction. (C) Severe obstruction. Note "scooping" of expiratory limb in obstructive flow-volume loops (B and C). (D) Variable extrathoracic upper airway obstruction as seen in inducible laryngeal obstruction or vocal cord dysfunction. Note blunting of inspiratory limb of flow-volume loop. (Modified from Miller MR, Hankinson J, Brusasco V, et al. Standardisation of spirometry. Eur Resp J 2005;26:319–38. Reproduced with permission of the © ERS 2019: Eur Resp J 2019;26(2):319–338; DOI: 10.1183/09031936.05.00034805. Published 1.08.05.

Methacholine challenge testing entails performing spirometry at baseline and after administration of increasing doses of methacholine until the FEV_1 decreases by 20% or the maximal recommended dose of methacholine is reached. The methacholine concentration at which the FEV_1 is decreased 20% below baseline is the provocative concentration (PC_{20}). More recently, the American Thoracic Society (ATS) recommends using a provocation dose (PD_{20}), which allows comparison of results using different nebulizers and inhalation times.[13] The relationship between level of airway responsiveness and asthma is quite complex, depending in part on the pretest probability of asthma. A detailed discussion of these concepts is beyond the scope of this chapter. However, in children, the degree of AHR correlates with asthma severity,[11,14–16] and, in general, the stratification outlined in Table 21.1 can be used to correlate PC_{20} and level of AHR. It is important to note that although bronchial hyperresponsiveness (BHR) is characteristic of asthma, it also can be present in children with allergic rhinitis and/or other chronic lung disease.[17] Additionally, there is evidence to suggest

TABLE 21.1	Level of Airway Hyperresponsiveness (AHR) Based on Provocative Concentration (PC$_{20}$)	
Classification*	**PC$_{20}$ (mg/mL)**	
Moderate to severe AHR	<1	
Mild AHR	1–4	
Borderline AHR	4–16	
Normal airway responsiveness	>16	

*The following assumptions are made: baseline airway obstruction is absent, spirometry is of satisfactory quality, and there is significant recovery of forced expiratory volume in 1 second (FEV1) after challenge.

Modified from Table 45.1 in Kercsmar CM, McDowell KM. Wheezing in older children: asthma. In: Wilmott RW, Deterding R, Li Albert, et al, editors. Kendig's disorders of the respiratory tract in children. 9th ed. Philadelphia, PA: Elsevier; 2019. p. 686–721. Used with permission.

that BHR in normal infants or children with chronic cough may predict asthma later in childhood.[18] A negative methacholine challenge has a high negative predictive value, meaning that in the face of such results, asthma is unlikely.[19] Methacholine challenge testing is safe to administer to children when performed in accordance with current guidelines and patients are monitored appropriately; thus, it has been used extensively in clinical trials and epidemiologic studies. There are data to suggest that although methacholine challenge is sensitive for detection of AHR, exercise provocation may be more specific than methacholine challenge for detection of asthma or confirmation of the diagnosis.[20,21] Medications that can decrease bronchial reactivity, such as long- and short-acting β agonists should be withheld before performing methacholine challenge testing. Guidelines for specific medications and the time frame to withhold before testing are available.[11] Inhaled and oral corticosteroids are typically not discontinued before performing a methacholine challenge; however, because the antiinflammatory effect of these medications can result in decreased airway responsiveness, their use should be taken into consideration when interpreting test results. Likewise, the presence of factors that increase BHR, such as recent respiratory infection, aeroallergen exposure, irritants, and pollution also should be considered.[11]

Exercise challenge testing can be easily and safely performed by older children and is useful for detecting exercise-induced bronchospasm. To perform an exercise test safely, the child must be able to run on a treadmill or ride a cycle ergometer. During an exercise challenge, spirometry is performed at baseline and after an exercise protocol. The child exercises at a speed and grade at which the he or she can maintain exercise at 80% to 90% of maximal heart rate for 4 to 6 minutes. This usually requires a total of 6 to 8 minutes of exercise. Spirometry is repeated 5, 10, 15, 20, and 30 minutes after cessation of exercise. A fall in FEV$_1$ of 10% to 15% after exercise is considered evidence of exercise-induced bronchospasm.[11] Alternatively, a cycle ergometer can be used with a protocol that elicits a target ventilation rate for 4 to 6 minutes of exercise. Some authors propose that exercise challenge using a treadmill is superior to that using a bicycle[22–24]; however, studies directly comparing the two methods are lacking. Children who participate in sports at highly competitive levels or who are extremely fit may require a more intensive challenge to trigger exercise-induced bronchospasm.

Impulse Oscillometry

IOS, although not as widely available as spirometry, is a noninvasive method of obtaining lung function during tidal breathing and therefore is easily performed by preschool children and others unable to perform spirometry.[25,26] However, a 2018 large multicenter study of inner city children at risk for asthma found that of 485 children who attempted lung function testing, a higher percentage were able to perform acceptable spirometry than IOS at ages 3, 4, and 5 years.[6] It is worth noting, though, that the study used FEV$_{0.5}$ rather than the more commonly used FEV$_1$ in determining acceptable and repeatable spirometry. An advantage of IOS, in addition to the ease with which it is performed in young children, is that it can measure airway resistance, which typically requires body plethysmography. During IOS, sound waves are transmitted into the airways, allowing measurement of pressure and flow in the airways over a range of frequencies. Obtaining pressure and flow measurements allows calculation of other important mechanical properties of the airways such as resistance and reactance. Reactance occurs in response to the sound wave and therefore is the energy echoed back to the system after, and out of phase with, the sound wave. Reactance can be thought of as the "stored energy" of the respiratory system or rebound energy that is generated in response to the sound wave moving through the lungs. It is composed, in large part, of the elastic recoil of the airways. Lower frequency sounds waves (those <15 Hertz [Hz]) have small amplitude and therefore are able to travel more distally into the airways. IOS measurements obtained at low frequencies reveal the characteristics of larger airways together with those of the peripheral airways. Because of their higher amplitude, higher frequency sound waves travel over shorter distances and thus traverse only the larger airways. Values acquired at frequencies of 20 Hz or greater will indicate properties of larger airways. Small-airway parameters are then derived by determining the difference between the low- and high-frequency measurements.

Although the measurements of reactance and resistance are determined over a range of frequencies in IOS, values are usually reported at 5, 10, and 20 Hz. Resistance is denoted by the letter R followed by the frequency at which the measurement was made. Similarly, reactance is represented by the letter X followed by the frequency at which the measurement was made. Thus, R5 and X5 are the resistance and the reactance, respectively, as measured at 5 Hz and indicate properties of the proximal and distal airways combined. R20 and X20 are the resistance and reactance of the large airways. Peripheral airway resistance is the difference between R5 and R20 and is represented by R5-R20. Values for R5 and R20 that are greater than 150% of predicted should be considered abnormal and are consistent with increased airway resistance. An R5-R20 value is considered elevated, and consistent with peripheral airway obstruction, if it is greater than 30% in children and greater than 20% in adults. When reactance is zero (X = 0), low-frequency and high-frequency reactance can be discriminated. This frequency is the resonant frequency (Fres). Fres is the dividing point between large and small airways based on the mechanical properties of the airways. It is important to realize that the distinction between large and small airways based on Fres is determined by the airway mechanics rather than the size or generation of the airway.[27] The value of Fres is higher in children than in adults and decreases with age.[28] Fres is also increased in airway obstruction.[29,30]

Reference values for IOS are more limited than those for spirometry and are derived from an ethnically homogeneous sample.

The equations are based almost exclusively on data obtained from white children of European descent.[31–34] However, a literature review by Galant and associates[35] and subsequent comparison of values obtained from diverse populations with commercially available regression equations revealed that predicted values in commercially available software are reasonable reference values for multiple races and ethnicities.

Impulse Oscillometry and Asthma

IOS has been studied extensively in asthma, including during acute exacerbations. Children with asthma have elevated resistance, specifically R5, and decreased reactance at baseline compared with children without asthma[36,37] (Table 21.2). R20 and Fres also have been shown to be increased in patients with asthma compared with healthy controls.[38–40] After administration of a bronchodilator, children with asthma demonstrate a decrease in resistance, both R5 and R5-R20. A concomitant decrease in reactance is also exhibited[36,41] (see Table 21.2). A decrease in R5 or X5 of 40% or greater after administration of a bronchodilator should be considered a positive response in pediatric asthma[35] (see Table 21.2). Even a response as low as a 20% decrease in R5 or R10 after bronchodilator differentiated preschoolers with asthma from those without asthma[42,43] (see Table 21.2). These studies demonstrated changes in IOS parameters even without concomitant change in spirometry, indicating that IOS may be more sensitive than spirometry in distinguishing asthma from healthy controls. Other authors have also reported IOS to be more sensitive than spirometry in distinguishing children with asthma from those who did not have asthma and in detecting small airway obstruction.[6,36,38,41,44] This is presumably because IOS reflects changes in the caliber of the small airways, where changes of asthma occur before the abnormalities in the larger airways, which are characterized by spirometry.[45] IOS also has been shown to be more sensitive than spirometry at detecting response to methacholine[45] and the degree of decrease in R5-R20 after bronchoprovocation correlates with asthma severity.[46] Other authors have demonstrated that IOS is more sensitive in identifying poorly controlled asthma,[47] loss of disease control,[48] and asthma exacerbations.[45] Thus, IOS may be more helpful than spirometry in detection of peripheral airway obstruction or severe disease and disease monitoring by providing opportunity for earlier intervention.

Infant Pulmonary Function Testing

Pulmonary function testing is available for infants using a technique of inflating the lungs to a set pressure and then rapidly compressing the thorax with an inflated vest. This technique (raised volume rapid thoracic compression [RVRTC]) causes the infant to forcefully exhale, creating a flow-volume loop similar to that produced by older children and adults during spirometry. Infants require sedation for measurement of flow-volume curves, lung volumes, and airway resistance in this fashion; thus, infant pulmonary function testing by the RVRTC method is performed only in pediatric hospitals by specially trained pulmonologists. The limited availability and need for sedation highlight that infant pulmonary function testing should be performed only in select high-risk patients in early infancy and toddlerhood. An additional consideration is that children older than 2 years of age have often outgrown infant pulmonary testing equipment. Appropriate candidates for infant pulmonary function testing would include infants who have not responded to therapy, and demonstration of abnormal lung function and/or bronchodilator response would aid in making a diagnosis.

Fractional Exhaled Nitric Oxide

FeNO is a marker of eosinophilic airway inflammation and can be measured noninvasively, making it a useful clinical tool in children to aid with the diagnosis and management of asthma. Nitric oxide (NO) is produced by respiratory epithelial cells, and production is increased in the presence of inflammatory cytokines.[49] NO is present in exhaled breath, and levels correlate with sputum eosinophil levels.[50] Thus, FeNO levels are elevated in most children with asthma and have been shown to differentiate children with asthma from those without.[51,52] Importantly, elevated FeNO levels can identify children who are likely to respond to therapy with inhaled corticosteroids (ICSs) and those who are likely to relapse after reduction of ICS dose.[53,54] Elevated FeNO levels early in life help predict which preschool children with wheezing are more likely to develop asthma[55] because eosinophilic airway inflammation may precede other criteria for the diagnosis of asthma.[56] However, there is more variability in the mean levels of FeNO reported among studies in healthy infants and toddlers than in older children and adults,[57–59] and larger studies are needed to determine normative values for healthy infants and preschoolers. Because FeNO can be easily measured in children and reflects eosinophilic airway inflammation, it has significant potential to be useful in the diagnosis and management of asthma in children, especially those too young to perform spirometry. Nonetheless, commercially available equipment for measuring FeNO requires respiratory maneuvers that are not easily performed by preschool children.

The ATS published an official Clinical Practice Guideline in 2011 addressing use of FeNO for diagnosis of eosinophilic airway inflammation.[55] An FeNO value greater than 50 parts per billion (ppb) is consistent with eosinophilic airway inflammation and an indication of responsiveness to corticosteroids; however, in children younger than 12 years of age, the cut-off may be as low as 35 ppb. An FeNO level less than 20 ppb is considered to be in the normal range and signifies the presence of little to no eosinophilic inflammation. Studies have demonstrated that using a level of less than 20 ppb as normal had a high sensitivity and specificity and positive predictive and negative predictive values.[60–62] Sivan and colleagues[52] reported a sensitivity of 80%, specificity of 92%, positive predictive value of 89%, and negative predictive value of 86%. An FeNO level of less than 15 ppb for the same cohort had a false negative rate of less than 5% and a level greater than 23 ppb had a false positive rate of less than 5%. Therefore, in patients who have symptoms consistent with asthma but nondiagnostic spirometric testing results, FeNO provides additional data that can help establish or refute the diagnosis of asthma.

Multiple factors influence FeNO values, including age, sex, height, atopy, smoking (active or passive exposure to tobacco smoke), exercise, consumption of nitrite-containing foods or caffeine,[63–65] and prematurity.[66,67] However, in younger children, from 1 to 5 years of age, height, weight, and sex have been shown not to affect FeNO.[59] Testing technique and analyzer type also can affect FeNO levels.[55] Prematurity has been shown to be associated with lower FeNO levels.[66,67] Furthermore, clinical information such as recent use of inhaled or systemic corticosteroids is important in interpreting the significance of FeNO, especially values in the intermediate range (those between 20 and 35 ppb).[67]

TABLE 21.2 Description, Abbreviations, and Normal Values for Common Impulse Oscillometry (IOS) Parameters

IOS Parameter	Symbol	Description	Reference Values
Respiratory impedance	Zrs	Impedance = Resistance + Reactance	
Respiratory resistance	Rrs	Airway + tissue + chest wall resistance	R5 normal if ≤150% predicted
	R5	Resistance at frequency of 5 Hz = Resistance of proximal and distal airways	R20 normal if ≤150% predicted
	R20	Resistance at frequency of 20 Hz = Resistance of proximal airways	None established but increase suggestive of elevated small airways resistance
	R5-R20	Value at R5 – value at R20 = Resistance of small airways	
Respiratory reactance	Xrs	Elastic + inertive properties of airways + lung tissue	
	X5	Reactance at frequency of 5 Hz. Increased value suggests small airway obstruction	Abnormal if X5 >150% predicted
Bronchodilator response		Decrease in R5 or X5 after administration of bronchodilator	Decrease by ≥40% is considered a positive response
Resonant frequency	Fres	Frequency at which elastic forces = inertive forces; X = 0. Increased value suggests peripheral airway obstruction	*Adults:* Normal <12 Hz, Abnormal >20 Hz; *Children:* Normal <20–25 Hz, Abnormal >25 Hz
Reactance area	AX	Area under the reactance curve bounded by Fres and X5. Increased value suggests peripheral airway obstruction	None established but increase suggestive of peripheral airway obstruction
Coherence	Co	Indicator of quality control. Assessment of reproducibility	*Test acceptable if:*
	Co 5	Coherence at 5 Hz	Co 5 Hz 0.7–0.9
	Co 20	Coherence at 20 Hz	Co 20 Hz 0.9–1.0

From McDowell KM. Recent diagnosis techniques in pediatric asthma: impulse oscillometry in preschool asthma and use of exhaled nitric oxide. Immunol Allergy Clin North Am 2019;39:205–219. Used with permission.

Fractional Exhaled Nitric Oxide and Diagnosis of Asthma

Although measurement of FeNO may be helpful in determining risk of developing asthma, it is important to remember that FeNO has been shown to be elevated in conditions other than asthma in both atopic and nonatopic children. In fact, it is difficult to differentiate asthma from atopy based on FeNO level alone. Patients with allergic rhinitis, but not asthma, have FeNO levels comparable to those of patients with allergic asthma.[68,69] FeNO level is significantly higher in children with recurrent wheezing for those who have a positive Asthma Predictive Index (API) compared with those with a negative API[70,71] and in comparison to children with no wheezing.[72] Similarly, FeNO is higher for children with allergic asthma compared with nonallergic asthma[73] and also in those who have allergic sensitization but not asthma.[73–75]

In spite of the overlap between atopy and asthma in producing elevated FeNO levels, many authors have found an association between high FeNO levels in childhood and subsequent asthma. In a large birth cohort of over 800 children from the Netherlands, the Prevention and Incidence of Asthma and Mite Allergy (PIAMA) study found that elevated FeNO level at 4 years of age is associated with physician diagnosis of asthma at age 7.[18] A prospective study by Singer and colleagues[76] demonstrated a similar finding. Regardless of atopic status, children with airway

hyperreactivity have elevated FeNO levels.[74,77] FeNO is also useful in differentiating wheezing phenotypes in early childhood. Gouvis-Echraghi and associates[78] examined wheezing and FeNO levels in 79 children younger than 3 years of age. Those with moderate to severe, uncontrolled nonatopic asthma had the highest exhaled NO levels, whereas children with viral-induced wheezing had the lowest levels. Children with allergic wheezing had values that were intermediate between the other two phenotypes. Although FeNO represents eosinophilic inflammation that is typically responsive to steroids, in this population, those whose asthma was uncontrolled despite use of high-dose ICSs had the highest FeNO levels. In a larger study that followed over 970 children, preschoolers with late-onset wheezing had the highest FeNO levels.[79] Among atopic children, those with transient wheezing had higher levels of exhaled NO. These associations were present by the age of 4 years but were even stronger at the age of 8. Clearly, preschool wheezing is complex, and further study is needed to fully understand the role of FeNO in younger children.

Management of Asthma Based on Fractional Exhaled Nitric Oxide Levels

Multiple studies have demonstrated that management of asthma based on FeNO levels is not of significant benefit, although the cut-off levels of FeNO for change in ICS dose and the outcome measures differ among studies. Smith and others[80] and Shaw and colleagues[81] found that use of FeNO-guided treatment in adults with asthma resulted in no difference in asthma exacerbations over the course of 1 year, although both studies reported a lower ICS dose in the FeNO group. Similar results were obtained by Szefler and associates,[82] who followed 546 children over a year, and de Jongste and co-workers,[83] who studied 151 children over 30 weeks. Both investigators found that using FeNO to adjust antiinflammatory treatment resulted in no difference in symptom frequency or symptom-free days, even though Szefler and associates[82] reported that children in the FeNO group required fewer courses of oral steroids. Although studies in adults have shown a reduction in ICS dose for those whose asthma was managed using FeNO, Fritsch and colleagues[84] found that higher doses of ICSs were used in children whose asthma treatment included FeNO. In sum, research has not demonstrated clear benefit in symptom burden, decrease in exacerbations, or ICS dose when FeNO level is used to guide asthma treatment.

Exhaled Breath Condensate

EBC is a noninvasive technique for measuring biomarkers of airway inflammation. EBC is composed of three components: (1) droplets that are aerosolized from the lining fluid of the airways, (2) water droplets that have condensed from the gas phase of the exhalant, and (3) water-soluble volatile compounds that are absorbed into the condensate as they are exhaled. Because EBC contains various-sized droplets derived directly from airway lining fluid, their content is presumed to mirror that of airway lining fluid.[85] The volatile compounds in EBC are water-soluble and present in high concentrations; thus, they are easily collected by cooling exhaled air. Increased levels of volatile organic compounds in exhaled breath have been reported in children with both allergic and nonallergic asthma.[86–88] Biomarkers associated with oxidative stress, such as acidity (pH), hydrogen peroxide, nitrates, nitrites, aldehydes, 8-isoprostane, and cysteinyl leukotrienes, also have been identified in EBC and have been shown to be elevated in pediatric asthma.[89,90] Additionally, multiple studies have demonstrated elevated markers of inflammation in EBC of children with asthma compared with healthy controls. Children with asthma have elevated levels of type 1 and type 2 T cell cytokines, cysteinyl leukotrienes, and multiple chemokines.[10] Airway pH as measured by EBC is lower in patients with asthma and is also associated with risk of asthma exacerbation and airway inflammation.[86] Children with asthma also may have lower antioxidant function, indicated by decreased levels of glutathione, a protective antioxidant found in the lungs.[10,91] Collection of EBC is a noninvasive technique for measuring biomarkers of airway inflammation. However, despite its promise as a clinical tool for diagnosing and monitoring asthma, use and interpretation of EBC is fraught with inconsistencies. It is often difficult to compare results among studies because of significant heterogeneity in study population, sample size, definition of asthma, and methodology for collecting and analyzing EBC.[92–94] Larger studies and further standardization are needed before EBC is ready for widespread clinical application.

Conclusions

A variety of lung function tests are useful in evaluating children with asthma or asthma symptoms. Spirometry is the mainstay of pulmonary function testing in children with asthma or suspected asthma, especially because documentation of reversible airway obstruction is seminal to establishing the diagnosis of asthma. However, in children who continue to demonstrate normal spirometry despite ongoing symptoms, challenge testing, such as methacholine challenge, may be helpful. For children too young or unable to perform spirometry, IOS can provide valuable information about airway obstruction and resistance (Box 21.1). IOS may be better than spirometry at discriminating children with asthma from those without and early detection of airway obstruction. Pulmonary function testing can be performed in infants; however, widespread use of infant pulmonary function testing is limited by the need for sedation of the child during testing. FeNO level is a reflection of eosinophilic airway inflammation and therefore can be helpful in identifying children with asthma who will respond to therapy with ICSs. Using longitudinal assessments of FeNO to guide asthma management has not shown benefit over clinical management. EBC is an evolving technique with promise as a noninvasive method for detecting asthma and distinguishing asthma phenotypes; however, further study and standardization are needed.

Disclosure: Dr. McDowell has no financial or commercial conflicts of interest regarding the material contained within this chapter. Dr. Guilbert reports personal fees from American Board of Pediatrics; Pediatric Pulmonary Subboard, GSK, Novartis/Regeneron, Aviragen, GSK/Regneron, and TEVA; grants and personal fees from Sanofi/Regeneron; grants from Astra-Zeneca and NIH, royalties from UpToDate outside the submitted work.

The reference list can be found on the companion Expert Consult website at http://www.expertconsult.inkling.com.

22

Infections and Asthma in Childhood

DANIEL J. JACKSON

KEY POINTS

- Wheezing viral respiratory illnesses are the most common initial presentation of childhood asthma.
- Once asthma is established, viral infections, most notably rhinovirus (RV), are the most frequent trigger of severe asthma exacerbations. RV-C appears to be a particularly pathogenic virus in young children with asthma.
- Evidence has emerged to suggest that bacteria may contribute to the expression of asthma. Ongoing studies are critical to our
- understanding of the role of the gut and airway microbiomes in asthma inception and exacerbation.
- Synergistic interactions between underlying type 2 inflammation and viral infections play an important mechanistic role in asthma inception and exacerbation and are an important therapeutic target.
- Novel therapies are needed to prevent and treat virus-induced wheezing and asthma exacerbations.

Introduction

Respiratory infections can cause wheezing illnesses in children of all ages and also influence the development and severity of asthma in several ways. First, viral wheezing episodes during infancy are a critical risk factor for asthma inception. Once asthma is established, viral respiratory tract infections are the most common trigger for acute exacerbations. Furthermore, a potential role for particular bacterial pathogens in the development of wheezing and asthma exacerbations has been identified. This chapter will review the relationships between infections and asthma inception and exacerbation. Additionally, mechanisms by which infections lead to lower respiratory inflammation and airway dysfunction will be discussed. Finally, treatment strategies for virus-induced wheezing and exacerbations of asthma will be reviewed.

Relationships Between Early Life Infections and Childhood Asthma Inception (Fig. 22.1)

Viruses

Viral respiratory illnesses leading to wheezing are one of the most common causes of hospitalization during infancy. Using multiple virus detection methods, including polymerase chain reaction, Jartti and colleagues[1] investigated the cause of wheezing illness in 293 hospitalized children. Of the 76 infants with virus detected, 54% had respiratory syncytial virus (RSV), 42% had picornaviruses (human rhinovirus [RV] and enterovirus) and 1% had human metapneumovirus (hMPV). In older children, respiratory

picornaviruses, most commonly RV, dominated (65% of children aged 1–2 years and 82% of children 3 years or older). Outpatient wheezing illnesses are also extremely common in young children, and viruses have been implicated in 67% to 90% of these episodes in different populations.[2,3]

Wheezing with viruses during infancy is often an early manifestation of asthma. Several large, long-term prospective studies of children have demonstrated that RSV bronchiolitis is a significant independent risk factor for recurrent wheezing, at least within the first decade of life.[4,5] A 2013 clinical trial comparing palivizumab (anti-RSV monoclonal antibody) to placebo in near-preterm infants demonstrated reductions in recurrent wheezing during the first year of life in the children treated with palivizumab.[6] This is the strongest level of evidence to date in support of a causal role for RSV infection in recurrent wheezing. However, longitudinal follow-up of this study did not show a reduction in asthma at 6 years of age.[7] These data suggest that although RSV infections contribute substantially to the risk of recurrent wheezing in early childhood, other co-factors (e.g., genetic, environmental, developmental) also contribute to the expression of asthma or modification of phenotypes over time.

With the development of molecular diagnostics, evidence has emerged to suggest that wheezing illnesses caused by RV identify children at highest risk for childhood asthma.[2,8] The Childhood Origins of ASThma (COAST) birth cohort study confirmed prior associations between RSV wheezing in the first 3 years of life and childhood asthma, but demonstrated that RV wheezing during the preschool years is associated with a 10-fold increased risk of childhood asthma.[2] Mechanisms by which recurrent RV infections may lead to wheezing and airway remodeling, particularly

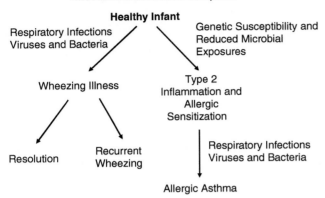

Infections and Asthma Inception

- **Fig. 22.1** Infections and asthma inception.

in susceptible hosts, have been described.[9] A new species of RV, RV-C, was discovered in the early 2000s[10,11] and has been shown to be an important cause of lower respiratory tract illnesses (LRTIs) and wheezing, particularly in children.[12,13] A longitudinal analysis within the COAST study demonstrated that both RV-A and RV-C were more likely than RV-B to cause moderate to severe respiratory illnesses in infants.[14] The Childhood Asthma Study in Australia identified RV-C wheezing episodes in early life as a stronger predictor of subsequent asthma than wheezing with other viruses.[15]

Molecular diagnostic techniques are not universally available to clinicians, so the question of whether the season in which wheezing occurs is helpful in delineating risk is an important one. Bronchiolitis during infancy is associated with an approximately 2-fold increased risk of early childhood asthma; however, this risk differs by the season in which the bronchiolitis occurs. Bronchiolitis occurring during RV-predominant months (spring and fall) was associated with an estimated 25% increased risk of early childhood asthma compared with RSV-predominant (winter) months. However, the overall proportion of bronchiolitis-associated asthma after winter season bronchiolitis is greater than RV-predominant months because of higher rates of bronchiolitis during the RSV season.[16] Season of birth also appears relevant: children born close to the onset of the winter virus season are most prone to the development of lower respiratory tract symptoms, likely because of a developmental component in relationship to the timing of the winter virus peak.[17,18]

Bacteria

It has been proposed that chronic bacterial infections or colonization with pathogenic bacteria could initiate chronic lower airway inflammation, impaired mucociliary clearance, increased mucus production, and ultimately asthma.[19,20] Organisms primarily implicated in this process include *Chlamydophila pneumoniae,*[21,22] *Mycoplasma pneumoniae,*[23,24] *Streptococcus pneumoniae, Haemophilus influenzae,* and *Moraxella catarrhalis.*[20] Studies of chronic *Mycoplasma* and *Chlamydophila* infection and asthma in children have yielded conflicting results, potentially in part because of the limitations of current diagnostics. Findings of diagnostic tests in the upper and lower airways are often not concurrent, and diagnosis of infection by serologic studies leads to inaccuracies. The role of these bacteria in acute wheezing in young children is unclear.

Several publications have suggested that pathogenic bacteria may play a role in both acute wheezing episodes and asthma inception in preschool children. First, Bisgaard and colleagues[20] found that neonates with *S. pneumoniae, H. influenzae,* or *M. catarrhalis* or with a combination of these organisms in their hypopharynx are at increased risk of recurrent wheeze early in life and the diagnosis of asthma at the age of 5 years. This original observation was made in infants of mothers with asthma, but the researchers were able to replicate some of these findings in an unselected cohort.[25] Further, these pathogens have been detected at higher rates in preschool children during acute wheezing episodes.[26] Interestingly, a similar predominance of *Proteobacteria* has been identified in the airways of older children and adults with established asthma.[27,28] Airway microbes also appear to modulate the risk of respiratory illnesses in infants and young children. In several more recent studies, detection of commensal organisms such as *Alloiococcus, Staphylococcus,* and *Corynebacterium* in the upper airway has been associated with lower risk of respiratory illnesses and wheezing.[15,29,30]

Both gut and environmental microbes have been implicated in early-life asthma risk. Two recent birth cohort studies examined the stool microbiome during infancy in relation to the development of allergic sensitization and wheezing.[31,32] These studies identify a high-risk gut microbial community depleted in particular bacteria and enriched for fungi in very young infants. Mechanistically, models using metabolic products from these microbial communities demonstrate plausible pathways for intervention in early life. In both human and animal studies, environmental exposure to "protective" bacteria appears to have the capacity to prevent the development of wheezing and/or asthma in young children.[33–36] These studies of the role of microbial exposures and the microbiome in asthma inception are intriguing, and additional studies are a high priority to establish causality/protection and the specificity of these observations to asthma pathogenesis and to define immunoinflammatory mechanisms contributing to these associations in both pediatric and adult patients.

Infections and Acute Exacerbations of Asthma

The relationship between viral infections and exacerbations of asthma has been clarified by the development of molecular diagnostic tests for viruses that are difficult to culture, including RV, hMPV, and bocaviruses. With the advent of these more sensitive diagnostic tools, information linking common cold infections with exacerbations of asthma has come from a number of sources. Prospective studies of children with asthma have demonstrated that up to 85% of exacerbations of wheezing or asthma in children are associated with viral infections.[37] Although many respiratory viruses can provoke acute asthma symptoms, RVs are most often detected, especially during the spring and fall RV seasons. In fact, the spring and fall peaks in hospitalizations because of asthma closely coincide with patterns of RV infections.[38] RV infections, most commonly RV-C, are frequently detected in children who present to emergency departments with acute wheezing and in children hospitalized for acute asthma.[12,13,39] Influenza and RSV are somewhat more likely to trigger acute asthma symptoms in the winter but account for a smaller fraction of total asthma flares. Other viruses that are less frequently associated with wheezing and exacerbations of asthma include bocavirus,[40] hMPV,[41] and coronaviruses.[42] Together, these studies provide evidence of a strong relationship between viral infections, particularly those associated with RV, and acute exacerbations of asthma.

It is interesting that individuals with asthma do not necessarily have more colds, but they do have greater lower respiratory tract symptoms associated with colds. A prospective study of colds in couples consisting of one individual with asthma and one healthy individual demonstrated that colds cause both greater duration and severity of lower respiratory tract symptoms in patients with asthma.[43] These findings suggest that asthma is associated with fundamental differences in the lower airway manifestations of respiratory viral infections. In addition to provoking asthma, RV infections can increase lower airway obstruction in individuals with other chronic airway diseases such as chronic obstructive pulmonary disease[44] and cystic fibrosis.[45] Thus, common cold viruses that produce relatively mild illnesses in most people can cause severe lower airway disease in susceptible individuals.

The role of respiratory viruses in exacerbations is particularly important in light of observations that severe asthma exacerbations may lead to progressive loss of lung function over time.[46,47] As seen in other chronic lung diseases, a paradigm by which recurrent severe exacerbations lead to progressive loss of lung function and enhanced disease severity over time is emerging in asthma. In fact, data from the Childhood Asthma Management Program showed that a significant portion of children with mild to moderate persistent asthma have impaired lung function growth and early decline by young adulthood.[48] Importantly, exacerbations were a risk factor for this phenotype, which was not modified by conventional asthma therapy.

Mechanisms of Infection-Induced Wheezing Illnesses

Clinical studies and in vitro studies have provided a number of insights into the pathogenesis of virus-induced wheezing illnesses and exacerbations of asthma (Box 22.1).

Spread of Infection From the Upper to the Lower Airways

Respiratory viruses such as RSV and influenza are well known to infect the lower airway and can cause bronchitis, bronchiolitis, and pneumonia. RV has traditionally been considered an upper airway pathogen because of its association with common cold symptoms and the observation that it replicates best at 33° to 35° C, which approximates to temperatures in the upper airway. In fact, lower airway temperatures are conducive to RV replication down to fourth-generation bronchi and exceed 35° C only in the periphery of the lung.[49] Moreover, some RV types, including RV-C isolates, replicate equally well at 33° and 37° C,[50] and RV appears to replicate similarly in cultured epithelial cells derived from either upper or lower airway epithelium.[51] Finally, RV has been detected in lower airway cells and secretions by several techniques after experimental inoculation.[52–54] Titers of infectious virus in lower airway sputum reach or exceed those found in nasal secretions in some individuals.[53] In addition to evidence from experimental infection models, RV is frequently detected in infants and children with lower respiratory tract signs and symptoms, including children hospitalized for pneumonia.[55,56] Collectively, these findings suggest that respiratory viruses, including RV, can cause wheezing illnesses and exacerbations of asthma mainly by infecting lower airways and causing or amplifying lower airway inflammation.

> ### • BOX 22.1 Key Concepts
> *Proposed Mechanisms of Virus-Induced Wheezing*
>
> - Viral infection spreads from the upper to the lower airway
> - Virus-induced damage to airway epithelium
> - Airway edema and transudation of serum proteins
> - Mucus hypersecretion
> - Cellular inflammation: Mononuclear cells and neutrophils
> - Neuroinflammation
> - Enhanced airway responsiveness
> - Interactions between respiratory viral infections and preexisting airway inflammation
> - Secondary bacterial infection

> ### • BOX 22.2 Key Concepts
> *Role of the Epithelium in Virus-Related Inflammation and Injury Pathogenesis*
>
> - Airway epithelial cells serve as hosts for viral replication.
> - Viral replication initiates the immune response to virus.
> - Interferon secretion inhibits inflammation and injury of neighboring cells.
> - Chemokine secretion recruits leukocytes into the airway.
> - Virus-induced epithelial cell damage can disrupt barrier function.
> - Viral infection induces mucus secretion and mucous metaplasia.

Virus-Induced Airway Inflammation

Viral infections damage airway epithelial cells and can cause airway edema and leakage of serum proteins into the airway. In addition, viral infections stimulate mucus secretion and can promote the formation of additional goblet cells (mucous metaplasia) that can enhance mucus secretion that can persist even after the acute infection has resolved. Virus-induced injury to the epithelium can disrupt airway physiology through a number of different pathways (Box 22.2). For example, viral infections can increase the permeability of the epithelium,[57] which may facilitate contact of irritants and allergens with immune cells, leave neural elements exposed, and promote secondary infection with bacterial pathogens. In addition, the combination of epithelial edema and sloughing together with mucus production can lead to airway obstruction and wheezing.

Role of Antiviral Immune Responses

Virus-induced immune responses are necessary to clear virus infections, but they can also contribute to airway dysfunction and symptoms by causing an influx of inflammatory cells that adversely affect lower airway physiology. Antiviral immune responses are initiated within the epithelial cell and amplified by resident and recruited leukocytes in the airway. For viruses such as RV that infect relatively few cells in the airway, virus-induced inflammation may be the primary mechanism for the pathogenesis of respiratory symptoms and lower airway dysfunction. Viral respiratory infections can also induce the synthesis of many of the factors that regulate airway and alveolar development and remodeling, including vascular endothelial growth factor (VEGF), nitric oxide (NO), metalloproteinases, and fibroblast growth factor (FGF).[58–60] How single or repeated bouts of virus-induced overexpression of these regulators of lung development and remodeling affect the ultimate lung structure and function is not known, but they could exert long-term effects on lung function and asthma after viral infection in infancy.

Epithelial Cells

The processes associated with viral replication trigger innate immune responses within the epithelial cell. Virus attachment to cell surface receptors can initiate immune responses. For example, RSV infection activates signaling pathways in airway epithelial cells through the innate immune system through Toll-like receptor (TLR)-4.[61] Furthermore, the development of oxidative stress during viral infections can activate epithelial cell responses. Inside the cell, viral RNA is detected by innate immune sensors on endosomal surfaces (i.e., TLR-3, TLR-7, TLR-8) and intracellular proteins, such as the dsRNA-dependent protein kinase and retinoic acid-inducible gene I (*RIG-I*), to activate the innate antiviral immune response.[62] Through these pathways, viral replication stimulates antiviral effector molecules such as RNase L and inhibition of protein synthesis within infected cells. In addition, innate antiviral responses induce chemokines (e.g., CXCL10) that recruit inflammatory cells into the airway and type I (interferon-alpha [IFN-α] and [IFN-β]) and type III (IFN-λ1 and IFN-λ2) IFNs that have autocrine and paracrine antiviral effects.

Leukocytes

Respiratory viruses activate monocytes, macrophages, and dendritic cells to secrete an array of proinflammatory cytokines such as IL-1, IL-8, IL-10, tumor necrosis factor (TNF)-α, and IFN-γ. In animal models, respiratory viral infections lead to a prominent expansion of mature dendritic cells in the lung.[63] Significantly, pulmonary dendritic cells express high levels of TLRs and secrete large amounts of IFNs in response to viral infection. Dendritic cell IFN responses are impaired in early life, which likely contributes to increased susceptibility to viral infections in infancy.[64]

Acute respiratory viral infections are often accompanied by pronounced neutrophilia of upper and lower respiratory secretions, and products of neutrophil activation contribute to airway obstruction and lower airway symptoms. For example, neutrophil elastase can up-regulate goblet cell secretion of mucus.[65] P2X7 is a cation channel expressed by leukocytes and airway epithelial cells that is important to pathogen control and neutrophilic inflammation. Attenuated P2X7 function, which is common in mild to moderate asthma, is associated with reduced recruitment of neutrophils to the airway during RV colds and an increased risk of acute asthma symptoms.[66]

Lymphocytes are recruited into the upper and lower airways during the early stages of a viral respiratory infection, and it is presumed that these cells help limit the extent of infection and to clear virus-infected epithelial cells. This is consistent with reports of severe viral lower respiratory infections in immunocompromised patients.[67] B cell responses to respiratory viruses also serve to limit duration and severity of illness, as indicated by the finding of frequent and prolonged viral illnesses in patients with X-linked agammaglobulinemia.[68]

Neuroinflammatory Mechanisms

Viral respiratory infections can induce inflammation through mechanisms involving neural mechanisms. These responses are difficult to study in humans, but studies in animal models have provided insights. For example, RSV infection in rodents leads to overproduction of nerve growth factor,[69] which promotes airway

inflammation. This observation has also been confirmed in studies of babies with RSV bronchiolitis.[70] In a guinea pig model, virus infection causes dysfunction of M2 muscarinic receptors on parasympathetic nerves, leading to overproduction of acetylcholine and airway hyperresponsiveness. These responses appear to be driven by virus-induced acute phase cytokines such as IL-1β and TNF-α.[71]

Mediators

Mediators that are produced in excess during respiratory illnesses include NO, leukotrienes, prostaglandins, kinins, and oxidative metabolites,[72–74] and inhibition of specific mediators can ameliorate some cold symptoms.[75] Histamine does not appear to play a role in common cold pathogenesis.[76]

Relationship of Cellular Antiviral Responses to Outcome of Viral Infections

Several studies have tested the hypothesis that individual variations in cellular immune responses and patterns of cytokine production are related to the outcome of respiratory infections. In clinical studies, reduced IFN-γ responses of blood mononuclear cells ex vivo are associated with a significant increase in viral respiratory illnesses during infancy.[77–79] In addition, several studies have found that asthma is associated with impaired virus-induced secretion of IFNs by airway and peripheral blood cells.[80–83] Together, these experimental findings suggest that individual variability in the cellular immune response to respiratory viruses, and IFN responses in particular, can influence the clinical and virologic outcomes of infection.

Interactions With Bacteria

It is well established that viral illnesses of the middle ear, sinuses, and lungs can promote secondary infections with bacterial pathogens such as *S. pneumoniae, M. catarrhalis,* and *H. influenzae.* As reviewed under "Bacteria," colonization with these bacteria in early childhood is also a risk factor for acute wheezing episodes and asthma.[20] In school-age children, these pathogens are more likely to be detected in association with a viral infection or just after a viral infection.[84] Furthermore, the risk of illness versus asymptomatic infection was greater in children who had both viruses and bacteria detected. Similarly, for children with asthma, moderate exacerbations were most likely to occur in viral infections in which *S. pneumoniae* or *M. catarrhalis* was also detected.[84] As discussed earlier, multiple studies in infants and children have identified microbial communities associated with enhanced or reduced risk of disease expression during viral infections.[15,29,30,85] These findings suggest that viruses and bacteria may work together to modulate airway pathologic conditions and respiratory symptoms.

Environmental Factors and Viral Illnesses

Environmental factors strongly influence the probability of wheezing exacerbations and appear to act together with viral infections in an additive fashion. As discussed later, allergy is a strong risk factor for the development of asthma after virus-induced wheezing episodes in infancy and is also closely associated with virus-induced exacerbations of asthma in older children and adults with asthma. Accordingly, the combination of allergy and exposure to a relevant allergen contributes to virus-induced exacerbations of asthma.[86] Similarly, exposure to greater levels of air pollutants such as nitrogen dioxide (NO_2) and sulfur dioxide (SO_2) also enhances the risk of exacerbations.[87,88]

Interactions Between Allergy and Infections

Allergic sensitization has been defined as a clear risk factor for the development of asthma.[89] Children with "multiple early sensitization" to aeroallergens have been identified as a phenotype at particularly high risk for asthma inception and severe exacerbations leading to hospitalization.[90] A sequential relationship whereby allergic sensitization precedes viral wheezing, most notably with RV, has been described.[91] Furthermore, children who develop both risk factors in early life are at highest risk for subsequent asthma.[2,92]

There is convincing evidence to implicate respiratory allergy as a risk factor for wheezing with common cold infections later on in childhood. Emergency department studies have identified detection of a respiratory virus, most commonly RV, positive allergen specific immunoglobulin E (sIgE) and presence of eosinophilic inflammation as important risk factors for the development of wheezing illnesses.[86,93,94] Notably, viral infections and allergic inflammation synergistically enhanced the risk of wheezing, and higher levels of allergen sIgE conferred the greatest risk. This synergism may be particularly notable for RV-C in early life.[13]

There are multiple mechanisms by which viral infections are thought to interact with allergic inflammation to lead to airway dysfunction, wheezing, and asthma exacerbations.[95] First, viral infections can damage the barrier function of the airway epithelium, leading to enhanced absorption of aeroallergens across the airway wall and enhanced inflammation; allergic inflammation may also lead to enhanced viral replication.[96] Furthermore, RV infection can enhance the release of interleukin 33 (IL-33) from airway epithelial cells to promote allergic inflammation.[97] Additionally, allergic inflammation enhances airway responsiveness to RV.[98] There is also evidence that patients with allergic asthma can have impaired antiviral responses, as noted earlier. Furthermore, allergen exposure and high-affinity IgE receptor cross-linking has been shown to impair virus-induced type 1 and 3 IFN production in peripheral blood cells.[99,100] This may lead to both enhanced viral replication and type 2 inflammation.[101,102]

Systems Immunology Approaches to Identify Mechanisms of Exacerbations

The majority of asthma exacerbations are associated with viral respiratory infections. However, even in children with moderate to severe asthma, a minority of viral infections actually progress to an exacerbation. The mechanisms underlying this observation are unclear. Over the last decade, systems immunology approaches have accelerated discovery in a wide array of diseases, including asthma. Early studies identified dysregulation of IFN-related pathways in the risk for exacerbation with a cold.[103] More recently, differential phenotypes of RV-induced exacerbations were identified based on interferon regulatory factor 7 (IRF-7) expression during episodes.[104] Addressing the fundamental question of what differentiates a "cold" from an exacerbation, the Inner City Asthma Consortium recently identified both common and distinct gene modules differentially regulated during viral and nonviral exacerbations.[105] These unbiased approaches are identifying novel

mechanisms and new potential therapeutic approaches to the prevention of exacerbations. Integration with additional "–omics" data sets will provide further insights and opportunities to modify disease.

Treatment of Infection-Induced Wheezing and Asthma

Virus-Induced Wheezing in Infancy

Acute LRTIs during the first year of life are usually termed "bronchiolitis" and are most likely due to infection with viral respiratory pathogens. The efficacy of various interventions for the treatment of the acute lower airway symptoms of wheezing, tachypnea, retractions, and hypoxemia that occur as a result of these infections has been controversial because of variations in study design, the inability to rapidly and conveniently measure pulmonary physiologic variables, the confounding of results by inclusion of children with a history of multiple wheezing episodes (i.e., asthmatic phenotypes), and the choice of outcome measures evaluated.[106] In a recent series of meta-analyses evaluating various therapies, the routine use of bronchodilators,[107] nebulized hypertonic saline,[108] anticholinergics,[109] and corticosteroids[110] have not been shown to be of consistent benefit.

Virus-Induced Wheezing in Preschool Children

Therapeutic approaches for virus-induced wheezing in preschool children (ages 2–5 years) are challenging because many children wheeze only with "colds" and are totally asymptomatic between these episodes, whereas others may have symptoms outside of colds as well. In addition, these episodes may range in severity from mild wheezing and coughing to severe respiratory distress that requires prompt medical intervention. Standard therapy for virus-induced wheezing in young children generally includes a stepwise addition of medications, typically commencing with a bronchodilator. If lower respiratory tract symptoms become increasingly severe or respiratory distress develops, oral corticosteroids are often added. Clinical trials in the management of these wheezing episodes also have included prophylaxis with daily low-dose inhaled corticosteroids (ICSs) and the intermittent use of high-dose ICSs and leukotriene receptor antagonists (LTRAs).

The Role of Oral Corticosteroids in Acute Exacerbations of Asthma in Young Children

Numerous studies have been undertaken to assess the role of oral corticosteroid therapy in acute episodes of asthma in children and adults.[111] Meta-analyses of these studies support the use of systemic corticosteroids in acute exacerbations based on a reduction in the admission rate for asthma and prevention of relapse in the outpatient treatment of exacerbations.[112,113] As a reflection of such information, the most recent National Heart, Lung, and Blood Institute Guidelines for the Diagnosis and Management of Asthma recommend the addition of systemic corticosteroids for asthma exacerbations unresponsive to bronchodilators.[114]

Unfortunately, the applicability of these recommendations to young children and infants whose acute wheezing episode is primarily related to viral respiratory tract infections has not been as thoroughly examined. Moreover, in studies that have been conducted in this age group, the results are conflicting.[115–119] Limitations of these studies involve the inclusion of multiple wheezing phenotypes,[117,119] relatively small sample sizes, poor adherence to study medication and protocol in outpatient studies,[116,119] and episodes of relatively mild severity in both outpatient and inpatient studies.[116,119] A randomized, double-blind, placebo-controlled trial compared a 5-day course of oral prednisolone with placebo in over 650 children between the ages of 10 months and 60 months hospitalized with acute viral wheezing. The primary outcome, the duration of hospitalization, was no different between the treatment groups.[117] An accompanying editorial for this published study challenged the clinical research community to conduct additional prospective trials to clearly establish the efficacy of oral corticosteroid treatment of these "asthma-like" episodes in preschool children.[120]

To address these concerns further, the Childhood Asthma Research and Education (CARE) network investigated whether oral corticosteroids reduced symptom scores during acute LRTIs in preschool children with recurrent wheeze. The investigators performed post hoc and replication analyses in two outpatient cohorts of children ages 1 to 5 years with episodic wheezing that had participated in previous CARE-conducted studies.[121] Comparisons were made of symptom scores during LRTIs that were or were not treated with oral corticosteroids, adjusting for differences in disease and episode severity. In both of the two cohorts studied independently, oral corticosteroid treatment did not reduce symptom severity during acute LRTIs as reflected by area under the curve of total symptom scores among the more severe episodes. Moreover, subgroups of children who might have been more likely to experience benefit, such as those with asthma risk factors (i.e., positive modified asthma predictive index, personal eczema, and/or family history of asthma), did not appear to have a greater benefit than those without such characteristics. The investigators emphasized, however, that these results generated hypotheses and needed to be confirmed in randomized prospective studies, which remain challenging to complete.[122] Taken together, these studies indicate that acute asthma-like episodes of airway obstruction in preschool children appear to respond less well to oral corticosteroid administration than do similar episodes in older children and adults.

The Role of Inhaled Corticosteroids in the Prevention and Treatment of Acute Wheezing Exacerbations

The CARE Network conducted a 3-year prospective trial in preschool children, all of whom had asthma risk factors reflected by a modified positive asthma predictive index.[123] Children 2 to 4 years of age were randomized to receive either fluticasone propionate 88 mcg twice daily or matching placebo. During the active treatment phase, children receiving an ICS had a significantly increased number of episode-free days and reduced exacerbations. Unfortunately, about 3 months into the observation period, there was no longer any significant difference in any of these outcome measures. These data indicate that continuous therapy with ICS in preschool children at high risk of developing asthma reduces lower respiratory tract exacerbations that are most frequently caused by respiratory pathogens in this age group.

Many preschool children wheeze only with respiratory tract pathogens and are asymptomatic between these episodes. Therefore, a 1-year randomized, double-blind comparison among intermittent treatment with high-dose ICS, an LTRA (montelukast), and scheduled albuterol (the standard of care) was conducted in preschool children with histories consistent with this type of

respiratory pattern.[124] Therapy was initiated by the family, based on the participant achieving a symptom profile threshold that the child had exhibited in the past that would usually foreshadow the development of more significant lower airway involvement. After 1 year of treatment, the three groups did not differ in proportions of episode-free days (primary outcome), oral corticosteroid use, healthcare usage, quality of life, or linear growth. However, during respiratory tract illnesses, both ICS and montelukast therapy led to modest reductions in trouble breathing and interference with activity scores compared with those children treated with only albuterol.

The observations that both the continuous[123] and intermittent[124] use of ICS had an effect on both the frequency and severity of exacerbations that were most likely related to a concomitant viral or bacterial respiratory tract illness provided the impetus for a third CARE network-initiated trial.[125] This trial studied 278 children between the ages of 12 and 53 months who all had positive modified asthma predictive indices, recurrent wheezing episodes with a low grade of interval impairment, and at least one exacerbation in the previous year. Children were randomly assigned to receive nebulized budesonide suspensions for 1 year as either an intermittent high-dose regimen (1 mg twice daily for 7 days starting at the onset of predefined respiratory tract illness symptoms) or a daily low-dose regimen (0.5 mg nightly) with corresponding placebos in both treatment arms. The two regimens were similar with respect to exacerbation frequency (primary outcome) and other measures of asthma severity, including the time to first exacerbation. The mean exposure to budesonide was 104 mg less with the intermittent regimen. These results indicate that, in preschool children with this type of preasthma phenotype, intermittent therapy versus continuous therapy is a therapeutic consideration.

Role of Leukotrienes Modifiers in Viral-Induced Wheezing

The cysteinyl leukotrienes have been identified as important mediators in the complex pathophysiologic processes of asthma.[126] Leukotrienes are detectable in the blood, urine, nasal secretions, sputum, and bronchoalveolar lavage fluid of patients with chronic asthma. In addition, leukotrienes are released during acute asthma episodes. As a result of the potential for these mediators to influence airway tone, inflammatory cascades, and mucus secretion, antagonists for their receptors have been developed and extensively studied. The cysteinyl LTRA montelukast has been the most frequently studied in both preschool and school-age children.

Robertson and associates[127] evaluated the intermittent use of montelukast in 2- to 14-year-old children with histories of intermittent asthma. The family was instructed to begin a 7-day treatment with montelukast (age-appropriate dose) at the onset of asthma symptoms or the first sign of an upper respiratory tract illness that had previously been associated with the subsequent development of lower airway asthma symptoms. Compared with placebo, montelukast treatment resulted in a modest reduction in acute healthcare resource usage, symptoms, time off from school, and parental time off work in children with intermittent asthma.

Bisgaard and colleagues evaluated the efficacy of 1-year daily treatment with montelukast in children with intermittent asthma in reducing exacerbations.[128] The primary efficacy endpoint was the number of asthma exacerbation episodes defined as any 3 consecutive days with symptoms and at least two treatments of β agonist per day, rescue use of oral/inhaled corticosteroids during 1 or more days, or a hospitalization because of asthma. Over

12 months of therapy, montelukast significantly reduced the rate of asthma exacerbations. Unfortunately, treatment did not reduce the necessity for oral corticosteroid administration. One of the remarkable aspects of this trial was the marked seasonal variation in exacerbation rates, with the summer months having less frequent exacerbations and no observed treatment effects. These data are an excellent documentation of the "honeymoon" period from asthma symptoms that many clinicians observe in their patients during the summer months, most likely related to reduced numbers of respiratory tract illnesses.

Because infections with RSV in early life have been associated with an increased risk of developing recurrent wheezing and later asthma, two studies have evaluated the effects of montelukast treatment on the development of subsequent wheezing. In the first pilot study,[129] children hospitalized with acute RSV bronchiolitis, were randomized into a double-blind, parallel comparison of 5 mg montelukast or placebo given for 28 days starting within 7 days of the onset of symptoms. Infants on montelukast were free of any symptoms on 22% of the days and nights compared with 4% of the days and nights in infants on placebo. Daytime cough was significantly reduced, as were exacerbations in those children on active treatment. In contrast, in a follow-up study in children 3 to 24 months of age conducted over a period of 24 weeks, montelukast treatment did not alleviate post–RSV-induced respiratory tract symptoms.[130]

In school-age children, montelukast has been shown to be less effective compared with ICS treatment in reducing the need for oral corticosteroid use and time to treatment failure over a 1-year period.[131] Both of these outcomes could be considered surrogates for respiratory pathogen–induced asthma exacerbations or worsening of overall asthma control.

Antiinfection Therapy

Therapy for infection-induced asthma could potentially include one or more of the following approaches: avoidance, nonmedicinal interventions, vaccination, antimicrobial drug therapy, and/or immunotherapy (monoclonal antibodies directed against the relevant pathogens). The ubiquitous nature of respiratory pathogens in the environment and the social nature of interactions in childhood (e.g., daycare, school, older siblings) make avoidance strategies unfeasible. Indeed, on average, children experience two to eight or more "colds" per year during their preschool years.

The cure for the common cold remains elusive; thus, a number of nonmedicinal interventions have been tried. Vitamin C has long been touted as common cold treatment; however, a meta-analysis of common cold treatment studies found no significant effects on either prevention or treatment.[132] A Cochrane review of clinical studies found evidence that zinc lozenges reduce common cold duration but have significant side effects, including bad taste and nausea.[133] Large-scale trials of Echinacea have provided no evidence of efficacy.[134,135] There is evidence that warm drinks, as recommended for generations, can provide symptomatic relief from malaise and nasal symptoms without troublesome side effects.[136] These approaches obviously are aimed at symptom reduction of the common cold, but their effects on asthma control or exacerbations have not been directly evaluated.

Given the close relationship between viral infections and wheezing illnesses in children, it would be attractive to apply antiviral strategies to the prevention and treatment of asthma, and both RV and RSV are obvious targets. Attempts at developing an RSV vaccine have so far been unsuccessful; however, recent data have provided renewed encouragement.[137] Although vaccination to prevent RV infection is even more challenging because of the large number of serotypes, recent advances in technologies provide hope for development of an RV vaccine.[138] Additionally, several types of antiviral agents are in development, and several compounds with activity against RV have been tested in clinical trials.

Improved knowledge of RV molecular virology has led to several attempts to develop antiviral agents. IFN-α has antiviral effects in vitro and shortens the duration and severity of colds, but topical application led to nasal irritation and bleeding.[139] Anti–intercellular adhesion molecule 1 (ICAM-1) and soluble ICAM-1 were developed to prevent binding of major group viruses to their receptor.[140] Capsid binding agents that bind to the VP1 pocket and inhibit viral binding and/or uncoating have shown modest antiviral effects and efficacy in clinical trials.[141] An inhibitor to the 3C protease (rupintrivir) also showed broad anti-RV activity in vitro and efficacy in clinical trials.[142] Unfortunately, these antiviral approaches have not led to development of a clinically useful medication. The molecules tested to date have been limited by combinations of modest efficacy, side effects, and/or drug interactions.[143]

Another new approach has been to boost antiviral defenses in the lung with inhaled IFN-β. In a randomized study, adults with persistent asthma and a history of exacerbations with colds were treated with either nebulized IFN-β or placebo within 24 hours of the onset of cold symptoms.[144] In the intent-to-treat population, there were no significant effects on the asthma symptoms scores (which was the primary outcome), but IFN-β treatment improved recovery of peak expiratory flow. Notably, IFN-β was well tolerated and also induced expression of innate antiviral effectors in the blood and sputum. In a subgroup analysis of study subjects with more severe asthma, colds were associated with increased symptoms in the placebo group but not in IFN-β–treated subjects. These findings have yet to be confirmed in follow-up study.

Trials evaluating the efficacy of monoclonal antibody therapy directed specifically against RSV and the allergic antibody, IgE, yielded interesting results. The first trial studied the anti-RSV monoclonal antibody palivizumab in a double-blind, placebo-controlled trial: 429 otherwise healthy preterm (33–35 weeks' gestational age) infants were randomly assigned to receive either monthly palivizumab injections or placebo during the RSV season. The prespecified primary outcome was the total number of parent-reported wheezing days in the first year of life. Nasopharyngeal swabs were taken during respiratory episodes for viral analysis. Palivizumab treatment resulted in a relative reduction of 61% in the total number of wheezing days during the first year of life. During this time, the proportion of infants with recurrent wheeze was 10% lower in patients treated with palivizumab (11% versus 21%). This approach prevented recurrent wheezing from RSV infections but not subsequent allergic asthma.[7]

The second trial evaluated the anti-IgE monoclonal antibody omalizumab, which specifically targets the Fc portion of IgE to prevent binding to the surface of cells. In a placebo-controlled study of guidelines-based asthma treatment compared with omalizumab added to standard therapy, omalizumab prevented the seasonal increases in exacerbations during the fall and spring, which are peak times for viral exacerbations.[145] Analysis of viruses in nasal secretions during a subset of exacerbations confirmed that the treatment group had fewer viral and nonviral exacerbations. This study provides direct evidence that IgE-mediated inflammation contributes to the risk of virus-induced exacerbations of asthma. Follow-up studies demonstrated that omalizumab enhances virus-induced IFN responses and reduces duration of RV infections in children with asthma.[146–148] These observations indicate that interactions among allergic sensitization, exposure, and viral respiratory illnesses play an important role in asthma control.

Use of Antibiotics in Asthma

Asthma guidelines both in the United States (http://www.nhlbi.nih.gov/health-pro/guidelines/current/asthma-guidelines/full-report.htm) and internationally (http://www.ginasthma.org) have not recommended the use of antibiotics to treat asthma exacerbations because the majority of the exacerbations have been considered to be triggered by viral respiratory tract infections. Nonetheless, oral antibiotics are frequently prescribed for wheezing illnesses in preschool children (650 antibiotic prescriptions/1000 wheezing children).[149] Furthermore, 28% of preschool children who make a physician visit for wheezing receive a prescription for an antibiotic within 2 days of the visit, and 77% receive a prescription for an antibiotic within 7 days. These prescriptions are dominated by azithromycin, the use of which increased 15-fold between 1995 and 2001.

As noted previously, bacteria (either alone or in combination with viral pathogens) have now been demonstrated to potentially play a role in acute wheezing episodes and increases in asthma symptoms in children.[26,84] Furthermore, certain antimicrobials have not only antibacterial properties but also antiviral and antiinflammatory properties.

As a class, macrolides have been demonstrated to provide clinical benefit in airway diseases such as cystic fibrosis[150] and diffuse panbronchiolitis,[151] possibly through mechanisms unrelated to antimicrobial activity. Viral infections, particularly those caused by RV, are associated with neutrophilic inflammation and increased CXCL-8 expression.[152] Neutrophils are the predominant inflammatory cell at the onset of most infections, including those with RV,[152,153] and although many chemoattractants participate in summoning neutrophils to the site of infection, CXCL-8 seems to play a central role. Interestingly, azithromycin has been demonstrated to attenuate immunoinflammatory responses and may reduce the ensuing destructive neutrophilic inflammation. In addition, azithromycin reduces RV replication and increases IFN gene expression in human bronchial epithelial cells.[154]

Two more recent studies in young children with recurrent wheezing suggested that azithromycin has the potential to prevent exacerbations when used preemptively[155] and shorten the duration of symptoms once a significant episode has developed.[156] Chronic use of azithromycin also has recently been shown to reduce the frequency of asthma exacerbations in adults with severe asthma.[157] It is unclear whether these benefits are due to antimicrobial or antiinflammatory effects or both of these. Furthermore, there are concerns about the repeated use of this approach in children and adults related to risks of antimicrobial resistance and potential impact on the gut and airway microbiome.

Conclusions

Infections play a critical role in the inception and exacerbation of asthma. Viral infections are the most common cause of wheezing in infants and children. Interactions between underlying allergy and virus infections lead to the greatest risk of asthma inception and exacerbation. New data indicate that the gut and airway microbiomes may play a critical role in modulating the response to respiratory viral infections, and virus-induced alterations in airway microbial populations likely also contribute to illness severity. Treatment of virus-induced wheezing and asthma exacerbations remains challenging, and novel therapies and approaches to the prevention of asthma and asthma exacerbations are needed.

The reference list can be found on the companion Expert Consult website at http://www.expertconsult.inkling.com.

23

Special Considerations for Infants and Young Children

RONINA A. COVAR, JOSEPH D. SPAHN

KEY POINTS

- The care of infants and small children with suspected asthma deserves special consideration because of the potential to modulate the disease process early on and alleviate the increased morbidity associated with uncontrolled asthma in this group.
- After confounders and masqueraders of asthma have been excluded, recurrent wheezing in infants and young children still comprises a heterogeneous group of conditions with different risk factors and prognoses.
- The diagnosis of asthma in infants and young children is often based on clinical grounds and complicated by the lack of clinically available tools that meet the criteria for the definition of asthma used in older children and adults such as airflow limitation, reversibility, bronchial hyperresponsiveness, and airway inflammation.

- Difficulties in the management of asthma in this age group include limited forms of medication delivery, complete dependence on the caregivers to carry out the treatment regimen, and limited selection of medications that have been studied or are completely devoid of adverse effects.
- A partnership approach with emphasis on education, monitoring, and training is key in the effective management of chronic cough or recurrent wheezing illnesses in very young children.
- Despite the high risk of morbidity and frequent healthcare usage from wheezing illnesses inherent in infants and young children, there are limited options for management of severe or uncontrolled asthma in this age group and even more limited interventions to prevent the development of asthma.

Introduction

From the National Center for Health Statistics Surveillance of Asthma[1] the prevalence of current asthma in children younger than 5 years of age was 4.4% compared with 8.8% and 11.1% in children aged 5 to 11 years and 12 to 17 years of age, respectively. However, the healthcare usage (i.e., ambulatory, emergency department visits, and inpatient hospital admissions) for children under the age of 5 years is much greater than that of other pediatric age groups.[2] Younger children with asthma are also more likely to be readmitted to the hospital for acute exacerbations.[3] Of children with asthma admitted to a community-based pediatric intensive care unit (ICU) over a 10-year period, as many as 75% were 6 years or younger.[4] The public health consequences of dealing with recurrent respiratory illnesses include the number of missed work days parents/guardians incur to care for an acutely ill child. Some studies have hinted that pulmonary development in infancy can be adversely affected by asthma, resulting in a decrease in lung function of approximately 20% by adulthood.[5]

Relevant clinical practice guidelines developed in recent years have addressed special challenges in the management of asthma in this age group.[6,7] Many issues are unique to this age group: identifying very young children with recurrent episodes of cough and wheeze associated with viral illnesses who will develop persistent

asthma later in life, presence of confounding factors or disease masqueraders, who needs controller therapy and when to start treatment, what medications to use, how best to deliver the medications, and how to monitor the response to treatment.

Phenotypes of Wheezing in Young Children

Recurrent wheezing in infants and young children comprises a heterogeneous group of conditions with different risk factors and prognoses. Various wheezing phenotypes have been derived from epidemiologic and longitudinal data, including phenotypes based on time of onset and outcome (e.g., transient or intermittent versus persistent wheezing).[8,9] Such phenotypes tend to be more helpful for prognostication and have only limited clinical utility. The Tucson Children's Respiratory Study cohort enrolled over 1000 newborns served by a large health maintenance organization to evaluate factors involved in early-onset wheezing in relation to persistent wheezing at 6 years of life.[9] About half of the children had at least one episode of wheezing by 6 years of age. Nearly one-third of the cohort had at least one episode of wheezing by 3 years of age. Only 40% of children who wheezed early had persistent wheezing at age 6 years. Of the total group, 20% had at least one episode of wheezing associated with a respiratory tract infection during the first 3 years of life but had no wheezing at 6 years (transient wheezing), 14% did not wheeze during the first 3 years of life but had wheezing at 6 years (late-onset wheezing), and 15% had wheezing at ages 3 and 6 years (persistent wheezing). Those with transient wheezing were more likely to have diminished airway function and a history of maternal smoking and were less likely to have atopia. Children with late-onset wheezing had a percentage of atopy similar to that in those with persistent wheezing and were likely to have mothers with asthma. Thus, there appears to be a similar genetic predisposition for the asthma phenotype characterizing both persistent and late-onset wheezing.

The clinical utility of these phenotypes based on pattern and timing of symptom occurrence is limited when a medical provider is actually faced with a young child with recurrent wheezing or chronic cough. Thus, other phenotypes may have greater relevance when management decisions must be made or clinical trials are undertaken. For example, symptom trigger–based classification (e.g., episodic, wheeze only in discrete periods, mostly associated with upper respiratory infection) versus multitrigger (e.g., symptom also occurs with activity, laughing, crying, or even at night outside of an acute illness) was first proposed by the European Task Force in 2008.[10] However, the clinical applicability of these phenotypes was recognized to be quite limited because this classification does not consider the frequency, seasonality, and severity of the episodes and perhaps they are more reflective of severity of disease rather than actual phenotypes.[11] Children can switch between the two categories at different times. Viral infections (e.g., respiratory syncytial virus, rhinovirus, coronavirus, human metapneumovirus, adenovirus, and parainfluenza virus) are usual triggers for wheezing in preschool-age children, even in those who will not later develop persistent asthma. A preschool child may have exercise-induced wheeze only when he or she is also having an acute episode or shortly after. During the late fall, winter, and early spring in most areas in the northern hemisphere, preschool children who are in regular contact with other children can develop back-to-back viral respiratory illnesses that can each last up to 2 weeks or even longer. A child with a viral illness requiring a hospital admission is in the same classification as a child whose viral-induced wheezing illness is treated with a bronchodilator alone.

It is not known if there is a unique immunopathologic difference that can affect treatment response between these phenotypes. Latent class analysis was used to identify groups among preschool-age children with recurrent wheezing illnesses with several categorical clinical features and how these classes relate to specific outcomes, specifically exacerbations and response to inhaled corticosteroid (ICS) treatment. In this study using data from four pediatric asthma trials, four latent classes were identified that were associated with varying degrees of allergen sensitization and exposures. Latent class 1 (minimal sensitization, 30% of the sample) were predominantly non-Hispanic white with low indicators of atopy (i.e., low prevalence of eczema, no aeroallergen or food sensitization, low serum immunoglobulin E [IgE]) or low peripheral eosinophils. Latent class 2 (aeroallergen sensitized and exposed to pet; 25% of the sample) were also predominantly male, non-Hispanic white, and had a lower parental history of asthma. They had the highest prevalence of pet ownership and elevated total serum IgE and blood eosinophils. They tended to have sensitization to at least one allergen and had the highest pet exposure. Latent class 3 (sensitized and exposed to tobacco smoke, 25% of the sample) were children who were nonwhite and had the highest percentage with parental asthma. They had the highest percentage of tobacco

smoke exposure and modest atopic characteristics. Pet exposure was lowest for this group. Latent class 4 (multiple sensitization with eczema, 20% of the sample) contained children who were older and predominantly contained males. They had the highest level of atopic features (i.e., percent with eczema and serum IgE) and blood eosinophils. Almost all had aeroallergen sensitization, with about three-quarters sensitized to at least three allergens, mostly indoor. Close to 90% had food sensitization. The risk of exacerbation was highest in latent classes 2 and 4. In addition, daily ICS treatment was associated with a much lower exacerbation rate reduction in these same latent classes.

Because these current proposed phenotypes reflect only limited facets of asthma characterization, clinical guidelines suggest starting treatment based on frequency of symptoms, severity of episodes, and presence of risk factors.

Predicting Who Is Likely to Develop Persistent Asthma

Factors or exposures early in life, such as prematurity; fetal nutrition, including vitamin D; duration of pregnancy; viral lower respiratory tract infections in the first years of life; acetaminophen and antibiotic exposure; cigarette smoke exposure; air pollution; postnatal nutrition; breastfeeding; family size; maternal age; socioeconomic status; and allergen exposure, have been implicated in causing persistent asthma to varying degrees. Observational studies have demonstrated an increased risk of asthma attributed to acetaminophen exposure during prenatal periods, infancy, childhood, and even adulthood.[12–15] Genetics, atopy, and prematurity appear to be the most important host risk factors in the development of asthma.

The Asthma Predictive Index (API), which uses a combination of clinical and easily obtainable laboratory data to help identify children 3 years of age or younger with a history of wheezing at risk of developing persistent asthma, was developed from the Tucson cohort.[16] Information on parental asthma diagnosis and prenatal maternal smoking status was obtained at enrollment, and the child's history of asthma and wheezing and physician-diagnosed allergic rhinitis or eczema, along with measurements of blood eosinophil count, were obtained at the follow-up visits. Two indices were used to classify the children. The stringent index required recurrent wheezing in the first 3 years plus one major (i.e., parental history of asthma or physician-diagnosed eczema) or two of three minor (i.e., eosinophilia, wheezing without colds, or allergic rhinitis) risk factors, whereas the loose index required any episode of wheezing in the first 3 years plus one major or two of three minor risk factors. Children with a positive loose index were 2.6 to 5.5 times more likely to have active asthma sometime during the school years. In contrast, risk of asthma increased to 4.3 to 9.8 times when the stringent criteria were used. In addition, at least 90% of young children with a negative loose or stringent index will not develop active asthma in the school-age years.

A modified version of the API (mAPI) incorporates inhalant allergen sensitization as an additional major risk factor and food allergen sensitization as an additional minor risk factor to take into account along with important findings from other longitudinal natural history asthma studies.[17] In the Berlin Multicenter Allergy Study, additional risk factors for asthma and bronchial hyperreactivity at age 7 years included persistent sensitization to foods (e.g., hen's egg, cow's milk, wheat, soy) and perennial inhalant allergens (e.g., dust mite, cat), especially in early life.[18,19] In a prospective randomized controlled study of food allergen avoidance in infancy evaluating the development of atopy at age 7 years in a high-risk cohort, egg, milk, and peanut allergen sensitization were risk factors for asthma.[20] With these additional considerations, the mAPI was used in an early-intervention study for young children with recurrent wheezing.[21] It was adapted by the National Asthma Education Prevention Program Expert Panel Report 3 (NAEPP EPR-3) asthma guidelines as a requirement, along with a history of four wheezing episodes per year lasting more than 24 hours, on which initiation of controller therapy should be considered.[6]

The Pediatric Asthma Risk Score (PARS) was developed from the Cincinnati Childhood Allergy and Air Pollution Study birth cohort and validated as a tool to predict development of asthma in children who were born to parents with atopy. In addition to the components included in the API, the tool also accounts for polysensitization to environmental or food allergens, early wheezing before the age of 3 years, and African American race. The scoring tool had a higher probability of predicting the development of asthma compared with the API (giving an 11% increase in sensitivity), especially in children with mild to moderate asthma.[22]

Essentially all of the current natural history studies have found that allergic disease and evidence of proallergic immune development are significant risk factors for persistent asthma.

Differential Diagnosis or Possible Confounders

The first practical consideration in the approach for the wheezing child is to ensure that an alternative diagnosis is not present. In addition, infants and small children have a greater degree of bronchial hyperresponsiveness (BHR), which may predispose them to wheeze.[23]

The differential diagnosis of wheezing in infants and young children includes conditions that result in airflow obstruction, such as foreign body aspiration, structural airway anomalies, congenital lobar emphysema, abnormalities of the great vessels (e.g., vascular rings), congenital heart disease, cystic fibrosis, recurrent aspiration, immunodeficiency, infections, ciliary dyskinesia, and mediastinal masses. Other clinical features, such as neonatal onset of symptoms, associated failure to thrive, diarrhea or vomiting, focal lung or cardiovascular findings, clubbing, constant wheezing, and hypoxemia outside of an acute illness, suggest an alternative diagnosis and require special investigations. Factors in addition to age at onset of symptoms that should be taken into consideration include triggers for the respiratory symptoms and aggravating conditions such as nighttime occurrences, environmental exposure, physical exertion, feeding, positioning, and infections. Clearly, making the correct diagnosis is essential because the treatment for these conditions can vary substantially.

Diagnosis of Asthma in Young Children

Preschool children present some diagnostic challenges inherent to their young age such that a confirmation of a diagnosis can be difficult. Infants and young children are often too young to reliably perform objective measures of disease activity. Furthermore, they are unable to provide their own history so clinicians must depend on the parents'/caregivers' report. Werk and colleagues[24] sought to determine the factors primary care pediatricians think are important in establishing an initial diagnosis of asthma. Questionnaires on asthma diagnosis consisting of 20 factors obtained from the National Heart, Lung, and Blood Institute (NHLBI), NAEPP

EPR-2 guidelines,[25] and an expert local panel of subspecialists were sent to 862 active members of the Massachusetts American Academy of Pediatrics. Over 80% of the respondents rated five factors as necessary or important in establishing the diagnosis of asthma: recurrent wheezing, symptomatic improvement after bronchodilator use, presence of recurrent cough, exclusion of other diagnoses, and suggestive peak expiratory flow rate findings. Of note, 27% of the respondents indicated that a child had to be older than 2 years; 18% indicated that fever must be absent during an exacerbation.

The following characteristics are suggestive of asthma: recurrent or episodic wheezing or difficulty breathing, persistent nonproductive cough that may be worse at night, or these symptoms occurring with exercise, laughing, crying, or exposure to tobacco smoke in the absence of a respiratory infection; reduced activity or interest in running or playing compared with other children, with easy fatigability during walks; presence of other personal allergic diseases (i.e., atopic dermatitis, food allergy, or allergic rhinitis) or family history of asthma in first-degree relatives; and response to either a therapeutic trial of a corticosteroid or a short-acting β agonist (SABA) as needed.[7]

For adults and older children, easily performed lung function measures and noninvasive markers of airway inflammation can be used to make the diagnosis of asthma, monitor asthma control, or guide therapeutic decisions. A more detailed discussion of lung function measurements is presented in Chapter 21. In preschool-aged children, limited tools to assess airflow limitation (particularly involving the peripheral or small airway) and bronchodilator response (using forced or impulse oscillometry, specific airway resistance using whole body plethysmography, or respiratory resistance using an interrupter technique)[26–29]; BHR (using hyperventilation induced by cold or dry air[30,31] or auscultative methacholine or exercise challenges); and airway inflammation (exhaled nitric oxide[32–35] and serum eosinophil cationic protein [ECP][36]) are available only in specialized centers and mostly applied in research. The difficulty in using these in clinical practice has to do with complexity (especially employing sedation in infant lung function testing using body box plethysmography), cooperation from the very young child, challenges with standardization of procedures (bronchial provocation challenges), and the considerable degree of variability and overlap in results between children with and without asthma, particularly in regard to baseline measurements and bronchodilator response.

Even in older children and adolescents, imaging (using chest x-ray or high-resolution computed chest tomography) and bronchoscopy with or without biopsy have limited clinical applicability, except when other pulmonary abnormalities are being considered. However, understanding the underlying pathophysiologic processes of the disease in young children may be important to identify processes that can be targeted by early interventions. Thickening of the bronchial epithelial reticular basement membrane (RBM) and eosinophilic airway inflammation are characteristic pathologic features of asthma found in children as young as 3 years of age, but typically occurring between the ages of 6 and 16 years.[37] It is unclear when airway thickening begins, because routine biopsy studies are not performed in infants.[38] Studies on bronchoalveolar lavage samples obtained from wheezing infants and preschool children revealed an overall increase in airway inflammation, though it is rarely eosinophilic. In one study in which bronchial biopsies were performed on symptomatic infants, there were no consistent relationships between RBM thickening and inflammation, clinical symptoms, and variable airflow

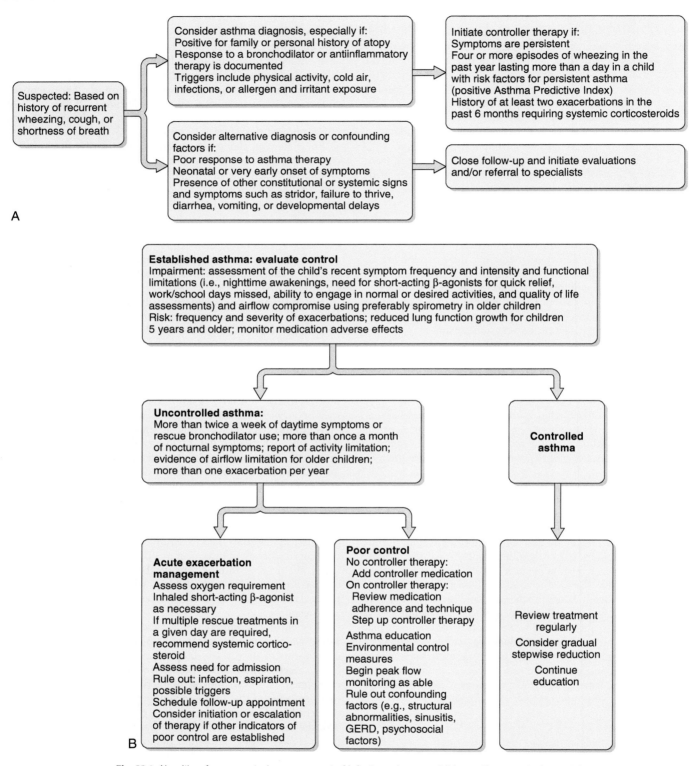

A

B

• **Fig. 23.1** Algorithm for suggested management of infants and young children with suspected or established asthma. *GERD,* Gastroesophageal reflux disease.

obstruction,[39] similar to findings from biopsy studies in older school-aged children with asthma.[40]

The use of sensitive, noninvasive physiologic and biologic markers is very limited in diagnosing young children with asthma and recurrent wheezing; therefore, a trial of treatment is often a practical way to make a diagnosis of asthma in young children (Fig. 23.1).

Management

The goals of asthma management—to attain good symptom control and allow normal activity levels, reduce exacerbations, optimize lung function, and minimize medication side effects—are not different between older children and preschool-aged children. Available asthma guidelines, such as the NAEPP EPR-3[6] and the Global

TABLE 23.1 **Classifying Asthma Severity and Initiating Treatment in Children Aged 0 to 4 Years** *Assessing Severity and Initiating Treatment for Patients Who Are Not Currently Taking Long-Term Control Medications*

COMPONENTS OF SEVERITY		CLASSIFICATION OF ASTHMA SEVERITY (0–4 YR)			
		INTERMITTENT	PERSISTENT		
		Mild	Mild	Moderate	Severe
Impairment	Daytime symptoms	≤2 days/wk	>2 days/wk but not daily	Daily	Throughout the day
	Nighttime awakenings	0	1–2×/mo	3–4×/mo	>1×/wk
	SABA use for symptoms (not EIB pretreatment)	≤2 days/wk	>2 days/wk but not daily and not more than once on any day	Daily	Several times per day
	Interference with normal activity	None	Minor limitation	Some limitation	Extremely limited
Risk	Exacerbations requiring systemic corticosteroids	0–1/yr	≥2 exacerbations in 6 mo requiring systemic corticosteroids, or ≥4 wheezing episodes/1yr lasting >1 day and risk factors for persistent asthma		
			Consider severity and interval since last exacerbation. Frequency and severity may fluctuate over time. Exacerbations of any severity may occur in patients in any severity category.		
Recommended step for initiating therapy		Step 1	Step 2	Step 3 and consider short course of oral systemic corticosteroids	
			In 2–6 weeks, depending on severity, evaluate level of asthma control that is achieved. If no clear benefit is observed within 4–6 weeks, consider adjusting therapy or alternative diagnoses.		

Notes:
- The stepwise approach is meant to assist, not replace, the clinical decision making required to meet individual patient needs.
- Level of severity is determined by both impairment and risk. Assess impairment domain by patient's/caregiver's recall of previous 2–4 weeks. Symptom assessment for longer periods should reflect a global assessment, such as inquiring whether a patient's asthma is better or worse since the last visit. Assign severity to the most severe category in which any feature occurs.
- At present, data are inadequate to correspond frequencies of exacerbations with different levels of asthma severity. For treatment purposes, patients who had ≥2 exacerbations requiring oral systemic corticosteroids in the past 6 months or ≥4 wheezing episodes in the past year and who have risk factors for persistent asthma may be considered the same as patients who have persistent asthma, even in the absence of impairment levels consistent with persistent asthma.

EIB, Exercise-induced bronchospasm; *SABA*, short-acting β₂-agonist use.

From National Asthma Education and Prevention Program. Expert Panel Report 3 (EPR 3): Guidelines for the diagnosis and management of asthma—summary report 2007. J Allergy Clin Immunol 2007;120(Suppl):S94–138, http://www.nhlbi.nih.gov/guidelines/asthma/asthgdln.htm.

Initiative for Asthma (GINA) global strategy[7] acknowledge the special challenges unique to the management of asthma in preschool children; thus, a specific approach and treatment recommendations for preschool children with asthma are presented. The NAEPP EPR-3 was last published over 10 years ago, whereas GINA has been updated about every 1 to 2 years based on new studies, with the most recent one from 2019. A comprehensive management plan is outlined in several components and/or sections and generally includes establishment of patient-doctor partnership and provision of education to enhance the patient's/family's knowledge and skills for self-management (appropriate use of devices and medications), identification and management of risk and precipitating factors and comorbid conditions that may worsen asthma, adequate assessment and monitoring of disease activity (including symptom monitoring by parent/caregiver), appropriate selection of medications to address the patient's needs, and management of asthma exacerbations (with provision of a written asthma action plan).

Key differences between the two clinical guidelines are noted with respect to assessment of disease severity and/or control and mechanics of a stepwise approach. The approach implemented by the NAEPP EPR-3 on starting controller therapy is based on the concept of asthma severity, which is the intrinsic intensity of disease and applicable for patients not receiving controller therapy.[6] The guidelines have a separate set of criteria for various age groups. Table 23.1 summarizes the classification of asthma severity for children 0 to 4 years old. The classification of asthma severity is contingent on the domains of impairment and risk, and the level of severity is based on the most severe impairment or risk component. Impairment includes an assessment of the child's recent symptom frequency (daytime and nighttime), need for SABA for quick relief, and ability to engage in normal or desired activities. Risk refers to an evaluation of the child's likelihood of developing asthma exacerbations. Of note, in the absence of frequent symptoms, persistent asthma should be considered and therefore long-term controller therapy initiated for infants or children who have risk factors for asthma (i.e., using the mAPI: any of parental history of asthma, physician-diagnosed atopic dermatitis, or sensitization to aeroallergens; or two of the following: wheezing apart from colds, sensitization to foods, or peripheral eosinophilia) and four or more episodes of wheezing over the past year that lasted longer than 1 day and affected sleep or two or more exacerbations within 6 months requiring systemic corticosteroids.

TABLE 23.2	Assessing Asthma Control and Adjusting Therapy in Children Aged 0 to 4 Years			
	COMPONENTS OF CONTROL	**CLASSIFICATION OF ASTHMA CONTROL (0–4 YR)**		
	Well Controlled		**Not Well Controlled**	**Very Poorly Controlled**
Impairment	Daytime symptoms	≤2 days/wk but not more than once on each day	>2 days/wk	Throughout the day
	Nighttime awakenings	≤1×/mo	>1×/mo	>1×/wk
	SABA use for symptoms (not EIB pretreatment)	≤2 days/wk	>2 days/wk	Several times per day
	Interference or limitations with normal activity	None	Some limitation	Extremely limited
Risk	Exacerbations requiring oral systemic corticosteroids	0–1/yr	2–3/yr	>3 yr
	Treatment-related adverse effects	Medication side effects can vary in intensity from none to very troublesome and worrisome. The level of intensity does not correlate to specific levels of control but should be considered in the overall assessment of risk.		
	Recommended action for treatment per NAEPP guidelines	Maintain current treatment Regular follow-up every 1–6 months Consider step down if well controlled for at least 3 months	Step up (1 step) and re-evaluate in 2–6 weeks If no clear benefit in 4–6 weeks, consider alternative diagnoses or adjusting therapy For side effects, consider alternative treatment options	Consider short course of oral systemic corticosteroids Step up (1–2 steps), and re-evaluate in 2 weeks If no clear benefit in 4–6 weeks, consider alternative diagnoses or adjusting therapy For side effects, consider alternative treatment options

Notes:
- The stepwise approach is meant to assist, not replace, the clinical decision making required to meet individual patient needs.
- The level of control is based on the most severe impairment or risk category. Assess impairment domain by caregiver's recall of previous 2–4 weeks. Symptom assessment for longer periods should reflect a global assessment, such as inquiring whether the patient's asthma is better or worse since the last visit.
- At present, data are inadequate to correspond frequencies of exacerbations with different levels of asthma control. In general, more frequent and intense exacerbations (e.g., requiring urgent, unscheduled care, hospitalization, or intensive care unit admission) indicate poorer disease control. For treatment purposes, patients who had ≥2 exacerbations requiring oral systemic corticosteroids in the past year may be considered the same as patients who have asthma that is not well controlled, even in the absence of impairment levels consistent with asthma that is not well controlled.
- Before step-up therapy:
  - Review adherence to medications, inhaler technique, and environmental control.
  - If alternative treatment option was used in a step, discontinue it and use preferred treatment for that step.

EIB, Exercise-induced bronchospasm; *NAEPP,* National Asthma Education and Prevention Program; *SABA,* short-acting β_2-agonist use.

From National Asthma Education and Prevention Program. Expert Panel Report 3 (EPR 3): Guidelines for the diagnosis and management of asthma—summary report 2007, http://www.nhlbi.nih.gov/guidelines/asthma/asthgdln.htm.

For preschool children already on a controller medication, medication adjustment is made on the basis of the child's level of control. As with the classification of asthma severity, assessment of asthma control is based on both impairment and risk (Table 23.2). The three levels of asthma control are well controlled, not well controlled, and very poorly controlled. Children whose asthma is not well controlled have daytime symptoms or need for rescue albuterol more than 2 days/week, have nighttime symptoms more than once a month but not more than once a week, have some limitation with normal activity, had two to three exacerbations in the past year, and have a forced expiratory volume in 1 second (FEV_1) of 60% to 80% of predicted (or FEV_1/forced vital capacity [FVC] ratio of 75%–80%) for children 5 years of age or older. Children with very poorly controlled asthma have symptoms throughout the day; have nocturnal symptoms more than once weekly; need rescue albuterol several times per day; have extreme limitations with normal activity; had three or more exacerbations in the past year; and for children at least 5 years of age, an FEV_1 of less than 60% of predicted or FEV_1/FVC ratio less than 75%. Using a validated questionnaire to monitor quality of life for older children is recommended. The pediatric version of the Asthma Control Test (cACT) has been validated for children as young as 4 years of age.[41] A five-item caregiver-administered instrument, the Test for Respiratory and Asthma Control in Kids (TRACK), has been validated as a tool to assess asthma control in young children with recurrent wheezing or respiratory symptoms consistent with asthma.[42] This questionnaire includes an assessment of both impairment and risk reflected in the NAEPP EPR-3 asthma management guidelines.[6] The items

TABLE 23.3   GINA Assessment of Asthma Control in Children 5 Years and Younger

A. Level of Symptom Control

In the past 4 weeks, has the child had:	Yes	No
Daytime asthma symptoms for more than a few minutes?		
Any night waking or coughing because of asthma?		
Reliever medication needed more than once a week (excludes reliever taken before exercise)?		
Any activity limitation because of asthma? (Runs/plays less than other children, tires easily during walks/playing?)		

Controlled (none of the above)

Partly controlled (1–2 of these)

Uncontrolled (3–4 of these)

B. Future Risk for Poor Asthma Outcomes

Risk factors for asthma exacerbations
- Uncontrolled asthma symptoms
- One or more severe exacerbations in previous year
- The start of the child's usual flare-up season (especially if autumn or fall)
- Exposures: tobacco smoke, indoor or outdoor air pollution, indoor allergens (e.g., house dust mite, cockroach, pets, mold), especially in combination with viral infection
- Major psychologic or socioeconomic problems for child or family
- Poor adherence with controller medication, or incorrect inhaler technique
- Outdoor pollution (nitrogen dioxide and particles)

Risk factors for fixed airflow limitation
- Severe asthma with several hospitalizations
- History of bronchiolitis

Risk factors for medication side effects
- Systemic: frequent courses of oral corticosteroids; high-dose and/or potent inhaled corticosteroids
- Local: moderate/high-dose or potent inhaled corticosteroids, incorrect inhaler technique, failure to protect skin or eyes when using inhaled corticosteroids by nebulizer or spacer with facemask

Modified from the Global Strategy for Asthma Management and Prevention 2019, http://www.ginasthma.org.

include four impairment questions (three on symptom burden and activity limitations over a 4-week period and one on rescue medication use over a 3-month period) and one risk question on oral corticosteroid use over a 12-month period. Each item has five descriptive ordinal responses that can be scored over a 5-point scale (0, 5, 10, 15, and 20; total score range 0–100). The screening ability of the entire scale showed areas under the receiver operating characteristic (ROC) curve of 0.88 and 0.82, respectively, in the development and validation samples, with a diagnostic accuracy of 81% and 78%, respectively. Based on the highest area under the ROC curve, a score of less than 80 provided the best cut-off between sensitivity and specificity for uncontrolled asthma for this group.

The GINA global strategy[7] uses an assessment of asthma control based on two components: respiratory status over the previous 4 weeks (current symptom control) and how asthma may affect the person in the future (future risk for exacerbations, fixed airflow limitation, and medication side effects). The criteria for current symptom control (well controlled, partly controlled, and uncontrolled asthma) according to the GINA global strategy are summarized in Table 23.3, based on a 4-week recall. Well-controlled asthma is characterized by at most daytime symptoms once a week, rescue/reliever treatment less than 2 times a week, absence of any activity limitation because of asthma, and no nocturnal cough or awakenings. Partly controlled asthma has one or two of the following: two or more daytime symptoms a week, 2 or more times of rescue bronchodilator use, any nocturnal cough/awakenings, or limitations of activities. Finally, uncontrolled asthma is defined as presence of three or all features characteristic of partly controlled asthma present in any week or exacerbation occurring once in any week. The risk assessment identifies factors for different adverse outcomes. Risk factors of having exacerbations in the next few months are uncontrolled asthma symptoms; 1 or more exacerbations in the previous year needing an emergency room visit, hospitalization, or oral corticosteroid burst; child's flare-up season; presence of smoking or outdoor or indoor air pollution; indoor allergen exposure (house dust mite, cockroach, pets, mold) especially with concurrent viral infection; major psychologic or socioeconomic problems; and inadequate ICS use (from lack of prescription, poor adherence, or incorrect inhaler technique). Risk factors for impaired lung function are severe asthma with multiple hospitalizations and history of bronchiolitis. Frequent oral corticosteroid use and long-term, high-dose and/or potent ICS use are risk factors for systemic medication side effects; whereas a moderate/high-dose or potent ICS, incorrect inhaler technique, and failure to protect the skin or eyes when using ICSs (by either nebulizer or spacer and facemask) are also risk factors for local side effects.

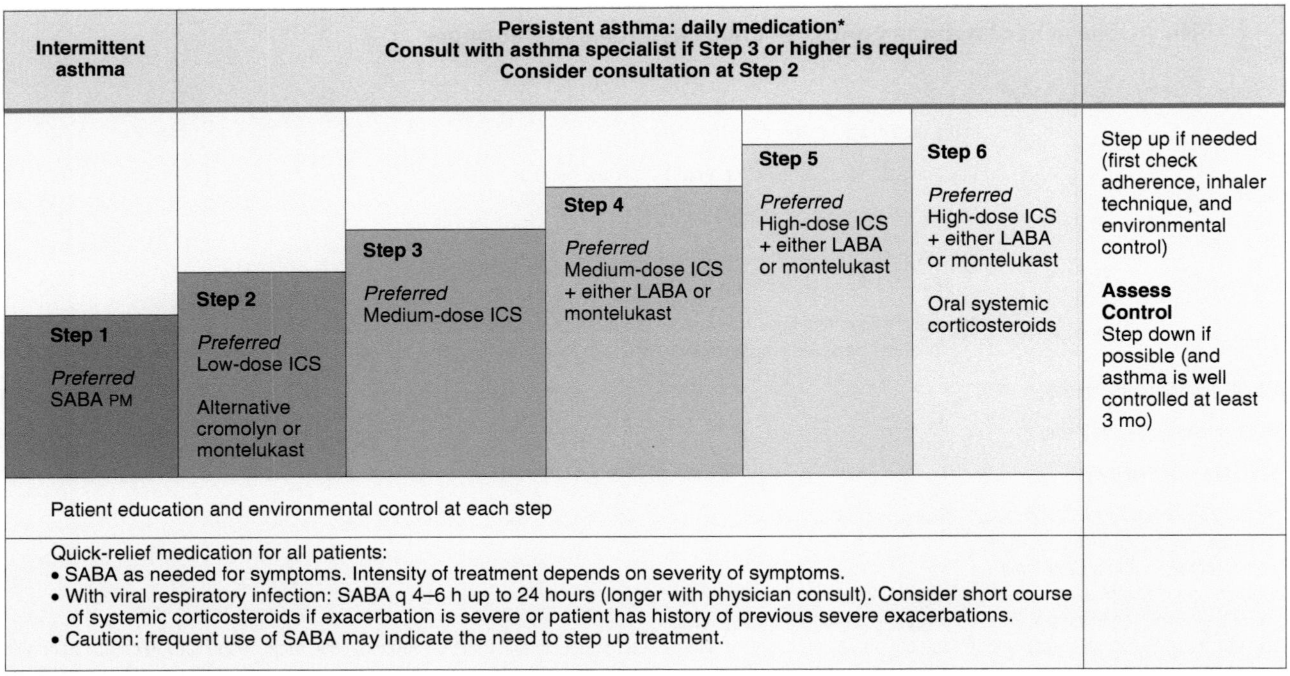

Intermittent asthma	Persistent asthma: daily medication* Consult with asthma specialist if Step 3 or higher is required Consider consultation at Step 2					
Step 1 *Preferred* SABA PRN	**Step 2** *Preferred* Low-dose ICS Alternative cromolyn or montelukast	**Step 3** *Preferred* Medium-dose ICS	**Step 4** *Preferred* Medium-dose ICS + either LABA or montelukast	**Step 5** *Preferred* High-dose ICS + either LABA or montelukast	**Step 6** *Preferred* High-dose ICS + either LABA or montelukast Oral systemic corticosteroids	Step up if needed (first check adherence, inhaler technique, and environmental control) **Assess Control** Step down if possible (and asthma is well controlled at least 3 mo)
Patient education and environmental control at each step						
Quick-relief medication for all patients: • SABA as needed for symptoms. Intensity of treatment depends on severity of symptoms. • With viral respiratory infection: SABA q 4–6 h up to 24 hours (longer with physician consult). Consider short course of systemic corticosteroids if exacerbation is severe or patient has history of previous severe exacerbations. • Caution: frequent use of SABA may indicate the need to step up treatment.						

• **Fig. 23.2** Stepwise approach for managing asthma in children aged 0 to 4 years.* Alphabetical order is used when more than one treatment option is listed within either preferred or alternative therapy.

NOTES:

• The stepwise approach is meant to assist, not replace, the clinical decision making required to meet individual patient needs.
• If alternative treatment is used and response is inadequate, discontinue it and use the preferred treatment before stepping up.
• If clear benefit is not observed within 4 to 6 weeks and patient/family medication technique and adherence are satisfactory, consider adjusting therapy or alternative diagnosis.
• Studies on children aged 0 to 4 years are limited. Step 2 therapy is based on Evidence A. All other recommendations are based on expert opinion and extrapolation from studies in older children. The stepwise approach is meant to assist, not replace, the clinical decision making required to meet individual patient needs.

ICS, Inhaled corticosteroid; *LABA,* inhaled long-acting β₂ agonist; *prn,* as needed; *SABA,* inhaled short-acting β₂-agonist.

National Asthma Education and Prevention Program. Expert Panel Report 3 (EPR 3): guidelines for the diagnosis and management of asthma—summary report 2007. J Allergy Clin Immunol 2007;120(Suppl):S94–138, http://www.nhlbi.nih.gov/guidelines/asthma/asthgdln.htm.

It also puts an emphasis on a shared-care approach using an effective patient–healthcare provider partnership that has been shown to improve outcomes and the process of assess, adjust treatment, and review response. Eliciting specific goals of treatment from caregivers and providing education are key elements in this partnership. The process of assessing (diagnosis, symptom control, risk factors, inhaler technique, adherence, and parent preference), adjusting treatment (medications, nonpharmacologic strategies, and treatment of modifiable risk factors), and reviewing response (medication effectiveness and side effects) is recommended on an ongoing basis.

Controller Therapy for Young Children With Persistent Asthma

Based on the NAEPP EPR-3 guidelines,[6] on establishing a diagnosis of asthma in young children, initiation of controller therapy is warranted for persistent asthma. The most important determinant of dosing is the clinician's judgment of the patient's presenting degree of severity. Initiation of long-term controller therapy also should be considered for infants and younger children who have risk factors for asthma (i.e., modified asthma predictive index: parental history of asthma, physician-diagnosed atopic dermatitis, or sensitization to aeroallergens; or two of the following: wheezing apart from colds, sensitization to foods, or peripheral

eosinophilia) and four or more episodes of wheezing over the past year that lasted longer than 1 day and affected sleep or two or more exacerbations in 6 months requiring systemic corticosteroids. As discussed earlier, medication dose adjustment is based on levels of asthma control.

The NAEPP EPR-3 provides an expanded stepwise treatment approach (Fig. 23.2) even for young children. The choice of initial therapy is based on assessment of asthma severity. For patients who are already on controller therapy, modification of treatment is based on assessment of asthma control and responsiveness to therapy. A major objective of this approach is to identify and treat all persistent and uncontrolled asthma with antiinflammatory controller medication. Management of intermittent asthma is a SABA as needed for symptoms and for pretreatment for those with exercise-induced bronchospasm (Step 1). The type(s) and amount(s) of daily controller medications to be used are determined by the asthma severity and control rating. Even for young children, the preferred treatment for persistent asthma is daily ICS therapy, with or without an additional medication. Alternative medications for Step 2 include a leukotriene receptor antagonist (LTRA; montelukast) or a nonsteroidal antiinflammatory agent (cromolyn). For young children (4 years of age or younger) with moderate or severe persistent asthma, medium-dose ICS monotherapy is recommended and combination therapy of medium-dose ICS plus either a long-acting β agonist (LABA) or montelukast is to be initiated only as a Step 4 treatment for uncontrolled asthma. Children with severe persistent asthma (treatment Steps 5 and 6) should receive a high-dose ICS, a LABA or montelukast, and an oral corticosteroid, if required. A rescue course of systemic corticosteroids may be necessary at any step.

The "step-up, step-down" approach was initially introduced in the earlier versions of the NAEPP guidelines[21] and slightly modified in the current iteration.[6] The NAEPP guidelines emphasize initiating higher level controller therapy at the outset to establish prompt control, with measures to step down therapy once good asthma control is achieved. Initially, airflow limitation and the pathologic process of asthma may limit the delivery and efficacy of ICS asthma control. Asthma therapy can be stepped down after good asthma control has been achieved and the ICS has had time to achieve optimal efficacy, by determining the least number or dose of daily controller medications that can maintain good control, thereby reducing the potential for medication adverse effects. If step-up therapy is being considered at any point, it is important to re-evaluate for asthma confounders and differential diagnostic conditions, check delivery device technique and adherence, implement environmental control measures, and identify and treat comorbid conditions.

The GINA global strategy also offers a stepwise approach in the long-term management of asthma in very young children based on asthma control (current asthma control and risk of poor outcomes) mentioned earlier[7] (see Table 23.3). Its stepwise approach has important differences from the NAEPP EPR-3,[6,7] in that although both are based on symptom patterns, it also incorporates identification of modifiable risk factors of future exacerbations, impaired lung function, and side effects. The need for long-term treatment should be assessed regularly.

For Step 1, as-needed inhaled SABA is recommended for children with infrequent viral wheezing, with few or no interval symptoms. Intermittent high-dose ICS is an alternative option if SABA treatment is not sufficient.[43,44] Intermittent high-dose ICS therapy given at the onset of a respiratory illness is further demonstrated to be as beneficial as maintenance therapy with an ICS in children with recurrent wheezing and risk factors for persistent asthma.[45] Because repeated high-dose ICS therapy has the potential to cause side effects if given quite often during the year, this should be considered for families who are able to use this intervention responsibly. Step 2 treatment is recommended for young children with a symptom pattern consistent with asthma and not well controlled, with three or more exacerbations per year or frequent wheezing episodes requiring a SABA three or more times per year. Similar to the NAEPP EPR-3 guidelines, the preferred medication is a daily low-dose ICS (for at least a 3-month trial) and the alternative option of using an LTRA. The GINA global strategy also includes an intermittent ICS for Step 2 as an alternative option. The Individualized Therapy for Asthma in Toddlers (INFANT) study compared differential response based on a composite measure of asthma control to daily ICS, daily LTRA, and as-needed ICS treatment co-administered with albuterol in children 12 to 59 months of age, administered in a randomized, double-blind, double-dummy, cross-over design. Of the participants, 74% had a differential response to any of the three treatments: daily ICS was associated with highest response (40% probability), and as-needed ICS and daily LTRA were nearly 20% each.[46]

For young children with frequent viral-induced wheezing and symptoms between these episodes, daily ICS should be used first. If there is still inadequate control, alternative options for Step 2 can be used (i.e., LTRA or intermittent ICS) before moving to Step 3.

Preferred Step 3 treatment is double low-dose ICS, indicated for children with established asthma not well controlled on low-dose ICS. The alternative option is low-dose ICS with an LTRA. Referral to a specialist is recommended. The highest step (Step 4) basically proposes a referral to a specialist for expert advice, and the best treatment for this group has not been established. Additional options include increasing the ICS dose and/or adding an LTRA, a LABA, theophylline, or intermittent ICS (if exacerbations are the main concern).

Through all of these previously discussed steps, before any changes in treatment in the event symptom control is not achieved with adequate controller therapy, assess for other confounders or an alternative diagnosis, appropriate inhaler technique, adherence, parent understanding and preference, and environmental exposures. The need for controller therapy should be evaluated and treatment adjusted because symptoms in this age group may remit at certain times of the year or even over time. Once therapy is decreased or discontinued, a close follow-up within 3 to 6 weeks is ideal, and caregivers should be provided with a written asthma action plan that incorporates early warning signs of worsening asthma control and what to do or whom to contact when the child's condition deteriorates.

Controller Medications Recommended for Young Children With Asthma

Inhaled Corticosteroids. ICSs are the preferred controller therapy for persistent asthma or asthma that is not controlled. They have been shown to improve symptoms, lung function, and overall asthma control; decrease exacerbations; and reduce chronic oral prednisone use.[47–51] Although multiple clinical trials with other ICSs have demonstrated favorable clinical effects, nebulized budesonide is the only ICS approved by the U.S. Federal Drug Administration (FDA) for children younger than 4 years of age. The efficacy of nebulized budesonide over placebo was consistently demonstrated with improvement in symptom scores, reduction in rescue medication use, and improvement in morning peak expiratory flow rates in patients who could adequately perform the procedure. Improvement in symptom scores occurred as early as 2 weeks after starting budesonide.[51] Twice-daily dosing of 0.5 mg appeared to be somewhat more effective than 1 mg administered once daily. The investigators suggested that a dose of 0.25 mg/day may be sufficient for mild asthma. Patients with moderate asthma should be treated with 0.5 to 1 mg/day, and those with severe asthma dependent on oral corticosteroids should be treated with 1 to 2 mg/day. No significant differences in basal cortisol levels or adrenocortico-tropin-stimulated cortisol levels were found among any of the active treatment groups and placebo.

Recommended doses of different ICS formulations for children 5 years and younger according to low, medium, and high doses in the NAEPP EPR-3 and low-dose formulations in the GINA global strategy are shown in Table 23.4.[6,7]

The type of patient who will respond favorably to ICS in this age group has been addressed. A study by Roorda and colleagues[52] using data from two large placebo-controlled studies evaluated the clinical features of preschool children likely to respond to fluticasone administered by a pressurized metered-dose inhaler

TABLE 23.4   Estimated Comparative Inhaled Corticosteroid Doses

Drug	NAEPP EPR-3* Low	Medium	High	GINA 2019† Low Daily Dose
Beclomethasone HFA, 40 or 80 mcg/puff	NA	NA	NA	100 mcg (ages ≥5 years)
Budesonide DPI 90, 80, or 200 mcg/inhalation	NA	NA	NA	
Budesonide pMDI + spacer	NA	NA	NA	Not sufficiently studied in this age group
Budesonide inhaled suspension for nebulization, 0.25-, 0.5- and 1-mg dose	0.25–0.5 mg	>0.5–1.0 mg	>1.0 mg	500 mcg
Ciclesonide HFA/pMDI, 80 or 160 mcg/puff				Not sufficiently studied in this age group
Flunisolide, 250 mcg/puff	NA	NA	NA	
Flunisolide HFA/pMDI, 80 mcg/puff	NA	NA	NA	
Fluticasone propionate HFA/pMDI, 44, 110, or 220 mcg/puff	176 mcg	>176–352 mcg	>352 mcg	50 mcg
Fluticasone DPI, 50, 100 or 250 mcg/inhalation	NA	NA	NA	
Mometasone furoate110, 220 mcg/inhalation	NA	NA	NA	110 mcg
Triamcinolone acetonide, 75 mcg/puff	NA	NA	NA	Not studied in this age group

HFA, Hydrofluoroalkane propellant; *NA*, not available; *pMDI*, pressurized metered-dose inhaler.

*Modified from the National Asthma Education and Prevention Program: Expert Panel Report 3 (EPR 3): Guidelines for the diagnosis and management of asthma—summary report 2007. J Allergy Clin Immunol 2007;120(Suppl):S94–138, http://www.nhlbi.nih.gov/guidelines/asthma/asthgdln.htm.

†This is not a table of clinical equivalence. Only low doses are given. A low daily dose is defined as the lowest approved dose for which safety and effectiveness have been adequately studied in this age group. Low-dose inhaled corticosteroids provides most of the clinical benefit for most children with asthma. Higher doses are associated with an increased risk of local and systemic side effects, which must be balanced against potential benefits.

Modified from the GINA Global Strategy for Asthma Management and Prevention 2019, http://www.ginasthma.org.

(pMDI) with holding chamber and facemask. The investigators identified two clinical features that predicted a positive response to ICS therapy: frequent symptoms (≥3 days/week) and a family history of asthma. The presence of eczema and the number of previous acute exacerbations were not associated with response to fluticasone. Eczema predisposes a child with recurrent wheezing to subsequent asthma,[16] but it does not appear to predict response to ICS therapy. It should be noted that a lack of response over a short course of treatment (12 weeks) does not necessarily mean that a response would not be seen over a much longer period (months to years). The INFANT study described earlier also evaluated predictors of response to different interventions, specifically daily ICS versus daily LTRA versus intermittent ICS, in preschool-aged children with persistent asthma and found that both aeroallergen sensitization and blood eosinophils predicted response to daily ICS.[46]

The clinical efficacy and safety of intermittent ICS or systemic corticosteroid for young children with associated upper respiratory tract infection or viral-induced wheeze remain controversial. A study that evaluated as-needed high-dose fluticasone propionate (750 mcg twice daily) given at the onset of an upper respiratory tract illness found lower rescue oral corticosteroid use in those on active treatment compared with placebo (8% versus 18%, respectively); however, this was accompanied by a statistically significant difference in height and weight gain.[43] In another study, oral prednisolone was found not to be superior to placebo with respect to duration of hospitalization, clinician and parent symptom severity assessment, and hospital readmission for preschool children presenting to a hospital with viral-induced mild to moderate wheezing.[53] A third study, which evaluated daily versus intermittent high-dose ICS therapy given at the onset of a respiratory illness in preschool-aged children with recurrent wheezing and atopic risk factors, found no difference between the two treatments with respect to prevention of severe exacerbations.[45]

ICSs and Growth in Small Children. Few published studies have evaluated the effects of ICSs on the linear growth of preschool children. Reid and associates,[54] in an open-label study, measured linear growth velocity in 40 children (mean age 1.4 years) before and during treatment with nebulized budesonide.[54] All of the children had "troublesome" asthma despite treatment with an ICS administered with a pMDI with spacer and facemask or nebulized cromolyn before entry into the study. They were then administered 1 to 4 mg/day of nebulized budesonide depending on their level of asthma severity. The median intervals of time for linear growth determinations during the run-in period and nebulized budesonide treatments were 6 months and 1 year, respectively. The height standard deviation scores (SDSs) for the group during the run-in period were –0.21, at baseline –0.46, and after at least 6 months of nebulized budesonide –0.17. The subjects were growing at less than an impaired rate before nebulized budesonide therapy, and the institution of nebulized budesonide did not result in further growth suppression. In fact, there was a trend toward improved growth velocity while on nebulized budesonide.

Skoner and associates[55] evaluated the growth of children enrolled in 52-week open-label extension studies of the three efficacy studies of budesonide.[49–51] The dose of budesonide was either 0.5 mg once or twice daily with a taper to the lowest tolerated dose, and conventional asthma therapy consisted of any available therapy, including ICSs in two of the studies; in total, 670 children participated. The investigators found a modest impairment in growth in only one of the three extension studies. The extension study in which a decline in growth was noted consisted primarily of young children with milder asthma who had not been on ICS before entry into the initial study. In contrast, the two extension studies that did not find growth impairment consisted of children with more severe disease and had allowed for ICS use as part of the conventional asthma therapy algorithm. The Skoner study suggests that modest growth suppression can occur in young children receiving nebulized budesonide who have not required ICS therapy in the past and that children with milder asthma may be at greater risk for growth suppression secondary to increased intrapulmonary deposition. Alternatively, the findings may be attributable to the fact that over twice as many children randomized to the conventional asthma therapy arm withdrew from the study because of poor asthma control.

The Prevention of Early Asthma in Kids (PEAK) and Inhaled Fluticasone in Wheezy Infants (IFWIN) studies, which used ICS by MDI with a holding chamber and facemask, have provided important findings on the adverse effects of long-term ICSs on growth in preschool children at risk for persistent asthma.[21,56,57] It is still uncertain if there is a potential for catch up or if the effects in very young children are cumulative. A follow-up study of PEAK participants 2 years after the clinical trial was completed showed no difference in growth between children who were on active ICS therapy and those who were randomized to placebo.[56] However, in a post hoc analysis, lower growth velocity was found among participants who were younger and weighed less, probably because of a relatively greater drug exposure. For young children with poor asthma control, the disease itself can negatively affect growth. The growth of 58 children (mean age 3.5 years for males, 4.4 years for females) with asthma was followed over a 5-year period.[58] Each child's asthma was classified as being in good, moderate, or poor control according to asthma symptoms during a 2-year observational period before the institution of ICS therapy. The group as a whole had diminished growth velocity to start the study, with a mean height velocity standard deviation (HVSD) score of –0.51. Children whose asthma was in good control had the least evidence for growth suppression before ICS therapy was instituted and continued to grow at the same rate as when on therapy (HVSD score –0.01 before treatment versus –0.07 during treatment). In contrast, the subjects whose asthma was poorly controlled grew poorly before and after institution of ICS therapy (HVSD score –1.50 pretreatment versus –1.55 during treatment). Of interest, those with moderately controlled asthma demonstrated improved growth velocity while on ICS therapy, with their HVSD score increasing from –0.83 to –0.49. The investigators concluded that poor asthma control adversely affects linear growth to a greater extent than ICS therapy.

Alternative and Potential Medications

The NHLBI NAEPP EPR-3 guidelines recommend cromolyn or montelukast as an alternative therapy for younger children with mild persistent asthma and combination therapy using an ICS plus either a LABA or montelukast for younger children with moderate to severe persistent asthma (Steps 4 and 5).[6] The GINA global strategy recommends an LTRA or increased or intermittent ICS therapy as alternative options for Step 2 and add-on options for Steps 3 and 4[7] and only indicates LABA as add-on Step 4 therapy, recognizing that no studies on LABAs for young children are available.

An interesting option to consider for infants and young children who develop severe episodes of lower respiratory tract illnesses with no persistent symptoms in between episodes is early administration of azithromycin, a macrolide, during an acute illness.[59] It is still not clear why children, regardless of their atopic risk, develop these severe symptoms during respiratory infections, regardless of cause. In children with asthma, the presence of bacteria and viruses in respiratory secretions can be associated with an increased likelihood of having an asthma exacerbation. Thus, it is quite possible that a drug with an antiinflammatory property in addition to antimicrobial profile might be beneficial and might justify why antibiotics (especially macrolides) are commonly used clinically during exacerbations associated with respiratory tract infections. Azithromycin has been shown to reduce interleukin 8 (IL-8) levels in nasal secretions during respiratory syncytial virus bronchiolitis. A randomized clinical trial was undertaken involving preschool children with a history of severe intermittent wheezing during respiratory tract infections to determine if early administration of azithromycin would prevent the progression of the subsequent episode.[59] Azithromycin started at the earliest signs of a respiratory illness was effective in significantly reducing the risk of experiencing a severe episode compared with placebo (hazard ratio [HR], 0.64 [95% confidence interval [CI], 0.41–0.98], $P = .04$; absolute risk for first respiratory tract illness: 0.05 for azithromycin, 0.08 for placebo; risk difference, 0.03 [95% CI, 0.00–0.06]) and reducing symptom severity. These favorable results were found regardless of atopic features; therefore, it could be a treatment option for young children even with low risk for persistent asthma. Over the duration of the study 16.7% versus 10.8% of children treated and not treated with azithromycin, respectively, had azithromycin-resistant organisms. Although this approach would benefit from additional study, including attention given to the risk of possible antibiotic resistance, it offers a potential option for a subgroup of infants and young children with severe intermittent respiratory illnesses.

Cromolyn. Cromolyn inhibits mediator release from mast cells. It inhibits both the early and late phase pulmonary components of the allergic response after inhalation of an allergen in sensitized patients. A few studies have shown no added benefit with the use of cromolyn over placebo in young children with more severe disease.[60–63] Several efficacy studies that have found cromolyn to have beneficial effects were short-term trials and employed small numbers.[64,65] A meta-analysis of 22 control studies evaluating cromolyn in childhood asthma found it no better than placebo.[66] A multicenter, randomized, parallel-group, 52-week, open-label study in preschool children found nebulized cromolyn (20 mg four times daily) (N = 335) to be inferior to nebulized budesonide suspension (0.5 mg daily) (N = 168) using several outcome parameters.[67] Children who received inhaled budesonide suspension had a reduced rate of asthma exacerbations per year, longer time to first asthma exacerbation, lower use of rescue medications. First use of additional long-term controller therapy nearly doubled improvements in nighttime and daytime symptom scores by the second week of treatment. Although there were no significant differences in the rates of hospitalization and emergency room visits between the two groups, significantly lower urgent care or unscheduled physician visits and oral corticosteroid use were found in children who received the ICS. However, mean height increases from baseline in children randomized to inhaled budesonide and inhaled cromolyn were 6.69 and 7.55 cm, respectively. This difference of 0.86 cm is similar to the difference in height measurements seen in other studies with ICS therapy after 1 year of treatment in both younger and older children.[21,68,69]

Leukotriene-Modifying Agents. Leukotrienes are potent proinflammatory mediators that induce bronchospasm, mucus secretion, and airway edema. In addition, they may be involved in eosinophil recruitment into the asthmatic airway.[70] Leukotriene modifiers (synthesis inhibitor or receptor antagonist) have beneficial effects in terms of reducing asthma symptoms and supplemental β-agonist use while improving baseline pulmonary function.[71–73] LTRAs prevent the binding of leukotriene D4 (LTD4) to its receptor. This class has a pediatric indication and includes both montelukast (given once daily; has been approved for treatment of chronic asthma for children 1 year and older) and zafirlukast (administered twice daily; approved for children 7 years and older).

Safety and efficacy studies with the 4-mg chewable montelukast tablet in children 2 to 5 years of age with asthma have been published.[74–76] Almost 700 children 2 to 5 years of age were enrolled to receive montelukast or placebo for 12 weeks in a double-blind, multicenter, multinational study at 93 centers worldwide.[74] Montelukast was well tolerated and was not associated with any significant adverse effects. It was superior to placebo in reducing daytime symptoms, including improvements in cough, wheeze, difficulty breathing, activity level, and nighttime cough. In addition, montelukast therapy was associated with a reduction in rescue β-agonist use and reduced need for prednisone for acute severe exacerbations.

Studies have been done to evaluate the long-term effects of an LTRA (continuous[75] and intermittent[76]) on the occurrence of exacerbations in young children. In a 12-month, double-blind, parallel study designed to investigate the role of montelukast in the prevention of viral-induced asthma exacerbations in children aged 2 to 5 years with a history of intermittent asthma symptoms, montelukast significantly reduced the rate of asthma exacerbations by 31.9% compared with placebo. Montelukast delayed the median time to first exacerbation by approximately 2 months and the rate of ICS courses compared with placebo.[75] In another study, 220 children ages 2 to 14 years were randomized to receive either intermittent montelukast or placebo at the onset of asthma or upper respiratory tract infection symptoms for a minimum of 7 days.[76] The montelukast group had 163 unscheduled healthcare resource usages for asthma compared with 228 in the placebo group (odds ratio [OR] = 0.65, 95% CI 0.47–0.89). There was a nonsignificant reduction in specialist attendances and hospitalizations, duration of episode, and β-agonist and prednisolone use. These studies suggest that intermittent or persistent therapy with montelukast for children with intermittent asthma symptoms is effective in reducing risk of exacerbations compared with placebo.

Long-Acting Inhaled β Agonists. LABAs are the alternative add-on therapy for children and adults with moderate and severe persistent asthma. The GINA global strategy mentions LABAs as additional therapy that can be added to Step 4 for very young children.[7] By itself, they are not viewed as rescue medications for acute episodes of bronchospasm. However, in combination with an ICS, they are included in GINA as relief and maintenance medications for older children and adults. Salmeterol has a prolonged onset of action with maximal bronchodilation approximately 1 hour after administration; formoterol has an onset of effect within minutes. Both medications have a prolonged duration of action of at least 12 hours. Therefore, they are especially well suited for patients with nocturnal asthma[77] and for individuals who require frequent use of SABA inhalations during the day to prevent exercise-induced asthma.[78] There is an added advantage to the use of these alternative therapies for preschool children who may deserve an extended bronchodilatory coverage for exercise because they are constantly active. Salmeterol delivered with the Diskus device is FDA approved for children as young as 4 years of age (50-mcg blister every 12 hours), whereas formoterol delivered with the Aerolizer is approved for use in children 6 years of age and older (12-mcg capsule every 12 hours). Both LABAs are also available as a combination pMDI with an ICS (salmeterol and fluticasone, budesonide and formoterol, and mometasone and formoterol). Although LABAs combined with ICS are recommended for young children in Steps 4 to 6 of the NAEPP EPR-3 guidelines (see Fig. 23.2), they have limited application.[6] The Diskus combination product is FDA approved down to 4 years of age, but its use requires adequate inspiratory effort to get an optimal delivery of the dry powder. Although the pMDI combination products can be used with a holding chamber, they are currently FDA approved for children older than 5 years of age (i.e., budesonide and formoterol). The efficacy and safety of LABA or combination products in younger children with asthma are still uncertain because of the lack of studies.

Treatment immediately before vigorous activity or exercise is usually effective. The combination of a SABA with either cromolyn or nedocromil is more effective than either drug alone. Montelukast may be effective for up to 24 hours. Salmeterol and formoterol may block exercise-induced bronchospasm for up to 12 hours. One study has evaluated single-dose bronchoprotective effects of salmeterol given through a Babyhaler spacer device using a methacholine provocation challenge in infants younger than 4 years with recurrent episodes of wheezing.[79] Originally, 42 preschool children (age range 8–45 months) received one of the 25-, 50- or 100-mcg doses of salmeterol and a placebo dose 2 to 7 days apart in a randomized, double-blind fashion, but only 33 completed the study. The investigators found a dose-dependent bronchoprotective effect of salmeterol measured by treatment-to-placebo methacholine dose ratios. Significant improvements from placebo were found only for the 50-mcg (2.5-fold) and 100-mcg (4-fold) doses.

Issues Related to the Delivery of Medications to Infants and Small Children

Unique challenges exist relating to the delivery of medications (both oral and inhaled) to infants and young children with asthma. Obviously, liquid preparations are tolerated by infants, but chewable tablets and pills can be consumed by toddlers. Montelukast is available as oral granules or chewable tablets, and prednisone and prednisolone come in either liquid formulations or orally disintegrating tablet preparations. With regard to inhaled medications, certain anatomic and physiologic characteristics of children younger than 6 years are worth considering. First, because infants display preferential nasal breathing and have small airways, low tidal volume, and high respiratory frequency, delivery of the drug to the lower airways is often inadequate.[80] Second, it is difficult if not impossible for young children to perform the maneuvers specified for optimal delivery of aerosol therapy, such as slow inhalation through the mouth with a period of breath-holding for pMDIs or rapid and forceful inhalation required in the case of dry-powder inhalers (DPIs). Third, delivery devices appropriate for the young child are limited to those that require minimum cooperation from the child and allow ease of administration for the caregivers. Although at present there are at least three inhaled aerosol delivery systems available for older children and adults, only two are used in this age group: the nebulizer and the pMDI with spacer/holding chamber and facemask. Because of the reliance on the patient's ability to generate a sufficient inspiratory flow and overcome the resistance required of DPIs, preschool-age children are unable to use them.

Within these two general types of delivery systems there are numerous products available that vary widely in performance. The pMDI with spacer or holding chamber is portable and inexpensive, takes less time to administer, and is likely to be better tolerated than delivery with a nebulizer. Dolovich and colleagues[81] published a comprehensive systematic review to determine if device selection affects clinical efficacy and safety. Randomized placebo-controlled trials that involved various devices for the delivery of β agonists, ICSs, and anticholinergic agents in different clinical settings (e.g., emergency department, inpatient, intensive care, and outpatient) and patient populations (i.e., pediatric and adult asthma, and patients with chronic obstructive pulmonary disease) were included. A meta-analysis comparing inhaled β-agonist nebulizer versus MDI with spacer/holding chamber in patients (0–17 years) seen in an acute care setting showed no significant differences between the two techniques for symptom scores or lung function measures. This, along with their other analyses using other medications in different settings and patient populations, indicated that the drugs delivered by different formats are equally effective. Appropriate technique, cooperation, and convenience determine which delivery may be best.

Asthma clinical guidelines mention the use of inhaled SABA by either pMDI or nebulizer as an initial asthma exacerbation home intervention.[6,7] The GINA global strategy recommends the use of SABA by pMDI (ideally with a spacer) for home management of mild, moderate, and severe exacerbations. GINA also recommends nebulized treatments for severe exacerbations at home and for hospital-based management of acute asthma.[7]

Data in young children clearly support the use of β agonists, at higher doses, administered with a pMDI with spacer for acute asthma.[82,83] In a study of 60 children between 1 and 5 years of age hospitalized for an asthma exacerbation, Parkin and co-workers[82] found salbutamol (400–600 mcg, 4–6 puffs, based on weight) and ipratropium bromide (40 mcg, 2 puffs), both delivered by pMDI with an AeroChamber and mask, to be as effective as nebulized salbutamol (0.15 mg/kg) and ipratropium bromide (125 mcg) administered over 15 minutes by facemask.[82] However, nearly one-third of the subjects randomized to MDI eventually required a nebulized β agonist.

Two studies have evaluated lower respiratory tract deposition of a radiolabeled salbutamol and albuterol mixture administered to young children. Tal and associates[84] showed that, on average, less than 2% of the nominal dose of the albuterol given by a pMDI with a spacer and mask to children younger than 5 years was deposited in the lower respiratory tract, with most of the drug remaining in the spacer.[84] Wildhaber and associates[85] compared the lung deposition of radiolabeled salbutamol from a nebulizer and a pMDI and spacer in 17 children with asthma ages 2 to 9 years. Both devices were delivering roughly 5% of the nominal dose to the lower airways. Because of the larger doses of salbutamol administered via the nebulizer (2000 mcg versus 400 mcg) than the pMDI, a larger amount of drug was deposited in the

airways using the nebulizer (108 mcg versus 22 mcg, respectively). In addition, both devices were approximately 50% less efficient in children younger than 4 years than in older children.

In general, β-agonist administration by nebulization is probably a more practical delivery system for most infants and young children with severe acute asthma because it requires the simple technique of relaxed tidal breathing, particularly if it is difficult to use a tight-fitting spacer and mask for a pMDI. In addition, oxygen can be used to power the nebulizer, providing β agonist and supplemental oxygen simultaneously, and it does offer the capability to administer a controller agent and rescue β agonist at the same time.

With respect to controller therapy, the only available inhaled drugs that are FDA approved for children under 4 years of age are cromolyn solution and budesonide suspension intended for nebulization. However, a pMDI with a spacer device is certainly more convenient and easier to administer for many children. The GINA global strategy prefers the administration of ICSs by a pMDI with a spacer and either a facemask (for 0–3 years of age) or a mouthpiece (for 4 years or older) for young children with asthma, but the dose delivered is variable between spacers.[7] These guidelines mention the use of nebulizers as an alternative delivery system for children who are unable to use the spacer device effectively. Because young children are expected only to perform tidal breathing, the optimal number of breaths to empty the spacer device varies with the tidal volume, dead space, and volume of the device. Important measures to maximize delivery of medication to very young children include enforcing a tight-fitting mask around the child's mouth and nose, encouraging immediate inhalation after actuation, allowing five or six breaths per single pMDI actuation, making sure that the spacer valve is moving when the child is breathing through the spacer, shaking the inhaler in between actuations, and using a lower volume spacer (<350 mL) in these very young children.

The Montreal Protocol, adopted in 1987, mandated a complete elimination of the chlorofluorocarbon (CFC) propellant because of concerns about its damaging effect on the ozone layer. Since 2008, pMDIs now contain hydrofluoroalkane (HFA). However, the pMDI HFAs (even rescue SABA) are approved for use only in children 4 years of age and older. There is no information available on the relationship between lung deposition from HFA pMDI and clinical efficacy or even long-term safety in small children. In addition, no studies exist comparing inhaled medications administered via nebulizer and HFA pMDI with a spacer and mask.

Additional factors that should be considered are the costs to the patient (including use of spacer attachments, which are not reimbursable) and the use of multiple delivery devices, which requires more time for the clinician staff to educate families on proper techniques. To address both issues, perhaps the same type of device can be used for all inhaled drugs for an individual patient. The decision should also incorporate which device the clinician is capable of teaching properly and what the patient/parent prefers. When a child presents with uncontrolled asthma, the assessment should first focus on technique and adherence.

Adherence

The issue of adherence in infants and small children is complicated because the child is entirely dependent on the caregiver to administer the medication. In an observational study of preschool children, Gibson and associates[86] sought to evaluate adherence with inhaled prophylactic medications delivered through a large-volume spacer using an electronic timer device. Adherence was only 50%, with a range of 0% to 94%. In addition, only 42% of the subjects received the prescribed medication on each study day, and reporting of symptoms in the diary cards did not correlate with good compliance with the prophylactic medication, nor was a correlation found between frequency of administration and adherence. In another study, parental reporting of symptom scores correlated with measured bronchodilator use in only 63% of preschool children.[87]

A few studies have attempted to determine why caregivers are unable to administer medications as prescribed. Lim and co-workers[88] asked parents why they were reluctant to administer prophylactic medications (such as ICSs) to their young children with asthma. Reasons cited included hesitancy to use medications for fear of dependence, side effects, and overdosage. Fortunately, patient education programs developed for parents of small children with asthma improve asthma morbidity and self-management outcome.[89,90]

Nonpharmacologic Intervention

Nonpharmacologic measures may be as important not only for young children with established respiratory symptoms, allergies, and passive smoke exposure but also in the primary and secondary prevention of asthma.[91–93] These interventions as they relate to prevention of asthma development are discussed in more detail in Chapter 29. The first and likely the most important step toward controlling asthma in sensitized children is to avoid or reduce the patient's exposure to the offending allergen(s). The environmental interventions that seem to hold the most promise are those that target reducing exposure to indoor allergens and tobacco smoke. Specific environmental control measures are covered in Chapter 15.

Yearly influenza immunization is also strongly recommended for children 6 months of age and older with chronic pulmonary diseases, including asthma. Kramarz and colleagues[94] evaluated the effectiveness of influenza vaccination in preventing influenza-related asthma exacerbations in children 1 to 6 years of age using a retrospective cohort study with the Vaccine Safety Datalink, which contains data on more than 1 million children enrolled in four large health maintenance organizations.[94] Of note, less than 10% of children with asthma were vaccinated against influenza in any of the years studied. Although the incidence rates of asthma exacerbation in those who were vaccinated were found to be higher in the vaccinated group than in those who were not vaccinated, the difference was thought to be largely confounded by asthma severity in the vaccinated group. Using a self-control analysis to correct for this confounder, the risks of asthma exacerbation during each of the influenza seasons were reduced by 22% to 41% with influenza vaccination.

Management of Asthma Exacerbations in Young Children

Exacerbations, also commonly referred to as *episodes* or *flare-ups*, are acute deterioration of asthma control characterized by increased wheezing or shortness of breath or coughing (especially while the child is asleep), sudden change in child's activity or performance (lethargy or lack of interest or exercise intolerance or feeding), poor response to or sudden increased need for rescue medication, and breathing difficulty or respiratory distress at its worst. In this age group, these are often preceded by upper respiratory tract symptoms or viral syndrome. From a post hoc analysis of diary data

obtained from children 2 to 5 years of age who participated in a 12-week trial for persistent asthma, the combination of increased daytime cough and wheeze, and nighttime inhaled rescue β-agonist use predicted 70% of exacerbations a day later (defined as requiring oral corticosteroid, emergency room or unscheduled visit, or hospitalization), with only 14% false positive rate.[95] The most effective approach in managing asthma exacerbations involves early recognition of warning signs and early treatment. An action plan should be provided to the family members or caregivers that includes information about what medications to give, medical provider's contact information and when to seek urgent medical attention (e.g., with signs of acute distress, symptoms unrelieved by bronchodilator, increased need for rescue treatment or repeated use of bronchodilator more often than every 3 hours, when relief period is becoming shorter, in children younger than 1 year of age, and repeated inhaled SABA rescue use over several hours).[7] A copy should also be given to daycare providers and school personnel.

Home Management

Early treatment of asthma exacerbations may prevent a life-threatening event or a hospital admission. Initial treatment should be with a SABA (e.g., albuterol or levalbuterol): 2 puffs (200 mcg albuterol) from an MDI via a spacer device with or without a facemask, which may be repeated every 20 minutes 2 more times, or a single treatment can be given by nebulizer (0.05 mg/kg [minimum dose, 1.25 mg; maximum, 2.5 mg] of 0.5% solution of albuterol in 2–3 mL saline; or 0.075 mg/kg [minimum dose, 1.25 mg; maximum, 5 mg] of levalbuterol).[6] If the response is good, as assessed by sustained symptom relief, the SABA can be continued every 3 to 4 hours for 24 to 48 hours. Patients should be advised to seek medical care once excessive doses of bronchodilator therapy are used or for prolonged periods (e.g., >6 puffs of inhaled SABA are used within the first 2 hours, >12 puffs/day for >24 hours, or if the child has not recovered after 24 hours).[6,7]

If the child does not completely improve with the initial therapy, the SABA should be continued, and the caregiver should contact the physician urgently. If the child experiences marked distress, the caregiver should give the SABA immediately and bring the patient to the emergency department or call 911 or another emergency number for assistance. Treatment with an oral corticosteroid initiated by family members can be considered, but evidence for its early use is debatable.[96] Doubling the dose of inhaled corticosteroids has not been proved sufficient to prevent worsening of exacerbations. However, studies in small children with viral-induced wheezing not on regular controller therapy have shown benefits of preemptive high-dose ICS at the early onset of a respiratory illness in preventing the need for systemic corticosteroid.[97] This should be considered only if the family can apply this judiciously and side effects can be monitored closely. One study has shown the efficacy of starting a short course of montelukast at the onset of a respiratory tract illness in small children with episodic wheezing with respect to reducing symptom burden, healthcare usage, and time off work.[76] However, in one trial, children 12 to 59 months of age who had at least two moderate to severe wheezing episodes requiring an urgent care visit and/or systemic corticosteroid course in the context of a respiratory tract illness within the past year were randomized to receive one of the following for 7 days at the onset of symptoms: budesonide inhalation suspension (1 mg twice daily), montelukast group (4 mg once daily), or conventional rescue bronchodilator therapy. Neither budesonide nor montelukast initiated at early signs of illness increased the proportion of episode-free days over a 1-year period, nor was there a differential effect on oral corticosteroid rescue, asthma healthcare usage, or quality of life.[98] Nevertheless, both budesonide and montelukast demonstrated modest reductions in symptom severity score (e.g., wheezing, trouble breathing, or activity limitation) relative to conventional therapy, particularly among children with positive API or prior oral corticosteroid use. Perhaps this benefit from a short course of an LTRA at reducing symptom burden may be expected only in young children who have atopic risk factors.

Management in the Emergency Department or Hospital

Clinical assessment is used, and scoring systems (e.g., Preschool Respiratory Assessment Measure [PRAM] and the Pediatric Asthma Severity Score [PASS]) have been developed to assess the severity of asthma exacerbations.[99] Severe exacerbations are characterized by any one of the following: altered mental state (e.g., agitated, confused, or drowsy), oxygen saturation less than 92%, tachycardia (i.e., >200 beats/min for 0–3 years old; >180 beats/min for 4–5 years old), retractions, cyanosis, and "silent" chest (i.e., wheeze inaudible).[7] Immediate transfer to a hospital is required when any of those features is found or there is lack of response to 6 puffs of inhaled SABA over 1 to 2 hours, or persistent tachypnea despite three doses of SABA, even if the young child shows other signs of improvement. Functional assessment of a young child's degree of airflow limitation is impractical, but oxygen saturation should be obtained. Chest radiographs are not recommended routinely but should be considered to rule out pneumothorax, pneumomediastinum, pneumonia, or atelectasis.

Initial treatment can be with a SABA by inhaler (albuterol, 2–6 puffs) or nebulizer (minimum dose 2.5 mg) every 20 minutes for 3 doses. If symptoms improve, albuterol 4-8 puffs MDI or 0.15-0.3 mg/kg up to 10 mg every 1-4 hours as needed can be given. Levalbuterol can also be used as an alternative short acting beta agonist bronchodilator treatment (nebulized minimum dose 1.25 mg) every 20 minutes for 3 doses, then 0.075-0.15 mg/kg up to 5 mg every 1-4 hours as needed. Oxygen should be given to maintain oxygen saturation above 93%.[6,7] For moderate to severe exacerbations, ipratropium bromide (80 mcg, 2 puffs or 0.25 mg by nebulizer), up to three doses in the first hour only. Adjunctive therapies include intravenous magnesium sulfate (single dose 40–50 mg/kg, maximum 2 g by slow infusion over 20–60 minutes).[7] The use of isotonic magnesium sulfate by nebulization (150 mg, three doses in the first hour) as an add-on treatment for children as young as 2 years of age with severe exacerbation was found beneficial for those with more severe presentation in the presence of oxygen saturation below 92% and with symptoms lasting less than 6 hours.[100]

For impending or ongoing respiratory failure, epinephrine 1:1000 (1 mg/ml, 0.01 mg/kg up to 0.3—0.5 mg every 20 minutes for 3 doses) or terbutaline (0.01 mg/kg every 20 minutes for 3 doses then every 2—6 hours as needed) may be administered subcutaneously. Per GINA 2019, if inhalation is not possible, an intravenous bolus of terbutaline (2 mcg/kg) may be given over 5 minutes, followed by continuous infusion of 5 mcg/kg/hour. Close monitoring is imperative and dose should be adjusted according to clinical course and adverse effects. Children may need ventilatory support with 100% oxygen, intravenous corticosteroids, and admission to an ICU. Further treatment is based on clinical response and objective laboratory findings.

If symptoms do not respond to the initial bronchodilator treatment, continuous albuterol nebulization (0.5 mg/kg/hour) can be started, and the patient should be admitted for closer observation.

If symptoms improve but recur within 3 to 4 hours, more frequent inhaled bronchodilator and oral corticosteroids should be given. The child should be observed in the emergency room.

If symptoms resolve quickly after initial bronchodilator treatment and remain stable for 1 to 2 hours, SABA every 3 to 4 hours can be administered. If symptoms persist beyond 24 hours, additional treatment such as inhaled or oral corticosteroids can be provided.[7]

For children who have already been prescribed maintenance therapy, the controller medication should be continued, and increasing the dose of ICS only during the episodes is not effective. For those who are not on controller medication, a medium- to high-dose ICS given for 5 to 10 days or even for a few weeks or months, may reduce oral corticosteroid requirement. Again, side effects should be monitored over time.

Systemic corticosteroids (oral prednisolone 1–2 mg/kg/day; maximum of 20 mg/day for <2 years of age, 30 mg for children 2–5 years of age or dexamethasone 0.6 mg/kg, or intravenous methylprednisolone 1 mg/kg every 6 hours)[7] should be instituted if the child responds poorly to therapy at 1 hour or continues to deteriorate, if symptoms recur within 3 to 4 hours, if symptoms persist beyond 1 day, or if the child has recently been on oral corticosteroids. Reduced risk of hospitalization when systemic corticosteroids are given in the emergency room setting and not in an outpatient setting was found. Usually a 3- to 5-day course of prednisolone or once-daily dose of dexamethasone for 1 to 2 days is sufficient.[101]

An intramuscular corticosteroid before emergency room discharge also may be given, particularly if the young child would not tolerate oral medications. Sensitivity to adrenergic drugs may improve after initiation of corticosteroids.

Hospitalization should be strongly considered for any child with a history of respiratory failure. It is also appropriate if symptoms improve by the first hour but still require at least 10 inhalations of SABA within a 3- to 4-hour period. The decision to hospitalize should also be based on presence of risk factors for mortality from asthma, duration, and severity of symptoms, course and severity of previous exacerbations, medication use at the time of the exacerbation, access to medical care, and home and psychosocial conditions and exposure. Maintenance fluids and electrolyte requirements (both corticosteroids and β_2 agonists can cause potassium loss) should be provided, especially because these young children are likely to have poor oral intake secondary to respiratory distress or vomiting. They require intensive monitoring because overhydration may contribute to pulmonary edema associated with high intrapleural pressures generated in severe asthma. Antibiotics may be necessary to treat co-existing bacterial infection.

Criteria for discharging young children home should include a sustained response of at least 1 hour to bronchodilator therapy. The child should also be ambulatory according to age expectation, comfortable, and able to retain food or liquids.[7] Before discharge the caregiver's ability to continue therapy and assess symptoms appropriately needs to be considered because children with a recent exacerbation are at risk of recurrent episodes. The caregiver should be given an action plan for management of recurrent symptoms or exacerbations, identification of triggers and how to avoid them, and instructions about rescue and controller medications and their proper use. Hospitalized patients should receive more intensive education before discharge. This is another opportunity to review inhaler technique. The inhaled SABA and oral corticosteroids should be continued, the latter for 3 to 7 days. Finally, the caregiver should be instructed about the follow-up visits, which should take place within 1 or 2 days and again within 1 to 2 months. Referral to an asthma specialist should be considered for all children with severe exacerbations or multiple emergency department visits or hospitalizations.

Conclusion

Chronic cough and recurrent wheezing, typical manifestations of asthma, are quite common in young children, yet these symptoms render different long-term outcomes and, acutely, can be quite concerning. For those with a more persistent pattern, controller therapy is indicated. A significant subset have a severe, intermittent course, and for these patients daily controller therapy may still be beneficial. However, recent studies have suggested the efficacy of as-needed high-dose inhaled corticosteroid started at the onset of a respiratory illness, particularly in very young children who have atopic risk factors. The development of persistent asthma and requirement for long-term controller therapy in a very young child can be predicted to a limited degree. Currently no clinically easily available objective and reliable measure of lung function, BHR, or airway inflammation exists that is applicable to this age group; thus, monitoring the effects of interventions or treatment on prevention of asthma inception, modulation of underlying inflammation, perhaps airway remodeling, prevention of deterioration in lung function over time, and induction of physiologic or immunologic remission is not feasible. The need to evaluate objectively the efficiency and safety of the various delivery devices and HFA formulation available for inhaled therapies to infants and young children remains. Only a few medications have been approved for use in this population, and especially for those with more severe disease that is more life threatening and requires healthcare use. Given that these young children have a shorter duration of disease, they may be more responsive to disease-altering interventions such as immunomodulators or biologic therapy.

Helpful Websites

The National Heart, Lung, and Blood Institute; website (http://www.nhlbi.nih.gov/guidelines/asthma/asthgdln.htm)

The Global Initiative for Asthma; website (https://ginasthma.org/gina-reports/)

The reference list can be found on the companion Expert Consult website at http://www.expertconsult.inkling.com.

24

Inner City Asthma: Strategies to Reduce Mortality and Morbidity

MEYER KATTAN

KEY POINTS

- Racial and ethnic minorities and children with low socioeconomic status living in urban communities have a disproportionate burden of asthma morbidity, mortality, and healthcare use.
- Successful interventions targeting inner city children with asthma must be multifactorial and take into account access to care, social, environmental, and behavioral factors.
- Community linkages, epidemiologic evaluation, self-management, decision support, and improved patient-provider communication are essential ingredients of asthma management programs.

- It is important to determine individual risks and tailor asthma interventions in the context of the physical and social environments.
- Translation of successful evidence-based interventions into practice presents a challenge that requires evaluation and feedback from those implementing these interventions at the community level.

Introduction

Wide variations exist in the prevalence of childhood asthma worldwide, ranging from less than 1% to as high as 37%.[1] The National Health Interview Survey in 2017 reported that the current asthma prevalence is 8.4% in children under 18 years of age in the United States. Small area analyses have demonstrated the asthma period prevalence rate in poor urban communities in the United States to be twice the national prevalence rate.[2] The current asthma prevalence rate of children living below 100% of the poverty level is 11.7% compared with 6.8% in children living 450% above the poverty threshold. There is variation in prevalence among ethnic groups. Puerto Rican children living in the Northeast United States reported some of the highest prevalence rates.

Interventions aimed at primary prevention of asthma in inner city children are lacking. Longitudinal birth cohort studies are underway that may drive novel interventions. These studies will increase our understanding of the interaction of prenatal factors, viral infections, environmental tobacco smoke (ETS), microbiome, epigenetics, obesity, and stress in the development of asthma.

Disparities in morbidity in addition to prevalence are evident. Hospitalization rates and emergency department (ED) visits are highest in poor urban areas.[3,4] Reviews of asthma disparities find that African American and Hispanic children who live in low-socioeconomic urban environments experience higher morbidity and mortality than white children.[5,6]

Racial and ethnic minorities that are socioeconomically disadvantaged and disproportionately affected by asthma live predominantly in densely populated urban areas.[7] These so-called "inner cities" are not uniform in many of their characteristics. The differences include housing stock, climate, environmental exposures, race, and ethnicity. As a result of the documented disparities in asthma morbidity, the inner cities have been the focus of studies to determine the characteristics of these areas that contribute to high prevalence and morbidity and develop interventions.

The relationship of race/ethnicity, environment, and socioeconomic status (SES) to asthma morbidity is complex. The hospital readmission rate for asthma is twice as high in African Americans than in whites. In an attempt to characterize the racial disparities, one study found that traditional SES measures coupled with financial and social hardship explained 50% of the readmission rate.[8] Behavioral factors and patterns of care also determine asthma outcome. Jones and colleagues[9] demonstrated that minority children with wheeze were nearly twice as likely as white children to have used urgent care for asthma, after controlling for disease severity, access to care, and environmental factors.[9] Puerto Rican children had more clinic visits for asthma but spent fewer days in the hospital for asthma than African American children.[10] Health beliefs may differ among various cultures. Ethnic minorities with low incomes might regard asthma as less serious than other pressing problems of life.[11] Low parental expectations and competing family priorities are associated with poor asthma control. In a multivariate analysis that included these factors in the analytic model, the association between race/ethnicity and poor asthma control was not significant.[12] In summary, a variety of interrelated factors contribute to morbidity, and multifaceted tailored interventions are more likely to succeed.

Challenges to Asthma Management

Despite the existence of effective disease control strategies and medications, asthma remains a major public health problem. Morbidity, direct and indirect healthcare costs, and mortality continue to impose a high burden. Individual asthma care is only one component of effective asthma control. Psychosocial and environmental factors are important determinants of asthma outcome. Interventions must identify breakdowns in multiple pathways to optimize outcomes (Fig. 24.1).

Evidence indicates that establishment of a successful asthma management program entails a logical progression through specific developmental stages, starting with political/stakeholder endorsement and commitment, followed by epidemiologic evaluation, evaluation of disease burden, evaluation of access to care and best therapy, and finally optimization and maintenance therapy for individual patients.[13,14] Applying a model embodying these concepts in an inner city setting for patients with chronically poorly controlled asthma resulted in sustained improvement in asthma control in adolescent patients. The interventions implemented included delivery system redesign to provide standardized and evidence-based care, productive interactions between informed patients and prepared

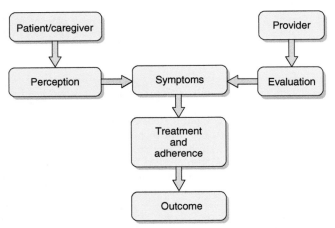

• **Fig. 24.1** Interaction between patient/caregiver and provider. Inaccurate reporting of symptoms or inadequate assessment can lead to suboptimal treatment and poor outcome.

clinicians, self-management support, community linkages, clinical information systems, and decision support.[15]

Factors Contributing to Morbidity in Inner Cities (Table 24.1)

Asthma Knowledge and Patterns of Care

Guidelines recommend that asthma self-management education should be integrated into all aspects of asthma care, but it is important to note that knowledge does not always translate into change in behavior. The National Cooperative Inner-City Asthma Study (NCICAS) found that although caregivers of inner city children had reasonably good asthma knowledge, they had difficulty giving responses that could be helpful in asthma management when they were given hypothetical vignettes.[16] Caregivers' expectations regarding their ability to manage the child's asthma are predictive of the child's functional status, suggesting that attitudes play a role in determining the child's asthma outcome.[17] Low parental involvement and delays in recognizing symptoms and initiating therapy are also associated with poor outcomes. Patients and caregivers tolerate poor symptom control and possess inadequate knowledge of correct drug usage.[18] Language barriers between provider and patient or caregiver contribute to underreporting of symptoms and suboptimal communication.[19]

Among urban minority children with asthma, lack of primary health care was associated with a higher risk of hospitalization compared with those children with a greater number of visits.[20] Difficulty finding care outside the ED for exacerbations despite having a usual source of primary care results in fragmented care.[21]

Adherence

Overall estimates for adherence to medications in children are about 50%[22,23] (Box 24.1). In urban minority adolescents, asthma prevention and management behaviors were suboptimal, with only 36% of those prescribed medication for persistent asthma reporting taking medications daily.[24] Adherence to an asthma management program involves use of controller medication, appointment keeping, and applying an emergency plan of action. Barriers to adherence may exist in any of these areas, leading to ineffective control of asthma.[25] Concern about side effects, cultural beliefs, and negative caregiver beliefs regarding efficacy of medications provide the rationale for limiting or discontinuing the use of medications.[25–27] Smith and associates[12] reported that suboptimal asthma control and controller medication underuse were highly associated with potentially modifiable risk factors,

TABLE 24.1	Factors Contributing to Asthma Morbidity in Children of Lower Socioeconomic Status				
Access to Care	**Environment**	**Host**	**Psychosocial**	**Adherence**
Underdiagnosis	Allergens	Genetics	Maternal factors	Child/caregiver
Undertreatment	Irritants	Obesity	Child factors	Healthcare provider
Availability of specialty care		Asthma knowledge	Stress	
Insurance			Violence	
			Housing	

• BOX 24.1 **Predisposing Factors for Poor Adherence**

- Insufficient asthma knowledge
- Inability to translate knowledge into practice
- Negative beliefs about medications
- Cultural beliefs about medications
- Low parental expectations for symptom control
- Competing priorities
- Suboptimal communication between parent and healthcare provider

---

especially low parental expectations for functioning and symptom control, discordant estimation of asthma control, lack of routines for administering medication, and concerns about asthma medications.[12] Complementary and alternative medicine use is highest in black, poor, lesser educated parents, and children with persistent asthma.[28]

The level of responsibility for asthma management increases with age.[16] However, older children may still be ill equipped to manage the illness independently.[29] A complicating factor is that there is discordance between the caregiver and the child regarding responsibility for the management of the child's asthma.[16]

Access to Care

Lack of adequate health insurance is an important barrier to healthcare services for children in the United States. Diagnosis and treatment of asthma are related to healthcare coverage.[30] However, some evidence suggests that asthma-related healthcare differences across groups might exist independently of financial barriers.[11,21] Access to care from asthma specialists is reduced for those who are poor and belong to an ethnic minority. Primary care physicians have been slower to adopt asthma guidelines than specialists.[31] Physicians under-prescribe controller medication for inner city children despite guidelines recommending the use of antiinflammatory medications for persistent asthma.[32] Furhman and colleagues[33] reported that children with asthma hospitalized for an exacerbation had experienced consistently poorly controlled asthma during the previous year. They were under-treated and insufficiently educated about asthma. However, physician adherence to guidelines will not translate into appropriate treatment without attention being paid to caregiver-physician communication.

Psychosocial Factors

Behavioral and psychosocial factors can affect asthma morbidity.[34] There are variations in asthma morbidity in neighborhoods with low SES. This indicates that asthma morbidity cannot be explained solely by economic factors and that community factors may be important. Exposure to violence was independently associated with asthma morbidity after simultaneous adjustment for income, employment status, caregiver education, housing problems, and other adverse life events, which suggests that exposure to violence is not merely a marker for these other factors. Increased exposure to violence predicts increased symptomatology in a graded fashion.[35] Children spend more time indoors because of fear of violence, which could potentially increase exposure to indoor allergens and irritants. Inner city school children with asthma whose primary caregivers perceived the neighborhood to be unsafe had an increased likelihood of poorly controlled asthma, increased use of rescue medication, more limitation in activity,

and more nighttime symptoms compared with participants living in safe neighborhoods.[36]

The mental health of children and caregivers is a significant factor in predicting asthma morbidity. In NCICAS, caregiver mental health as assessed by the Brief Symptom Inventory revealed that children of caregivers who had psychological symptoms were almost twice as likely to be hospitalized for asthma.[37] In inner city adolescents, stressful life events and anxiety were associated with morbidity and quality of life independent of environmental exposures and sociodemographic factors.[38,39] Interventions that do not address psychosocial issues may have limited impact.

Indoor Environmental Exposures

Attention to the indoor environment is of particular importance because children living in urban areas spend approximately 70% of their time indoors, where they are exposed to irritants, pollutants, allergens, and endotoxin.[40]

Exposure to ETS in children with asthma living in inner cities is high. Studies in inner cities report that more than half of children with asthma have one or more smokers in the household and over one-third of primary caregivers of children with asthma are smokers.[21] Measurement of cotinine levels in children reveal even higher levels of personal exposure ranging from 38% to 69%.[21,41,42] African American children are more likely to be exposed than Latino children.[41,42] A conceptual model developed to investigate pathways explaining asthma severity in inner city children reported a significant effect of ETS exposure on asthma severity.[43]

Particulate matter (PM) is a major source of indoor air pollution in inner city homes. Indoor concentrations of PM are related to combustion products and variation in ventilation and air filtration.[44,45] Penetration of particles from outdoor sources contributes about 25% of the indoor concentration.[46] In the Inner-City Air Pollution (ICAP) study the mean indoor value of fine PM ($PM_{2.5}$) in smoking homes was 46.5 $\mu g/m^3$ compared with 17.8 $\mu g/m^3$ in nonsmoking homes. Frying, smoky cooking events, burning incense, and cleaning activities such as sweeping are additional sources of PM.[45] Indoor PM is associated with an increase in asthma symptoms and rescue medication use.[47–49]

Nitrogen dioxide (NO_2) is a by-product of combustion sources. Household appliances fueled by gas such as gas stoves or kerosene heaters are the major sources of indoor NO_2.[50] Gas stoves are commonly found in inner city homes.[51] Ventilating with exhaust fans reduces indoor NO_2 levels significantly, but the majority of households in the NCICAS did not have proper venting. Measurements in inner city households demonstrate high indoor concentrations of NO_2, often exceeding the U.S. Environmental Protection Agency outdoor standard (53 ppb).[51,52] Asthmatic children exposed to NO_2 indoors are at risk for increased asthma morbidity.[51–53] NO_2 increases the risk of asthma exacerbations after respiratory infections, even at relatively low levels of exposure.[54]

Allergens can be produced from pests (e.g., mites, cockroaches, rodents), pets (e.g., cats, dogs), plants (i.e., pollen), and fungi (i.e., mold spores). Cockroach, mice, and mold are prevalent in urban areas, but there are geographic variations in exposures and sensitization.[55–57]

Exposure to indoor allergens among sensitized patients with asthma is associated with greater asthma severity and increased healthcare utilization. In sensitized children, indoor exposures to total fungi and to *Penicillium* spp. were associated with significant increases in unscheduled visits, even after controlling for outdoor fungal levels.[58] Children exposed and sensitized to cockroach had more days of wheeze, unscheduled doctor visits, and hospitalizations compared with those children who were only exposed, only sensitized, or neither exposed nor sensitized.[59] Among those who were sensitized and exposed to both cockroach and mouse, mouse appeared to be the stronger driver of worse asthma.[60] Cat, cockroach, rodent, and house dust mite exposure in children has been associated with asthma exacerbations in a dose-dependent fashion.[59,61]

Outdoor Environmental Exposures

Higher levels of ambient air pollutants are associated with increased asthma morbidity.[62,63] PM (<10 μm [PM_{10}] and <2.5 μm in aerodynamic diameter [$PM_{2.5}$]) is a collection of mostly inorganic pollutants that has been associated with adverse respiratory effects and exacerbations of asthma. $PM_{2.5}$ can penetrate deep into the lung. Ozone, NO_2, and $PM_{2.5}$ can induce airway inflammation and airway hyperresponsiveness. Wu and co-workers demonstrated that near-roadway PM produced higher levels of inflammatory cytokines interleukin 6 (IL-6), IL-8, and tumor necrosis factor-alpha (TNF-α) than urban background PM.[64]

Many children in inner cities live in close proximity to highways and businesses that rely on high volumes of truck traffic. Exacerbations of childhood asthma were attributed to exposure to pollutants related to road traffic. There is an increasing risk of adverse respiratory outcomes and asthma exacerbations with increasing exposures to diesel exhaust emissions related to road traffic in children with asthma.[65]

Obesity

There has been a parallel rise in the prevalence of obesity and asthma over the last few decades. Blacks and Hispanics experience higher rates of obesity than whites. Low SES is also associated with higher rates of obesity.[66,67] Studies show an association between obesity and asthma prevalence and severity. Over one-third of children with asthma living in inner cities were obese compared with 17% of the general population of children in the United States.[68] In a longitudinal study, obesity was associated with poorer asthma control in females.[68] Lu and colleagues[69] reported that in an urban, predominantly African American population, the effects of indoor $PM_{2.5}$ and NO_2 exposure on asthma symptoms were greater in overweight and obese than children and adolescents of normal weight.[69]

Interventions

Interventions have been developed and implemented in a variety of settings, including EDs, hospitals, clinics, schools, and home. The approaches include educational interventions aimed at patients and their families or healthcare providers, specific medical interventions, case management, and environmental control strategies. The limitations of studies of interventions are that the majority have not been subjected to randomized controlled clinical trials, have small sample sizes, are not culturally sensitive, or do not examine the cost-effectiveness. The importance of a proper study design to assess new interventions is underscored by the fact that there is a significant improvement in outcome in children with asthma enrolled in control arms of these trials.[70] Therefore,

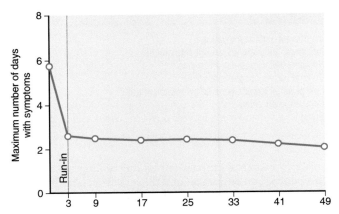

• **Fig. 24.2** Response to guideline-based care. The graph shows symptom days per 2 weeks averaged over 1 year in adolescents in a control arm of a study given guideline-based care. (Modified from Szefler SJ, Mitchell H, Sorkness CA, et al. Management of asthma based on exhaled nitric oxide in addition to guideline-based treatment for inner-city adolescents and young adults: a randomised controlled trial. Lancet 2008;372(9643):1065–72.)

caution needs to be exercised in interpreting results of efficacy studies that use a pre-post study design.

Medical Intervention

Currently available medications for the management of asthma used according to published guidelines and with good adherence and follow-up are highly effective in controlling asthma symptoms in inner city children. A guideline-based approach improved asthma control in several studies enrolling subjects with moderate to severe asthma.[71,72] For example, Fig. 24.2 demonstrates that adolescents in a control arm of a study receiving guideline-based care improved quickly and maintained control over the course of the 1-year treatment period. Some children and adolescents continue to experience exacerbations, particularly during the fall months, despite good control of symptoms indicating the need for novel and personalized approaches. The Asthma Phenotypes in Inner-City study found that the most symptomatic children with asthma receiving high Step–level treatment had the highest total serum immunoglobulin (IgE) level, blood eosinophil count, and allergen sensitizations. Knowledge of phenotypes may help guide therapy as new drugs for asthma become available.

Immunomodulatory therapy such as omalizumab (anti-IgE), dupilumab (IL–4 and IL–13 antibody), mepolizumab (anti–IL–5), and benralizumab (IL-5 receptor antibody) is an important approach to treatment, particularly in those with an allergic asthma phenotype. Omalizumab is the only one of these medications that has been studied in an inner city population.[73] The Inner-City Asthma Consortium (ICAC) demonstrated that omalizumab added to guidelines-directed treatment started before the start of the school year and continuing for only 4 months reduced the frequency of viral-induced asthma exacerbations in the fall.[74] Given the high cost of biologics, this short-term therapy may provide a more cost-effective approach in children as young as 6 years of age. A limitation of omalizumab is that dosing is based on a combination of IgE level and weight. The prevalence of obesity and elevated IgE is high in inner city communities. In ICAC, 27% of children were ineligible to receive the medication because they were outside the recommended dosing range.[73]

Dupilumab was shown to reduce asthma exacerbations, improve symptom scores, and improve lung function, and mepolizumab was shown to reduce asthma exacerbations but not symptoms.[75,76] Benralizumab improved asthma symptoms and lung function and reduced exacerbations.[77] The data on the use of these biologics in children are limited.

Emergency Department Interventions

Use of the ED for children with asthma living in inner cities is high. Previous ED visits are strong predictors of subsequent ED visits.[78] Interventions targeting these high-risk children might be expected to have an impact on asthma morbidity. Several strategies have been studied, but the results have been conflicting.

A three-part ED-based intervention, including asthma screening, viewing an educational video addressing beliefs, and a mailed reminder, did not improve follow-up or outcomes.[79] A randomized trial by Teach and colleagues[80] evaluated a single comprehensive follow-up visit after ED discharge that included education, initiating controller medications, and scheduling a follow-up visit with a primary care provider. The intervention improved asthma treatment adherence, symptom control, quality of life, and healthcare use in this population of urban, largely disadvantaged, and minority children. It decreased the rate of unscheduled visits for asthma during the entire 6-month follow-up period. There was no effect of the intervention on follow-up with the primary care provider. A review of studies comparing usual care for asthma to more intensive educational programs concluded that asthma education aimed at children and their caregiver who present to the ED for acute exacerbations resulted in lower risk of future ED visits and hospital admission. It remained unclear as to what type, duration, and intensity of educational packages were the most effective in reducing acute care utilization.[81] A Joint Task Force Report reviewing ED interventions recommended among other things that patients seen in the ED should have a follow-up appointment with a primary care physician or asthma specialist made before leaving the ED and if possible get a telephone reminder.[82]

School-Based Interventions

Various strategies have been used in school-based interventions, but few have been subjected to randomized controlled clinical trials. Many programs have had trouble fully implementing their plans because school staff, healthcare providers, and parents find it difficult to commit sufficient time and effort to establish new patterns of cooperation. The success of school-based programs for asthma depends on a partnership with families and the healthcare system.[83,84] Individual schools have different capabilities to deal with school health in general and with asthma in particular. The strategy to improve asthma outcomes that is most likely to succeed in a particular school will be dependent on the resources that each component of the partnership can contribute.[85,86]

In a randomized study evaluating supervised asthma therapy in urban schools, Gerald and colleagues[87] reported improved asthma control among urban school children in a predominantly African American population in Alabama. A modified program did not improve asthma control compared with usual care in a predominantly Mexican American population.[88] In addition to administering medication in school, Halterman and co-workers[89] made guideline-based dosage adjustments and gave a home-based ETS reduction program for smoke-exposed children.[89] Compared with usual care, the program improved asthma symptoms and decreased exacerbations.

Another strategy is to focus on self-management skills. Evans and associates[90] provided self-management education in inner city elementary school children. The program emphasized the child's responsibility for recognizing symptoms and taking appropriate management steps. Children in treatment schools had increased management skills, fewer symptoms of asthma, and improved school performance. A school-based intervention for adolescents used both group and tailored individual sessions and included education for their medical providers. Relative to control subjects, students in the intervention group reported more confidence to manage their asthma; taking more steps to prevent symptoms; greater use of controller medication; and fewer symptoms, acute care visits, hospitalizations, and school absences because of asthma.[91]

School-based mobile clinics have been used in several cities in the United States. The model attempts to reduce barriers to delivering effective care to underserved children with asthma. The mobile clinics are staffed by specialty trained asthma providers and integrate strategies for case identification, community outreach, continuity of care, structured healthcare encounters, and patient tracking. Comparison of pre-year and post-year data for subjects enrolled in the program for at least 1 year revealed reductions in the percentage of patients reporting ED visits, hospitalizations, and missed school days.[92]

Provider-Targeted Interventions

Despite the findings that adherence to guidelines by providers is suboptimal, there are few rigorously designed trials of interventions aimed at providers in inner cities. A systematic review of provider interventions concluded that decision support tools, feedback and audit, and clinical pharmacy support were most likely to improve provider adherence to asthma guidelines, as measured through healthcare process outcomes.[93]

Training of staff in clinics providing care to inner city minority children coupled with administrative support for change in practice behavior increased the number of patients with asthma receiving continuing care and improved the quality of care they received compared with control clinics.[94] Health outcomes were not reported. Easy Breathing is an asthma management program instituted in primary care clinics serving inner city communities. The program had a positive effect on clinicians' knowledge and adherence to asthma guidelines as evaluated using a pre-post study design.[95]

The Inner City Asthma Study (ICAS) evaluated a decision support system with feedback to providers.[96] An automated computer program provided information regarding current symptoms, unscheduled visits for exacerbations, and medication use to the child's primary care physician along with guideline-based treatment recommendations. Children whose primary care physicians received these computerized letters had more follow-up care visits, received increased treatment more rapidly when warranted, and had fewer ED visits.

A computerized decision support tool for pediatric asthma management that standardizes assessment and treatment steps can improve control among high-risk inner city children enrolled in clinical trials and can be clinically adapted to the electronic health record.[97]

Environmental Interventions

Asthma guidelines recommend reducing exposure to relevant allergens and irritants to reduce inflammation, symptoms, and need for medication. Environmental control represents a financial and practical burden for both patients and society. Successful approaches need to set realistic goals that account for limitations imposed by the inner city setting. Necessary resources may not be available for optimal environmental control. For example, only 38% of homes in NCICAS had functioning vacuum cleaners.[98] Current approaches include integrated pest management, which consists of filling cracks with copper mesh, vacuuming, putting away or disposing of food, rodent traps, and application of low-toxicity pesticides to control cockroach and mice infestation, fitting impervious mattress and pillow encasings, or running an air filter.[99,100]

Krieger and associates[101] used community health workers to provide in-home environmental assessments, education, support for behavior change, and resources. The intervention reduced asthma symptom days and urgent health services use while improving caregiver quality-of-life score.

The ICAS implemented a multifaceted home-based environmental intervention for inner city children with asthma. Intervention was tailored to each patient's sensitization and environmental risk profile, using a series of modules to reduce home allergen exposure.[102] In this randomized trial, the individualized intervention reduced exposures to cockroach, mouse, and dust mite allergens and resulted in significantly fewer symptom days during the intervention year and during the year after intervention.[71,103] A multifaceted allergen avoidance study by Carter and colleagues[104] studied the effect of avoidance of dust and cockroach in a group of inner city children with asthma. Although there was no overall improvement in the intervention group compared with the control group, significant reduction in acute visits for asthma was demonstrated for mite-allergic children who had a significant decrease in exposure to mite allergen. DiMango and colleagues[105] demonstrated that environmental control measures in allergen-exposed and sensitized individuals effectively reduced levels of all measured household allergens (i.e., roach, mouse, dust mite, cat, and dog), but did not lead to stepping down asthma controller therapy compared with a control group receiving a home visit that did not target allergies and asthma. The Mouse Allergen and Asthma Intervention Trial (MAAIT) compared professional integrated pest management and education to education alone in inner city children exposed and sensitized to mouse.[106] The trial found no significant difference in symptom days between the intervention and control groups. However, in both the DiMango and MAAIT trials, participants in control and intervention groups had reduction in allergen exposures and symptoms that could have resulted in an underestimation of the benefits of the interventions. Of note, across both intervention and control groups, both studies showed a dose-response relationship between mouse allergen reduction and asthma control.

Rabito and co-workers[107] reported a simpler approach targeting cockroach infestation with bait insecticide. This resulted in sustained cockroach elimination and improved asthma outcomes, suggesting that a single allergen intervention may be an alternative to multifaceted interventions.

Butz and associates[108] randomly assigned children with asthma residing with a smoker to interventions consisting of air cleaners only, air cleaners plus a health coach, or a control group receiving delayed air cleaner. The use of air cleaners resulted in a reduction in indoor PM concentrations and an increase in symptom-free days but did not reduce air nicotine or urine cotinine concentrations.

Technology-Based Interventions

Interactive computer applications for asthma have met with limited success. A review of studies using these applications concluded that the applications improve knowledge but do not change behavior or asthma outcomes.[109] Emerging health information technologies designed to improve patient-physician communication have been used in inner city populations. Among children and adolescents in a low-income, urban population, a text messaging intervention compared with usual care was associated with a modest improvement in the rate of influenza vaccination.[110] Smartphone applications to monitor peak flow or asthma symptoms are available, but their use has not been evaluated in controlled clinical trials. The technologies are developing rapidly and have the potential of delivering targeted interventions to individuals.[111] An important barrier to overcome with interventions requiring daily monitoring or daily diaries is decreased compliance with monitoring over time that has been observed in inner city children with asthma.[112]

Multifactorial Interventions

A Cochrane review suggested that culture-specific education programs for children from minority groups are effective in improving asthma-related outcomes of quality of life, asthma knowledge, and rate of asthma exacerbations and asthma control.[113] The first phase of NCICAS demonstrated that multiple factors are responsible for asthma morbidity, including adherence, access to care, and physician undertreatment. Other risk factors involve the living conditions, social welfare, and mental health issues of the family. These risk factors may interfere with the ability of the family to give enough attention to the child's asthma. It also became apparent that asthma management was not the responsibility solely of the physician but of the family as well. For an intervention in the inner city to succeed, it must address a variety of risk factors, not all of which would be the same among individuals.

The asthma counselor intervention program developed by NCICAS used social workers to empower families to increase asthma self-management and improve their communication with primary care providers. A risk profile was prepared for each child based on assessments of skin test sensitivities, environmental exposures, psychosocial factors, difficulty accessing care, exposure to pets or smoking, and other factors. The multifactorial intervention was tailored to each child using specific modules, each of which addressed specific risk factors. This tailored intervention approach was found to be highly effective in reducing asthma symptoms among the children.[114]

Walders and associates used an interdisciplinary intervention consisting of a written asthma treatment plan, asthma education, an asthma risk assessment, problem-solving, and access to a 24-hour nurse advice line.[115] The intervention group did not show evidence of reduced asthma symptoms or improved measures of quality of life beyond the changes demonstrated by the comparison group. However, the interdisciplinary intervention group had less frequent healthcare usage for asthma over the course of the 1-year follow-up period.

Home-based educational interventions may improve asthma outcomes among inner city children. A home-based intervention using asthma counselors modeled after the NCICAS intervention and culturally adapted for Puerto Rican families found no significant differences in symptom-free days between the intervention and control groups, although significant reductions were observed in symptom-free nights, ED visits, and hospitalizations.[115] Otsuki and colleagues[116] demonstrated that multiple home visits by trained asthma educators reviewing medications, identifying barriers, and discussing beliefs and concerns led to improved adherence and decreased morbidity compared with usual care.

Asthma coaching by lay workers increased asthma monitoring visits but were not associated with fewer ED visits. The heterogeneity of outcomes in inner city populations may be due to intervention design or the background of the individuals providing the counseling and education. Maintaining contact can be a challenge, but the use of text messaging rather than telephone contact has become a more efficient method of reaching families. Accommodating parent and child schedules can also enhance retention in education programs.

Community-Wide Asthma Coalitions

Community-wide asthma coalitions are collaborative efforts at the local level to achieve asthma control by bringing together diverse stakeholders that include healthcare providers, grassroots groups, voluntary and government agencies, and business and industry who collectively implement strategies to improve asthma outcomes. The results are mixed.

Fisher and co-workers[117] evaluated a neighborhood asthma coalition in St. Louis, Missouri. The coalition included educational programs for parents and children, promotional activities, and individualized support provided by trained neighborhood residents. Acute care rates decreased for both the coalition and control groups from the year before intervention to the last year of intervention but with no significant differences between the coalition and control groups.

Allies Against Asthma is a group of community-based coalitions working to improve asthma outcomes in vulnerable children. The evaluation of the program indicated that mobilizing diverse stakeholders and focusing on policy and system changes can generate significant reductions in healthcare use for vulnerable

children with asthma.[118] What is evident is that results from the asthma coalitions are not instantaneous but become evident over the long term.

Conclusions

The management of asthma in inner cities presents a challenge that requires participation of multiple stakeholders. Major challenges to preventive asthma care are encountered by inner city children and include family and patient attitudes and beliefs, lack of access to quality medical care, and psychosocial and environmental factors. The myriad factors contributing to morbidity are interdependent. It is evident that a "one size fits all" approach is unlikely to be successful. There are lessons to be learned from the characteristics of successful interventions. It is important to assess individual risk factors. Programs require flexibility so that elements can be tailored to the individual. Guideline-based care will not succeed unless attention is paid to psychosocial and societal issues that are barriers to care. For example, a family with good asthma knowledge may not be able to overcome barriers such as no access to after-hours clinics or lack of insurance coverage for spacers.

The interventions outlined in this chapter demonstrate that positive outcomes can be achieved. The challenge is to translate research into practice. An attempt to disseminate the NCICAS asthma counselor model at 22 sites across the country by the Centers for Disease Control and Prevention exemplifies some of the difficulties. Implementation varied among sites. Retention was related to type and location of the sites, ease of obtaining written plans, language and ethnicity of the asthma counselor, and availability of onsite allergy testing.[119] A report from the Merck Childhood Asthma Network discussed the adaptation of evidence-based interventions at five sites and documented the site-to-site variations in fidelity to the original interventions.[120] More real-world data on implementation and barriers are needed from those implementing community interventions, to refine programs and reduce morbidity.[121]

The reference list can be found on the companion Expert Consult website at http://www.expertconsult.inkling.com.

25

Asthma in Older Children: Special Considerations

JEFFREY R. STOKES, LEONARD B. BACHARIER

KEY POINTS

- Childhood asthma is increasing in prevalence because of a combination of genetic and environmental factors.
- Pulmonary function testing is essential in managing children with asthma.
- Asthma may not be optimally controlled if comorbid conditions such as sinusitis, allergic rhinitis, gastroesophageal reflux disease, and vocal cord dysfunction are not effectively managed.
- The current management profile focuses on the most effective therapies in reducing asthma exacerbations and achieving asthma control.

- For school-age children with mild persistent asthma, a daily inhaled corticosteroid (ICS) is the preferred therapy, whereas adolescents can use either daily ICS or as-needed ICS with formoterol.
- For children with moderate and severe asthma, ICS with a long-acting β agonist (LABA) medications are the first-line therapy.
- In addition to medium- to high-dose ICS/LABAs, the patient with severe asthma may require biologic therapy or tiotropium to reduce asthma exacerbations.

Epidemiology and Etiology

Prevalence of Childhood Asthma

Asthma is the most common chronic lung disease of childhood in the United States, affecting over 6 million children. In the United States, from 1980 to 2016, asthma prevalence in the general population increased from 3.1% to 8.3%, with increases noted among children 5 to 11 years of age to 9.6% and children 12 to 17 years of age to 10.5%.[1] In 2016, nearly 54% of children with asthma had experienced at least one asthma exacerbation, with 16.7% making an emergency department (ED) or urgent care visit and 4.7% requiring hospitalization.[1]

Factors Influencing the Cause of Asthma

A general pattern of multiple factors influencing development of asthma seems to be emerging, including family history and genetics, smoking, diet, obesity, and inactivity, all of which influence the development of asthma and disease outcomes (Table 25.1).

Socioeconomic Status

Income is a determinant of access to health care and frequently the quantity and quality of health care available. Persons who have low income, regardless of race or ethnicity, are more likely to be underinsured or uninsured, to encounter delays in receiving or be denied care, to rely on hospital clinics in EDs for health services, and to receive substandard care.

Many clinical and population studies have reported substantially higher rates of asthma prevalence, morbidity,

hospitalization, and mortality among racial and ethnic minorities. However, asthma is also more common among low-socioeconomic groups regardless of race. One potential factor is exposure and sensitization to allergens common in urban environments. Litonjua and colleagues[2] concluded that a large proportion of the racial/ethnic differences in asthma prevalence can be explained by factors related to income, area of residence, and level of education. Similarly, Fitzpatrick and associates[3] noted that racial differences in ED use for asthma were minimized when other factors, such as community factors, family socioeconomics, and environmental exposures were considered.

Genetics

The genetic basis of the well-known heritability of asthma has been extensively studied and, although the genetic basis of asthma remains incompletely understood, studies are yielding some understanding[4,5] (see Chapter 3). There is no currently established genetic pattern that predicts the development of asthma or defines its severity.

Allergy

Studies of school children in Melbourne, Australia, by Williams and McNicol[6] have indicated increases in both the incidence of asthma and asthma severity with increases in number of positive skin tests and total serum immunoglobulin E (IgE). The relationship between allergy and asthma has been highlighted by the importance of aeroallergen sensitivity in the progression of frequent intermittent wheezing to persistent

TABLE 25.1	Factors That Influence Disease Development and Severity	
Factor	Disease Development	Disease Severity
Atopy	++++	++++
Allergen exposure	++	++++
Rhinitis	++	++
Sinusitis	?	+++
Infection (viral)	++	++++
Gastroesophageal reflux	–	++
Environmental factors		
Intrauterine tobacco smoke	++	?
Passive tobacco smoke	+	++
Air pollution	+	++
Psychological factors (including stress)	+	++++
Socioeconomic status	++	++++
Adherence	–	++++
Obesity	Adolescent females	++
Diet	?	?
Exercise	?	++*
Drugs (including ASA/NSAIDs)	–	++†

*Although exercise is a common precipitant of asthma symptoms, improved physical conditioning can reduce asthma severity.

†Consider in the context of asthma, nasal polyposis, and severe sinus disease.

ASA, Acetylsalicylic acid (aspirin); NSAIDs, nonsteroidal antiinflammatory drugs.

asthma in young children.[7] Several large epidemiologic studies have clearly indicated the importance of aeroallergen sensitization in asthma development among populations at risk. In particular, the importance of early-life allergic sensitization to multiple aeroallergens as a risk factor for subsequent asthma has been demonstrated among children in the Manchester Allergy and Asthma Study and the Wayne Tri-County Health & Environmental Allergy Longitudinal Study (WHEALS) cohort.[8,9]

Demographic and Environmental Factors

Studies comparing the populations of East and West Germany showed the prevalence of hay fever and asthma to be significantly higher in West German children, suggesting that environmental factors may explain the difference in prevalence in these ethnically similar populations.[10] Early exposure to infections (e.g., being in a daycare environment early in life) or exposure to endotoxin or other bacterial products (e.g., growing up on a farm with close exposure to the farm animals) is associated with a lower prevalence of asthma. In contrast, growing up in an urban environment or generally with a higher standard of living is associated with an increased prevalence of asthma.[11]

Gene and Environment Interaction

Genetic factors alone cannot explain the temporal rises in asthma prevalence, morbidity, or mortality.[12] However, a small change in the prevalence or extent of relevant environmental exposures could explain a significant rise in disease prevalence among genetically susceptible individuals. Gene and environment interaction, defined as the co-participation of genetic and environmental factors, is particularly relevant to the cause of asthma morbidity, particularly in individuals who experience a disproportionate burden of environmental exposures, and may exert its effect through epigenetic mechanisms.[13,14] Relevant exposures include smoking, stress, nutritional factors, infections, allergens, and occupational exposures.

Stress

Evidence for a link between stress and asthma has been gained from temporal studies, because experiencing an acute negative life event increased children's risk for an asthma attack 4 to 6 weeks after the occurrence of the event.[15] Moreover, the combination of chronic and acute stress plays a role in the temporal association. Experiencing an acute life event among children who had ongoing chronic stress in their lives shortened the time frame in which they were at risk for an asthma attack to within 2 weeks of the acute event. Further, high levels of stress have been associated with detrimental biologic profiles, such as greater inflammatory responses after antigen challenge or in vitro stimulation of immune cells among children with or at risk for asthma.[16,17]

Obesity

Obesity is linked with the development and severity of asthma in both children and adults, and weight reduction improves asthma severity and symptoms.[18,19] The relationship between obesity and asthma observed in adults also has been most often observed in adolescent females, but not in males. Girls who were overweight or obese at age 11 years were more likely to have current wheezing at ages 11 and 15 years but not at ages 6 to 8 years. The relationship between obesity and asthma is strongest among females beginning puberty before the age of 11 years. Females who become overweight or obese between 6 and 11 years are seven times more likely to develop new asthma symptoms at ages 11 and 13 years.[20] The mechanism of increased asthma with obesity is not clear. The strong gender differences observed suggest that overweight status itself does not produce the asthma, because a direct effect of weight is not seen in both boys and girls.[20,21]

Infection

Viral respiratory infections are present in up to 85% of children with exacerbated asthma.[22] In addition to worsening asthma, there may be a more fundamental relationship between infection and the development of asthma. Infants hospitalized with respiratory syncytial virus bronchiolitis are at increased risk of asthma at school age, and this risk appears to persist to early adulthood.[23–26] In addition, wheezing in the context of rhinovirus infection during the preschool years is also a significant risk factor for asthma at school age[27] (see Chapter 22).

Natural History of Asthma

Persistence and Progression of Disease into Adulthood

The course of asthma through childhood and adolescence is variable (see Chapter 2). Among children with mild to moderate asthma during the school-age period, 26% may experience clinical

TABLE
25.2

TABLE 25.2 Differential Diagnosis for Asthma

Condition	Clinical Features
Bronchopulmonary dysplasia	Premature birth, symptoms since birth
Primary ciliary dyskinesia	Recurrent upper and lower airway infections, ~50% dextrocardia
Congenital heart disease	Cardiac murmur
Chronic upper airway cough syndrome	Sneezing, nasal congestion, post-nasal drip
Cystic fibrosis	Excessive cough and mucus production, gastrointestinal symptoms, chronic sinusitis
Bronchiectasis	Productive cough, recurrent infections
Inhaled foreign body	Sudden onset of symptoms
Vocal cord dysfunction	Dyspnea, stridor

remission by early adulthood.[28] More severe asthma is likely to persist from childhood into adulthood without remission, with only 15% of children with severe asthma experiencing remission by 50 years of age.[29] Another important tendency in the natural history is for symptoms to markedly improve or remit in adolescence only to return again in adulthood. In general, the amount of wheezing in early adolescence seems to be a guide for severity in early adult years, with 73% of those with few symptoms at 14 years of age continuing to have little or no asthma at age 28 years.[30] Although many children become asymptomatic in adolescence, pulmonary function deficits associated with asthma and wheeze increase throughout childhood.[31] A longer duration of asthma was associated with lower levels of lung function in children with mild to moderate asthma aged 5 to 12 years.[32] Lung growth, as reflected by forced expiratory volume in 1 second (FEV_1), is affected by even mild to moderate asthma, because approximately 75% of such patients experience abnormal lung growth through reduced growth and/or early decline in lung growth, with evidence of significant airflow obstruction by early adulthood.[33]

Differential Diagnosis of Asthma

The differential diagnosis of cough and wheeze is extensively reviewed in Chapter 27. Common conditions such as with recurrent cough and wheeze in school-age children and adolescents are listed in Table 25.2.

Evaluation

Fig. 25.1 presents an algorithm for evaluation of a school-age child or adolescent who presents with chest symptoms of recurrent cough, wheeze, shortness of breath, chest tightness, or chest pain.

History

Historical elements should include specific symptoms, their frequency and severity, triggering factors, and response to therapy. Age of onset of symptoms is important, because 80% of patients with asthma experience symptoms within the first 5 years of life. Because asthma is a disorder characterized by repeated episodes of at least partially reversible airflow obstruction, failure of symptoms to improve with treatment, including bronchodilators and corticosteroids, should prompt evaluation for other processes, either a nonasthma diagnosis or a comorbid condition complicating underlying asthma.

Additional history should focus on identification of other comorbid conditions that may worsen asthma severity and symptom burden, including allergen exposure, rhinitis, sinusitis, and gastroesophageal reflux. Furthermore, an assessment of underlying psychosocial factors and adherence to the medical regimen may provide valuable clues as to barriers in delivery and receipt of asthma care.

A short series of questions focusing on recent symptom frequency is extremely informative in assessing the child with asthma. Validated questionnaires, such as the Asthma Control Test (ACT), Childhood Asthma Control Test (c-ACT), and Asthma Control Questionnaire (ACQ), serve this purpose and when completed at each follow-up asthma visit can serve as a rapid appraisal of asthma control over time (Box 25.1).[34,35]

Physical Examination

Outside of periods of acute symptoms or exacerbations, many patients with asthma have normal chest examinations. Findings may include an increased anteroposterior chest diameter in severe disease and expiratory wheezes and prolongation of the expiratory phase during exacerbation. Presence of nasal polyposis should prompt an evaluation for cystic fibrosis, regardless of the age of the child, because cystic fibrosis remains the leading cause of polyps in childhood. The primary focus of the examination should include careful evaluation to ensure absence of findings suggestive of other diseases, such as the presence of crackles, digital clubbing, and hypoxemia, and to uncover factors that worsen disease, including nasal and sinus disease.

Laboratory Evaluation

Peripheral blood eosinophilia and/or elevated serum IgE levels are often found in children with asthma and may be helpful in the evaluation of severe disease. A cross-sectional analysis of a birth cohort of 562 children studied at 11 years of age found that bronchial hyperresponsiveness significantly correlated with higher levels of total serum IgE.[36] Burrows and co-workers[37] found a close relationship between total serum IgE and both the severity and persistence of bronchial responsiveness in a longitudinal study of adolescents and adults.[37] Laboratory evaluation is helpful in excluding entities that make up the differential diagnosis of asthma. Serum immunoglobulin levels (i.e., IgG, IgM, and IgA) and specific antibody responses may be helpful in evaluating for defects in humoral immunity predisposing to recurrent lower respiratory tract illness. Sweat chloride or *CFTR* mutation analysis is required to exclude cystic fibrosis. Children with bronchiectasis along with chronic otitis media and sinusitis may warrant an evaluation of ciliary structure and function. A purified protein derivative (PPD) skin test is helpful in excluding mycobacterial infection.

Assessment for Allergic Sensitization

Evaluation for allergen-specific IgE by either percutaneous skin testing or in vitro testing should be part of the evaluation of all children with persistent asthma, because proper identification of allergic sensitivities and instruction in environmental control measures may provide significant clinical benefit.

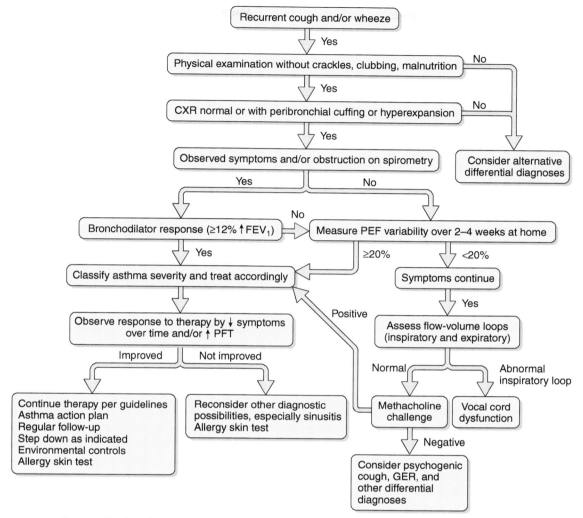

• **Fig. 25.1** Algorithm for establishing diagnosis in children with recurrent cough and wheeze. *CXR,* Chest x-ray; *FEV$_1$,* forced expiratory volume in 1 second; *PEF,* peak expiratory flow; *PFT,* pulmonary function test; *GER,* gastroesophageal reflux.

Exposure and allergic sensitization to cockroach allergen was associated with a significantly greater risk of asthma hospitalization and greater healthcare usage among 476 children aged 4 to 9 years who participated in the National Cooperative Inner-City Asthma Study.[38] Allergic sensitization to the mold *Alternaria* has been identified as a significant allergen in terms of increasing airway hyperresponsiveness and was associated with a nearly 200-fold increased risk of respiratory arrest because of asthma, emphasizing the importance of determining underlying allergic sensitivities in patients with asthma and providing patients with accurate and practical advice on allergen avoidance techniques.[39,40]

The Childhood Asthma Management Program, comprising 1041 children ages 5 to 12 years with mild to moderate asthma, found that allergic sensitization to tree pollen, weed pollen, *Alternaria* spp., cat dander, dog dander, or indoor molds was associated with greater airway hyperresponsiveness to methacholine, although only sensitivity to dog and cat dander and the outdoor fungus *Alternaria* spp. had independently significant relationships.[41] Together these findings further the importance of identifying and controlling these allergens in attenuating asthma symptoms.

Radiology

All children with recurrent episodes of cough and/or wheeze should have a chest radiograph (anteroposterior and lateral views) to aid in exclusion of other diagnostic entities. Although many children with asthma have normal chest radiographs, radiographic findings that may be seen with asthma include hyperexpansion, increased anteroposterior diameter, peribronchial cuffing, and/or areas of atelectasis (any lobe or subsegment can be involved). Findings of chronic changes, including bronchiectasis, should lead to further evaluation of alternative diagnoses.

Pulmonary Function Tests

With the help of well-trained and experienced pulmonary function technicians, children as young as 3 to 4 years of age should be capable of performing spirometry. Spirometry measures forced vital capacity (FVC), FEV$_1$, the ratio of FEV$_1$/FVC, and other measures of airflow, including the forced expiratory flow between 25% and 75% of FVC (FEF$_{25-75}$). The FEV$_1$ is the most commonly used and reproducible measure of pulmonary function, whereas the FEF$_{25-75}$ demonstrates much more intrapatient variability. Standards are widely available for most spirometric measures and allow for correction for patient age, gender, race, and height. The FEV$_1$/

Childhood Asthma Control Test (c-ACT)

- Ages 4 to 11
- Maximum score 27
- Seven questions: four for child and three for parent
- Review of the last 4 weeks
- Score of 19 or less: not well controlled re-evaluate asthma therapy
- Score of 20 or greater: greater-controlled asthma
- Minimally important cut-off (scores that reflect meaningful change for the patient): 2

Asthma Control Test (ACT)

- Age 12 years and older
- Maximum score 25
- Five questions for patient
- Review of the last 4 weeks
- Score of 19 or less: not well controlled re-evaluate asthma therapy
- Score of 20 or greater: greater-controlled asthma
- Minimally important cut-off (scores that reflect meaningful change for the patient): 3

Asthma Control Questionnaire (ACQ)

- Age 12 years and older
- Five, six, or seven questions (three different versions)
- Review of the last week
- Each question 0 to 6 scale (0 = asymptomatic)
- Mean score 1.5 or greater: re-evaluate asthma therapy
- Mean score 0.75 or less: well-controlled asthma
- Minimally important difference (scores that reflect meaningful change for the patient): 0.5

FVC ratio is an indicator of airflow obstruction and may be more sensitive in identifying airflow abnormalities in asthma than the FEV_1, because most children with asthma have an FEV_1 within the normal range, even in the presence of severe disease.[42]

Asthma is characterized by airflow obstruction that is at least partially reversible by a bronchodilator. Thus, spirometry is often performed before and 15 to 20 minutes after administration of a bronchodilator such as albuterol. An increase in the FEV_1 of at least 12% is considered to represent a significant change and exceeds that seen in individuals without asthma, although evidence suggests that lower levels of bronchodilator response ($\geq 8\%$) may be more appropriate cut-offs in identifying asthma in children.[35,43] It should be noted that many children with asthma do not demonstrate a bronchodilator response when well (i.e., outside of periods of exacerbation), and thus the absence of such a response does not exclude asthma as a diagnosis.

Particular attention should be given to the inspiratory and expiratory flow-volume loops because they are extremely helpful in excluding other patterns of airway obstruction.[44,45] For example, fixed airway obstruction (abnormalities on both the expiratory and inspiratory loops) can be seen with a mediastinal mass compressing a large airway or variable extrathoracic airway obstructive processes (i.e., abnormalities just on the inspiratory loop) is seen with vocal cord dysfunction (VCD). Asthma produces variable intrathoracic obstruction (i.e., abnormalities on just the expiratory loop). Patients with VCD without asthma do not demonstrate intrathoracic airway obstruction but may show blunting or truncation of the inspiratory loop consistent with variable extrathoracic obstruction. Variability between spirometric trials is not uncommon in patients with VCD, often consisting of normal and abnormal inspiratory loops during a single session.

In addition to spirometry, other tests of pulmonary function may aid in the evaluation of the child with asthma that is difficult to diagnose or control (see Chapter 21). Patients with asthma generally demonstrate normal total lung capacity (TLC) on lung volume testing by plethysmography but may demonstrate evidence of air trapping, as shown by elevated residual volumes (RV) and RV/TLC ratio. Measurement of diffusing capacity of carbon monoxide (DL_{CO}) is normal in patients with asthma, and abnormalities in DL_{CO} should prompt evaluation for interstitial lung diseases.

Fractional exhaled nitric oxide (FeNO) is a noninvasive marker related to eosinophilic airway inflammation, as reflected by bronchial wall inflammation, sputum eosinophilia, and airway hyperresponsiveness. FeNO levels increase as asthma control deteriorates and decrease with treatment with agents that reduce airway inflammation, including inhaled corticosteroids (ICSs) and leukotriene receptor antagonists (LTRAs).[46–55]

Challenge Testing

Some children present with atypical features of asthma and may pose greater challenges in confirming an asthma diagnosis. Thus, use of bronchial challenges with agents that provoke bronchoconstriction (including methacholine, exercise, or inhalation of cold dry air) may be helpful in the diagnosis and management in the child with atypical symptoms, poor response to asthma medications, or lack of response to a bronchodilator during spirometry. Challenge studies should be performed in laboratories familiar with such procedures.

Bronchoscopy

In children with particularly severe disease, with atypical features such as chronic sputum production, or with poor response to conventional therapy, direct visualization of the airways along with bronchoalveolar lavage (BAL) may provide important clinical information. Such examinations may reveal the presence of previously undiagnosed foreign body aspiration or other intrinsic airway mass, infection, extrinsic airway compression, evidence of chronic aspiration or infection, and indicators of airway inflammation (such as eosinophilia or neutrophilia).

Comorbid Diseases

Rhinitis

Rhinitis is common in children with asthma, with estimates of up to 80% of patients with asthma reporting upper airway symptoms. Whereas most rhinitis that worsens asthma is allergic, perennial rhinitis in individuals without atopy can be a risk factor for more severe asthma.[56] Topical nasal corticosteroid therapy for allergic rhinitis has been shown to attenuate the increase in bronchial hyperresponsiveness during the grass pollen season and decrease the risk of ED visits or hospitalizations for asthma.[57–59] Thus, treatment plans for patients with asthma and allergic rhinitis should consist of optimal management of concomitant allergic rhinitis (see Chapter 24).

Sinusitis

Sinusitis is often implicated in the search for factors responsible for an overall worsening of asthma unexplained by changes of environment or other obvious historical features. Although many patients present with symptoms of upper airway disease along with asthma, some have sinusitis as a significant contributor to difficult-to-control asthma but with a paucity of symptoms suggestive of sinusitis.

Gastroesophageal Reflux

Gastroesophageal reflux (GER) is common among patients with asthma. In adults with asthma, the estimated prevalence of GER approaches 80%.[60] Most children and adolescents with GER do not report symptoms classically associated with GER in adults, including heartburn, chest pain, dysphagia, or hoarseness. In fact, children rarely complain of symptoms even in the presence of significant GER demonstrated by pH probe studies. Studies of the prevalence of GER in pediatric patients with asthma are limited, but a reported 43% incidence of a positive pH probe study in a group of 115 children with asthma without symptoms of GER suggests that asymptomatic GER also may be present among children with asthma.[61] However, a trial in children with persistent asthma without symptoms of GER did not demonstrate a benefit of gastric acid suppression with omeprazole in terms of asthma symptom control, even among children with evidence of GER by pH probe study.[61]

Environmental Exposures (Including Tobacco Smoke)

Passive exposure to tobacco smoke is a clear exacerbating factor in asthma, with increases in asthma prevalence and asthma severity among children exposed to parental smoking.[62] Maternal smoking is associated with small but statistically significant, and probably clinically important, deficits in pulmonary function among school children. Most smokers begin smoking during the adolescent years; therefore, active personal tobacco smoke exposure must be considered in all adolescents with asthma, especially when the clinical course becomes more severe. Cigarette smoking has been reported to be associated with mild airway obstruction and slowed growth of lung function in adolescents without asthma.[63] Furthermore, asthma has been linked to an accelerated rate of decline in FEV_1 over time, and this rate is even greater among asthmatic individuals who smoke.[64]

Vocal Cord Dysfunction

VCD, a functional respiratory tract disorder resulting from paradoxical adduction of the vocal cords, complicates the diagnosis and management of common respiratory tract problems, including asthma.[65] The recognition of VCD in a patient with atypical or difficult-to-control asthma is critical in minimizing symptoms and potential side effects associated with treatment of severe asthma. The symptoms of VCD are not unique to the disorder and include cough, wheeze, stridor, dyspnea, hoarseness, and choking. Some patients report difficulty swallowing or tightness in the chest or throat. Patients with VCD often report difficulty "getting air in" because of paradoxical adduction of the vocal cords during inspiration, in contrast to difficulty with exhalation as reported by patients with asthma. However, patients with significant exacerbation of asthma do have diffuse airway narrowing and can have significant inspiratory limitation, which can dominate their perception of breathing difficulties. Cough is a common feature of VCD and must be differentiated from cough because of asthma or from postnasal drainage resulting from rhinosinusitis. Patients with VCD frequently complain of tightness in the throat and/or chest and may speak in a hoarse voice. Nocturnal symptoms are uncommon in uncomplicated VCD, but may occur in patients with both VCD and asthma. Exercise is a frequent precipitant of both VCD and asthma. In our experience, a combination of speech therapy and psychological evaluation is necessary for successful therapy for VCD. Maintenance therapy for VCD includes minimization of medication use for comorbid conditions frequently confused with VCD (i.e., asthma).

Psychological Factors

Psychological factors may be as, or even more, important than medical factors in determining outcomes of asthma, particularly in children with more severe asthma. School performance and gross and fine motor coordination, although generally in a normal range overall, correlated with psychological functioning but not the medical characteristics of the asthma.[66,67] Depression symptoms, cigarette smoking, and cocaine use occurred more frequently in youth reporting current asthma than in youth without asthma.[68] These results indicate a need to screen adolescents with asthma for depression.

Poor Adherence to the Medical Regimen

Most patients receive suboptimal benefit from any given prescribed asthma regimen. This is often reflected as inadequate asthma control and often leads to prescription of higher doses or additional controller medications based on the assumption that the medication prescribed accurately reflects the medication the patient actually takes. However, because most patients miss substantial amounts of medications, even when participating in research studies examining medication adherence, practitioners must focus on patient education regarding the importance of asthma medication use as directed and provision of a written plan of action that is practical for the patient.[69] Thus, the action plan for each child must be individualized based on the child's developmental stage. Although children begin to acquire basic asthma decision-making abilities by the age of 8 years, they remain unable to manage their asthma independently until about 16 years of age. Promoting adherence and effective self-management of asthma is discussed in detail in Chapter 28.

Obesity

Weight reduction in obese patients with asthma has been associated with improvement of lung function and other indicators of lung status.[70] Recognition that obesity may produce respiratory symptoms that mimic, but do not actually represent, asthma is essential to avoid inappropriate and unnecessary escalations of asthma therapy.[71]

Exercise

Exercise-induced asthma (EIA) may lead to decreased participation in physical activities because of either exertional limitation or fear of symptom development. This may explain the finding that children with asthma are less physically fit than their peers without asthma.[72] Despite these facts, asthma should not be perceived as a limitation on physical fitness, as evidenced by the prevalence of asthma among Olympic athletes approximating twice that of the general population.[73] Increased aerobic fitness decreases EIA because better conditioned individuals require smaller increases in heart rate and ventilation for a given task.[72]

Goals of Asthma Care

The goals of asthma care are to achieve asthma control, reflected by a minimization of symptom burden (including the frequency of daytime and nighttime symptoms, reliever medication, and activity limitation), attain optimal lung function, and reduce the future risk of adverse outcomes such as exacerbations or medication side effects. Asthma symptoms such as cough, wheeze, shortness of breath, chest tightness, and exertional limitation can vary in frequency and intensity. Validated tools, such as the c-ACT, ACT, and ACQ, can be used to identify and monitor the level of asthma control and track response to therapy over time[74,75] (see Table 25.1).

Prevention of exacerbations should remain a focus of management because exacerbations can be severe and occasionally fatal.

Risk factors for exacerbations include uncontrolled asthma symptoms, short-acting β agonist (SABA) use of three or more canisters per year, having one or more exacerbations in the previous 12 months, history of intubation for asthma, low baseline lung function, greater bronchodilator reversibility, and poor adherence to controller medications.[76]

When asthma is not well controlled, consideration of factors such as inhaler technique, medication and treatment regimen adherence, potential comorbidities, and barriers to care should occur before altering therapy. Most patients (up to 80%) do not use their inhalers correctly, and at least 50% of patients do not take controller medications as prescribed.[77] Improvement in symptoms for most controller medications begins within days of treatment, whereas peak benefit may take 3 to 4 months to achieve. Children should be seen every 1 to 3 months after starting or modifying therapy and every 3 to 12 months thereafter. It is important to review response to therapy and assess the patient at each visit, adjusting medications, either increasing or decreasing, depending on the overall assessment of control and other relevant factors such as season of year.

Medication efficacy and safety may differ by age; thus, it is important to base recommendations on robust controlled trials conducted in the appropriate age group, when applicable. For school-age children and adolescents, asthma therapy is described in a stepwise fashion, with the lower numbered steps representing milder (or easier to control) disease[8] (see Figs. 25.2 and 25.3).

Step 1

Controller Therapy. Step 1 therapy is intended for patients who present with symptoms or albuterol use less than twice monthly with no risk factors for exacerbations. Step 1 therapy has historically consisted of as-needed SABA, with no regular controller medications. However, an emerging base of evidence highlights that patients with mild asthma still experience severe exacerbations, and the overuse (or overreliance) of SABAs has been associated with adverse outcomes.[79]

Two 2018 studies (Symbicort given as-needed in mild asthma: SYGMA 1 and 2) cast a new light on the management of mild asthma and highlight the potential risks of SABA-only therapy even at this level of disease.[80,81] These studies examined as-needed use of an ICS plus a rapid-acting LABA (ICS with formoterol) for mild asthma. In the SYGMA 1 study of 3849 adolescents and adults with mild asthma, treatment with as-needed ICS with formoterol (without daily controller therapy) was superior to SABA alone in indicators of both asthma control and reducing severe exacerbation rates.[81] Compared with as-needed SABA use, as-needed ICS with formoterol decreased the rate of severe exacerbations by 64%. Regular ICS use was more effective than as-needed ICS with formoterol in overall asthma control (although the magnitude of the differences was clinically quite small) but was comparable in terms of exacerbations. Patients receiving as-needed ICS with formoterol were exposed to only 17% of the dose of ICS over 52 weeks compared with the regular ICS use group. The SYGMA 2 study included 4215 adolescents and adults with mild asthma and found that as-needed ICS with formoterol was noninferior to regular ICS in terms of the rate of severe asthma exacerbations over 52 weeks of treatment.[80] Improvement in asthma control was again statistically superior (but clinically small) with regular ICS use compared with as-needed ICS with formoterol, although the median daily ICS exposure with ICS with formoterol as-needed therapy was 25% of that experienced by the maintenance ICS group. Based on these findings, along with the documented

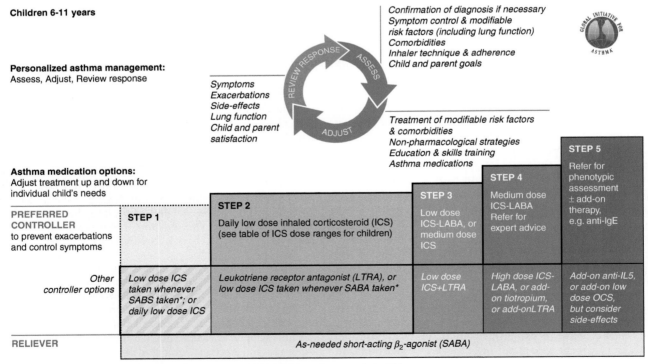

* Off-label: separate ICS and SABA inhalers; only one study in children

• **Fig. 25.2** Management of asthma in 6- to 11-year-old children. (With permission from Global Initiative For Asthma: Global Strategy for Asthma Management and Prevention © 2019 Global Initiative for Asthma (GINA); Box 3.5B; p. 48.)

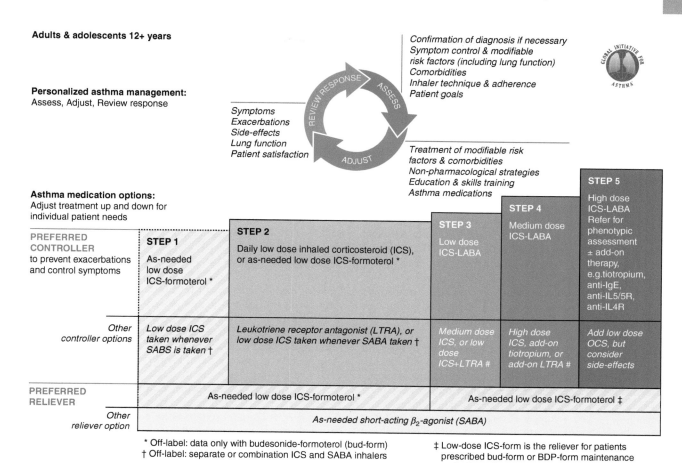

Adults & adolescents 12+ years

Personalized asthma management:
Assess, Adjust, Review response

Symptoms
Exacerbations
Side-effects
Lung function
Patient satisfaction

Confirmation of diagnosis if necessary
Symptom control & modifiable
risk factors (including lung function)
Comorbidities
Inhaler technique & adherence
Patient goals

REVIEW RESPONSE — ASSESS — ADJUST

Treatment of modifiable risk
factors & comorbidities
Non-pharmacological strategies
Education & skills training
Asthma medications

Asthma medication options:
Adjust treatment up and down for
individual patient needs

	STEP 1	STEP 2	STEP 3	STEP 4	STEP 5
PREFERRED CONTROLLER to prevent exacerbations and control symptoms	As-needed low dose ICS-formoterol *	Daily low dose inhaled corticosteroid (ICS), or as-needed low dose ICS-formoterol *	Low dose ICS-LABA	Medium dose ICS-LABA	High dose ICS-LABA Refer for phenotypic assessment ± add-on therapy, e.g.tiotropium, anti-IgE, anti-IL5/5R, anti-IL4R
Other controller options	Low dose ICS taken whenever SABS is taken †	Leukotriene receptor antagonist (LTRA), or low dose ICS taken whenever SABA taken †	Medium dose ICS, or low dose ICS+LTRA #	High dose ICS, add-on tiotropium, or add-on LTRA #	Add low dose OCS, but consider side-effects
PREFERRED RELIEVER	As-needed low dose ICS-formoterol *			As-needed low dose ICS-formoterol ‡	
Other reliever option	As-needed short-acting β₂-agonist (SABA)				

As-needed low dose ICS-formoterol *

As-needed low dose ICS-formoterol ‡

As-needed short-acting β_2-agonist (SABA)

* Off-label: data only with budesonide-formoterol (bud-form)
† Off-label: separate or combination ICS and SABA inhalers

‡ Low-dose ICS-form is the reliever for patients prescribed bud-form or BDP-form maintenance and reliever therapy
# Consider adding HDM SLIT for sensitized patients with allergic rhinitis and FEV >70 % predicted

• **Fig. 25.3** Management of asthma in patients 12 years and older. (With permission from Global Initiative For Asthma: Global Strategy for Asthma Management and Prevention © 2019 Global Initiative for Asthma (GINA); Box 3.5A; p. 47.)

potential adverse outcomes associated with as-needed SABA-only therapy, the Global Initiative for Asthma (GINA) 2019 modified Step 1 recommendations in adolescents 12 years of age and older and adults such that the preferred controller therapy for Step 1 is as-needed low-dose ICS with formoterol, rather than SABA alone.[79] It is noteworthy that this approach has not been approved by the U.S. Food and Drug Administration, thus representing an off-label recommendation. GINA also identifies daily use of low-dose ICS therapy as an alternative for Step 1 controller therapy and acknowledges that many patients with such mild disease may not be highly adherent to daily therapy.

There is much less evidence available to determine the optimal management in Step 1 for children 6 to 11 years of age. At the present time, SABA-only therapy remains an acceptable treatment strategy for such children. Although the strategy of as-needed ICS with formoterol has not been studied in children 5 to 11 years of age, the approach of using a low-dose ICS when SABA is needed has been examined in one clinical trial including this age group. In the Treating Children to Prevent Exacerbations of Asthma (TREXA) trial of 288 children 5 to 18 years of age with mild asthma previously well-controlled on low-dose ICS therapy, the use of ICS with a SABA as a reliever medicine (without concomitant daily controller) was compared with SABA alone and daily low-dose ICS alone.[82] In this four-arm study, patients were randomized to receive either maintenance low-dose ICS or placebo and their reliever was either ICS with SABA or SABA alone.

Compared with SABA alone, all three ICS-containing arms experienced reduced frequencies of exacerbations requiring oral corticosteroids and had fewer treatment failures. There was less linear growth in children receiving daily ICS compared with the SABA use alone group. This decrease was not seen in the as-needed ICS with SABA group. Children with allergic markers, such as increased total IgE level and positive testing for aeroallergens, were more likely to benefit from an ICS-containing regimen compared with SABA alone.[83] Thus, consideration of low-dose ICS used when SABA is needed may be considered as a controller option for children 6 to 11 years with Step 1 mild asthma.

Reliever Therapy. Consistent with the approach described previously for all steps, the preferred reliever in adolescents is a low-dose ICS with formoterol combination inhaler, as supported by the SYGMA trials mentioned earlier. Bisgaard and colleagues[84] studied 341 children 4 to 11 years of age in a 12-month randomized, double-blind, controlled trial evaluating ICS with formoterol as reliever medicine compared with SABA in children on maintenance ICS with formoterol or high-dose ICS. The use of ICS with formoterol as both maintenance and reliever prolonged the time to first severe exacerbations 45% to 47% compared with ICS-formoterol or high-dose ICS with SABA reliever. Among adolescents, low-dose ICS with formoterol is the preferred reliever therapy for patients at all steps of care, with as-needed SABA as another reliever option.

For children 6 to 11 years of age, the use of ICS with formoterol as needed has not been adequately evaluated, so at this time SABA remains the preferred reliever in this age group at all steps of care.[84]

Step 2

For children and adolescents who experience infrequent asthma symptoms but have risk factors for asthma exacerbations or those with symptoms or SABA use at least twice a week, Step 2 therapy would be the initial treatment.[85] In addition, those who fail to achieve control with Step 1 treatment should be advanced to Step 2 after reassessment. At Step 2, for children 6 to 11 years of age, the preferred controller is daily low-dose ICS, whereas in adolescents 12 years of age and older, preferred options include therapy of daily low-dose ICS or as-needed low-dose ICS with formoterol. These recommendations are based on several lines of evidence. The Inhaled Steroid Treatment as Regular Therapy in Early Asthma study (START) consisted of over 7000 patients with mild asthma 5 to 66 years of age who were treated with either ICS or placebo early in the course of their disease.[86] The use of daily ICS reduced oral corticosteroid use, improved lung function, and reduced asthma symptoms, even among patients who had infrequent symptoms (0–1 days per week).[86,87] In the Pediatric Asthma Controller Trial (PACT), three therapies (ICS, LTRA, and ICS with LABA) were compared in 285 children (6–14 years old) with mild to moderate asthma.[52] Regular low-dose ICS and low-dose ICS with LABA (with LABA given once daily) were comparable in asthma control days, but low-dose ICS alone was more effective in improving lung function. In children with mild to moderate persistent asthma, low-dose ICS had lower cost and higher effectiveness compared with an LTRA, especially in those with a higher FeNO and greater airway hyperresponsiveness to methacholine.[88] As noted in the SYGMA trials the use of ICS with formoterol may offer a unique use of this specific ICS with LABA medication. A systematic review of randomized controlled trials in children with mild to moderate persistent asthma identified 214 studies and evaluated 8 comparing ICS to LTRA, finding four studies favoring ICS and the other four demonstrating no significant difference.[89] Based on the current data the preferred controller options at Step 2 for adolescents are either as-needed low-dose ICS with formoterol, based on the SYGMA 1 and 2 trials, or daily low-dose ICS, whereas other controller approaches include daily LTRA or use of low-dose ICS when as-needed SABA is required. For school-age children, daily low-dose ICS is the recommended treatment. In some children, LTRA monotherapy may be effective as an alternative controller therapy option and, as noted in the TREXA study, use of a low-dose ICS when SABA taken is another controller option for school-age children.

Step 3

Children with troublesome asthma symptoms, such as those occurring most days or waking up because of asthma symptoms once a week or more, especially with risk factors for exacerbation, or those whose asthma remains symptomatic despite Step 2 therapy, should receive Step 3 therapy. Any time the apparent need to step up therapy arises, it is essential to reevaluate adherence, inhaler technique, and comorbidities before escalating therapy. For both children 6 to 11 years of age and adolescents 12 years and older, a preferred approach is an escalation in therapy to low-dose ICS with LABA because this approach is associated with reduced exacerbation risk and improved lung function.[79] However, as noted later, in children 6 to 11 years of age, increasing the ICS dose to the medium dose range is also considered a preferred approach for Step 3. Furthermore, in some children and adolescents, the addition of an LTRA to low-dose ICS is an alternative therapy option.

In the Best Add-on Therapy Giving Effective Responses (BADGER) trial, 182 children 6 to 17 years of age with asthma uncontrolled on low-dose ICS were randomized in a triple-crossover design evaluating a composite of three outcomes (i.e., exacerbations, asthma control, and lung function).[90] Children were treated in random order for 16 weeks each with medium-dose ICS, low-dose ICS with LABA, and low-dose ICS with an LTRA. The proportion of patients who had a better response to the addition of a LABA was 52% compared with adding an LTRA at 34% and to medium-dose ICS at 32%. Overall, adding a LABA was most likely to produce the best response, but in substantial proportions of patients, adding an LTRA or increasing the ICS dose was likely to result in better outcomes, including exacerbations, asthma control, and lung function. In addition, step-up therapy with the addition of a LABA was more effective in children without eczema. In a follow-up post hoc analysis of the BADGER data, higher impulse oscillometry reactance, indicative of peripheral airway obstruction, favored the addition of LABA over an increase in ICS therapy, whereas higher urinary leukotriene E4 levels marginally favored LTRA over LABA step-up therapy.[91] In contrast to these findings, in a double-blind, placebo-controlled study of 158 children 6 to 16 years of age with asthma symptoms despite low-dose ICS, no difference was noted between increasing the dose to medium-dose ICS or changing to low-dose ICS-LABA in regard to lung function, exacerbations, and symptom-free days.[92]

The safety of the addition of LABA in children as young as 4 years is supported by a trial conducted in over 6000 children 4 to 11 years of age that demonstrated that the use of a fixed-dose ICS with LABA had rates of serious asthma-related adverse events similar to those of ICS monotherapy.[93] Similar safety findings have been demonstrated in adolescents and adults.[94,95]

Step 4

For children whose asthma is not well controlled with Step 3 care and who appear to warrant Step 4 or 5 therapy, it is strongly recommended that an asthma expert (allergist or pulmonologist) be involved in the care of the child. Better outcomes are associated with the care of asthma by an expert compared with other specialists.[96] It is important to realize that young children are more susceptible to side effects of increased ICS doses, such as growth effects, weight gain, and hypothalamus-pituitary-adrenal axis suppression, so the need for higher doses of ICS needs to be thoroughly and continuously re-evaluated. Before escalating therapy, a careful and comprehensive review of modifiable comorbidities and barriers to effective care must be completed. Once these have been adequately addressed, augmentation to therapy to Step 4 is indicated.[79] Among children 6 to 11 years of age, there are no specific data in this age group on the relative efficacies of the suggested step-up approach (i.e., medium-dose ICS with LABA). Alternative approaches include the addition of a long-acting muscarinic antagonist, such as tiotropium bromide by soft mist inhaler, or adding an LTRA to a medium-dose ICS. In children 6 years of age and older, add-on therapy with tiotropium to moderate- to high-dose ICS in patients with uncontrolled moderate to severe asthma improved lung function and asthma control and was well tolerated.[97–100] A final option is to increase the dose of ICS to the high-dose range.

Step 5

For those children and adolescents with severe asthma requiring Step 5 care, treatment recommendations are limited by a relative lack of data for many therapies in this age and severity group. Adolescents may benefit from an increase in ICS to allow for high-dose ICS with LABA therapy.

The need for Step 5 therapy also warrants a phenotypic evaluation of asthma, including measurement of relevant biomarkers. Based on these evaluations, several biologic agents are currently available (see Chapter 27). These therapies target a T helper cell type 2 (T_H2) cell high-phenotype of disease, which may manifest as allergic and/or eosinophilic asthma.

For children 6 years and older with allergic asthma with sensitization to a perennial aeroallergen, the addition of omalizumab to Step 4 care should be considered. Omalizumab is an anti-IgE monoclonal antibody that binds to free IgE, preventing it from binding to the high-affinity IgE receptor on mast cells and basophils and markedly reducing free IgE levels. Omalizumab has been effective in reducing asthma exacerbations, is corticosteroid sparing, and improves asthma control in children with perennial allergic asthma.[101–106] This is particularly effective among children requiring the highest doses of ICS with LABA.[107]

For adolescents with an eosinophilic asthma phenotype, three other biologics are FDA approved for management of uncontrolled asthma despite Step 4 care. Mepolizumab is an anti–interleukin 5 (IL5) antibody that is administered subcutaneously every 4 weeks and is FDA approved for children 12 years and older. Ortega and colleagues[108] evaluated the use of mepolizumab in over 500 patients, including children 12 years and older and noted that adolescents had a reduction in the rate of exacerbations that trended in favor of mepolizumab. Benralizumab is a monoclonal antibody that binds to the IL-5 receptor α chain and is also FDA approved for children 12 years of age and older. The SIROCCO and CALIMA studies evaluated over 2000 patients with asthma, including 108 adolescents. Patients treated with benralizumab experienced a significant reduction in exacerbations, with those patients having a higher baseline blood eosinophil count and history of more frequent exacerbations having a greater response.[109–111] Initial dosing is every 4 weeks subcutaneously for the first three doses, followed by dosing every 8 weeks. Dupilumab is an antibody that binds to the IL-4 receptor α subunit, thus blocking the effects of both IL-4 and IL-13. It is FDA approved for use in patients with asthma ages 12 years of age and older. It is administered subcutaneously every 2 weeks. A 52-week study including 1902 subjects, with 107 adolescents 12 years of age and older, demonstrated dupilumab therapy led to improvement in FEV_1 and a significant reduction in exacerbations.[112]

Management of Exercise-Induced Asthma and Bronchoconstriction

Exercise-induced asthma or bronchoconstriction (EIB) describes acute airway narrowing that occurs as a result of exercise. Exercise is a very common trigger of asthma symptoms reported by children and adolescents, and thus the prevention and management of exercise-triggered symptoms should be a prominent part of all asthma treatment regimens. SABAs are the most effective at short-term protection of airway narrowing when taken by inhalation 5 to 20 minutes before exercise; this strategy typically provides clinical protection for 2 to 4 hours.[113] LABAs are not recommended for use as monotherapy in the management of EIB because of tachyphylaxis and loss of bronchoprotection. The regular, daily use of β agonists, even in the context of concomitant ICS, can lead to tolerance and reduction in duration of protection or recovery from EIB.[114] Leukotriene modifiers can be used intermittently or as maintenance prophylaxis for EIB; however, protection may be incomplete.[114]

For patients whose EIB remains symptomatic despite pretreatment with SABA or LTRA therapy, or who require multiple doses for pretreatment each week, the regular use of ICS can decrease the severity and frequency of EIB. Use of short-acting antimuscarinic antagonists also reduces EIB, especially in the setting of increased vagal tone as is often seen in highly competitive athletes. Warm-up before exercise has been shown to reduce airway responsiveness by approximately half in 50% of patients with EIB.[114]

Management of Asthma Exacerbations

Asthma "flare-ups," or exacerbations, are acute or subacute increases in asthma symptoms with worsening lung function from the patient's normal status. Asthma exacerbations occur frequently and may occur even in the context of regular use of long-term controller therapy. Most exacerbations, especially those that are mild, can generally be managed without difficulty at home. However, success in outpatient care of acute asthma demands excellent preparation, including a written set of instructions to help guide the patient and his or her family. The asthma action plan is the central component for home asthma management. It would describe their usual medications, when to increase their medications or start oral corticosteroids, and when to access medical care when needed. Patients must be instructed as to the early and accurate recognition of changes in asthma status, because early intervention is likely to lessen the severity and rate of progression of the episode. An algorithm that serves as the basis for the action plan and allows for telephone triage and recommendations is shown in Fig. 25.4.

At the onset of asthma symptoms, including cough, chest tightness, wheeze, or shortness of breath, or with a decline in peak expiratory flow (PEF) below 80% of personal best, initial therapy should include administration of a rapid-acting bronchodilator such as albuterol, by either a metered-dose inhaler (with a spacer device) or a nebulizer. This treatment may be repeated up to three times in the first hour, with PEF measured before and after each albuterol administration. Patients who demonstrate rapid improvement after this intervention should be closely followed over the ensuing hours and days for signs of recurrence of symptoms, with a particular attention to nocturnal awakenings.

The approach to ICS dosing in the setting of loss of asthma control has been an area of uncertainty for many years, and the impact of this approach may vary by patient age and baseline ICS dose. Jackson and associates[115] examined a 5-fold increase in ICS dosing among 254 children 5 to 11 years of age with mild to moderate asthma receiving baseline low-dose ICS and who had experienced at least one exacerbation in the last year.[115] This 5-fold increase in ICS when asthma control began to deteriorate did not decrease the rate of exacerbations requiring oral corticosteroids compared with maintaining the low-dose ICS, and the strategy of a 5-fold increase was associated with adverse effects on growth. In contrast, a recent open-label randomized trial among adolescents and adults with asthma and at least one exacerbation in the previous year while receiving a wide range of ICS therapies found that increasing ICS dosing 4-fold when asthma control deteriorated modestly decreased the risk of exacerbation requiring oral corticosteroids, with a number needed to treat of 15 and with higher rates of glucocorticoid side effects among the group receiving the increased ICS dose.[116]

Failure of this rescue approach to markedly reduce symptoms and improve PEF to greater than 80% of personal best should lead to institution of systemic corticosteroids. Several protocols for administration of oral corticosteroids are commonly used. One

Follow this plan for after hours patients only. Nurse may decide not to follow this home management plan if:
• Parent does not seem comfortable with or capable of following plan
• Nurse is not comfortable with this plan, based on situation and judgment
• Nurse's time does not allow for callbacks
In all cases, tell parent to call 9-1-1 if signs of respiratory distress occur during the episode
NOTE: If action plan has already been attempted without success, go to "RED ZONE—poor response" or
"YELLOW ZONE—incomplete response" as symptoms indicate.

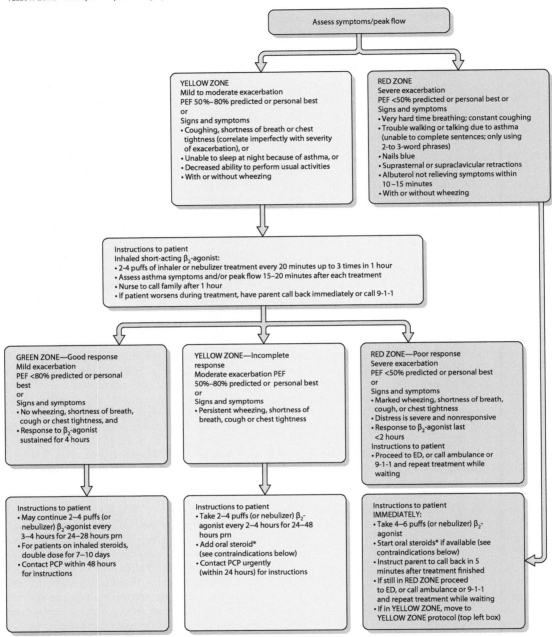

Documentation faxed or given to PCP within 24 hours; phone or verbal contact sooner as indicated.
*Ask patient about preexisting conditions that may be contraindications to oral steroids (including type 1 diabetes, active chickenpox, chickenpox exposure or varicella vaccine within 21 days, MMR within 14 days). If so, nurse to contact PCP before initiating steroids. Oral steroid dosages: Child: 2 mg/kg/day, maximum 60 mg/day, for 5 days.

Date: _____

Signature: _____

• **Fig. 25.4** Algorithm for treatment of acute asthma symptoms. *PEF,* peak expiratory flow; *ED,* emergency department; *MMR,* mumps, measles, and rubella; *PCP,* primary care physician. (Courtesy BJC Health System/Washington University School of Medicine, Community Asthma Program, St. Louis, MO; January 2000.)

BOX 25.2   Clinical Pearls

- Rhinovirus-induced wheezing during preschool years is a significant risk factor for developing asthma.
- About one-fourth of children with mild to moderate asthma may experience remission by adulthood.
- Aeroallergen sensitization to cockroach and mold is associated with asthma in children.
- A normal physical examination and baseline forced expiratory volume in 1 second (FEV_1) does not rule out asthma.
- Vocal cord dysfunction may be playing a role in children whose asthma is atypical or difficult to control.
- For children 12 years and older on Step 1 of asthma therapy the preferred treatment is as-needed low-dose ICS with formoterol; for the younger child 6 to 11 years of age as-needed SABA remains the preferred treatment.
- Step 2 therapy for mild persistent asthma, the preferred controller is daily low-dose ICS for children 6 to 11 years of age, whereas in adolescents 12 year of age and older, preferred options include therapy daily low-dose ICS or as-needed low-dose ICS with formoterol.
- For Step 3 in both children 6 to 11 years of age and adolescents 12 years and older, the preferred treatment is low-dose ICS and LABA.
- For children with moderate to severe asthma, Steps 4 and 5, it is recommended that an asthma expert be involved in the care of the child, especially with the use of biologics.

such approach is to give prednisone 2 mg/kg/day (up to 60 mg) for 5 days. The approach used in the Childhood Asthma Management Program (CAMP) trial, 2 mg/kg/day (up to 60 mg) for 2 days followed by 1 mg/kg/day (up to 30 mg) for 2 days, resulted in decreased overall steroid exposure, and the program was very effective in resolving exacerbations in patients with mild to moderate asthma.[117] This should be accompanied by frequent reassessment of clinical status and PEF and albuterol every 4 to 6 hours or more frequently if needed. Patients who do not improve with this approach are experiencing moderate to severe exacerbation and may need further evaluation and intervention, generally in the physician's office or in the ED. Signs of worsening respiratory distress should prompt emergent evaluation and therapy.

Conclusions

Asthma can have a significant impact on the quality of life of both children and their families. Careful attention to the details of determining severity and applying an appropriate therapeutic regimen can control asthma symptoms in almost all children (Box 25.2). In determining severity and applying the appropriate regimen, it is essential to establish good communication about the goals of therapy and to understand the family dynamics to ensure the family can adhere to the therapeutic regimen prescribed. Ongoing evaluation based on communication of current symptoms, with regular assessment of the family's ability to adhere to therapeutic recommendations and the appropriateness of recommendations, is necessary for long-term control of the disease and minimization of side effects of medications. Review of actions to take during exacerbation, using the asthma action plan as the central mechanism of communication, is part of regular visits for asthma.

The reference list can be found on the companion Expert Consult website at http://www.expertconsult.inkling.com.

26

Collaborating With Schools to Support Children With Asthma

MELANIE GLEASON, LISA CICUTTO, STANLEY J. SZEFLER

KEY POINTS

- Healthcare providers have a vital role in managing asthma and preparing children for success at school.
- Along with the essential asthma management tools (asthma care plans and access to quick relief inhalers), improved communication among the family, school and provider is key to successful asthma management.

- Schools are an important point of contact for large numbers of children and make good partners for expanding quality asthma care.

Introduction

Asthma is a leading cause of health disparities in children and one of the most common causes of school absences.[1,2] Poorly controlled asthma can lead to poor sleep quality and difficulty concentrating in school and may ultimately have an impact on academic success.[1] Children who experience frequent asthma symptoms are more likely to miss more days of school, turn in fewer assignments, and have lower quality academic work.[3] This disparity is magnified for students living in poverty and who are from a racial/ethnic minority, thereby widening the academic achievement gap.[3]

The link between good health and school success is well established.[4,5] Asthma is one of the health conditions most often cited as having an impact on academic achievement. Despite this body of knowledge, the health and education sectors tend to operate in silos, thus missing the opportunity to coordinate efforts and effectively change the course of poor health and subsequent impact on academic achievement.

Given the vital role that the provider plays in managing asthma and preparing children and youth for success at school, the purpose of this chapter is to provide the busy clinician with practical tips to support patients and their families in managing asthma at school, focusing on those who are at greatest risk for asthma burden and education disparities.

Impact of Asthma on School Performance

Goals of Asthma Treatment for School-Aged Youth

The National Asthma Education and Prevention Program guidelines highlight the goals for pediatric asthma as follows: control

asthma by reducing impairment through prevention of troublesome symptoms; reduce the need for quick-relief medication; maintain near-normal lung function; and maintain normal activity levels, including physical activity and attendance at school.[6]

The patient-centered goals are simply to sleep, learn, and play (Fig. 26.1). Despite many advancements in asthma management over the past decade, the basic goals for asthma therapy are not being achieved for large numbers of school-aged youth, particularly those living in poverty and from minority populations.[7,8]

The Impact of Asthma on School Performance

A missed school day is a lost opportunity to learn.[9] Missing as few as 2 days of school per month adds up and places a child at risk of chronic absenteeism, which is defined as missing 15 or more days of school per year.[10] This is a critical amount of school loss and is a predictor of poor school performance and subsequent academic failure. Therefore, it is important to identify this trend early and intervene with appropriate strategies to prevent the occurrence of chronic absenteeism.

Since passage of the Every Student Succeeds Act[11] in 2015, increased attention has been given to school absences. It is a focal point for multidisciplinary organizations and stakeholders who are invested in reducing health disparities and closing the academic achievement gap. The American Academy of Pediatrics (AAP) is doing its part as observed in a recent policy statement[12] linking good health to education. The AAP urged pediatricians to work with schools to help reduce school absences by implementing a tiered approach to encourage attendance. Recommendations in this policy are applicable and can be tailored for children with asthma. For example, providers can educate and

Goals of care for school-aged children with asthma

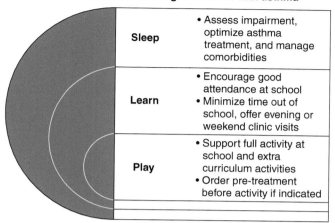

Sleep	• Assess impairment, optimize asthma treatment, and manage comorbidities
Learn	• Encourage good attendance at school • Minimize time out of school, offer evening or weekend clinic visits
Play	• Support full activity at school and extra curriculum activities • Order pre-treatment before activity if indicated

• **Fig. 26.1** Patient-centered asthma treatment goals.

collaborate with school professionals about appropriate reasons for exclusion, avoid writing excuses for school absences when the absence was not appropriate, and avoid contributing to school absences by offering extended office hours and encouraging families to make preventive appointments for times outside of regular school hours.[12]

Poor health can affect learning in ways that are not well understood. The association between persistent asthma symptoms and poor school performance independent of school absences was demonstrated in two 2019 studies. In a carefully evaluated sample of urban youth ages 7 to 9 years old with persistent asthma, Koinis-Mitchell and colleagues[3] found that children who had more daily symptoms were significantly more likely to have worse quality of work, worse math scores, and more school absences than those with well-controlled asthma. These associations were stronger in Latino children, who appeared to be at heightened risk for poorer academic performance. Persistent asthma symptoms are also associated with low reading levels, as observed in a New Zealand study that evaluated reading levels in children after the first year of school.[13] Children with asthma were on average 4 months behind on learning to read compared with their peers without asthma. Further, children with persistent asthma symptoms performed at the lowest reading level compared with those whose asthma improved. Taken together, these findings highlight the importance of achieving and maintaining asthma control to prevent learning difficulties that may lead to poor academic performance.

Providers have a unique opportunity to help youth with asthma reach their goals of symptom control, regular school attendance, and health equity. These goals are best accomplished through coordinated asthma care among the provider, the family, and the school.

The School Setting: Facilitators and Barriers of Asthma Management

Conditions exist in schools that can either facilitate or create barriers for successful asthma management. Common barriers to asthma management include insufficient school health team staff; poor communication among child/youth, family, school, and asthma healthcare provider; and exposure to environmental triggers. Facilitators include easy access to high-quality health services;

opportunities for asthma education for those with asthma, their families, and the school community; and a supportive and asthma-friendly school environment.

School Health Team Staffing

The presence of a school nurse makes the school an important point of care for children with asthma. School nurses provide direct care to help manage asthma and facilitate care coordination among the family, school, and healthcare provider. Because school nurses are on the front line, they can identify early signs of asthma worsening, activity limitation, and impact on school attendance. When this information is shared among the family and provider, early intervention can prevent progression and avoid poor outcomes.

Insufficient health team staffing is one of the major barriers to asthma management in schools. Less than 40% of U.S. schools staff a full-time nurse, and 25% do not have a school nurse at all.[14] Competing priorities influence school administrators' allocation of funding and frequently result in shortage of school nurses. In the absence of a full-time school nurse, the school health office may be staffed by unlicensed assistive personnel. These individuals are not medically trained, but through delegation they work under the supervision of a school nurse and may perform tasks traditionally carried out by school nurses.

Asthma Self-Management Education

The school setting is ripe for promoting health education because children in school are primed and ready to learn. School is often the first place outside of the home in which a child must navigate complexities of asthma self-management without the support of a close family member.[15] Children, especially those in early school years may be shy, embarrassed, or intimidated and therefore afraid to ask for help. Furthermore, they do not want to be seen as different and thus often ignore symptoms in an effort to fit in and keep up with their peers.[16] Asthma education, whether in a formal small group class such as the American Lung Association's Open Airways for Schools (https://www.lung.org/lung-health-and-diseases/lung-disease-lookup/asthma/asthma-education-advocacy/open-airways-for-schools/about-open-airways.html)[17,18] or one-on-one education with the school nurse, is an effective strategy and can help children master the skills necessary for proper asthma self-management.

Environmental Triggers

Children spend a significant part of their day at school for most of the calendar year where they may encounter an array of triggers (including allergens, pollutants, bacteria, and viruses). Children are more vulnerable than adults to the effects of environmental hazards because they breathe more air per pound and are less likely to be aware of and thus avoid environmental hazards.[19] In some instances, the school environment may pose more risks of exposure to triggers than a child's home environment.[20,21] This makes the school an important consideration for environmental control interventions.

Of the triggers encountered in inner city schools, in which much of the work has been done, mouse antigen is significantly higher in schools compared with homes.[20,21] In these studies, high levels of mouse antigen were associated with asthma morbidity, including increased days with asthma symptoms and decreased lung function.[21,22] Animal dander is also a common occurrence even in classrooms that do not allow pets. Presumably, the dander is brought in on the clothing of students, staff, and visitors. Additional asthma triggers for schools include mold, dust, air fresheners, art, cleaning supplies, and outdoor air pollutants from nearby roadways or idling vehicles parked near intake ducts.[19–24] The predominating environmental exposures will vary geographically because of differences in climate and socioeconomic conditions.[22]

Communication and Care Coordination

A major obstacle to successful asthma management at school is the lack of communication and care coordination among the school, family, and provider. School nurses report that poor parental support and lack of provider involvement are barriers to successful school asthma management.[25] Communication, when it does occur, is often fragmented or ineffective, with parents primarily responsible for transmitting information between school nurses and healthcare providers.[25]

Poor communication is also a result of school nurses' and providers' hesitancy to speak to each other, citing concern for violations with Health Insurance Portability and Privacy Act (HIPPA) and Family Educational Rights and Privacy Act (FERPA). Under FERPA, school nurses are prohibited from sharing school records, including student health records, without parental consent. There are two exceptions to this rule: to clarify an existing treatment plan and to share necessary information to protect the student or others during an emergency posing eminent danger.[26] For this reason, schools often obtain prior written permission from a parent/guardian at the beginning of the school year.

To address the communication abyss, the following recommendations are offered by Snieder and his team,[25] who conducted focus groups and interviews with schools, caregivers, and providers: (1) establish formal communication channels between schools and providers to increase the efficient and prompt transmission of information about change in a youth's asthma management; and (2) integrate technology such as a shared electronic medical records, texting, or secure emails that are compliant with both HIPAA and FERPA and fit into existing workflows.

Essential Components of an Asthma-Friendly School

Asthma Action Plans and Quick Relief Therapy

Two essential elements for successful asthma management in the school setting are (1) a completed school asthma action plan and (2) provision of a quick-relief medication that is easily accessible at school. In general, the written asthma action plan provides individualized prevention and management steps developed by the healthcare provider for the school nurse or the designated school personnel to follow. It serves as a type of medical order for youth to take quick-relief asthma medication at the school. Despite the obvious benefits of having this important document to guide complex and sometimes life-threatening asthma episodes, rates for having an individualized asthma action plan at school are surprisingly low. Barriers for providers include the lack of availability or consistency of asthma action forms that are acceptable to different schools. Parents/guardians will often omit the form if it is too inconvenient to obtain from the provider. Harmonization and standardization of asthma action plans reduce some of the barriers, as does having the standardized form accessible in electronic medical record systems.

Similarly, there is a lack of access to quick-relief therapy at schools, especially in under-resourced communities.[27] Tragically, asthma deaths have occurred in the school setting that might have been prevented with easy access to quick relief therapy.[28] Providers can help support access to inhalers at school by requesting that the pharmacy dispense two inhalers, one for home and one designated for school use.

Clinical Pearl

- Keep label for quick relief inhaler consistent with directions on the asthma action plan.

Asthma Resources for School Asthma Management

Several excellent resources are available to help guide asthma care coordination between providers and schools. Box 26.1 is a quick reference guide to some of these resources. One of the more pertinent resources for asthma providers is the School-Based Asthma Management Program (SAMPRO) published in 2016.[29,30] This initiative was developed by the American Academy of Allergy, Asthma & Immunology with additional support from the National Association of School Nurses, who convened an asthma summit with multiple stakeholders to create a central resource. The SAMPRO workforce identified four components essential to creating an effective partnership between providers and schools centered around asthma care: (1) creating a circle of support to facilitate communication among the family, clinician, school nurse, and community; (2) asthma management plans that include both an asthma emergency treatment plan and an asthma action plan; (3) a comprehensive asthma education plan for all school personnel; and (4) a plan for assessment of the school environment and remediation of school-based asthma triggers.

SAMPRO includes a prototype asthma action plan (Fig. 26.2) that may be adapted by school systems and providers. This action plan is unique because it integrates both home and school plans into a single document. It includes key features that facilitate communication for multiple users, is efficient for providers to complete, and is consistent across multiple settings. Importantly, the SAMPRO asthma action plan includes HIPPA-compliant and FERPA-compliant permissive language that allows for bidirectional communication and facilitates care coordination.

Practical Tips for Providers to Support Asthma Management at School

Basic Steps Recommended for All Children/Youth With Asthma

The following steps should be considered for all children/youth who have asthma:

AAAAI American Academy of
www.aaaai.org Allergy Asthma & Immunology

Asthma Action Plan for Home & School

Name: **Birthdate:**

Asthma Severity: ☐ Intermittent   ☐ Mild Persistent   ☐ Moderate Persistent   ☐ Severe Persistent
☐ He/she has had many or severe asthma attacks/exacerbations

☺ **Green Zone**	Have the child take these medicines every day, even when the child feels well.

Always use a spacer with inhalers as directed.
Controller Medicine[s]: _____
_____
Controller Medicine[s] Given in School: _____
Rescue Medicine: Albuterol/Levalbuterol _____ puffs every four hours as needed
Exercise Medicine: Albuterol/Levalbuterol _____ puffs 15 minutes before activity as needed

☺ **Yellow Zone**	Begin the sick treatment plan if the child has a cough, wheeze, shortness of breath, or tight chest, Have the child take all of these medicines when sick.

Rescue Medicine: Albuterol/Levalbuterol _____ puffs every 4 hours as needed
Controller Medicine[s]:
☐ Continue Green Zone medicines: _____
☐ Add: _____
_____
☐ Change: _____
If the child is in the **yellow** zone more than **24** hours or is getting worse, fallow **red** zone and call the doctor right away!

☹ **Red Zone**	If breathing is hard and fast, ribs sticking out, trouble walking, talking, or sleeping, **Get Help Now**

Take resucue medicine(s) now
Rescue Medicine: Albuterol/Levalbuterol _____ puffs every _____
Take: _____
_____

If the child is not better right away, call 911
Please call the doctor any time the child is in the red zone.

Asthma Triggers: (List)

School Staff: Follow the Yellow and Red Zone plans for rescue medicines according to asthma symptoms.
Unless otherwise noted, the only controllers to be administered in school are those listed as "given in school" in the green zone,
☐ Both the asthma provider and the parent feel that the child <u>may carry and self administer their inhalers</u>
☐ School nurse agrees with student self administering the inhalers

Asthma Provider Printed Name and Controal Information:	Asthma Provider Signature:
	Date:

Parent/Guardian: I give written authorization for the medications listed in the action plan to be administered in school by the nurse or other school members as appropriate, I consent to commuication between the prescribing health care provider/clinic, the school nurse, the school medical advisor and school based health clinic providers necessary for asthma management and administration of this medication.

Parent/guardian signature:	School Nurse Reviewed:
Date:	Date:

Please send a signed copy back to the provider listed above

• **Fig. 26.2** SAMPRO asthma action plan.

1. Engage youth and family in routine asthma care that includes a back-to-school asthma checkup.
2. Assess asthma self-care skills, including inhaler technique, at each visit and retrain as necessary. Inhaler technique is inherently challenging. There are multiple reasons for inaccurate inhaler technique, including gaps in skills of providers and or the lack of attention given to training the child how to properly take inhaled medications.[31,32] Be aware that students may get different messages regarding inhaler technique from various healthcare providers. To reinforce this important skill, have all office staff trained using a standardized approach and provide the family with clear, easy to follow written instructions for home and school use.
3. Provide asthma education tailored at a level that is understandable and culturally appropriate to meet the needs of the child and caregiver. When asked about preference, caregivers report that they need and would like more asthma education but point out barriers to education, including (1) insufficient time during the office visit, (2) ineffective educational practices such as feeling "lectured to" by the healthcare provider that leads to feelings of guilt, and (3) provision of too much information, especially at a time of crisis.[33]
4. Proactively complete an asthma action plan for school and home and make provision for an easily accessible quick-relief inhaler at school.
5. Encourage school attendance and provide clear guidance on when it is appropriate to miss school because of asthma. Minimize time out of class for routine follow-up appointments by scheduling these visits during times when school is not in session, such as evening or weekend hours.

Additional Steps for Children and Youth With More Severe or Difficult to Control Asthma

For children with difficult to control asthma, the provider should address the usual causes for poor control, including comorbidities, poor adherence, and social determinants of health. Asthma comorbidities such as allergic rhinitis, eczema, and sleep disordered breathing can make asthma worse and contribute to poor sleep and difficulty concentrating, both of which disrupt the ability to learn. Medication nonadherence is a major obstacle to achieving and maintaining asthma control. Effective strategies to improve adherence include shared decision making for treatment regimens and motivational interviewing techniques.[34–36] Electronic medication monitoring devices that track patterns of medication use also show promise for improving adherence.[37]

Strategies to Support Youth Who Have Severe or Difficult to Treat Asthma

The following strategies should be considered in support of youth with severe asthma or who have asthma that is difficult to treat:
1. Review and potentially step up asthma therapy before returning to school. Seasonal asthma exacerbations frequently occur soon after the return to school. This may occur for a variety of reasons, including suboptimal therapy, underlying asthma severity, and exposure to viral and seasonal allergens. The "September spikes"[38] in exacerbations early in the school year contributes to school absences and disrupts learning at a critical time. One successful strategy in reducing seasonal exacerbations and associated asthma morbidities for youth with severe/exacerbation-prone asthma is to initiate treatment with a biologic agent before starting the school year.[39]
2. Direct observation of controller therapy at school. For students who have continued nonadherence with therapy and poorly controlled/exacerbation-prone asthma, determine whether a school nurse is available and willing to provide direct observation of controller medication. This strategy has demonstrated effectiveness in some children with asthma.[40–43]
3. Assess social determinants of health and provide referrals to appropriate community resources and agencies. Social determinants of health include nonmedical factors, such as lack of stable housing, food insecurities, and stressful life events, that have an impact on health. Enlist the help of patient navigators or community health workers who are adept at linking patients to needed services.
4. Collaboration among members of the medical neighborhood (i.e., primary care, specialty providers, hospitals, and nonclinical entities such as schools) is increasingly critical to reach optimal health outcomes, especially in under-resourced communities. The Centers for Disease Control and Prevention's Whole School, Whole Community, Whole Child model[44]; the National Association of School Nurses' Framework for 21st Century School Nursing Practice[45]; and SAMPRO's Circle of Support[29] are all models of expanded patient-centered care that provide complete and coordinated care. Communication and clear delineation of roles of the interdisciplinary team are required for this level of coordination.

• **BOX 26.1** **School-Based Asthma Resources for Busy Clinicians**
Websites to Access Key Resources

- American Academy of Allergy Asthma and Immunology
  - School-Based Asthma Management Program SAMPRO: https://www.aaaai.org/conditions-and-treatments/school-tools/SAMPRO
- American Academy of Pediatrics School Health: http://www.schoolhealth.org
  - Schooled in Asthma: www.aap.org/schooledinasthma
- American Lung Association
  - Asthma Friendly Schools Initiative Toolkit: http://www.lung.org/lung-disease/asthma/creating-asthma-friendly-environments/asthma-in-schools/asthma-friendly-schools-initiative/
- Centers for Disease Control
  - School and Childcare Providers: http://www.cdc.gov/asthma/schools.html
  - Creating an Asthma Friendly School: http://www.cdc.gov/HealthyYouth/asthma/creatingafs/
  - Strategies for Addressing Asthma within a Coordinated School Health Program: http://www.cdc.gov/healthyyouth/asthma/strategies/asthmacsh.htm
- National Association of School Nurses
  - Asthma resources and tools: https://www.nasn.org/ToolsResources/Asthma
- U.S. Environmental Protection Agency
  - Creating Healthy Indoor Environments in Schools. Tools for Schools: http://www.epa.gov/iaq/schools/
  - Managing Asthma in the School Environment: http://www.epa.gov/iaq/schools/managingasthma.html

Level 1 Essential Elements for All Students With Active Asthma:

1. Encourage family to complete school health records annually and to inform the school about the diagnosis of asthma.
2. Schedule checkup visit before the start of school.
3. Assess and train child on asthma self-management skills (avoiding triggers, recognizing symptoms, taking quick relief medication, assess and train on inhaler technique).
4. In collaboration with the family, complete a zone-based Asthma Action Plan for school that provides information on what medication to give, dose and frequency, and what to do if the child does not respond. Use standardized form provided by school if available.
5. Determine need for activity pretreatment to prevent exercise-induced asthma.
6. Prescribe quick relief inhaler and valved-holding chamber designated for use at school.
7. Encourage and stress importance of school attendance.

Level 2 Additional Support for Children With Uncontrolled or Exacerbation Prone Asthma:

All of the above plus the following tailored to the child's needs:

1. Evaluate and address comorbid conditions and adherence with controller medications.
2. Inquire about asthma support services at the school (health office staffing, asthma education, access to quick relief medication).
3. Reinforce asthma care skills and trigger avoidance.
4. Engage in care coordination and communication with the school health team (obtain parental HIPAA and FERPA* authorization).

Level 3 Intensified Support for Children Who Continue to Have Significant Asthma Morbidity and Associated School Impairment:

1. Screen for social determinants of health and provide referrals.
2. For persistent adherence issues enlist help from school nurse with direct observation of controller therapy.
3. Provide documentation and support needed for IEP[†] and 504 plans.[‡]
4. Schedule a meeting with family, school nurse, and or administrator to formulate a plan for supporting the student with difficult-to-control asthma.
5. Identify additional resources to work with the family such as a health navigator or community health worker.
6. Refer to school-based health clinic or consider engaging in telehealth visits at the school.

*The Family Educational Rights and Privacy Act (FERPA) is federal legislation in the United States that protects the privacy of students' personally identifiable information. The act applies to all educational institutions that receive federal funds and includes school health records.
†The Individualized Educational Plan (IEP) is a plan or program developed to ensure that a child who has a disability identified under the law and is attending an elementary or secondary educational institution receives specialized instruction and related services.
‡The 504 plan is a plan developed to ensure that a child who has a disability identified under the law and is attending an elementary or secondary educational institution receives accommodations that will ensure their academic success and access to the learning environment.

5. Children with physical or mental impairments, including severe asthma, may qualify for additional protection under Section 504 of the U.S. Rehabilitation Act of 1973[46] and the Individuals with Disabilities Education Act (IDEA 2004).[47] The goal of 504 plans is for students to be educated in regular classrooms along with the services, accommodations, or aids they may need. Examples of accommodations in 504 plans include excused lateness, absences, or missed classwork; preapproved nurse office visits and accompaniment to visits; and modified activities. As part of the IDEA, an Individualized Education Program (IEP) is developed for the child with special needs to set goals and arrange any special support needed to help them achieve them. The providers' role is to support the child, family, and school nurse by providing necessary documentation. The provider may also make a referral for evaluation if a concern is identified.

School-Based Asthma Programs

For over 30 years, school-based asthma programs have attempted to improve the quality of asthma care through a variety of strategies. Poor and underrepresented minority children who experience disproportional asthma morbidities are typically targeted to receive these services. Because of limited capacity, competing priorities, and financial constraints, schools do not typically lead these initiatives on their own. Rather, an outside agency, such as a coalition or a medical or community health organization, drives the design, implementation, evaluation, and funding of school-based asthma programs. A drawback for schools is that most of these programs tend to be short-lived and disappear when the funding runs out. Fortunately, schools that serve as active partners in these initiatives have the ability to put in place sustainable policies and procedures that support evidence-based asthma management to reap the benefit of these programs.[48]

A variety of strategies have been evaluated and typically involve some degree of partnership among school personnel, community health providers, and families. The focus of these interventions was to increase the quality of asthma care, but the process to achieve this goal varied from direct asthma service provision, case management, and care coordination to asthma self-management educational programs and creating supportive school environments.

Human Resource Supplementation of the School Health Team

To address the shortage of trained health professionals onsite at schools, strategies evaluated have included adding physicians and other community healthcare providers and extending the hours of school nurses to full time. Healthcare provider support can be brought into the school through school-based health centers. These centers provide onsite care delivered by physicians, physician assistants, or nurse practitioners for students at school. Two studies focusing on improving asthma care through school-based health clinics demonstrated improvements in the need for emergency department visits, hospitalizations, and school absenteeism.[49,50] Bringing a mobile health clinic to the school to provide healthcare staff, diagnostics, and regularly scheduled visits is an alternative strategy to improve asthma outcomes, again leading to improvements in reducing hospitalizations, emergency department visits, asthma symptoms, rescue inhaler use, and school absenteeism.[51–53]

Directly Observed Therapy

Because adherence to asthma medications is typically below 50%, it is an important factor in achieving asthma control. Several studies have evaluated the benefits of directly observed asthma maintenance therapy (primarily inhaled corticosteroids) by school nurses that involved the partnership and coordination of care among school nurses, primary care providers, and families.

These studies have typically observed improvements in medication adherence and asthma-related outcomes such as symptoms-free days, asthma control, reduced number of exacerbations, and school absenteeism.[40–43]

Case Management and Care Coordination

Care coordination and case management activities include an initial assessment of service needs; development of a comprehensive, individualized plan; coordination of services required to implement the plan; monitoring of the client and family to assess the plan's effectiveness; and re-evaluation and revision of the plan as necessary. Case management strategies applied through schools to higher risk students with asthma hold promise. Many of the school-centered interventions evaluated have included case management as an element of the intervention.[40–43,51–59] The case management activity most frequently reported was working with the family followed by contacting healthcare providers. Extensive care coordination and case management services are typically needed only by students who continue to experience poorly controlled asthma despite having the usual support systems. Benefits observed included improved asthma control, reduced use of healthcare services related to asthma exacerbations, and reduced school absenteeism.[40–43,51–59]

Information Technology Infrastructure

Information technology that permits data sharing is an important component of an infrastructure to promote coordination of care across schools, families, and healthcare providers to achieve successful asthma management. A project in the Charlotte Mecklenburg Schools suggests that databases maintained by nurses, asthma program staff, and school personnel can be successfully integrated into a single asthma program evaluation database. Benefits reported as a result of their shared database included an ability to identify students with an elevated level of need to receive priority care status from the asthma education program, and an ability to evaluate program outcomes that were not possible before, such as academic performance, school attendance, school behavior, and quality of life.[60]

Interventions to Improve Asthma Self-Management Skills

The National Heart, Lung and Blood Institute Expert Panel Guidelines for the Diagnosis and Management of Asthma stress the need for asthma education and the development of asthma management skills to achieve successful disease control.[6] A number of studies have assessed the effectiveness of providing asthma education in schools.[61–72] These educational programs incorporate health education theories and asthma practice guidelines. Most school-based educational programs have focused on building skills for elementary school–aged children and have demonstrated improvements in asthma knowledge, confidence/self-efficacy, asthma management skills and associated asthma morbidity outcomes, such as improved quality of life and reduced symptoms, emergency department visits, urgent care visits, hospitalizations, and school absenteeism.[61–72]

Studies in adolescents, an identified difficult-to-reach group, have demonstrated acceptance, involvement, and retention by this age group: over 75% of those eligible participated and over 70% were retained.[73,74] Benefits observed included improved self-confidence in asthma management skills; appropriate use of controller and quick-relief asthma medications; fewer days with symptoms and activity limitation; fewer interrupted nights because of asthma; decreased hospitalizations, emergency department visits, and school absenteeism; and improved quality of life.[73–77]

Although results across studies have not been consistent, systematic reviews suggest school-centered asthma education has positive clinical, humanistic health, economical, and academic outcomes.[71,72] Adding to this body of knowledge, a 2019 Cochrane review of school-based self-management interventions for asthma concluded that this strategy is effective in reducing days of restricted activities, reduces the frequency of asthma-related ED visits, and has moderate effectiveness in reducing hospitalizations.[78] However, in the studies evaluated there was uncertainty as to whether school-based asthma programs have an impact on reducing school absences. The Building Bridges for Asthma Care program, which focused its intervention on students with the most severe asthma, demonstrated significant improvement in asthma knowledge and clinical outcomes and an overall 22% decrease in percentage of school absences.[58] Although asthma self-management was a component of this program, the success in reducing school absence is likely the result of the intensified care coordination and communication among the school, family, and provider.[58,59]

How Can Healthcare Providers Get Involved in School-Based Asthma Programs?

Schools are willing and make excellent partners for community providers interested in working with them to implement high-quality, supportive programs that enhance the school's primary mission of education. Future implementers of school-based asthma programs are encouraged to review the literature for lessons learned[79] and to draw from evidence-based strategies that can be transferred to the school setting. The latter strategy refers to implementation research in which the goal is not to acquire new knowledge but rather to determine how to transfer that knowledge into the real world. In a rostrum on this topic, Hollenbach and Cloutier[80] describe the value of applying the implementation research framework to school-based asthma interventions. Included in this framework is the importance of building trust and strong partnerships and engaging the primary care clinician. Box 26.3 includes these key activities and other important "building blocks" to help providers get started in school-based asthma programs.[80–82]

Conclusions

Pediatric asthma care providers have a critical role in helping children and youth meet their asthma goals. Second to home, youth spend the largest portion of their wakeful time at school. Therefore, providers are encouraged to integrate key questions and recommendations that support school-based asthma management into their practice. An essential key to well-managed asthma is quality communication among the family, school nurse, and provider. Each member of this asthma care team has valuable information to contribute and roles and responsibilities to fulfill in caring for the child with asthma. Children who are fully able to participate in school activities, including educational, social, emotional, and physical activities, are more likely to be successful in school and in life. In addition to caring for

Step 1: Identify a community or school district to partner with. Identify and engage key stakeholders (school nurses, administrators, clinicians, families). Build trust.

Step 2: Conduct a needs assessment to identify gaps and strengths in existing asthma management. With input from key stakeholders select an evidence-based intervention that is meaningful and resonates with the community. Be mindful of available resources and funding. Adaptations of the program may need to be made.

Step 3: Form a leadership team. The team will set up goals, objectives, and expectations. It is important to do this in a collaborative way, for example, co-leadership with representation from the medical center and the schools. Identify team members and assign roles.

Step 4: Set goals for each component and build capacity to implement the program. The medical center can provide the asthma expertise and train the school nurses to make sure they are up to date with current concepts around asthma management. The schools can identify an asthma champion, usually a school nurse, who leads the day-to-day management of the program. Selecting a person who is interested in asthma and has leadership skills is ideal. Each group should make some commitment with personnel and resources to make it work.

Step 5: Start small. A school readiness questionnaire can help with asking the key questions to see who is on board and what resources are available. Pick a few schools to start with, so that you can set up the working model and measure success. It will help identify the challenges as well.

Step 6: Identify students who have asthma. This information is collected from the caregivers, usually at the beginning of the school year. Assess

the level of impact of asthma on each student. Obtain additional information through questions that ask about impairment and risk. This information helps gauge the severity of asthma and identifies which students may require closer review.

Step 7: You can now begin to place students in tiers to identify the level of support needed. Tier 1 might be those that have inactive asthma. Less attention is needed for this group. Tier 2 would be those with active asthma who may need some level of monitoring to ensure they are maintaining control. Tier 3 might be those with active asthma who need a support system to maintain asthma control. Tier 4 are those students who have persistent symptoms and multiple exacerbations and may have certain circumstances that factor into their level of support, such as family disarray, multiple caregivers, low health literacy, etc.
Establish asthma friendly policies. Check to see that each student with active asthma has an asthma action plan and quick relief inhaler at the school.

Step 8: Build in continuous quality improvement. This is accomplished through regular and frequent program evaluation of process and outcome measures. It is good to set up regular meetings with the medical center and school leaders to review process measures, identify barriers and make necessary adjustments.

Step 9: Set up a communication system. The system will include participating families, care providers, school nurses, and program implementers. Communication must be multidirectional, meaningful, and responsive. Periodically include focus groups and interviews with key stakeholders to understand if program changes are needed.

Step 10: Build in steps for program sustainability. Seek additional sources of funding to sustain and grow the program with the ultimate goal of establishing sustainable funding sources.

---

individual children with asthma, providers have the potential to improve the quality of asthma care for large numbers of youth with asthma by partnering with schools. Evidence supports school-based asthma programs, particularly those that target under-resourced youth as an effective strategy to reduce asthma

morbidities and improve self-management skills, school attendance, and overall school performance.

The reference list can be found on the companion Expert Consult website at http://www.expertconsult.inkling.com.

27

Refractory Childhood Asthma: Assessment and Management

ANDREW BUSH, LOUISE FLEMING

KEY POINTS

- Apparent problematic severe asthma includes wrong diagnosis (not asthma at all), asthma with extrapulmonary comorbidities (asthma plus), difficult asthma (social and environmental comorbidities), and true severe, therapy-resistant asthma (which is rare). Patients whose intractable symptoms truly are due to asthma should first undergo an initial detailed protocolized multidisciplinary assessment, rather than have treatment escalated uncritically.

- More than 80% of children referred to tertiary centers with problematic severe asthma in fact will be well controlled if basic management is optimal; however, some have refractory asthma plus (e.g., obesity with failed weight loss) and refractory difficult asthma (e.g., persistent poor adherence despite multiple efforts). Children with refractory asthma should be considered for airway phenotyping and, if they have ongoing type 2 inflammation, be treated with biologic agents.

- Invasive investigation should be considered in children with apparent severe, therapy-resistant asthma to determine whether there is discordance between symptoms and inflammation, whether there is an unusual pattern of inflammation, whether the child is steroid responsive and to what extent, and whether there is fixed airflow limitation. Depending on the airway pathology condition, these children also should be considered for biologic agents.

- Asthma attacks are a sign of management failure. A severe asthma attack is a strong predictor of future attacks and should lead to a focused response to try to prevent it happening again.

- We need to move from phenotypes (e.g., airway eosinophilia) to endotypes, specific pathophysiological pathways responsible for different asthma subtypes, especially so that we can specifically match the burgeoning numbers of biologics to the right patient, to maximize benefits.

- It is disappointing that there is so little evidence about safety and efficacy of the anti–T helper cell type 2 strategies in children and virtually no evidence-based treatments for pediatric non-eosinophilic asthma.

Introduction

Most school-age children with asthma respond to low-dose inhaled corticosteroids (ICSs; 200 mcg/day fluticasone equivalent) when properly administered, sometimes requiring a second controller such as long-acting β_2 agonists (LABAs) or leukotriene receptor antagonists (LTRAs).[1] Therefore, in the apparently nonresponding child, before escalating therapy up the "evidence-based" stepwise guidelines, the pediatrician should investigate why the child is not responding to simple, low-dose therapies. Assuming the child truly has asthma, the answer will lie in (1) a refractory airway pathologic condition, which is rare; (2) more usually, unaddressed social or environmental factors; or (3) extrapulmonary comorbidities.[2] Truly severe disease probably accounts for less than 5% of all pediatric asthma.[3] However, this group accounts for huge morbidity and healthcare costs and even mortality and thus is important.[4] This chapter describes the current Royal Brompton Hospital approaches to the child referred with apparently severe asthma.

Nomenclature

We use the term *problematic severe asthma* (or, better, *problematic severe respiratory symptoms unresponsive to asthma therapy*) to describe children who, despite apparently optimal asthma management and maximal therapy, have ongoing chronic symptoms or acute attacks (Box 27.1).[5–8] Traditional definitions of severe asthma have been based on (arbitrary) levels of pharmacotherapy and asthma control; however, the 2019 National Review of Asthma Deaths in the United Kingdom[9] reported that, by this definition, 60% of those who died did not have severe asthma. Any modern definition therefore also must include domains of risk irrespective of levels of medication prescribed; these include

Criteria for Problematic Severe Asthma (More Than One of These Scenarios May Be Encountered in the Same Child[12])

- *Chronic symptoms:* Defined as the use of short-acting β_2 agonists (SABAs) on at least 3 days a week for at least 3 months, despite inhaled corticosteroid (ICSs; beclomethasone dipropionate equivalent 800 mcg/day) and the use of any combination of long-acting β_2-agonists (LABAs), leukotriene receptor antagonists (LTRAs), and low-dose theophylline (or failed trials of at least two of these add-on therapies).
- *Severe asthma attacks:* Any or all of one admission to pediatric intensive care, the need for more than two intravenous treatments in the previous year, and the use of two or more prednisolone bursts in the previous year. This attack-prone pattern is not inevitably associated with poor background control.
- *Airflow limitation:* Forced expiratory volume in 1 second (FEV_1) of less than 80% after SABA withhold, or an FEV_1 of less than 80% despite a trial of systemic steroids and acute administration of SABA (persistent airflow limitation).
- *Disconnect of symptoms:* Strictly, the child presenting with a multitude of symptoms with no objective evidence of uncontrolled disease may belong in a separate disease category and certainly is not managed by severe asthma guidelines. Because the means of addressing this scenario are so very similar, inclusion in this group is pragmatically justified. The reverse scenario, underreporting of symptoms, is also considered.

failure to attend routine reviews, multiple emergency department visits, underuse of ICSs and overreliance on short-acting β_2 agonists (SABAs).[10,11] There is a joint responsibility on families and professionals to understand the reasons for these failings and address them. From an initial referral with problematic severe asthma the child is placed in one of six categories,[12] which are discussed in turn (Fig. 27.1). This chapter aims to develop an individualized treatment plan for the child.

Approach to the Child With Problematic Severe Asthma

Does the Child Actually Have Asthma or Is There Another Diagnosis?

The first step is, as always, obtaining a full history and performing a physical examination. Close attention should be paid to the nature of the symptoms. In particular, the word *wheeze* is used very imprecisely, including being applied to crackling noises, upper airway noises, and even stridor.[13–17] The possibility that the child does not in fact wheeze should be considered unless and until a reliable, trained healthcare professional has heard wheeze with a stethoscope.[18] Cough-variant asthma is overdiagnosed, and most children who cough do not have any disease.[19] Classic

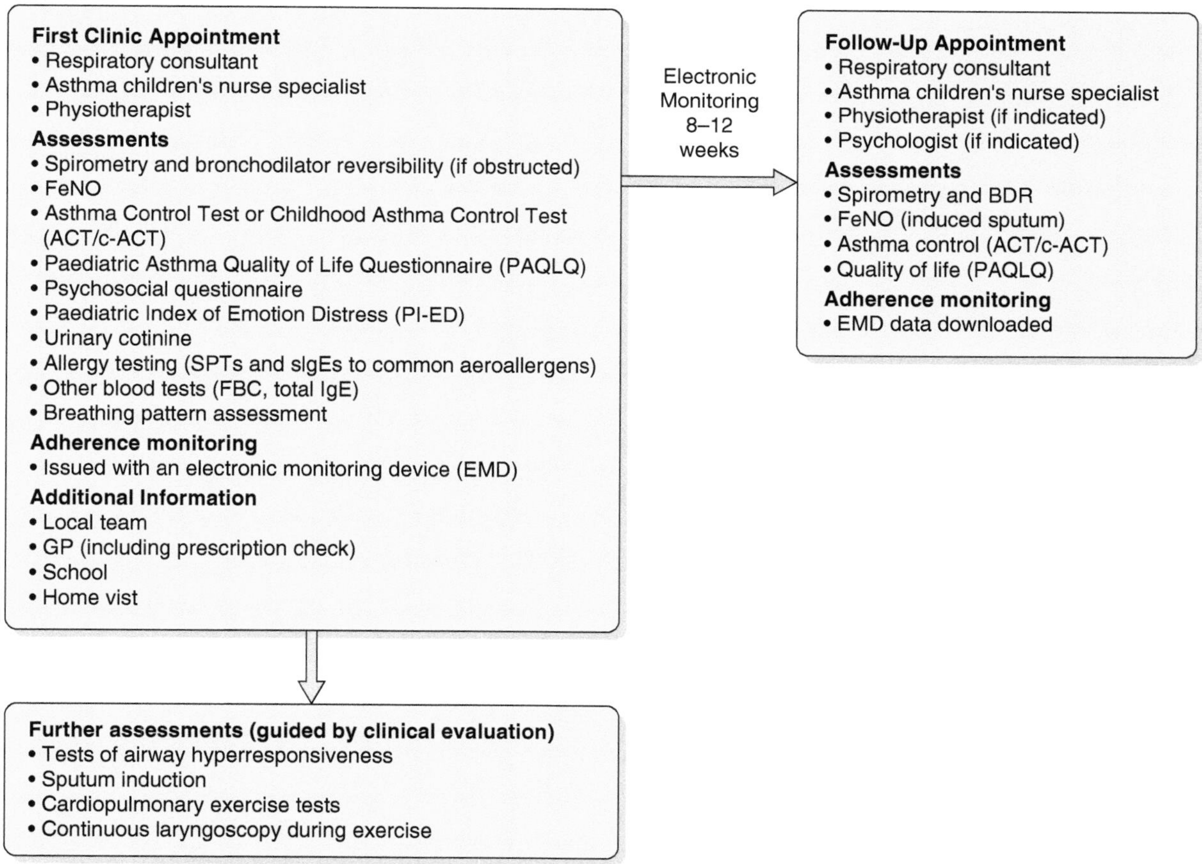

First Clinic Appointment
- Respiratory consultant
- Asthma children's nurse specialist
- Physiotherapist

Assessments
- Spirometry and bronchodilator reversibility (if obstructed)
- FeNO
- Asthma Control Test or Childhood Asthma Control Test (ACT/c-ACT)
- Paediatric Asthma Quality of Life Questionnaire (PAQLQ)
- Psychosocial questionnaire
- Paediatric Index of Emotion Distress (PI-ED)
- Urinary cotinine
- Allergy testing (SPTs and sIgEs to common aeroallergens)
- Other blood tests (FBC, total IgE)
- Breathing pattern assessment

Adherence monitoring
- Issued with an electronic monitoring device (EMD)

Additional Information
- Local team
- GP (including prescription check)
- School
- Home vist

Electronic Monitoring 8–12 weeks

Follow-Up Appointment
- Respiratory consultant
- Asthma children's nurse specialist
- Physiotherapist (if indicated)
- Psychologist (if indicated)

Assessments
- Spirometry and BDR
- FeNO (induced sputum)
- Asthma control (ACT/c-ACT)
- Quality of life (PAQLQ)

Adherence monitoring
- EMD data downloaded

Further assessments (guided by clinical evaluation)
- Tests of airway hyperresponsiveness
- Sputum induction
- Cardiopulmonary exercise tests
- Continuous laryngoscopy during exercise

• **Fig. 27.1** Assessments performed at the multidisciplinary hospital visit. *BDR,* Bronchodilator reversibility; *GP,* general practitioner; *IgE,* immunoglobulin E; *sIgE,* specific IgE; *SPTs,* skin prick tests.

errors are failure to document physician-heard wheeze and failure to document airflow obstruction that changes over time or with treatment. Furthermore, breathlessness is often uncritically attributed to asthma and treatment escalated, when in fact more than half of such children (and not just the obese) are deconditioned.[20] The *Lancet* commission[21] has highlighted the need to base management of objective diagnosis of treatable traits such as airway eosinophilia (i.e., induced sputum eosinophil count, peripheral blood eosinophil count, exhaled nitric oxide [FeNO], usually measured at a flow rate of 50 mL/s [fractional FeNO {$FeNO_{50}$}] supported by the documentation of atopy) and airflow obstruction with bronchodilator reversibility (i.e., acute administration of a SABA, a short period of home peak flow monitoring, or a field exercise test). The decision as to whether to investigate further and what tests to perform is driven by findings on history and examination. Finally, the diagnostic process should not end at this stage; the possibility of a wrong diagnosis always should be at the forefront and further testing considered in the presence of a surprising finding such as airway neutrophilia (see later discussion).

Numerous conditions mimic asthma (Table 27.1). The most likely mimics will vary by age and across the world. Important clues to a nonasthma diagnosis include neonatal onset of symptoms, chronic productive cough for more than 4 to 8 weeks, and evidence of systemic disease. The nonatopic child with apparently severe asthma always should be carefully assessed for alternative diagnoses. A review of diagnostic testing for all the conditions listed in Table 27.1 is beyond the scope of this chapter, but as a general principle, testing should be done in a logical and focused manner.

The Next Step: Assessment by the Entire Multidisciplinary Team for the Initial Management Plan

Once it is clear that the child truly has an airway disease and that a diagnosis other than one of the asthmas is unlikely, a full assessment is performed, focusing on comorbidities and possible social or environmental factors involved. This is because most school-age children (in contrast to preschool children exhibiting wheezing) with asthma have an airway disease that is usually easy to treat.[1] We perform a comprehensive assessment over two clinic visits,[6,8,21–23] with the primary aims of formulating an individualized management plan and deciding on other appropriate investigations and interventions (see Fig. 27.1). The information gained at these visits is supplemented by insights from the local team, general practitioner (including prescription record), and school and home visits.

Are There Significant Comorbidities to Address?

A thorough history is obtained and clinical examination performed, including the evaluation of comorbidities. These have been reviewed in detail.[24] Children with one or more comorbidities that do not improve on standard management (including because the parents are unable or unwilling to implement management strategies) are put in the category "refractory asthma plus"; we now argue[12] that these children too should be candidates for biologic therapies (see later discussion).

Allergic Rhinitis

Upper airway disease worsens quality of life and should be treated on its own merits in any context.[25,26] There is increasing evidence that treating allergic rhinitis may be beneficial at least in mild to moderate asthma.[27] The mechanisms of any benefit remain conjectural.[28,29] In our series, severe allergic rhinitis is unusual in severe asthma.

Obesity

Complex interactions exist between asthma and obesity. Obesity may cause breathlessness and wheezing without evidence of any airway disease, potentially leading to inappropriate treatment escalation. However, it is clear that children with true asthma complicating obesity have a severe phenotype. Although obese children are not immune from atopic, type 2–driven asthma,[30] generally, obese asthma is not the same as lean asthma, represents a different endotype,[31] and may be steroid resistant.[32] There may be airway growth (normal forced expired volume in 1 second [FEV_1], above-normal forced vital capacity [FVC], and reduced FEV_1/FVC ratio, implying abnormally long airways) that is associated with more severe disease.[33] The airway may be the target of interleukin 6 (IL-6)-mediated systemic inflammation, independent of type 2 inflammation.[34] Asthma (by reduced exercise performance) and its treatment (prednisolone bursts or long-term therapy) may cause or contribute to obesity. Therefore, particular care is necessary before escalating therapy for suspected asthma in

TABLE 27.1 Differential Diagnoses of Severe Asthma

Class of Diagnosis	Examples
Local immunodeficiency	Cystic fibrosis, primary ciliary dyskinesia, persistent bacterial bronchitis
Systemic immunodeficiency	Any, including B cell and T cell dysfunction
Intraluminal bronchial obstruction	Foreign body, carcinoid, other tumor
Intramural bronchial obstruction	Tracheobronchomalacia, complete cartilage rings, intramural tumor
Extraluminal bronchial obstruction	Vascular ring, pulmonary artery sling, congenital lung cyst, enlarged lymph nodes because of tumor or tuberculosis, other mediastinal masses
Direct aspiration	Bulbar or pseudobulbar palsy; laryngeal cleft
Aspiration by direct contamination	H-type fistula
Aspiration secondary to reflux	Any cause of gastroesophageal reflux, including hiatus hernia and esophageal dysmotility
Complications of prematurity	Bronchomalacia, structuring secondary to intubation, vocal cord palsy secondary to surgery for patent arterial duct
Congenital heart disease	Bronchial compression from enlarged cardiac chambers or great vessels; pulmonary edema
Interstitial lung disease	Any not presenting with neonatal respiratory failure
Dysfunctional breathing	Exercise-induced laryngeal obstruction, hyperventilation syndromes

the obese child with respiratory symptoms. Weight reduction is always beneficial in the obese child but may be difficult to achieve. It is associated with better symptom control,[35] but often it is not clear that any improvement is due to change in airway disease status. Bariatric surgery may be indicated in the very obese.[36]

Airway Obstruction and Sleep-Disordered Breathing

The literature on asthma and obstructive sleep apnea (OSA) is increasing.[37,38] Although there are associations in at least mild to moderate asthma, OSA is very rare in our cohort except in the presence of concomitant obesity (see earlier discussion). We do not routinely perform polysomnography on children with severe asthma who are not obese and do not have symptoms of OSA. OSA was reported to be associated with sputum neutrophilia rather than eosinophilia in one study[39]; this inflammatory pattern rarely if ever occurs in true severe, therapy-resistant asthma and, if seen, should prompt a diagnostic reevaluation.

Dysfunctional Breathing

Exercise-induced laryngeal obstruction (EILO) and other forms of dysfunctional breathing are common in asthma,[40] although not all groups report this.[41] Failure to diagnose EILO frequently leads to inappropriate escalation of asthma therapy. There is much less work in children than in adults.[42–44] Of the children investigated after our protocol, 15% had evidence of dysfunctional breathing,[45] including hyperventilation and EILO. Clues include the absence of symptoms at night, symptoms during rather than after exercise, and often stridor rather than expiratory noises. An experienced respiratory physiotherapist should be asked to assess and treat any abnormal breathing patterns, although currently there is no randomized controlled trial evidence of benefit.[40] Parental video-recording of an attack may be illuminating.[46] In older children, direct laryngoscopy during an exercise test enables direct demonstration of the problem.[47] Dyspnea perception has been little studied in severe pediatric asthma,[44] but adults with severe asthma do not become as dyspneic as those with mild asthma during bronchoconstriction.[48] The possibility of poor perception of airflow obstruction as a cause of an apparent sudden catastrophic deterioration should be borne in mind.

Food Allergy

Atopy is common in severe pediatric asthma, but patients with asthma and food allergy are overrepresented.[49,50] Whether food allergy is causative of the problem or a marker is unclear; certainly anaphylaxis enters the differential diagnosis of acute severe asthma and always should be considered because it is treatable. Food allergy should be properly documented if exclusion diets are proposed; blind dietary exclusions are frequently tried and in our experience are of no benefit. We do not routinely perform double-blind food challenges unless there is a strongly suggestive history, in which case we refer to a specialist allergy service. Children with an unclear history of possible allergy may also benefit from such a referral to document whether a putative allergy in fact exists.

Gastroesophageal Reflux

Gastroesophageal reflux is common in severe asthma, but treatment does not improve asthma outcomes.[51–53]

Characterizing Asthma in the Individual Child: Are There Significant Social and Environmental Factors?

The effects of social and environmental factors are extremely common in children with severe asthma. Evaluation of these factors

involves input especially from respiratory nurse specialists and clinical psychologists and includes hospital, home, and school evaluation.

Atopy

We evaluate allergic sensitization by both skin prick tests and specific immunoglobulin E tests, because there is imperfect concordance (76%–83%) between them.[54,55] This includes fungal sensitization,[54] because severe asthma with fungal sensitization (SAFS) (Table 27.2) has different treatment options (see later discussion).

Airway Inflammation. $FeNO_{50}$ is routinely measured; it indirectly measures airway eosinophilia but is neither fully sensitive nor specific[56]; it is also elevated in atopic children without airway[57] disease. However, a normal or low $FeNO_{50}$ in a very symptomatic child would militate against type 2 inflammation–driven asthma as a cause for the child's symptoms. FeNO also can be measured at multiple flow rates as an indirect assessment of proximal (J_{NO}) and distal (C_{ALV}) airway inflammation.[58] Although there is evidence that distal inflammation may be important in severe asthma (see later discussion), variable-flow FeNO is largely a research technique and indeed many children cannot perform satisfactory maneuvers, so this is no longer part of our routine clinical assessment.

Spirometry, Bronchodilator Responsiveness, and Bronchial Challenge Testing. Spirometry poorly discriminates between asthma of different severities in children; however, it can be useful in the individual.[59–61] Spirometry is part of clinical monitoring, particularly to monitor progression of lung growth (see later discussion). The acute response to a SABA may be used diagnostically. Airway challenge testing is generally used only in children with normal spirometry but reported severe symptoms and in whom a negative challenge would make uncontrolled asthma unlikely. In such children, a combined protocol of hypertonic saline challenge and sputum induction[62] may be useful; in genuine severe asthma, the need for albuterol pretreatment before sputum induction as a

TABLE 27.2	Diagnostic Criteria for Severe Asthma With Fungal Sensitization	
Adult Criteria	**Proposed Pediatric Criteria***	
Treatment with 500 mcg fluticasone/day or continuous oral corticosteroids, or 4 prednisolone bursts in the previous 12 months or 12 in the previous 24 months, *and*	Meets criteria for problematic severe asthma (see Box 27.1)	
IgE <1000 (exclude ABPA)	No IgE exclusion	
Negative IgG precipitins to *Aspergillus fumigatus*	No IgG exclusion	
Sensitization (SPT, sIgE) to at least one of *Aspergillus fumigatus, Alternaria alternata, Cladosporium herbarum, Penicillium chrysogenum, Candida albicans, Trichophyton mentagrophytes,* and *Botrytis cinerea*	As adult criteria	

*There is no agreed definition in children, but given the rarity of ABPA in children with asthma, we have proposed to eliminate the total IgE and IgG criteria from the diagnostic criteria.
ABPA, Allergic bronchopulmonary aspergillosis; *IgE,* immunoglobulin E (IgG); *sIgE,* specific IgE; *SPT,* skin prick test.

safety measure precludes this approach. Methacholine and exercise challenges also can be used; again, a negative challenge is most useful to rule out asthma in a symptomatic child.

High-Resolution Computed Tomographic Scanning. High-resolution computed tomographic scanning (HRCT) may on occasion be performed as part of the diagnostic workup if, for example, the patient is nonatopic or bronchiectasis is suspected, but in children HRCT is not a useful biomarker in severe asthma. Furthermore, HRCT scans are unable to distinguish severe asthma from obliterative bronchiolitis.[63]

Home Visit. The nurse-led home visit is a key part of the workup.[45] Clinicians in the office do not actually know what is really occurring in the patient's home. Five areas are explored: adherence, tobacco and e-cigarette exposure, allergens, psychosocial issues, and asthma education. If the patient has been referred from a distant center, the home visit may be performed by a local specialist nurse after discussion with our own team. This approach may not be feasible everywhere, but in our hands, it allows the identification of significant and potentially reversible factors in more than half of those referred with problematic severe asthma. It is certain that relying purely on a hospital-based assessment by a pediatrician will lead to many mistakes.

Adherence. The home visit is discussed in detail in Chapter 28. We found that fewer than half of patients had collected more than 80% of their required prescriptions, and nearly one-third had picked up less than 50%.[45] We also enumerate the collection of excessive prescriptions for SABAs; collecting six or more prescriptions per year is associated with a poor outcome.[10]

It was common to find that medication was past its expiry date; in nearly 25% of cases a complete set of in-date medications could not be produced when the nurse did a planned home visit. Other issues were total inaccessibility of any medications and medications unopened in their original wrapping, neither of which inspired confidence that medications were actually being taken.[45] Electronic monitoring of adherence over a 3-month period using a smart inhaler is now a routine part of assessment. The child and family know that adherence is being monitored. The results are often very illuminating[64] (Table 27.3, Fig. 27.2). Of course the devices only measure activation, not inhalation, and may overestimate adherence.[65] A pilot study has shown that using a cell phone to record the child taking treatment and a Bluetooth technology–equipped smart inhaler to send the data to the center is feasible; of concern, however, was that despite multiple teaching sessions at the hospital, it took 5 weeks before inhaler technique was correct.[66]

Parental Supervision. In one study, even young children (20% of 7 year olds, 50% of 11 year olds) were left to take asthma medications unsupervised.[67] Often parents think they are supervising treatment, but do not in fact actually witness their child take the therapy, instead merely calling out reminders to their child who is in a different room in the home. This situation requires sensitive exploration. In older adolescents it is important that they take more responsibility for their own health and well-being and are provided with appropriate asthma education and support to achieve greater autonomy as they transition to adult care.

Use of Inhaler Devices. Inhaler devices are often wrongly used, and regular instruction in their use may lead to improvements.[66–68] However, even multiple teaching sessions are not enough to ensure good inhaler technique[66]; all of the children in our series had repeated instruction in specialized centers and yet still many had poor technique. A common issue is using pressurized metered-dose inhalers without spacers, because spacers are considered babyish; this omission guarantees minimal airway deposition of medications. We also frequently see children inappropriately using spacers and masks. From 2 or 3 years of age most children should be able to use a spacer with a mouthpiece. Assessment of technique with an inhalational device by an experienced respiratory nurse is essential if the best device is to be found for an individual patient

Environmental Tobacco Smoke and Other Irritants. Active smoking by adults with asthma causes steroid resistance,[69–73] and it appears likely that passive smoke exposure (including exposure to vaping, which the authors consider to be potentially more harmful than tobacco[74]) has the same effect. Passive smoke exposure is common in children with asthma[75–77]; the prevalence of active smoking is unknown, but unlikely to be low. We found that 25% of children with problematic, severe asthma were exposed to tobacco smoke.[45]

The mechanisms of tobacco smoke–induced steroid resistance have been researched mainly in adults[78]; the phenotype is neutrophilic. In children with severe, therapy-resistant asthma,[79] parental smoking reduced histone deacetylase protein expression and activity and induced in vitro steroid resistance. Bronchoalveolar

TABLE 27.3	**Summary of Results of Electronic Monitoring**	
Symptom/Test Results	**Interpretation**	**Actions**
FEV_1 and FeNO abnormal at start of monitoring, adherent during monitoring, tests normalize and symptoms improve	Previously nonadherent, became adherent during monitoring	Intervention to support adherence
FEV_1 and FeNO abnormal at start of monitoring, adherent during monitoring, tests remain abnormal, still symptomatic	Severe, therapy-resistant asthma	Invasive airway phenotyping
FEV_1 and FeNO abnormal at start of monitoring, nonadherent during monitoring, tests remain abnormal, still symptomatic	Either refractory severe asthma; or severe, therapy-resistant asthma who stopped medications because they do not work	Ascertain response to DOT; if no response, invasive airway phenotyping. If responds, refractory difficult asthma, consider simplifying regimens or biologic agents
Poorly adherent on monitoring, but actually remains well with normal FEV_1 and FeNO	Previously overtreated	Wean asthma treatment

DOT, Directly observed therapy; *FeNO,* fractional expired nitric oxide; *FEV_1,* forced expiratory volume in 1 second.

Results of electronic monitoring

- Adherence good, ACT & FEV_1 improve, FeNO falls = problematic severe asthma, disappearing when medications taken (24%, see right panel)

- Adherence poor, no improvement = refractory severe asthma or disillusioned STRA, (32%)—WHAT HAPPENS WHEN TREATMENT TAKEN?

- Adherence good, no change in asthma control or attacks – true STRA, go to invasive assessment of airway (18%)

- Poor adherence, good control—likely overtreated (32%)

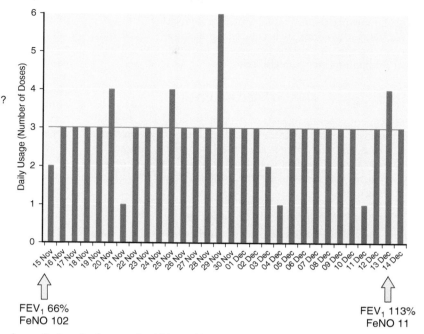

FEV$_1$ 66%
FeNO 102

FEV$_1$ 113%
FeNO 11

• **Fig. 27.2** Interpretation of electronic monitoring of adherence in children with apparently severe asthma. *ACT,* Asthma Control Test; *FeNO,* fractional exhaled nitric oxide; *FEV$_1$,* forced expiratory volume in 1 second; *STRA,* severe, therapy resistant asthma.

lavage (BAL) showed higher IL-8 concentrations and neutrophil counts, and the children had lower Asthma Control Test (ACT) scores compared with nonpassive smoke-exposed children. Additionally, it is also likely that symptoms are exacerbated by a direct irritant effect of smoke.

Other environmental irritants sometimes encountered include incense or joss sticks and the extensive use of air fresheners and other aerosol sprays. Environmental pollution is also important but is difficult to modulate except at the level of public health.

Allergen Exposure. Allergen exposure is discussed in detail elsewhere. Allergen exposure in the home combined with evidence of sensitization is all too common[45] and has been clearly implicated in the cause of asthma attacks.[80] Reduction of mold exposure may be particularly important if SAFS is suspected. Allergen exposure in school also may be important,[81] but this is an even more difficult area in which to intervene.

Psychosocial Issues. Acute and chronic stress may trigger asthma exacerbations[82–84]; there may be quite complex time relationships between the two. Stress has been shown to amplify the airway eosinophilic response to allergen challenge.[85] Psychosocial issues are common, especially anxiety and depression.[45,86] Most issues emerged only during discussions in the home.[45] It is not productive to try to determine whether anxiety and depression are the cause or result of severe asthma; both are treated on their individual merits.

Asthma Education. Some adherence issues relate to basic misunderstandings of the purpose of treatment, and these are also addressed. If the child does not have a detailed asthma plan, this is put in place and communicated to the school. It is to be hoped that all this will have been done previously, but any gaps are sought and closed. All children are issued with an updated personal asthma action plan at each visit.

Lesson Learned the Hard Way

School Visit

Despite the best efforts of our specialist respiratory nurses, we have made many mistakes. The importance of contact with the school cannot be overemphasized. Teachers are an important resource; they are experienced in assessing children and spend many hours each day with them. If there is any suspicion that symptoms are being overcalled by the parents, speak with the teacher. In one particularly egregious case (details modified to preserve patient confidentiality) a girl with so-called severe asthma was in fact the captain of the field hockey team and had the nickname "the Greyhound"; her teachers did not know she even had asthma, let alone keep a reserve supply of SABA for her.

Management of Asthma Attacks

The implications of asthma attacks are discussed in detail later. In theory, treatment is based on objective measurements of severity. In practice, the history is influential. When assessing the child with apparent multiple severe attacks, it is essential to determine what (if any) objective assessments were carried out before instituting treatment and whether the level of treatment was objectively justified. One child under our care was started on intravenous albuterol despite being fully saturated on room air when she was in fact hyperventilating. Episodes such as this should be taken seriously, but the answer is not escalating asthma treatment.

Parental Doublespeak

The basic tenet of pediatrics is to believe the parents. On occasion, parents deliberately not telling the truth may be the underlying problem and may be difficult to detect. This is distinct from the effect of an understandable parental anxiety leading to exaggeration of symptoms. Motivation for the former may include access to financial and other benefits as a result of having a "sick" child, right up to deliberate fabrication of symptoms (Munchausen by proxy). Unfortunately, the result is often a long delay in diagnosis. We frequently admit such children to hospital[87] for directly observed therapy and detailed observation, usually including a formal cardiopulmonary exercise test.

Multidisciplinary Team Discussion

The assessment generates a mass of detailed information, and this is next assessed in a dedicated, multidisciplinary team meeting. We aim to determine whether the child has difficult asthma, for which the basic management steps need to be addressed, or potentially severe, therapy-resistant asthma, which justifies further invasive investigations.

What Sort of Asthma Does the Child Have?

In more than 80% of the children, no further investigations are undertaken, or, at least, invasive testing is deferred pending other interventions. This unfortunately does not mean the problem is necessarily solved; for example, it is one thing to identify poor adherence as an issue, but quite another to address it. Often, the child's poor adherence to medication has not been appreciated by the parents, and identification of the problem leads to them finding a solution, such as setting up text reminders. It may be appropriate to use the MART regimen (budesonide/formoterol once or twice daily and as needed), which has been shown to be helpful.[87] At least theoretically, a once-daily, long-acting ICS/LABA combination such as fluticasone furoate/vilanterol might help adherence in eligible children. We have sometimes used directly observed therapy at school, on the basis that 5 days of treatment a week is better than none; if this is put in place, it is essential to check that the direct observation is actually happening. One child told us that the school nurse was always working at a desk with her back to the child when supposedly directly observing therapy. It is also necessary to ensure the inhaler is not empty or out of date.

Deferring investigations for psychological intervention is common. Psychological interventions may be effective.[88] In general, individualized plans work best.[89–91] Of course, these may be combined with the other interventions outlined previously and also with invasive investigations.

Addressing allergen exposure in the home is notoriously difficult, especially if the allergen concerned originates from a much-loved family pet (the English disease). Frequently, the cat will be sent away for a short time and then allowed to return because the child's asthma has not improved; however, at least a year without the presence of the cat is necessary substantially to reduce the allergen load.

The fact that many children with apparent severe asthma just need to have basic management handled correctly has been reported by others and has been an issue in intervention study design; those with apparently severe asthma tend improve considerably when proper, protocol-driven management is put in place.[92] Those thought at this stage to have true, therapy-resistant asthma proceed to airway phenotyping (see later discussion); no physiologic or inflammation measurement at baseline is clinically useful to distinguish them from the other groups.[93,94] The remainder are followed to determine if intervention has been successful.

Follow-Up: Has Intervention Worked?

Many patients assigned to the group with asthma that was difficult to control[93] were able to reduce their prescribed dose of ICS

(although perhaps in reality they were actually taking it for the first time) while increasing their FEV_1 and having fewer prednisolone bursts than the children with severe, therapy-resistant asthma, similar to findings in multifaceted intervention studies reported in those with less severe asthma.[95,96] However, some remain with poor outcomes despite all treatment attempts by the multidisciplinary team. These are children with refractory difficult asthma, or refractory asthma plus. We used to argue that treating nonadherent children with very costly biologic agents was unjustified; however, we now use them because children in this group are at particular risk of severe attacks and death.[12]

Research Implications. This differentiation of true severe, therapy-resistant asthma has important implications for the interpretation of research studies, such as genetic association studies. Cohorts of children with supposed severe asthma who have not gone through a detailed filtering process will be diluted by at least 80% with children for whom the basics have simply not been addressed and therefore may not be comparable to those with truly therapy-resistant asthma.[21] This is the most likely explanation for recent findings that there is substantial genetic overlap between mild to moderate and severe asthma.[97,98]

Protocol: Invasive Investigation of Severe, Therapy-Resistant Asthma

Typically children with severe, therapy-resistant asthma are phenotyped invasively to answer four key questions (Box 27.2).[99] Children with severe, therapy-resistant asthma differ from adults; there is no female predominance, but a strong atopic history is common[93,99] (85% atopy with a total median IgE of 386 [115–1286]), and we rarely see neutrophilic asthma.[98] Indeed, although in adult asthma, submucosal neutrophils are associated with a worse outlook, in children, neutrophils that are intraepithelial are associated with *better* asthma outcomes.[100] The children are also not more obese. An individualized treatment plan is devised on the basis of the answers to these questions in Box 27.2.

The child is assessed invasively and noninvasively on the same day. Noninvasive investigations are symptom assessment, spirometry, and acute response to bronchodilator, sputum induction, and FeNO. The child then undergoes a bronchoscopy under a general anesthetic, with performance of BAL and endobronchial biopsy, and often bronchial brushings as a research procedure.[99] The key requirement for the safe performance of bronchoscopy in these children is a skilled anesthetist. The child may be premedicated with SABAs. Adverse events are very rare. Close postbronchoscopy

---

> • **BOX 27.2** **Four Key Questions Answered by Invasive Investigation of Children With Severe, Therapy-Resistant Asthma**
>
> 1. Is there phenotype discordance: a disconnect between symptoms and airway inflammation? Antiinflammatory medication is not escalated if the airway is not inflamed and is intensified in an exacerbating child if there is airway inflammation when the child is asymptomatic.
> 2. Is the airway inflamed at all, and, if so, what is the pattern of inflammation?
> 3. Is the child partially or totally steroid responsive or steroid resistant?
> 4. Does the child have persistent airflow limitation? Therapy for airflow obstruction is not escalated if the child has reached the plateau of the dose-response curve.

monitoring of the child is essential. We administer a single dose of intramuscular triamcinolone (40–80 mg depending on the size of the child). The child is kept in hospital overnight. The child is then seen again 4 weeks later, and all the noninvasive measurements are repeated to assess steroid response.

Assessment of Airway Inflammation

Induced sputum, BAL, and endobronchial biopsy are either eosinophilic or, in some children, pauci-inflammatory. There tends to be agreement between induced sputum and BAL, but discordance exists between these luminal compartments and the airway wall histologic findings.[101] It is not clear which is most relevant to disease pathophysiologic processes. The relationship between FeNO and airway eosinophilia is discussed later. Many have an eosinophilic phenotype, and a T helper cell type 2 (T_H2) cytokine profile would be expected, but two pediatric severe asthma studies have failed to confirm this. We found scant evidence of the T_H2 signature cytokines IL-4, IL-5, and IL-13.[99] The Severe Asthma Research Program (SARP) group also failed to find evidence of T_H2-driven inflammation[102] and showed that the cytokines that best discriminated between severe asthma were GRO (CXCL1), RANTES (CCL5), IL-12, interferon-gamma (IFN-γ), and IL-10. Gene expression studies demonstrating T_H2 high and low groups in adults have so far not been performed in children.[103] Whether those few children in whom T_H2 cytokines are detectable are in fact T_H2 high is unknown. Periostin, a useful serum biomarker in adults for the T_H2 high phenotype, is not useful in children because it is released from growing bone.

The findings of these two studies do not necessarily show that T_H2 cytokines are unimportant in the pathophysiologic processes of severe asthma. All children with severe, therapy-resistant asthma are by definition prescribed high-dose ICSs, and it may be that the T_H2 component of their disease is abrogated by this therapy. What these studies do suggest is that the factors driving ongoing disease in children are different from those in adults. Attention is shifting to the epithelial-derived cytokines (IL-25, IL-33, thymic stromal lymphopoietin [TSLP]) as possible candidates, perhaps interacting with innate lymphoid cells.[104–106] We have shown that IL-33 promoted collagen synthesis by fibroblasts from pediatric patients with severe asthma.[107] We also showed that increased cellular expression of IL-33, but not IL-13, was associated with increased reticular basement membrane thickness in endobronchial biopsies. IL-33 also stained strongly in the endobronchial biopsy samples. In addition, a 2014 study of a monoclonal antibody (AMG 157) that prevents TSLP interacting with its receptor led to marked attenuation of both the early and late phase allergen response in adults with mild asthma,[108] a surprising finding given that only a single cytokine was blocked.[109]

The T_H17 pathway has been considered another candidate, at least in adults, but it possibly more likely drives a neutrophilic phenotype and thus is an unlikely candidate in children. However, eosinophil chemoattraction by IL-17 has been reported, at least in animal models.[110,111] A 2013 trial of the monoclonal anti–IL-17 receptor antibody brodalumab in adults was disappointing, perhaps because neutrophilic asthma was not an entry criterion.[112] Further work is clearly needed to delineate the proinflammatory mechanisms driving pediatric severe, therapy-resistant asthma.

There is an important implication of the previously described findings. Randomized, controlled studies of anti-T_H2 cytokine monoclonal agents have recruited only very few children aged 12 years and older and even fewer younger than 12 years.[113] It is essential that the results in these trials are not uncritically extrapolated to children and that pediatric trials are performed.

TABLE 27.4	Domains and Definition of Steroid Responsiveness	
Modality	**Response**
Symptoms	ACT >19/25 or 50% increase
Spirometry	FEV_1 >80% predicted or 15% increase
$FeNO_{50}$	Falls to <24 ppb
Sputum eosinophils	Falls to <2.5%

ACT, Asthma Control Test; *FeNO₅₀*, fractional exhaled nitric oxide; *FEV₁*, forced expiratory volume in 1 second; *ppb*, parts per billion.

Assessment of Steroid Responsiveness

It is likely that steroid responsiveness is a continuum; true steroid unresponsiveness is likely confined to rare cases of mutations in the corticosteroid receptor. The widely accepted definition of adult steroid response in adults[114,115] is 15% or greater predicted increase in FEV_1 in patients with bronchodilator reversibility of 12% or greater from baseline and an abnormal FEV_1 (≤80%) before the trial. There is no accepted definition in children, and the adult definition cannot be applied to around half of our pediatric patients with severe, therapy-resistant asthma, mainly because their baseline spirometry result is not sufficiently abnormal before the trial.[99] There is no consensus on the dose and duration of corticosteroids for the trial. We opted to use triamcinolone intramuscularly to ensure adherence. We use a multimodality definition of steroid responsiveness (Table 27.4).[116] Most children are partial responders, about 10% are total nonresponders and 10% are completely responsive in all domains. Some children who were nonresponsive according to the adult definition were partial responders in the multidomain assessment. Additional doses of triamcinolone do not change the category of responsiveness (unpublished, 2019). Although the clinical utility of this approach has yet to be confirmed, it might serve as a useful template for current research; so, for example, an intervention with an antiinflammatory medication might be expected to primarily affect the inflammatory domain.[117]

Assessment of Persistent Airflow Limitation. The definition of persistent airflow limitation (PAL) is relatively easy; FEV_1 less than 80% (or better, –1.96 Z [standard deviation] scores) despite a trial of systemic steroids and acute administration of SABAs. However, the dose, duration, and route of administration of steroids still has to be agreed upon, as has the dose of SABAs. We have shown that neither 40 mg of prednisolone for 2 weeks[118] nor a single dose of triamcinolone combined with 1 mg albuterol inhaled from a large volume spacer[119] is adequate to determine whether the child has PAL. Thus, we have taken the pragmatic decision that PAL should be at least provisionally diagnosed after a single dose of triamcinolone and albuterol as described earlier, which is supported by 2017 data published in abstract.[120]

Treatment of Pediatric Severe, Therapy-Resistant Asthma and Refractory (Nonadherent) Difficult Asthma

The treatment options, with the exception of the use of the biologic agents, are largely anecdotally based.[121] The following scheme is suggested:

- *Are biologic agents indicated?* Much of the evidence for omalizumab is inevitably in less severe asthma,[122–131] but if the child meets national guidelines for asthma *and* has been assessed in detail, as discussed earlier, and found to have persistent eosinophilic airway inflammation and aeroallergen sensitization, we recommend a 16-week trial of omalizumab, with detailed monitoring of the response. Omalizumab also may be used as a trial in the rare child without atopy with IgE in the range for which it is indicated.[132] If after 16 weeks there is no benefit, as assessed by symptoms, including asthma attacks, lung function, and airway inflammation (FeNO, induced sputum eosinophils), we discontinue therapy. Mepolizumab is now licensed in the United Kingdom for children of 6 years and older, despite the absence of efficacy and safety data.[113] It is the preferred option in children who have a blood eosinophil count greater than 150/µL or direct evidence of eosinophilic airway inflammation. It may be especially valuable in children with an IgE level above the dose range for omalizumab. The advantage of these approaches is that adherence is ensured by the parenteral administration of biologic agents, and also there have to be regular hospital visits allowing asthma assessments to take place. There is an increasing number of other biologic agents targeting the T_H2 pathway that are licensed in adults (e.g., benralizumab, which blocks IL-5 binding to its receptor; reslizumab, which binds to IL-5; and dupilumab, which blocks IL-4 and IL-13 signaling); undoubtedly these will be licensed in children in the future. Current indications in adolescents and adults recently have been summarized.[133]

- *Should standard medications be used in novel ways?* Options are high-dose ICSs, fine particle ICSs, oral prednisolone, and intramuscular triamcinolone; the MART regimen (a single combination ICS and LABA device, usually a Symbicort Turbohaler); and low-dose theophylline (antiinflammatory dose) if not already used before referral. The increasing use of omalizumab and mepolizumab mean theophylline and systemic steroids are rarely used. For most children, the plateau of the ICS dose response curve is 100 mcg twice daily of fluticasone,[1] and escalation of dosing risks increased side effects. However, a small minority of children with asthma may benefit from increasing the dose to as high as 2000 mcg/day.[134] However, if there is no response to dose escalation, it is essential that the ICS is promptly stepped down to the lowest possible dose. There is evidence from adult studies that some patients with asthma may have very distal inflammation on transbronchial biopsy.[135–137] These studies have not been performed in children because of the risks of transbronchial biopsy. There is also physiologic evidence from alveolar nitric oxide (NO) concentration (C_{alv}) measurements of distal airway inflammation in adults with asthma, with response both symptomatically and physiologically to fine particle ICSs or systemic steroids.[138,139] There is too much variability in C_{alv} for it to be used as a biomarker in individual children,[58] and there is no evidence for this approach in severe, therapy-resistant asthma. However, a trial of fine particle ICS may be worth considering, with its discontinuation if there is no benefit, although it is arguable how much actually reaches the target site if there is peripheral airway disease. Finally, it is interesting to speculate whether distal airway inflammation is related to poor peripheral deposition of ICS and might respond to low-dose oral prednisolone, delivering steroid by the blood-borne rather than the airborne route. We use the MART regimen both in severe, therapy-resistant asthma and in nonadherent children.[140] The risk of this strategy is that it relies on adequate symptom perception, which may not always be the case in children with severe asthma (see previous discussion).

- *Long-acting muscarinic agents.* The treatment of non-T_H2 and pauci-inflammatory phenotypes is a challenge. There is preliminary evidence from adult studies that ICSs are not effective.[141] Azithromycin reduced asthma attacks in neutrophilic asthma in an adult study.[142] Most data on antimuscarinic agents are in adults[143–145] and showed some nonconclusive evidence for reduction in asthma attacks. Clinical trials in children have for the most part been in relatively mild disease and shown safety without dramatic efficacy,[146–149] usually without phenotyping the children treated.

- *Does the child meet criteria for SAFS (see Table 27.2)?* Results of treatment trials of antifungals in adults are conflicting.[150,151] Fungal sensitization in children may be associated with a more severe phenotype,[152] but there are no randomized controlled trials of treatment in children. Our approach to the child who meets criteria for SAFA is first to minimize environmental fungal exposure in the home, including checking any nebulizer the child may have for fungal contamination and banning visits to stables before considering any antifungal therapy. Azoles interact with ICSs, leading to iatrogenic Cushing's syndrome.[153–155] Anecdotally, antifungals have been helpful in some children, but side effects and the high cost should be remembered and treatment discontinued if there is no clear benefit.

- *Should nonstandard medications be used?* Immunosuppression, intravenous immunoglobulin as an immunomodulator, and continuous subcutaneous infusion of terbutaline have virtually no place in the management of pediatric asthma since the institution of better assessment, especially of adherence, and the availability of biologics. Macrolide antibiotics may be indicated for the rare child with noneosinophilic asthma or if an atypical infection is suspected.[156,157] One study comparing azithromycin with montelukast as add-on therapy ended in futility[158] because only 55 of the 292 who were symptomatic while prescribed ICSs and LABAs could be randomized; most of the rest were nonadherent or did not have asthma at all, underscoring the need for detailed evaluation of these patients before uncritical acceptance of the diagnosis of severe asthma. However, in the small group who were actually studied, the results were not encouraging.

A Difficult Specific Problem: Asthma Attacks

Elsewhere it has been argued that acute deteriorations are attacks not exacerbations[159,160]; they have serious short-term (morbidity, death) and long-term (impaired lung growth[161,162]) effects. Asthma attacks and loss of baseline control are not the same thing; loss of baseline control is characterized by wide diurnal peak expiratory flow variation and acute attacks by a steep decline in peak flow with no increased variability.[163] Children may have good control but still have attacks.[164] A systematic review synthesized the evidence on prediction of attack risk, and, unsurprisingly, the single biggest factor was a previous asthma attack.[165–167] Other factors included poor control,[165] overuse of SABAs, underuse of ICS, and, in the United States, poor access to care.

In older children, the combination of respiratory viral infection and both sensitization and exposure in the home to high allergen levels is strongly predictive of an attack.[80] These patients are typically characterized acutely by mixed eosinophilic and neutrophilic or pure neutrophilic inflammation.[168–170] At the other extreme, very high allergen exposure can cause acute attacks (e.g., thunderstorm asthma[170] and the Barcelona soya bean epidemic asthma[171]), and thunderstorm asthma at least is characterized by airway eosinophilia.[172]

It is essential that an asthma attack is seen as a never event, a sign of failure of management. It should lead to a focused response to prevent the next (potentially fatal) attack.[173] There is no place for a standard 3- or 5-day course of prednisolone with no follow-up. All aspects of the child's asthma management should be addressed. Adherence to ICS and use of a SABA should be checked by prescription uptake as a minimum and inhaler technique assessed. The asthma plan should be scrutinized. Was it followed? Should it be modified? Attention should be paid to the environment and reduction of tobacco or allergen exposure. In one study, children aged 3 to 17 who were admitted to hospital with an asthma attack and were sensitized to house dust mite were randomized to mite-impermeable or placebo bedding covers. The mite-impermeable group had fewer asthma attacks in the succeeding year.[174] The effect was relatively modest, and this might have been improved if the intervention had been more multifaceted[175,176]; for example, exposure to pet allergen was not tackled. However, this study is proof of the concept that a postattack environmental intervention may be of benefit. There is evidence that guiding therapy by FeNO levels and, to a lesser extent, induced sputum eosinophils may reduce attack frequency.[177] However, longitudinal studies in children show that spontaneous and unpredictable changes in sputum cellular phenotype common in all severities of pediatric asthma and were not predictable,[178] unlike in adults who have stable sputum phenotypes over time.[179] The relationship between sputum eosinophil count and FeNO is highly variable in severe, therapy-resistant asthma: 148 samples were concordant (eosinophil positive, FeNO positive = 77; both negative = 71) and 49 (25%) were discordant (eosinophil positive, FeNO negative = 25; eosinophil negative, FeNO positive = 24). Fifty-nine children produced at least two sputum samples. Of these, 31 (53%) were consistently concordant, 24 (41%) were discordant in one sample but concordant on at least one other occasion (one showed discordance in both directions and concordance in a third sample), and only 4 (7%) demonstrated consistently discordant levels.[180] Thus, FeNO and sputum eosinophilia cannot be used interchangeably. Certainly in adult studies, evidence of persistent airway eosinophilia is a risk of asthma attacks.[181–183]

Other potentially beneficial strategies in the attack-prone child include using the MART regimen.[70] Indeed, given the evidence that overuse of SABA and underuse of ICS are important factors in asthma attacks, it could be argued that after a bad attack, it is negligent to prescribe SABAs at all; a view supported by 2018 and 2019 data in adults.[184–187] Another strategy is omalizumab for allergic children at Global Initiative for Asthma (GINA) stage 5 who are having attacks and mepolizumab if there is evidence of ongoing airway eosinophilia. Interestingly, there is evidence that omalizumab has antiviral effects as well as binding to the high-affinity IgE receptor.[188] The hospital treatment of acute attacks is beyond the scope of this chapter.

Monitoring Treatment Benefit and Risks in the Child With Severe, Therapy-Resistant Asthma on Treatment

The focus has moved from solely measuring asthma control to measurement of risk, especially in the domains of risk of asthma attack, risks of side effects of medications, and risk of a poor lung growth trajectory.

Assessing the Risk of an Asthma Attack

Children may have apparently well-controlled asthma but be at high risk of an asthma attack, especially if there is uncontrolled type 2 airway inflammation. Ideally, residual inflammation would be measured directly, but probably the best that can be done in routine clinical practice is measurement of FeNO. Obviously, children with poorly controlled asthma and previous bad asthma attacks are at high risk. Risk prediction scores have been developed and need to be used more in clinical practice. One such is the Asthma Exacerbation Clinical Score (AECS), which uses 17 questions related to symptoms, medication, healthcare usage, and medical history, and was able to predict asthma attacks up to 1 year later with a sensitivity of 0.69. A risk score (Risk Score for Asthma Exacerbation [RSE]) was developed in 7446 adult patients using five dominant baseline predictors for a severe attack, and predicted the risk of uncontrolled asthma within 3 months and severe asthma attacks within 12 months with high sensitivity.[189] The role of these or other indices in routine clinical practice and also in low and middle income settings merits further work.[190]

Assessing the Risk of Side Effects of Medications

The main risk is of cumulative inhaled and systemic corticosteroid side effects, in particular growth failure and adrenal suppression. Also coming to the fore is that ICSs may lead to mucosal immunosuppression[191] and an increased risk of pneumonia,[192] tuberculosis,[193] and nontuberculous *Mycobacterial* infection,[194] at least in adults. Every effort should be made to minimize the dose of ICS and minimize systemic absorption by using a large-volume spacer. There is some evidence that giving more ICS than is needed to control inflammation, rather than the absolute prescribed dose, may be responsible for side effects. A study in adult normal volunteers and subjects with asthma showed that both groups cleared an intravenous dose of fluticasone equally rapidly, but there was much greater systemic absorption of an inhaled dose in the normal controls than the subjects with asthma.[195] In addition, in terms of monitoring, most recommend a Synacthen test for children on high-dose ICSs, but the level of ICS, the dose of adrenal corticotrophin, the sampling protocol, and the frequency at which the test is performed are still controversial. We currently recommend that growth is monitored in all children at clinic visits, preferably with a calibrated stadiometer. Children prescribed 500 mcg/day of fluticasone propionate or equivalent or prescribed multiple courses of systemic corticosteroids (arbitrarily, at least 4 per year) have an assessment of adrenal function using the low-dose Synacthen test. We also perform bone mineral density (DEXA) scans at least once, with follow-up examinations depending on the initial results. We do not routinely refer children with no visual symptoms for ophthalmology assessment.

Monitoring Growth Trajectories

Numerous birth cohort studies have highlighted (1) that for most, if not all, children spirometry tracks from the preschool years to late middle age[196–199]; (2) impaired spirometric growth to the normal plateau age of 20 to 25 years is a strong risk factor for chronic obstructive pulmonary disease[200]; and (3) childhood asthma is a strong risk factor for an adverse lung function trajectory.[197,201] Thus, there is an increasing focus on using spirometry not merely as a guide to present health status but also measuring trajectories for future prognosis.[190] The present difficulty is that we have no strategies to reverse a bad trajectory. Worryingly, even individuals with good symptom control exhibit abnormal airway growth over time,[162,202,203] especially in children with asthma attacks.[162,203] That catch-up may be possible is shown by a proof of concept study that those who have a delay in puberty exhibit a catch up in spirometry.[204] At the moment, all we can do is strongly recommend general health measures such as avoidance of tobacco and pollution, exercise, and immunizations. Of note, given that a low FEV_1 is associated with increased all cause (including cardiovascular and metabolic) morbidity and mortality,[205,206] attention should be given to more general issues such as obesity, diabetes, and hypertension prevention, which may be more amenable to modulation.

Role of an Annual Assessment?

There is a strong case to be made for a structured annual assessment in all children with severe, therapy-resistant asthma. This should include a re-evaluation of adherence, which notoriously deteriorates over time and allergen exposure, as well as screening questionnaires at least for psychological morbidity. Spirometry and acute bronchodilator responsiveness, sputum induction, and FeNO should also be part of the evaluation. The annual assessment also provides the opportunity to evaluate side effects with measurements of height and weight, blood pressure, urinalysis, and the performance of a Synacthen test. After this reassessment, a multidisciplinary planning meeting is held, with the aim of updating the treatment plan.

Severe, Therapy-Resistant Asthma: The Future?

A phenotype is the set of observable characteristics of an individual resulting from the interaction of its genotype with the environment. Asthma phenotyping has a very long history. An early protagonist was the late Dr. Harry Morrow-Brown,[207] who in the 1950s used his medical student microscope to show that only those with eosinophils in the sputum were steroid responsive, thus preventing the most effective treatments for eosinophilic asthma being cast into a therapeutic dustbin. We have moved back to phenotyping, with the concept of treatable traits such as airway eosinophilia treated with ICS, and, although this has been beneficial, it is still not sufficient. We need to move to endotypes, defined as a subtype of a condition, which is defined by a distinct functional or pathobiologic mechanism. This is particularly important as a greater range of biologics largely targeted at type 2 inflammation become available. First, not all airway eosinophilia is necessarily T_H2 cytokine driven.[99,102,208] Second, we must find a way of matching the right patient to the right biologic, rather than performing a series of N-of-1, unfocused trials of treatment. Measurements of –omics platforms and gene expression using induced sputum or upper airway cells[209] or exhaled breath analysis with devices such as the electronic nose[210] are needed to achieve this. We may be able to follow the example of oncologists, who are now looking for tumor gene expression signatures and matching these to medications that reverse these changes. This approach has identified sodium valproate as a possible treatment for triple-negative breast cancer,[211] not an immediately obvious compound in this context. Of course, this innovative approach risks reversing what is a protective change, but must surely replace putting steroids in the tap water to control asthma.

A huge unmet need in children (and adults) is pauci-inflammatory and non–type 2 asthma. Little is known about the pathophysiology, and there are tantalizing hints from adult studies that ICS may not be necessary or effective,[212] but azithromycin or tiotropium may be useful. One can hope that repurposing medications and modern –omics studies may shed light on this challenging area.

Summary and Conclusions

Severe asthma is one of the great challenges of pediatrics. Mismanagement may result in a dead child. This chapter has proposed a systematic approach, trying to optimize basic management by a skilled multidisciplinary team. We still do not really understand the underlying pathophysiology of very severe asthma and hence have no targeted treatments. It is not safe to assume that adult and pediatric severe asthma is the same disease; compared with adults, in children with severe asthma, atopy is much more prominent, there is no gender difference or increased prevalence of obesity, and eosinophilic not neutrophilic airway inflammation is the rule. Furthermore, pediatric eosinophilic asthma may not be T_H2 driven, meaning that the successful use of anti-T_H2 strategies in adults may not be replicated in children. We need mechanistic studies and randomized controlled trials of biologic agents in well-characterized groups of children with severe asthma, but these will be possible only once there is multinational and multicenter cooperation in adopting standardized assessment protocols.

The reference list can be found on the companion Expert Consult website at http://www.expertconsult.inkling.com.

28
Promoting Adherence and Self-Management

BRUCE G. BENDER

KEY POINTS

- Patients typically use less than half prescribed controller medication for asthma, and nearly half stop taking their medication altogether.
- Nonadherence in turn undermines asthma control.
- Brief communication strategies backed by evidence from randomized trials can help providers improve adherence. These include:
  1 Take steps to build a relationship to establish trust.
  2. Ask open-ended questions and listen carefully to your patient's goals for the visit.
  3. Use shared decision making to collaborate with your patient to establish a treatment plan.
  4. Follow up. Many providers are developing innovative approaches to follow up include employing digital communication technology.

Adherence to Asthma Treatment

Patients with asthma typically take less than half of prescribed controller medication.[1–4] Individual adherence fluctuates greatly over time, often with periods of time during which patients take no medication for varying periods, often for days or weeks at a time.[5] Decreasing inhaled corticosteroid (ICS) adherence is followed by worsening asthma symptoms.[6] Because most adherence research is conducted on patients who volunteer to participate in studies and know that their adherence is being monitored, these numbers may be inflated. One medication refill study, reflecting the behavior of 5500 adult and pediatric patients using a national pharmacy chain, found mean ICS adherence of 22.2% over 12 months.[7]

Impact of Nonadherence

Treatment nonadherence is a major contributor to poorly controlled asthma.[8] Depending on the duration of action and the drug side effects profile, periods of nonadherence may have several potential consequences, including waning drug action, hazardous rebound effects when administration stops abruptly, and overdose effects when administration of full-strength drugs suddenly resumes.[5] In studies of metered-dose inhaler use among children with asthma, inhalers were not used on 48% of study days and abandonment of medication typically occurred for several consecutive days.[9] The consequences of such start-and-stop adherence patterns are unknown. Time to onset of the effectiveness of ICSs in the treatment of mild to moderate asthma is about 3 weeks, with faster impact (3 days) reflected on morning peak expiratory flow values in patients with severe asthma.[10] It remains to be determined how varying patterns of adherence translate into asthma control and whether, for example, control in patients with relatively high adherence who fail to use their medication for 1 week or longer is poorer than in patients who use less total medication but with better regularity.[11]

Diagnostic and Treatment Confusion

Poor adherence can contribute to misdiagnosis and mistreatment. If patients use less medication than prescribed and do not reveal that fact to their clinician as they present with inadequately controlled symptoms, clinicians may assume that the medication is ineffective at the prescribed dose and increase the dose or change to a different medication. That picture of poor control may lead clinicians to conclude that these patients have steroid-resistant asthma and may require therapy with biologic agents. Unless these clinicians have a means to screen patient adherence as part of the process of determining eligibility, patients who do not require treatment escalation may nonetheless receive it, adding unnecessary healthcare cost and potentially greater risks of side effects.[12]

Communication Strategies to Change Patient Behavior

Numerous strategies to improve patient adherence have been tested, many in carefully conducted randomized clinical trials.

Although most of these interventions have been able to change patient or parent behavior, changes are often small and difficult to sustain. Further, effective interventions are often costly and require large amounts of healthcare provider or supplementary staff time. A Cochrane collection meta-analysis of 69 randomized trials of adherence interventions, covering a large range of ages and diseases, reported that 4 of 10 produced an effect on adherence and at least one clinical outcome. All involved complex interventions combining components such as providing information, reminders, self-monitoring, reinforcement, counseling, psychological therapy, crisis intervention, and telephone follow-up.[13] A meta-analysis of 70 controlled studies of interventions to improve adherence across various chronic pediatric conditions, including asthma, diabetes, cystic fibrosis, cancer, sickle cell disease, and gastrointestinal disorders, revealed moderate effect size in multicomponent behavioral interventions and small effect size from interventions limited to education and instruction.[14] Multicomponent behavioral programs again included a variety of interventions such as behavioral reinforcement, social support, computer- and technology-based components, homework assignments, and family and individual psychological counseling.

One consensus report from a group of 20 internationally recognized experts on adherence emphasized the essential importance of identifying simple, brief interventions that could be delivered by healthcare providers during the course of routine office care.[15] The challenge, then, becomes one of identifying interventions that are not costly, do not require a large amount of healthcare provider time, and can be implemented during routine office visits. Do such interventions exist and are they evidence-based? A considerable amount of evidence indicates that key communication strategies exist that can change parent and patient behavior and are evidence-based, time efficient, and teachable to busy healthcare providers.

A Four-Step Communication Strategy for Changing Patient Behavior

Behavioral scientists have long adopted a translational research approach to understanding and changing health behaviors. Much like "bench" research, the process begins with studies that document frequencies, predictors, and moderators of health behaviors. This information is used to build models, or theories, that explain health behaviors. Such models of behavior change are used in turn to translate theory to the "bedside" by allowing behavioral scientists to develop and test interventions that change peoples' health behavior.[16] Strategies to change patient behavior have been rooted in a number of health behavior change frameworks. These include *patient-centered care, motivational interviewing, readiness to change,* and *shared decision-making.* Each has produced evidence of the effectiveness of very specific communication strategies. However, shared decision-making has emerged as a communication strategy that is particularly helpful, time-efficient, capable of being adopted into individual practice settings,[17–19] and specifically recommended by the Global Initiative for Asthma (GINA).[20] A set of four core elements of shared decision-making can guide provider behavior during patient visits to increase treatment effectiveness and outcomes. Further, these strategies can enhance satisfaction from the encounter for both the family and the healthcare provider.

• BOX 28.1   **Key Elements of the Initial Visit That Help Build a Positive Relationship**

- A warm smile moves mountains
- Greet and express interest in your patient
- Use tone, pace, eye contact, and posture to show care and concern
- Use simple language and basic concepts
- Do not overload the patient or parent
- Be sensitive to cultural differences

From Bayer-Fetzer Conference on Physician-Patient Communication in Medical Education. Essential elements of communication in medical encounters: the Kalamazoo Consensus Statement. Acad Med 2001;76:390–3.

Build a Relationship

Promoting strong adherence begins with the development of patient trust in the provider-patient relationship. Patients and parents are more likely to increase and accurately report their adherence levels and to express satisfaction with their care if healthcare providers demonstrate thorough information sharing, interpersonal sensitivity, and partnership-building.[21] *Patient-centered care* embraces the concept that trust is established when the provider demonstrates genuine interest in and concern about the patient and considers the family's cultural traditions, personal preferences and values, current situations, and lifestyle.[22] Trust begins with communication, including listening and exploring concerns. The first moment of interaction when the provider and patient come together sets the tone for the communication that will follow. Consensus recommendations indicate that very basic elements of communication that establish this foundation include adopting a friendly tone; greeting the family with a smile; and being aware of tone, pace, eye contact, and other elements of nonverbal communication that establish genuine interest in the patient (Box 28.1).[23] Further, patients will be more adherent when physicians provide more information and are nonjudgmental, supportive, and understanding.[24] Patient-centered care has been shown to improve health outcomes for some disorders, including diabetes,[25] hypertension,[26] obesity,[27] and asthma.[28]

Demonstration of interest and concern includes asking questions that allow the patient or parent to tell the physician about their worries, symptoms, and hopes for the visit. In a survey study, 865 patients from three primary care practices completed a questionnaire inquiring about what the patient desired in a consultation with his or her physician. Factor analysis of the results identified three primary domains: (1) communication, which included listening, exploring concerns, and providing information with clear explanations; (2) partnership, which included discussion with the physician to achieve common ground and mutual agreement about the problem and treatment; and (3) health promotion, which included information and encouragement to maintain health and reduce risks of future illness.[29] A systematic review of relevant literature revealed that physician questioning is an important part of effective communication that can exert positive influence on the patient's emotional well-being, symptom resolution, and functional and physiologic improvement.[30] This approach has advantages for both the family and the provider. Taking the time to ask and answer patient questions is associated with greater physician job satisfaction and higher rates of adherence to medical treatment[31] and lower rates of medical errors.[32]

The National Asthma Education and Prevention Program (NAEPP, 2007) Guidelines for the diagnosis and management of

- What worries you about your child's asthma?
- What do you want to accomplish at this visit?
- What do you want to be able to do that you cannot do now because of your asthma?
- What do you expect from treatment?
- What medicines have you tried?
- What other questions do you have for me today?

From National Asthma Education and Prevention Program. NAEPP Guidelines for the diagnosis and management of asthma, Expert Panel Report 3, 2007.

- Establish open communications.
- Identify and address patient and family concerns about asthma and asthma treatment.
- Identify patient, parent, and child treatment preferences regarding treatment and barriers to its implementation.
- Develop treatment goals together with patient and family.
- Encourage active self-assessment and self-management of asthma.
- Encourage adherence by:
  - Choosing a treatment regimen that achieves outcomes and addresses preferences that are important to the patient and parent.
  - Reviewing the success of the treatment plan with the patient/parent at each visit and making adjustments as needed.
- Tailor the asthma self-management teaching approach to the needs of each patient.
- Maintain sensitivity to cultural beliefs and ethnocultural practices.

From National Asthma Education and Prevention Program. NAEPP Guidelines for the diagnosis and management of asthma, Expert Panel Report 3, 2007.

asthma provide examples of questions that can be asked in the initial visit and help set the stage for positive communication (Box 28.2).

Focus on Listening

Healthcare providers who want to be helpful to their patients by sharing important information about an illness, test results, and treatment plans are often well-practiced at giving information but may not always be as cognizant of the importance of listening. When time pressures add to the sense that the encounter must be brief and efficient, there is a tendency to ask questions that that can be answered "yes" or "no" to limit discussion, and there is a desire to move briskly toward completion of the visit. The result may be that the family's concerns are not heard. The family's unheard concerns often undermine adherence. In the context of the Health Beliefs Model, the parent's decision about whether to follow a treatment plan is largely influenced by their perception of the risks associated with the disease and the risks and benefits introduced by the treatment.[33] For patients or parents of patients with asthma, concerns often include fears about medication side effects, a perception that the medication is not helping, concerns about long-term dependence on the medication, and the cost of the medication.[34] In a study of parents of 67 children with asthma, increased concerns about risks of taking asthma medications were associated with lower adherence; fewer concerns combined with a perception of benefit from the child's medication were associated with higher adherence.[35] When the patient or parent voices concerns, the healthcare provider has an opportunity to discuss these concerns and perceptions, to provide more information, and to discuss treatment options. Essential to this process is the physician's willingness to ask questions that invite patients and families to openly share questions and concerns.[36] When the discussion leads to a shift in the family's perception of the relative benefits of the medication over its risks, increased adherence is likely to follow.[35,37]

Collaborate on the Treatment Plan

Patient-centered care presumes that providers are willing to put aside a paternalistic approach in which patients are told what is wrong with them and what they need to do and instead work toward a partnership in which patients are heard, discussion occurs, and the two parties agree on both the goals of treatment and the treatment itself.[38] To accomplish this partnership, providers must engage and listen to patients and parents, showing sensitivity, interest, concern, and comprehension of the family's

message.[39] Differences in goals and expectations must be discussed and resolved before the treatment plan is finalized. The partnership approach is favored by many patients. For example, a survey of patients after a consultation showed increased satisfaction if physicians were "interested in what I think the problem is," "interested in what treatment I want," and would "discuss and agree with me on treatment."[29] The NAEPP guidelines emphasize the importance of this relationship and provide recommendations toward establishing a partnership with the patient and family (Box 28.3).

Establishing a partnership between the provider and family necessarily reflects a shift of authority within which the physician takes into account patient concerns and preferences before making treatment recommendations. Medication complexity is one of the treatment factors that can have an impact on adherence,[40] and thus the family's tolerance for more complex regimens must be included in the discussion. The degree to which the provider defers to the patient or parent will depend on both the physician and family. Many physicians are most comfortable maintaining control of the treatment plan and may do so while still adopting a sensitive patient-centered focus. Other physicians may be comfortable taking the partnership a step further, allowing the patient more control over the choice of treatment plan. This approach is adopted in the *shared decision-making* model, a communication approach that attempts to increase concordance about treatment choices and goals by promoting greater involvement of the individual patient in deliberations about treatment options.[41,42] One study evaluated the effectiveness of shared decision making in improving outcomes in adults aged 18 to 70 years with poorly controlled, mild to moderate persistent asthma. Healthcare providers were randomly assigned to one of three training conditions: (1) usual care (no training), (2) management by guidelines (training in following the evidence-based guidelines), and (3) shared decision making (training in guidelines combined with shared decision making). In the group of 170 patients of providers trained in shared decision making, controller medication adherence improved from 40% at baseline to 70% after the intervention, significantly more than for the 331 patients in the other two conditions.[43] In another study, 808 women with asthma were interviewed about their healthcare experiences. Those who reported that their provider had entered into a negotiated treatment plan with the patient reported greater adherence and lower oral steroid use at follow-up.[44] Not all patients may prefer a shared decision-making approach. In a study in which patients evaluated videos of two different types of consultations with a physician, one shared decision making and one in which the physician was more directive, the directed approach was often preferred by older patients and the shared decision-making approach was often preferred by younger patients and those with higher education levels.[45] Although shared decision making has not been studied as extensively in children, one matched-control study with 746 children with asthma found that those in the shared decision-making group had a longer time to exacerbation than those in the control group.[46] Consistent with a shared decision-making approach, the GINA 2018 guidelines recommend that providers (1) focus on the development of the partnership; (2) accept that this is a continuing process; (3) share information; (4) adapt the approach to the patient's level of health literacy; (5) fully discuss expectations, fears, and concerns; and (6) develop shared goals.[20]

Wrap Up and Follow-Up

Providers have limited opportunity to influence patient behavior once patients leave the office. However, if strong communication in the office has set the stage for motivating health-promoting behavior, follow-up contact can reinforce this motivation. Follow-up interventions may include return visits to the clinic, telephone calls, and other media-based interventions.

The NAEPP guidelines recommend follow-up visits at 2 to 6 weeks after the initiation of controller medication therapy, and intervals of 1 to 6 months for asthma well-care visits. Because a large number of patients are almost immediately nonadherent after initial controller therapy prescription,[7] investment of efforts to increase adherence at the point of initiation of controller treatment may yield the greatest return. Each follow-up visit provides an opportunity for discussion of the family's perceptions and concerns about treatment and, if necessary, renegotiation of the treatment plan. NAEPP guidelines include recommendations for questions that can be asked at follow-up visits that invite increased communication, provider-patient collaboration, and treatment adherence (Box 28.4).

Evidence indicates a strong potential for the employment of telecommunication technology to reach out to patients and encourage adherence. The rapid uptake of telecommunication technology has penetrated every demographic subgroup of the American public, which in turn means that the interest and opportunity to use technology exist to engage patients. Evidence is mounting to support adherence-enhancing strategies that include leveraging email,[47,48] text messaging,[49] and interactive voice recognition technology[50,51] to activate patients and encourage better disease self-management. In a randomized study of a computerized speech recognition program designed to call patients with asthma to inquire about disease control and promote adherence, patients who received the calls were

---

• BOX 28.4 **Monitoring Patient-Provider Communication and Patient Satisfaction**

- "What questions have you had about your child's asthma daily self-management plan and action plan?"
- "What problems have you had following the daily self-management plan? The action plan?"
- "How do you feel about making your own decisions about therapy?"
- "Has anything prevented you from getting the treatment you need for your asthma from me or anyone else?"
- "Have the costs of your child's asthma treatment interfered with your ability to get asthma care?"
- "How satisfied are you with your asthma care?"
- "How can we improve your asthma care?"

From National Asthma Education and Prevention Program. NAEPP Guidelines for the diagnosis and management of asthma, Expert Panel Report 3, 2007.

significantly more likely to use their ICS and to have a routine asthma follow-up visit.[51] A similar system has been developed to promote diabetes self-management.[52]

Conclusions

A large proportion of patients with asthma take less than half of their prescribed controller medication, and surprisingly many stop taking their controller medication altogether after an initial filling at their pharmacy. Decreasing use of ICSs has been linked to worsening asthma symptoms and increased risk of hospitalization and death. Many interventions to improve patient adherence have been tested in controlled clinical trials. Whereas some interventions increase adherence, many are complex, costly, time consuming, and nearly impossible to adopt in independent primary care and allergy practices. Nonetheless, four decades of behavioral research and modeling have produced communication strategies that may be used by healthcare providers to effectively change health behavior. From these, four key communication strategies with significant empirical support have been extracted and are presented here. These include (1) build a relationship, (2) focus on listening, (3) collaborate on the treatment plan, and (4) follow-up. These communication strategies do not require a large amount of healthcare provider time, can be implemented during routine office visits, and can change patient behavior. Realistically, these strategies will not transform every nonadherent patient into an effective illness self-manager, but employment of these strategies will improve adherence in many families. Furthermore, they can be used to affect change in other health behaviors, such as smoking cessation or weight loss. Finally, beyond behavior change, enhanced communication has been repeatedly shown to improve satisfaction in the interaction for both the family and the provider.

The reference list can be found on the companion Expert Consult website at http://www.expertconsult.inkling.com.

29

Strategies for the Primary Prevention of Asthma

FERNANDO D. MARTINEZ

KEY POINTS

- A variety of approaches for the prevention of childhood asthma have been tested in well-conducted clinical trials. None have provided definitive evidence of success and, therefore, there is currently no therapeutic approach that can decrease the incidence of asthma during the first years of life.

- Currently, the most promising strategy for asthma prevention seems to be the identification of surrogates of the microbial exposures that have been found to be associated with markedly diminished risk of asthma in children raised on farms.

Introduction

Primary prevention of a disease implies intervening through avoidance or reduction of exposures or active therapies before the first manifestations of the disease occur. Although at first sight determining onset may appear straightforward (albeit never easy) in the case of acute illnesses, it is usually much more difficult to define the precise point at which a chronic illness starts. This is particularly true for asthma, which is a heterogeneous condition identified mainly based on clinical manifestations and for which there is no definitive diagnostic or laboratory test. In the vast majority of cases, a variety of exposures and even emotions can trigger asthma symptoms. In a minority of patients with asthma, a single specific exposure elicits most symptoms and abolishing this exposure, for example, in the workplace, may be sufficient to prevent further manifestations of the disease. This would be an example of secondary prevention: a measure taken after the disease first appeared.

Primary Prevention and the Natural History of Asthma

Asthma can start at any age, but there is now solid epidemiologic evidence suggesting that in the majority of cases of asthma the first symptoms occur during the preschool years.[1] Moreover, a significant proportion of persons with bona fide adult-onset asthma, identified through longitudinal birth cohorts devoid of recall bias, had bronchial hyperresponsiveness and lung function deficits at or before the age of 6 years.[2] It is thus reasonable to surmise that in many cases of asthma the prodromal phase for the development of disease occurs in utero and/or during early postnatal life and that the most successful interventions will be those targeting this age range. Elsewhere in this text, we describe the data available

supporting this contention. Here, we will review the most important primary prevention strategies that have been or are currently being tested in clinical trials (Box 29.1).

Asthma and the House Dust Mite

In most coastal areas, a large proportion of children with asthma have positive skin tests or circulating immunoglobulin E (IgE) antibodies against house dust mites of the genus *Dermatophagoides*.[3] Moreover, a well-performed clinical trial showed that in children with severe asthma and who were sensitized against mites the risk of a severe exacerbation requiring a hospital visit decreased by 45% in children who used mite-impermeable bed encasings compared with those using a placebo treatment.[4] These results prompted the hypothesis that exposure to mites caused asthma[5] and that reduction of mite exposure starting in utero and during early life could prevent the development of the disease.

Two major trials were conducted in the Netherlands and Australia. In the double-blind Dutch Prevention and Incidence of Asthma and Mite Allergy (PIAMA) study, pregnant allergic women were randomized to either an intervention arm consisting of mite–impermeable polyester–cotton mattress and pillow covers for the parental bed and the child's bed or to the placebo arm, which received cotton placebo covers.[6] The intervention resulted in a dramatic, persistent decrease in mite allergen concentration in the child's mattress dust; at age 8 years, beds from the intervention group had 69% lower mite levels than those from the placebo group. However, there was no evidence of a decrease in the prevalence of asthma, wheezing, or allergic sensitization to mites or other allergens during the first 8 years of life between the active and placebo arms.[6] The Childhood Asthma Prevention Study (CAPS) in Sydney, Australia, randomized antenatally 616 children with parental asthma into a 5-year mite reduction regimen, consisting of either allergen-impermeable

Randomized Clinical Trials Are Available or Could Be Undertaken

- Reduction of exposure to house dust mites and other aeroallergens
- Food allergen avoidance
- Comprehensive approach (most often combination of aeroallergen reduction and food allergen avoidance)
- Fatty acid intake
- Vitamin D supplementation during pregnancy
- Respiratory syncytial virus prophylaxis
- Probiotic administration
- Bacterial extract administration
- Mediterranean diet

Randomized Trials Are Unfeasible or Unethical

- Reduce maternal smoking during pregnancy and exposure to environmental tobacco smoke postnatally
- Reduce exposure to air pollution
- Increase breastfeeding
- Reduce incidence of overweight status
- Reduce stressful events during pregnancy and childhood
- Reduce incidence of prematurity

mattress and pillow covers and washing of all bedding every 3 months in an acaricidal detergent, or no intervention.[7] This unblinded intervention regimen was also highly successful in decreasing mite exposure. However, at 11.5 years, there was no difference in the prevalence of asthma or allergic sensitization between the two arms.[8]

These results clearly indicate that the level of mite reduction attained with the methods used in these studies is not effective by itself in the primary prevention of asthma and cannot be recommended based on current evidence. Mite reduction may be effective in decreasing symptoms in patients with asthma who are allergic to mites. If more radical mite reduction or mite reduction in combination with reduction of other allergens could prevent asthma is unclear (see later discussion).

Asthma Prevention Through Food Allergen Avoidance

Longitudinal studies have shown that children who develop food allergy before the age of 4 years are more likely to have asthma during the school years.[9] Results are available for three trials testing food allergen avoidance in early life as a strategy for asthma prevention during the school years. In a first study, published two decades ago, children of patients with atopy were randomized to an aggressive food allergen avoidance regimen and delayed introduction of solid foods during pregnancy and the first year of life.[9] The control group was given standard advice. Approximately half of the randomized children were assessed at a mean age of 7 years; there was no difference in the prevalence of asthma, bronchial hyperresponsiveness, lung function, or nasal eosinophils between the active and control arms at that age. In 2016, results became available for the long-term follow-up of the double-blind German Infant Nutritional Intervention study, in which newborns with a family history of allergies who needed breast milk substitutes were randomized to either hypoallergenic formulas or usual standard cow's milk's formula.[10] Between ages 6 and 15 years, prevalence of asthma was not different between any of the hypoallergenic formulas and standard formula. Interestingly, some of

the hypoallergenic formulas did show preventive effects on atopic eczema. A very similar study from Australia, in which follow-up reached age 7 years, also failed to find any association between milk allergen avoidance during weaning from or replacement of breastfeeding and subsequent development of asthma.[11] Finally, in the opposite direction, early introduction of peanuts to the diet did not alter asthma risk.[12]

These results strongly suggest that food allergen avoidance and possibly early introduction of food allergens are not effective and should not be recommended for the prevention of asthma.

Combining Mite Reduction With Food Allergen Avoidance

Two additional studies supplemented allergen reduction with other preventive methods. The Isle of Wight Prevention Study randomized prenatally 120 children at high risk to either a prophylactic strategy consisting of mite reduction and either breastfeeding with the mother on a low-allergen diet or administration of an extensively hydrolyzed formula. The control group was provided standard advice. The study was not blinded. There was a significant 49% reduction in asthma prevalence from ages 1 to 18 years, but prevalence of atopy was not significantly different between the two groups.[13] In the Canadian Childhood Asthma Prevention Study, 545 children with a family history of asthma and allergies were randomized into an intervention group in which reduction of house dust, pets, and environmental tobacco smoke exposure; encouragement of breastfeeding; and delayed introduction of solid foods was started prenatally and during the first year of life or a control group who received usual care; the study was not blinded. At the age of 7 years, 380 participants were assessed[14] and there was a 56% reduction in "allergist diagnosed asthma" in the active compared with the control group, but there was no difference in the prevalence of skin test reactivity to allergens or in bronchial hyperresponsiveness between groups.

It is challenging to reach definitive conclusions from these two studies. Although they showed significant effects on asthma prevalence up to ages 18 and 7 years, respectively, neither was blinded, and the potential for biases created by this design is unknown. In addition, the biologic mechanism underlying a synergistic effect between two interventions that separately have not been shown to be effective (i.e., mite reduction and food allergen avoidance), and without affecting allergen sensitization, is unknown. Given these limitations and the results of studies showing that active introduction of food allergens in early postnatal life has strong protective effects on the development of IgE-mediated responses against these allergens,[15] combined mite reduction and dietary avoidance interventions are not currently advisable.

Fatty Acid Intake and Asthma Prevention

Observational studies performed in the 1990s suggested that fish consumption more than once a week was associated with a 30% to 70% decrease in bronchial hyperresponsiveness.[16] A large case-control study using a food frequency questionnaire and an exercise challenge test showed that children who did not eat fish were three times more likely to have asthma than those who ate fish regularly.[17] These results were supported by studies showing that a diet rich in marine fatty acids (fish oil) may have beneficial antiinflammatory effects. The potential antiinflammatory effects of fish oil appear to derive from a high content of the omega-3 (also called n-3) series fatty acids, which competitively inhibit the metabolism of arachidonic acid.[18] Based on this evidence, two randomized controlled trials have tested the hypothesis that diet supplementation with fatty acids could prevent the development of asthma.

The CAPS study cited earlier used a factorial design in which participants were randomized to a control arm and a mite reduction arm and to two additional arms: one that received canola-based oils and spreads, which are low in omega-6 fatty acids, and tuna oil capsules, which contain omega-3 fatty acids; and a fourth one, which performed allergen reduction and received these fatty acids.[8] In addition, both the mite reduction arm and the control arm received masked polyunsaturated oils and spreads, containing 40% omega-6 fatty acids, and oil capsules low in omega-3 fatty acids. At age 11.5 years, there was a significantly lower prevalence of atopy in the omega-3 supplementation intervention than in the control arms, but there was no difference in the prevalence of asthma between these two comparison groups.[15] In the Copenhagen Prospective Studies on Asthma in Childhood 2010 pregnancy cohort, women at 24 weeks of pregnancy were randomly assigned to receive either 2.4 g/day of n-3 long-chain polyunsaturated fatty acids (LCPUFAs) or placebo in the form of olive oil, containing 72% n-9 oleic acid and 12% n-6 linoleic acid.[19] Results showed a significant 30.7% relative reduction in the risk of persistent wheeze or asthma by age 5 years in the treatment arm compared with the placebo arm. There was no difference in the cumulative incidence of atopy between the two groups. There is currently no explanation for the different results obtained by these two well-conducted studies. The formulations used in both trials contained similar proportions of the putatively active ingredients in fish oil, eicosapentaenoic acid (EPA) and docosahexaenoic acid (DHA), which competitively inhibit the metabolism of arachidonic acid. Adherence to the intervention was actively monitored in both trials. Results of the continued follow-up of children enrolled in the Copenhagen trial should shed light on the persistence of the observed protective effect beyond the preschool years.

Asthma Prevention and Vitamin D Supplementation

Observational studies performed during the first two decades of this century suggested that maternal intake of vitamin D was associated with a decreased incidence of wheezing episodes in preschool children and, less often, with a diagnosis of asthma during the school years.[20] These observations were supported by studies showing significant effects of maternal vitamin D deficiency on lung development and immune responses[21] in the offspring. These results prompted the hypothesis that vitamin D insufficiency during pregnancy could play a major role in the increases in asthma prevalence observed during the last three decades.[22] Two clinical trials were undertaken to determine whether vitamin D supplementation given to mothers during pregnancy could prevent the development of asthma and wheezing in their children.

As part of the Copenhagen study quoted earlier, vitamin D_3 (2400 international units [IU]/day) was given to 315 pregnant mothers and matching placebo to 308 mothers from pregnancy week 24 to 1 week postpartum. Outcomes were assessed initially by the age of 3 years[23] and subsequently at 6 years.[24] There was no significant difference in the incidence of persistent wheeze by age 3 or in the prevalence of asthma at age 6 between the two arms of the trial. In the Vitamin D Antenatal Asthma Reduction Trial

(VDAART), 881 pregnant women at high risk of having children with asthma were randomized at 10 to 18 weeks' gestation to receive either daily 4000 IU vitamin D or a placebo.[25a] Through the age of 3 years, 24.3% of the children in the active arm and 30.4% in the placebo arm had parental report of physician-diagnosed asthma or recurrent wheezing, and this difference did not quite reach statistical significance. A follow up at age six years of the VDAART cohort showed no difference in the prevalence of asthma at age 6 years between the active and placebo arms.[25b] Data from VIDAART and from the Copenhagen trial up to the age of 3 years were combined in a meta-analysis that showed that vitamin D supplementation during pregnancy significantly reduced the incidence of asthma or recurrent wheeze through age 3 years by 25%.[26]

Based on the results of these two trials, it is reasonable to conclude that vitamin D supplementation during pregnancy cannot be recommended for the prevention of childhood asthma during the school years. The data suggest that this supplementation can reduce the frequency of recurrent wheezing during the preschool years, but this effect disappears by the school-age years. It has been argued that the trials should have been designed differently and that the analyses should have been made a priori conditional on baseline levels of vitamin D in the mothers and adjusted for co-nutrients.[27] In support of this contention, subgroup analyses of the combined data from both trials showed stronger effects on prevention of recurrent wheezing by the age of 3 years in mothers with a maternal 25-hydroxy-vitamin D (25[OH]D) level of 30 ng/mL or greater at trial entry than in those with levels less than that threshold.[28] With the evidence at hand, it is reasonable to recommend that mothers are prescribed vitamin D supplements during pregnancy that can keep their 25(OH)D levels at 30 ng/mL or greater. This approach will promote better health in both mother and offspring and could decrease the risk of recurrent wheezing during the first 3 years of life.

Asthma Prevention and Respiratory Syncytial Virus Prophylaxis

Long-term longitudinal studies have shown that children who had lower respiratory tract illnesses (LRIs) as a result of RSV during the first 3 years of life are more likely to have subsequent recurrent wheezing than those who do not have such illnesses.[29,30] It is still unclear whether this risk persists beyond the early school years[30] or is limited to preadolescents.[29] What determines the association between RSV-LRI and subsequent recurrent wheezing is unknown. One possibility is that, in predisposed individuals, RSV may cause airway damage or alterations in immune responses and these changes in turn may predispose for subsequent wheezing. It is also possible that, because only a minority of young children who are infected with RSV develop lower respiratory symptoms, RSV-LRI is just the first clinical manifestation of an increased susceptibility to develop inappropriate responses to viral respiratory infections. In the latter case, RSV would not cause any direct injury to the developing airway, but simply trigger the expression of a preexisting vulnerability.

Several clinical trials have tested the hypothesis that RSV prophylaxis using humanized, monoclonal anti-RSV antibodies produced by recombinant DNA technology can not only prevent RSV-LRI but also decrease the incidence of subsequent recurrent wheezing. Two such preparations have been used: palivizumab, which is sold for RSV prophylaxis worldwide, and motavizumab, an experimental drug that was never commercialized. Because of the current indications for RSV prophylaxis, most of these studies were done in preterm infants. The Committee on Recurrent Wheezing (CREW) study was a prospective, multicenter, observational cohort study performed in Japan that compared the incidence of recurrent wheezing up to 3 years of age in preterm children (33- to 35-weeks' gestational age) who had and had not received palivizumab prophylaxis during their first RSV season.[31] The study was thus not a double-blind, placebo-controlled, randomized trial. At age 3 years, recurrent wheezing was observed in 6.4% of infants in the treated group (n = 349) and 18.9% of infants in the untreated group (n = 95), and this difference was highly significant statistically. At the age of 6 years, there was no difference in the prevalence of atopic asthma between the two groups in this same study population, but prevalence of recurrent wheezing was twice as likely in the untreated than in the treated group.[32] It is plausible to surmise that wheezy children with more severe illnesses are more likely to be assigned the label of asthma, and epidemiologic studies have shown that children with atopy are at increased risk of having more severe episodes during the school years.[33] The data thus suggest that RSV prophylaxis may prevent the development of milder wheezing episodes but not of asthma during the school years.

A randomized, double-blind, placebo-controlled trial that enrolled 429 infants born prematurely at 32 to 35 weeks was conducted in the Netherlands. The trial was initially designed to investigate the potential causal role of RSV illnesses in the pathogenesis of wheezing illness during the first year of life,[34] but it was subsequently extended as a single-blind (researcher) study up to age 6 years.[35] The results were quite analogous to those of the CREW trial: compared with the placebo arm, treatment with palivizumab resulted in a significant 61% reduction in the incidence of recurrent wheezing during the first year of life. When participants were followed to the age of 6 years, the primary outcome was "current asthma," a composite defined as parentally reported wheeze in the past 12 months, use of asthma medication in the past 12 months, or both. There was a significant reduction in current asthma at age 6 in the active arm compared with the placebo arm, but the difference was mainly the result of a difference in infrequent wheeze (one to three episodes in the past year), which was twice as likely in the placebo arm than in the active arm. There was no difference in the prevalence of frequent wheeze (>3 episodes) between the two groups. These results support the conclusion that RSV prophylaxis may be more effective in preventing subsequent mild recurrent wheezing than in preventing more severe cases.

The only study performed in term children yielded results that contradict those in infants born prematurely. A double-blind, placebo-controlled, randomized trial enrolled healthy Native American infants who were born after at least 36 weeks' gestation in the southwestern United States. The active drug in this case was motavizumab, and 2127 infants were allocated to active drug and 710 to placebo.[36] Motavizumab was highly effective in preventing acute, severe RSV-LRI requiring hospitalization, but there was no difference in the incidence of recurrent wheezing between ages 1 and 3 years between the two arms.

The factors that determine the different results obtained using motavizumab compared with those using palivizumab for the prevention of subsequent wheezing are not known. It is unlikely that the differences are attributable to the drug used, because they were equally effective in preventing acute RSV-LRI. It is possible that there are different mechanisms linking RSV-LRI to subsequent asthma in premature compared with term children and between mostly white and Asian children and compared with Native American children.

Even if the results of the studies in preemies could eventually be replicated in term children, the fact that palivizumab was effective only in preventing infrequent wheezing through the early school years raises important issues regarding the relative financial and societal costs of purchasing and repeatedly administering a monoclonal antibody to infants versus those of treating older children with mild episodes of wheezing. With the information available today, there does not appear to be a major role that RSV prophylaxis can play in the primary prevention of asthma.

Asthma Prevention and Microbial Exposure in Utero and in Early Postnatal Life

A major advance in our understanding of the pathogenesis of asthma and allergic diseases came from landmark epidemiologic studies showing that children living in locales that exposed them to a higher dose of environmental microbes were protected against the development of these diseases. Only a brief summary of these studies will be provided here. Starting in the early 2000s, cross-sectional and longitudinal surveys of populations living in rural areas of Europe demonstrated that children living on single-family animal farms and in close contact with these animals during their mother's pregnancy and in the first years of life were less likely to have asthma and atopy than those living in the same rural communities but away from farms.[37] Subsequent reports indicated that there was a strong, inverse correlation between the concentration of bacterial and fungal products in dust obtained from these rural homes and the risk for asthma and wheezing in children living in these homes.[38] Doubts remained, however, because it was possible that parents susceptible to farming exposures could prefer to live in town, away from farms, but these were addressed by a study among the Hutterites and Amish.[39] These two inbred U.S. populations are genetically very similar, they live only in rural areas, and most members work on animal farms. However, whereas Hutterites have adopted modern animal husbandry, Amish have conserved the traditions of single-family farms and therefore live very close to the animals. Analogous to the results of the European studies, Amish children have four times less asthma than Hutterite children and are much more heavily exposed to microbes at home from an early age. Similarly, other studies showed that children living in homes with dogs have decreased risk of having asthma and wheezing,[40] and oral administration of dust from homes with dogs protected mice from the development of allergen-associated airway inflammation and against severe infection with RSV.[41] A specific gut commensal microbe, *Lactobacillus johnsonii,* was found to, at least in part, mediate these protective effects. These findings suggested the possibility that a cogent strategy for the prevention of asthma could be oral administration of potentially protective microbes to young children, either alive or in the form of extracts, for the prevention of asthma.

Asthma Prevention and Probiotics

First attempts to test this hypothesis leveraged on the well-demonstrated tolerability of probiotics, even in very young infants. Support for this approach came from experimental studies showing that human probiotic bacteria such as *Lactobacillus rhamnosus GG* and their products exerted immunomodulatory effects in mouse models of asthma.[42] A thorough meta-analysis identified nine trials of prenatal and postnatal administration of probiotics that enrolled 3257 infants and in which asthma was one of the outcomes.[43] Incidence of physician-diagnosed asthma at the last assessment available was 11.2% among participants randomized to receive probiotics and 10.2% among those receiving placebo, a difference that was not statistically significant. As is often the case for meta-analyses, there were limitations that precluded definitive conclusions: the trials were conducted in heterogeneous populations randomized to different probiotic bacteria and widely different doses, and with timing ranging from prenatal administration to 1 to 25 months of postnatal supplementation. In 2017 the Trial of Infant Probiotic Supplementation (TIPS) study was conducted in the United States.[44] A total of 184 children of parents with asthma were randomized to 6 months of supplementation with either *L. rhamnosus GG* or placebo. At the age of 5 years, there was no significant difference in the cumulative incidence of asthma between the two arms.

Taken together, these studies suggest that probiotics given prenatally or in early life are not effective in preventing the development of asthma. Parallel studies of the microbiota present in stools of the children enrolled in the TIPS study may provide an explanation for these negative results. Children who will go on to develop asthma have stool microbial communities in early life that differ from those of nonasthmatic children.[45] Supplementation with *L. rhamnosus GG* reprogrammed the composition of the gut microbiome toward one that is associated with reduced asthma incidence, but it did not reverse the delay in bacterial species accumulation observed in infants at high risk for asthma.[46] Interestingly, as described earlier, *L. johnsonii* by itself mimicked the protective effects of dust from homes with dogs, but these effects were not as strong as those observed with the use of the whole dust extract.[41] Taken together, these results support the contention that more than a single microbe is needed to activate the molecular mechanisms that putatively mediate the protective effects of microbial exposure. This creates an additional challenge: administering communities of live bacteria to young infants, even if these bacteria are known to be innocuous for most children, increases the possibility that they could not be well tolerated by a minority of children with undiagnosed immunodeficiencies. Thus, administration of live bacteria is still a highly promising avenue for asthma prevention, but more preclinical work is needed before this approach can be successfully tested in young children.

Asthma Prevention and Bacterial Extracts

The promise and challenges of an approach to asthma prevention based on the epidemiologic evidence of protections provided by microbial exposures prompted the search for alternatives to the administration of live bacteria to young children. Extracts of pathogenic respiratory bacteria have been used empirically for decades for the prevention of respiratory illnesses. The most frequently used oral formulations are made up of lyophilized bacterial lysates of *Haemophilus influenzae, Diplococcus pneumoniae, Klebsiella pneumoniae, Klebsiella ozaenae, Staphylococcus aureus, Streptococcus pyogenes, Streptococcus viridans,* and *Neisseria catarrhalis.* The apparent initial rationale for the use of these extracts was that of a vaccine; administration of these extracts was supposed to activate immune mechanisms against the bacteria they contain.[47] Numerous randomized clinical trials have been published using these extracts for the prevention of respiratory illnesses, and although meta-analyses have concluded that there is evidence for their effectiveness, most trials identified were considered of limited quality.[48]

Experimental studies from 2011 have suggested the possibility that these extracts could play a role in the prevention of asthma. When given orally to allergen-sensitized mice, bacterial extracts decrease airway inflammation and bronchial hyperresponsiveness and interact with dendritic cells in the gut to promote the activation of regulatory T cells, which migrate to the airways and apparently mediate their protective effects.[49,50] These experimental studies were recently extended to oral administration of bacterial extracts during pregnancy, which reduced susceptibility of their offspring to development of allergic airway inflammatory disease.[51] As with the postnatal model, offspring mice showed enhanced dendritic cell–dependent airway mucosal-homing of regulatory T cells in response to local inflammatory challenge. In addition, one double-blind, randomized clinical trial showed significant reduction in the frequency of wheezing episodes in preschool children with a previous history of such episodes treated with Broncho-Vaxom, a lyophilized bacterial lysate, compared with those treated with placebo.[52]

The results of a small randomized, placebo-controlled primary prevention trial of severe LRIs in preschool children using Broncho-Vaxom were reported.[53] Fifty-nine children aged 6 months with a family history of asthma and allergies were recruited and randomized to either active drug or placebo, which was administered for 2 consecutive years, during the first 10 days of each month, for 5 months (April to August, the viral respiratory season in Brisbane, Australia). The study was negative for the primary outcome (i.e., the frequency of severe LRIs over the first two winters of the child's life). However, the time to the first severe LRI was significantly longer for children receiving Broncho-Vaxom than for those receiving placebo. A second, much larger randomized, placebo-controlled prevention trial, the Oral Bacterial Extracts (ORBEX) for the Prevention of Wheezing Lower Respiratory Tract Illness Study, performed in the United States, was still enrolling participants when this chapter was written (NCT02148796). This study is randomizing 926 children aged 6 to 18 months who either have eczema or have a parent or sibling with asthma to a 2-year treatment with Broncho-Vaxom or placebo. The primary outcome is the time to the occurrence of the first wheezing LRI episode in the third observation year while not receiving study drug.

Conclusions

This review of objective evidence based exclusively on randomized, controlled clinical trials leads to the conclusion that there is currently no strategy that has been unequivocally shown to be effective for the primary prevention of asthma, as defined at the beginning of this chapter. There are potential approaches that are not amenable to a clinical trial and not reviewed here that could certainly decrease the risk of development of the disease (Box 29.2). Observational studies have strongly suggested that maternal smoking during pregnancy and postnatal exposure is associated with subsequent asthma,[54] especially during early childhood.[55] Discouraging caregivers from smoking should thus decrease the risk of asthma in children who would otherwise be exposed to tobacco smoke products. Higher levels of air pollution are weakly associated with increased prevalence of childhood asthma, especially when symptoms start in early life[56]; in children living in contaminated areas, the marked improvement in air quality in California during the last half century occurred parallel with a concomitant improvement in spirometric airway function, a strong predictor of asthma risk.[57] Societal efforts to improve air quality could thus decrease the burden of asthma worldwide.

The role of breastfeeding in asthma prevention is controversial, and long-term birth cohorts have suggested that, although associated with protection against recurrent wheeze early in life, breastfeeding may be associated with an increased risk of asthma, atopy, and recurrent wheeze beginning at the age of 6 years, but only for children with parents with asthma or atopy.[58,59]

Prematurity, and particularly very preterm birth, is associated with increased incidence of asthma-like symptoms[60] and increased prevalence of bronchial hyperresponsiveness[61] during childhood. Effort to decrease the incidence of prematurity are likely to result in decreases in the prevalence of childhood asthma.

Maternal stress and depression are associated with subsequent increased incidence of asthma in the offspring,[62] as are stressful events during postnatal life.[63] Although there are cogent biologic mechanisms that could explain the link between stress and asthma incidence, it is not possible to exclude the possibility that unmeasured maternal characteristics and co-exposures postnatally may confound the association. Unfortunately, clinical trials that could shed light on this association do not seem currently feasible.

Finally, a large number of epidemiologic studies have shown a strong association between overweight or obese status during early childhood and the subsequent development of asthma.[64] There are, however, reports suggesting that a diagnosis of asthma is associated with subsequent increased incidence of obesity.[65] No available randomized diet trials aiming at decreasing the incidence of obesity have had asthma as an outcome. Observational studies have suggested that a Mediterranean diet during pregnancy, consisting of elevated intake of plant foods such as fruits and vegetables, bread and cereals (primarily wholegrain), legumes and nuts, with low to moderate amounts of dairy products and eggs and only small amounts of red meat, may be protective against the development of childhood asthma.[66] Although asthma prevention trials comparing Mediterranean diet with more typical Western diets have been proposed,[67] such trials are likely to be prolonged in time and difficult to implement practically.

At present, the most promising strategy for the primary prevention of asthma seems to be the identification of therapeutic surrogates of the specific microbial exposures that have been shown to mediate the protective effects against asthma of microbe-rich environments in early life.

The reference list can be found on the companion Expert Consult website at http://www.expertconsult.inkling.com.

30

Mucosal Immunology: An Overview

DANIEL LOZANO-OJALVO, M. CECILIA BERIN

KEY POINTS

- The gastrointestinal (GI)-associated lymphoid tissue protects the vast surface of the GI tract from pathogens while remaining tolerant to antigens from food and commensal microbiota.
- Immune tolerance to luminal antigens from food and commensal microbiota captured by dendritic cells and macrophages is induced by the generation and expansion of regulatory T cells.

- Secretory immunoglobulin A (IgA) provides an immune barrier by excluding antigens from uptake, but antibodies, including IgA, IgG, and IgE, can function as antigen uptake mechanisms across the intestinal epithelium.
- Breakdown in the induction of oral tolerance to dietary proteins based on a failure of regulatory T cell response results in the IgE-mediated sensitization to antigens and the development of food allergy.

Introduction

The gastrointestinal (GI) tract is the largest immunologic organ in the body. The small intestine itself has the largest surface area in the GI tract because of structural features, including villi and microvilli. The purpose of this extensive surface is to facilitate nutrient absorption from ingested foods. From the stomach to the rectum, a single layer of columnar epithelial cells separates the external environment of the GI lumen from the body proper. The lumen contains a myriad of microorganisms and dietary components. In the small intestine, the main antigenic load is from ingested food. Along the proximal to distal axis the food antigen load decreases as it is digested and absorbed, but the microbial load increases. In the intestine, there are 10^8 to 10^{11} microorganisms per gram of luminal contents.[1] The challenge from an immune perspective is to guard the extensive surface area of the GI tract from breaches by microorganisms, in particular pathogenic microorganisms. In addition, the intestinal immune system must remain nonreactive or tolerant to food antigens because a breakdown in this state of unresponsiveness leads to sensitization to food proteins and the development of food allergy. These functions are accomplished by the GI-associated lymphoid tissue (GALT), which has adapted to its unique environment.

Structure of the Gastrointestinal Associated Lymphoid Tissue

The GI tract has several types of organized lymphoid tissue composing the GALT. Underlying the intestinal epithelial cell (IEC) layer is a loose connective tissue stroma, the lamina propria (LP), containing a resident population of T lymphocytes, plasma cells, macrophages, dendritic cells (DCs), eosinophils, and mast cells. The LP of the small and large intestine is drained via lymphatics that empty into the mesenteric lymph nodes (MLNs). Antigens are taken up by migratory DCs in the LP and delivered to the MLNs that are typical secondary lymph nodes with organized B cell follicles and paracortical T cell areas. Peyer's patches (PPs) are organized lymphoid structures found within the mucosal wall overlaid by specialized epithelial cells, the membranous or microfold cells.[2] PPs are large and visible by eye as bulges on the serosal surface of the intestine. In addition, the intestine contains smaller lymphoid structures, the isolated lymphoid follicles (ILFs), each containing a single B cell follicle with an overlying follicular epithelium. Mouse intestine contains an abundance of these small organized structures.[3] An immature form of the ILF is the cryptopatch, comprising clusters of lymphocyte precursors. Antigenic signals promote the enlargement of the ILFs through the recruitment of B cells.[4]

Together MLNs, PPs, and ILFs compose the inductive sites in the GI tract. Finally, T lymphocytes are normally found between epithelial cells (intraepithelial lymphocytes [IELs]). These IELs are predominantly CD8$^+$ T cells in the small intestine and have an oligoclonal repertoire. The immune cells of the LP and IELs make up the effector cells of the GALT, and they are responsible for both the maintenance of tolerance to harmless antigens and immunity against pathogens. Fig. 30.1 shows a schematic of the structure of the GALT.

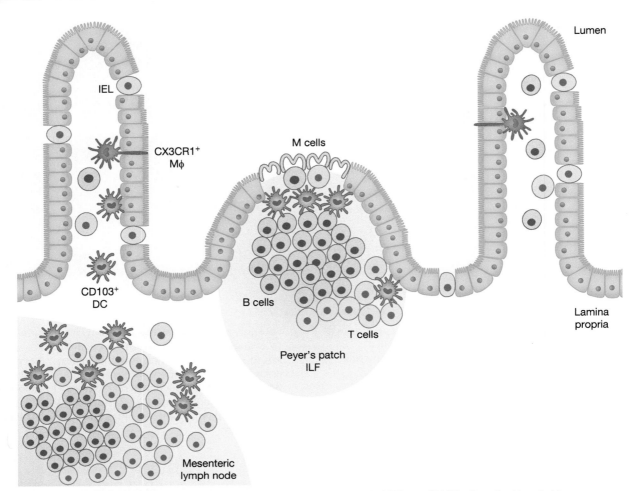

• **Fig. 30.1** Structure of the Gastrointestinal-Associated Lymphoid Tissue (GALT). Organized lymphoid structures in the gastrointestinal (GI) tract include the mesenteric lymph nodes (MLNs) that drain the mucosa via the lymphatics. Peyer's patches and isolated lymphoid follicles *(ILFs)* are present within the mucosal wall and are covered by specialized antigen sampling cells called microfold *(M)* cells. Dendritic cells *(DC)* continuously migrate from the lamina propria into the MLNs to present antigen. Organized lymphoid structures contain B cell follicles surrounded by T cell areas. Within the lamina propria are scattered T cells, B cells, macrophages *(MΦ)*, and DCs. A population of intraepithelial lymphocytes (IELs) is also found through the GI. A single layer of columnar epithelium separates the mucosal immune system from the luminal contents.

Mechanisms of Antigen Sampling in the Intestinal Mucosa

Food proteins are digested by a combination of gastric acid, pancreatic proteases, and brush border peptidases, resulting in a mixture of amino acids and dipeptides and tripeptides, which are then absorbed by the IECs. Dietary antigens that escape proteolysis in the lumen can be taken up by the intestine in various ways (Fig. 30.2). Soluble antigens are transported by transcellular or paracellular routes. In the transcellular route, IECs sample antigens by fluid phase endocytosis by the microvillous membrane; the antigens are then transported in small vesicles and larger phagosomes and digested when lysosomes combine to form phagolysosomes. Although some antigens can be directly deposited in the basolateral space, partially degraded antigens within endocytic vesicles can be loaded onto major histocompatibility complex II (MHCII) molecules and released from the basolateral membrane to interact with DCs.[5,6] In the paracellular route, antigens cross the epithelial barrier through tight junctions between adjacent IECs. An increased transport of intact antigen by the paracellular route has been related to its allergenic activity.[7,8] Goblet cells also have been identified as significant portals for the uptake of soluble antigens, delivering these antigens to subepithelial DCs.[9]

Particulate antigens are poorly sampled by enterocytes, at which the glycocalyx provides a barrier to even relatively small particles. Microfold cells that overlie PPs have a reduced glycocalyx layer and shortened microvilli, which allows for binding of particles that cannot adhere to enterocytes. Microfold cells have a sparse, flattened cytoplasm and enhanced endocytic activity, allowing rapid antigen delivery into the subepithelial dome region of the PPs, which is rich in DCs that process and present antigen to T cells or transfer antigen to B lymphocytes.

In addition to transport through the epithelium, the intestinal mucosa is densely populated with a network of phagocytes such as macrophages and DCs that extend dendrites between IECs and sample antigen without disrupting tight junctions between

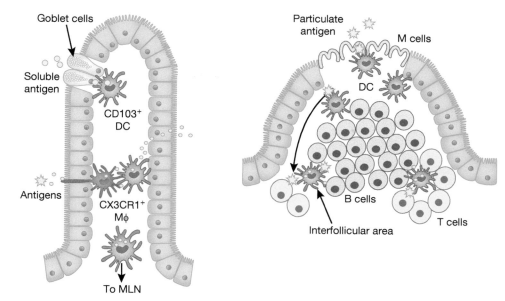

• **Fig. 30.2** Antigen Uptake in the Intestine. In the intestinal villus *(left)*, antigen can reach subepithelial dendritic cells *(DCs)* by several routes. Macrophages *(MΦ)* can send extensions between enterocytes to sample particulate antigens directly from the lumen and transfer these antigens to DCs. Alternatively, soluble antigens can be taken up by fluid phase endocytosis by enterocytes and be deposited in the lamina propria for uptake by MΦs or DCs. Goblet cells can also function as conduits for delivery of antigen to DCs. DCs migrate from the lamina propria to the mesenteric lymph nodes *(MLNs)*, where antigen can be presented to naïve T cells. In the Peyer's patch *(right)*, microfold *(M)* cells are specialized for uptake of particulate antigens that are delivered to DCs in the subepithelial space. These DCs can then traffic to the interfollicular areas of the Peyer's patch for presentation to T cells *(green)* or interacting with B cells *(blue)*.

cells.[10,11] Macrophages are the most abundant resident phagocytes in the small and large intestinal LP and form a band of cells directly beneath the surface epithelium.[12]

Resident macrophages send protrusions through the IECs to sample soluble antigens from the intestinal lumen in a mechanism that depends on the expression of CX_3CR1.[10,13] By contrast, CD103+ DCs are less efficient in sampling soluble antigen, although they have been shown to capture bacteria by using intraepithelial dendrites.[10,14] Like DCs, macrophages can take up antigen and present it to T cells; however, CX3CR1high macrophages do not migrate to the MLNs under steady-state conditions, and a cooperation between CX3CR1high macrophages and migratory CD103+ DCs is required.[10] After antigen uptake, CX3CR1+ macrophages transfer peptide-MHCII complexes by gap junctions to CD103+ DCs, which migrate to the MLNs and present antigen to naïve T cells. In addition, CD103+ DCs acquire antigen after it has been transported across enterocytes or goblet cells as outlined previously and carry antigen to draining lymph nodes to prime naïve T cells. Fig. 30.2 outlines these major pathways of antigen uptake.

Tolerogenic Response to Antigens Encountered Through the Gastrointestinal Tract

Food contains a diverse mix of antigens that are capable of stimulating immune responses if administered by other routes. Administration of antigens by the oral route is one of the most effective means of inducing tolerance. The process of oral tolerance was first defined experimentally in laboratory rodents that displayed systemic unresponsiveness to immunization with antigens to

which they had previously been fed. Tolerance can be transferred to a naïve animal by transferring T cells,[15,16] demonstrating that this is an active immune-mediated process. Oral tolerance also has been demonstrated experimentally in humans by feeding a neoantigen.[17,18]

Natural thymic-derived regulatory T cells (TREGs) are characterized by the expression of CD4, CD25, Foxp3, and a naïve phenotype and are not required for oral tolerance induction. Feeding mice with oral antigen induces a population of peripheral antigen-specific TREGs that express markers similar to those of thymic-derived TREGs (CD25+, Foxp3+, and CTLA-4) and mediate regulatory responses in a mechanism dependent on transforming growth factor-beta (TGF-β) secretion and independent of interleukin 10 (IL-10).[19,20] These peripherally induced Foxp3+ TREGs have been shown to be necessary for the induction of tolerance to oral antigens.[20] Indeed, mutations in the Foxp3 locus are associated with a loss of peripheral tolerance and development of severe food allergy in humans,[21] and specific depletion of peripherally induced Foxp3+ TREGs abrogates oral tolerance.[22]

Other TREG populations have been described in the context of oral tolerance induction, including CD4+ T helper 3 (TH3) cells and CD4+ TREGs type 1 (TR1). TH3 cells are identified by surface expression of latency-associated peptide (LAP) and have suppressive functions mediated by TGF-β secretion.[20,23] TR1 cells represent another subset of TREGs characterized by expression of the lymphocyte activation gene 3 *(LAG-3)* and CD49b in the face of absent Foxp3 and CD25 expression.[24] Their role in oral tolerance induction has been related to the suppression of immune responses via IL-10 production.[25] However, some studies indicate that IL-10 is dispensable for the induction of oral tolerance to foods, although they are critical for the suppression of inflammatory responses initiated by the intestinal microbiota.[26,27]

Naïve T cells must be instructed to become regulatory in phenotype rather than becoming effector T helper 1, 2, and 17 cells (Th1, Th2, and Th17, respectively). There is growing evidence that the milieu in which food antigens are presented to the naïve T cells by DCs is a critical factor promoting the development of regulatory T cells in the intestine.

The Role of Intestinal Dendritic Cells and Macrophages in Oral Tolerance and Immunity

Oral tolerance is initiated in the LP by CD103+ DCs that capture antigen and migrate to the MLNs, where they induce differentiation of naïve T cells into T_{REG}s, through a mechanism dependent on the release of retinoic acid and TGF-β production.[28,29] In addition, CD103+ expresses high levels of indoleamine 2,3-dioxygenase (IDO), an enzyme involved in tryptophan catabolism that enhances the induction of Foxp3+ T_{REG}s.[30] In this context, migratory CD103+CD11b− DCs have shown the highest capacity to induce Foxp3+ T_{REG} compared with other intestinal DC subsets such as CD103+CD11b+ and CD103+CD8α+CD11b^{low} DCs, because of their enhanced ability to express retinaldehyde dehydrogenase 2 (RALDH2) and TGF-β2.[31] The expression of the TGF-β receptor 1 (TGF-βR1) by intestinal CD103+ DCs has been shown to have an indispensable role in their generation, which may explain the tissue-specific development of this unique DC subset. Thus, the deletion of TGF-βR1 is accompanied by a significant reduction of CD103+CD11b+ DCs together with a reduced generation of antigen-specific Foxp3+ T_{REG}s.[32] Furthermore, the regulatory activity of CD103+ DCs is enhanced by environmental local factors. Microbial-derived production of granulocyte-macrophage colony-stimulating factor (GM-CSF) by type 3 innate lymphoid cells (ILC3s) acts on intestinal DCs, promoting the accumulation of T_{REG}s and intestinal homeostasis.[33] Mucins produced by goblet cells such as MUC2 also imprints a regulatory phenotype on CD103+ DCs through the induction of TGF-β, retinoic acid–synthesizing (RALDH) enzymes, IL-10 expression, and suppression of inflammatory cytokines, thus promoting oral tolerance.[34]

During oral antigen exposure, macrophages and monocyte-derived cells of the LP are dispensable in the peripheral induction of Foxp3+ T_{REG}s.[31] However, although resident macrophages do not have access to naïve T cells in the MLNs to initiate T_{REG} differentiation, they have an important role in the expansion of T_{REG}s during the generation of oral tolerance to fed antigens. It has been shown that CX3CR1+ macrophages express high levels of IL-10, which is necessary for expansion of T_{REG}s in the LP, and failure of this tissue T_{REG} expansion impairs the development of oral tolerance.[22] On the other hand, resident macrophages function as a secondary barrier after the epithelium in preventing the influx of microbes from the gut lumen into the body proper. Macrophages from the intestinal mucosa of mouse and human are nonresponsive to microbial stimuli compared with monocytes or macrophages from other sites.[35,36] This was shown to be due to TGF-β released from the intestinal stroma in humans[36] or autocrine effects of IL-10 in the mouse.[35] IL-10 is clearly important for immune homeostasis in the intestine as mice lacking IL-10 develop spontaneous colitis,[37] as do mice lacking IL-10 receptor specifically in macrophages.[38]

Homing of Lymphocytes to the Intestine

Lymphocytes that differentiate in the inductive sites of the GALT into effector T cells (T_H1, T_H2, and T_H17, among others), T_{REG}s, or antibody-secreting B cells home preferentially to the intestinal LP to carry out their function.[39,40] Targeted homing of lymphocytes is determined by expression of specific adhesion molecules and chemokine receptors.[41] Homing to the intestine is mediated by the adhesion molecule α4β7 binding to mucosal addressin cell adhesion molecule (MAdCAM) on high endothelial venules.[42] In addition, the chemokine receptor CCR9 promotes migration to the small intestine, where constitutive expression of the ligand CCL25 is found.[43,44] In the MLNs, retinoic acid produced by CD103+ DCs[28] and stromal cells[45] is required to program newly induced tolerogenic Foxp3+ T_{REG}s to home to the intestine through expression of CCR9 and α4β7.[46] A limited migration of antigen-specific T_{REG}s has been shown in mice deficient in β7 integrin and CCR9-deficient mice, resulting in impaired oral immune tolerance.[47]

Intestinal Humoral Immune Responses

Naïve B cells in the MLNs and PPs are activated by binding to their antigen, proliferate, and with T cell help differentiate into antibody-secreting cells or memory B cells. GALT DCs promote the differentiation of B cells into antibody-secreting cells, and up-regulate CCR9 and α4β7 on B cells to promote homing of cells to the LP.[40] CCR10 is also expressed on a subset of antibody-secreting B cells and contributes to homing to the large intestinal mucosa.[48,49] The intestinal mucosa is a rich site of antibody production, particularly secretory IgA. Immunoglobulins play an important role in neutralization of pathogens and function together with epithelial-expressed receptors as specific antigen sampling mechanisms in the intestinal mucosa.

In human and mouse, daily production of IgA outpaces that of all other immunoglobulin isotypes combined.[50] It is estimated that 75% to 80% of the antibody-secreting cells express IgA in the gastric mucosa, duodenum, and jejunum and 90% in the colon.[51] IgA in plasma occurs primarily as monomers, but IgA in mucosal secretions is composed of polymeric IgA (2–4 molecules) joined at the Fc region by a joining "J" chain and secretory component that is a fragment of the polymeric immunoglobulin receptor (pIgR). pIgR is expressed on the IECs and transports polymeric IgA (bound to pIgR through the J chain that connects the IgA subunits) from the basolateral face into the intestinal lumen. Each molecule of pIgR can perform only one transport of immunoglobulin because the extracellular portion is cleaved to form secretory component. Secretory IgA has been shown to selectively bind to microfold cells by the interaction of constant domains with Dectin-1.[52] Antigen sampling by microfold cells has been associated with induction of IgA production, which contributes to immune exclusion by neutralizing antigens in the lumen.[53] Antigens tagged to IgA are taken up by microfold cells and delivered to DCs in the PPs,[54] where they induce an immunoglobulin response. Thus, IgA may selectively allow for controlled entry of antigens into the PPs while preventing broad access to the remaining intestinal mucosa.[55]

There is also evidence for a significant contribution of IgG to host defense against enteropathogens.[56,57] IgG-expressing B cells have been reported to represent 13% of antibody-secreting cells in the gastric mucosa and 3% to 4% in the small intestine and large bowel.[51] The neonatal Fc receptor for IgG (FcRn) is expressed in the intestine before weaning and facilitates the transfer of passive immunity from the mother by colostrum. In mice, the induction of tolerance in the neonate by antigen exposure by IgG-containing breast milk has been shown to be mediated by FcRn-facilitated uptake and delivery to DCs.[58] In addition, a mouse model of food allergy has revealed that administration of allergen-specific IgG can act to induce and sustain immunologic tolerance to foods by preventing the development of IgE antibodies, T_H2 responses, and anaphylactic responses through their effects on mast cell function.[59] In humans, passive immunity is delivered by the placenta, but FcRn is expressed in the intestine and is maintained throughout adult life. This suggests a function for FcRn beyond transfer of passive immunity. In addition, IgG is secreted into the intestinal lumen by FcRn, where it binds to its antigens and can be recaptured by FcRn and transported into the intestinal LP.[60] Antigen is then delivered to subepithelial DCs that can generate an effector T cell response.

Food Allergy: Altered Oral Tolerance to Dietary Proteins

During allergic sensitization, the normal oral tolerance response to dietary proteins is altered and T_{REG} development is thought to be compromised and replaced by the generation of an effector immune response deviated toward a T_H2 phenotype characterized by IL-4 production. This cytokine is required for B cell class switching, synthesis of antigen-specific IgE, and the expansion of allergic effector cells.[61] Fig. 30.3 summarizes the main events underlying sensitization to dietary antigens and food allergy development.

Epithelial cytokines (IL-33, IL-25, and thymic stromal lymphopoietin [TSLP]), released by IECs in response to innate triggers or external insults, are central regulators of type 2 immune polarization and play a key role in the mucosal induction allergic responses.[62] Intestinal secreted IL-33 promotes sensitization to food antigens through the activation of ILC2s that produce large amounts of IL-4, suppressing the generation of Foxp3+ T_{REG}s in the small intestine.[63] In addition to the effects on T_H2 priming, IL-33 also promotes acute clinical reactions to food by acting directly on mast cells and enhancing IgE-mediated activation.[64] IEC-derived cytokine IL-25 is also overexpressed in the intestine of a transgenic experimental model of food allergy, whereas mice lacking the IL-25 receptor are resistant to IgE-mediated food sensitization.[65,66] Ingested antigens induce IL-25 and the secretion of type 2–related cytokines that promote ILC2-derived IL-13, which amplifies rather than initiates a T_H2-mediated response.[66] TSLP is a third IEC-derived cytokine that contributes to food allergy development, promoting sensitization to dietary antigens through DCs and basophils.[65,67] TSLP promotes IL-3–independent basophil hematopoiesis and eliciting a population of functionally distinct basophils that promote T_H2 cytokine-mediated allergic inflammation.[68] Altogether, it has been shown that all IEC-derived alarmins (IL-33, IL-25, and TSLP) may be required to induce sensitization to dietary antigens, whereas the single production of any of these cytokines can maintain an established food allergy.[69] Uric acid, another alarmin released after cellular damage, also shows adjuvant activity that promotes T_H2 responses.[70] In addition, IECs have been reported as a major source of eotaxin in the gut, and this epithelial-derived eotaxin regulates the recruitment of eosinophils in the gut during the effector phase of allergic response and thus the severity of intestinal manifestations to food antigens.[71]

In mouse models, to mimic food allergic sensitization, it is necessary to break the oral tolerance response by the use of exogenous adjuvants. Oral administered cholera toxin (CT) induces the expression of OX40L expression on CD103+ DCs and their migration to the MLNs, which results in T_H2 cell skewing.[72,73] Up-regulation of OX40L depends on IL-33 production by IECs in response to CT, but independent of IL-25 and TSLP.[73] Induction of T_H2 responses to food antigens in the presence of CT is associated with suppression of antigen-specific T_{REG}s in the GI tract.[74] In response to antigen feeding and CT, eosinophils can also contribute to activation and migration of CD103+ DCs by releasing eosinophil-specific granule protein (EPO), thus promoting T_H2 polarization and allergic sensitization.[75] The use of staphylococcal enterotoxin B as an adjuvant also promotes maturation of intestinal DCs and enhances expression of TIM-4, which is required to induce T_H2 polarization.[76] Taken together, the use of adjuvants in mouse models of food allergy has revealed the key role played by CD103+ DCs and how variations in their tolerogenic phenotype drive a suppression of antigen-specific T_{REG}s and prime naïve CD4+ T cells toward T_H2 responses to food antigens.

Production of IL-4 by primed T_H2 cells is required for B cell class-switching and synthesis of antigen-specific IgE. IL-4 also can be produced by T follicular helper cells (T_FH) and, in a mouse model of food allergy, ST2−CXCR5+ T_FH cells have been reported as necessary for IgE production and development of peanut allergy.[77] In addition, under the influence of chronic allergic inflammation, emerging evidence indicates that T_{REG}s could lose their suppressive functions and be redirected toward a pathogenic T_H2-like phenotype.[78] The reprogramming of allergen-specific T_{REG}s has been shown in mouse models and in food-allergic patients and is characterized by the expression of T_H2 master transcription factor GATA3 and IL-4 secretion, while retaining their Foxp3 expression. Reprogrammed T_{REG}s lose their ability to control the effector T_H2 response and mast cells expansion, impairing oral tolerance and promoting food allergy.[78,79]

Production of allergen-specific IgE is central to the development of food allergies. After sensitization to the dietary antigens, maintained antigen-specific IgE production may be caused by long-lived IgE+ plasma cells[80] and persistent memory B cells.[81] The development of IgE in the gut is poorly described, although secreted IgE antibodies are detectable in intestinal juice and stools of subjects with food allergy, suggesting antibody production by local IgE+ plasma cells. The low-affinity IgE receptor CD23 is constitutively expressed by IECs and has been shown to function as a bidirectional transporter of allergen-specific IgE across the intestinal epithelium in mouse[82] and human gut.[83] However, most of the antigen-specific IgE secreted by plasma cells binds to the high-affinity receptor FcεRI expressed on the surface of basophils and mast cells. The cross-linking of the IgE bound to these cells induces the release of preformed and newly synthesized mediators that are responsible for allergic symptoms.

Mast cells residing in the LP are not only implicated in the effector phase of food allergy but also play a key role in the sensitization to food proteins. Activation of mast cells through IgE leads to a suppression of antigen-specific T_{REG} generation and amplification of T_H2 responses.[84] In addition, a population of mast cells producing high amounts of IL-9 and IL-13 (MMC9) was identified in response to an orally administered dietary antigen. MMC9 is induced by T_H2 cells, and depletion was shown to suppress the development of food allergy and transfer of MMC9 restored allergic responses.[85]

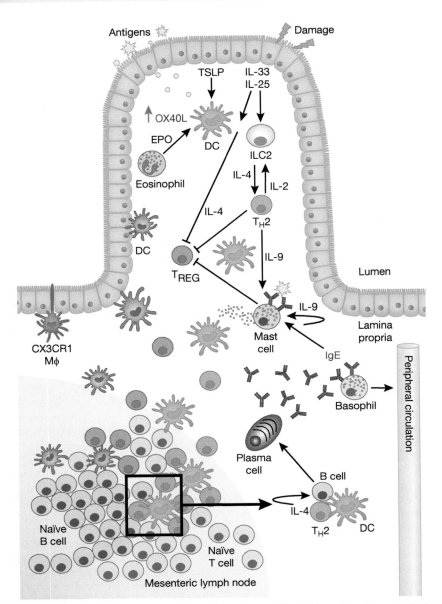

• **Fig. 30.3** Mechanism of Sensitization to Dietary Proteins and Food Allergy Development. In the presence of adjuvants and epithelial damage, the induction of epithelial-derived cytokines (interleukin 33 *[IL-33]*, *IL-25* and thymic stromal lymphopoietin *[TSLP]*) and other alarmins (such as uric acid), food allergens, transfered by macrophages (MΦ) or directly captured by dendritic cells (DCs), promote DC activation and maturation. Eosinophil-specific granule protein *(EPO)* also promotes DCs activation. In the mesenteric lymph nodes (MLNs), DCs prime naïve T cells toward a T helper 2 (T$_H$2) phenotype able to produce *IL-4,* which promote immunoglobulin E *(IgE)* class-switching on B cells and suppression of regulatory T cells (T$_{REG}$). T$_F$H cells can also contribute to B cell IgE class-switching. T$_H$2 cells act on mast cells via *IL-9* production. Epithelial cytokines also induce type 2 innate lymphoid cell *(ILC2)* activation, which contributes to T$_H$2 polarization and T$_{REG}$ suppression.

Environmental Factors and the Regulation of the Mucosal Immunity

Role of the Microbiota in Mucosal Immunity

The GI mucosa is often described as being in a state of "physiologic inflammation." In mice, the genetic deletion of a wide range of immunoregulatory genes results in colitis, a phenotype that is commonly absent if the mice are raised in germ-free conditions.[86] Although microbial signals can induce inflammation and tissue damage if not appropriately controlled, these signals are also

necessary for the health of the organism. Our intestinal microbiota contributes locally to the digestion of nutrients, regulates the epithelial barrier, and is essential for maturation of the mucosal immune system in addition to having systemic effects on metabolism and the neuroendocrine system.[87]

Several studies support the role of commensal microbiota in the regulation of oral tolerance to dietary antigens by T$_{REG}$ generation and expansion.[88] Germ-free mice have a reduced capacity for the generation of oral tolerance and conversely show increased susceptibility to allergic sensitization through the oral route.[89] In fact, germ-free and antibiotic-treated mice have poorly developed lymphoid structures in the GI tract and have shown a lack of T_{REG} generation in the colonic LP that is restored after bacterial colonization.[90–92] Different organisms have differing effects on the development of effector and regulatory responses in the GI tract. Segmented filamentous bacteria that are in intimate contact with mouse intestinal epithelium promote the development of T_H17 responses in the GI tract.[93] *Bacteroides fragilis,* some *Bifidobacterium* spp., and several *Clostridia* strains promote the development of T_{REG}s, enhance regulatory tone of the host immune system, and suppress allergic sensitization.[89,94,95] The gut microbiota also induces a subset of RORγt⁺ T_{REG}s that specifically suppress T_H2 immune responses.[96] Toll-like receptor 2 (TLR2), TLR4, and TLR9 are host receptors that have been shown to contribute to tolerogenic effects of the intestinal microbiota.[97–99] In addition, MyD88 signaling in T_{REG}s is essential to be able to sense commensal microbiota and to induce mucosal tolerance.[92] Humoral immunity, such as IgA production, is carefully regulated by the commensal microbiota, and the specificity of the IgA response adapts to respond to changes in intestinal microbial populations.[100] Intestinal colonization by *Clostridia* and *Bacteroides* spp. promotes induction of IgA, which can reduce allergen transportation across the epithelial barrier based on a blocking effect.[89] Commensal-derived signals also regulate IgE production. Germ-free mice have reduced levels of all isotypes of antibodies with the exception of IgE that is uniquely elevated.[101] The presence of microbiota limits serum IgE and circulating basophils by a mechanism dependent on MyD88 expression by B cells.[102] Because cellular and humoral immune responses in the GI tract are influenced by the commensal microbiota, it is unsurprising that the microbiota is a key factor in the development of tolerance or allergy in the GI tract.

Metabolic products of the microbiota are increasingly being recognized as an essential part of human physiology, with profound effects on immune function and dysfunction.[103] Short-chain fatty acids, derived from the fermentation of the dietary fiber, promote a tolerogenic tone in the intestine.[104] They have been proven to enhance tolerogenic function of CD103⁺ DCs via metabolism of vitamin A[105] and induce the expansion of functional Foxp3⁺ T_{REG}s.[106–108] In addition, degradation of dietary proteins by intestinal microbiota promotes generation of amino acid–derived metabolites with immunomodulatory properties. Tryptophan-derived metabolites activate hydrocarbon receptors, which have been associated with suppression of sensitization to food allergens by the generation of tolerogenic CD103⁺ DCs and Foxp3⁺ T_{REG}s.[109,110]

Although the microbiota has generally been shown to be tolerogenic, susceptibility to food allergy has been shown to be transmissible in mice.[111] In humans, although early childhood appears to be critical for the colonization of a diverse microbiota

necessary for the induction and maintenance of oral tolerance,[112] many specific bacterial signatures associated with food allergy have been identified.[113,114]

Influence of Diet on Mucosal Immunity

In addition to the changes that diet can induce in the intestinal microbiota,[115] dietary components can have direct effects on the host immunity through interaction with the mucosal immune system. Deficiency of dietary vitamin A has been associated with breakdown of oral tolerance through a decreased expression of RALDH2 in CD103⁺ DCs.[116] The vitamin A metabolite retinoic acid is best known for promoting generation of T_{REG}s and is required for the efficient generation of RORγt⁺ T_{REG}s in response to microbial signals.[96] However, the impact of retinoic acid is not always regulatory, because in the presence of the inflammatory cytokine IL-15, retinoic acid can amplify inflammatory responses and in this way has been shown to contribute to intestinal damage in a murine model of celiac disease.[117] Vitamin D promotes homing of lymphocytes to the GI tissue and suppresses IL-17 production.[118] Vitamin D insufficiency results in significant reduction of a unique population of regulatory IELs bearing the marker CD8αα.[119] In addition, vitamin D deficiency exacerbates allergic reactions mediated by increased levels of antigen-specific IgE and reduced induction of Foxp3⁺ T_{REG}s.[120,121] On the other hand, although intake of n-3 polyunsaturated fatty acids (PUFAs) has been found to reduce specific IgE and prevent sensitization to cow's milk,[122] consumption of n-6 PUFAs was shown to promote allergic response to whey proteins.[123] Furthermore, a high-fat diet can have proinflammatory effects by altering cytokines from innate lymphoid cells that regulate epithelial barrier function.[124]

Conclusions

The mucosal immune system is tightly regulated to prevent inappropriate immune reactions to food antigens or the commensal flora and is responsible for guarding a vast surface area against pathogenic entry. Antigens can gain access to the mucosal immune system by a number of different mechanisms, including direct DC uptake and antibody-facilitated antigen uptake. The normal response to food antigens is an active tolerance response mediated by regulatory T cells and induced by intestinal DCs and macrophages. Microbiota and diet are critical factors in the maintenance of GI immune homeostasis.

The reference list can be found on the companion Expert Consult website at http://www.expertconsult.inkling.com.

31

Evaluation of Food Allergy

SCOTT H. SICHERER, HUGH A. SAMPSON

KEY POINTS

- A *food allergy* is an adverse health effect arising from an immune response that occurs reproducibly on exposure to a given food, whereas a *food intolerance* is an adverse effect as a result of a nonimmunologic response (e.g., metabolic, pharmacologic, or toxic).
- Food allergies may be immediate (immunoglobulin E [IgE] mediated) or delayed (non–IgE mediated) in onset and induce a variety of symptoms involving the skin, respiratory or gastrointestinal tracts, and/or cardiovascular system.
- A thorough and detailed history is the most important part of the evaluation and determines which laboratory tests should

be ordered, which food challenges and treatments may be required, and the education that will be needed regarding the results.
- Skin prick tests and food-specific IgE levels, including tests measuring IgE against component proteins of foods, confirm sensitization and provide some evidence on the probability of clinical allergy, but alone are not adequate to make the diagnosis of food allergy.
- The oral food challenge remains the gold standard for diagnosing food allergy.

Introduction

Food allergy is common, affects quality of life, and can result in severe and even fatal allergic reactions.[1] In a guideline developed by an expert panel convened by the National Institute of Allergy and Infectious Diseases[2] and in a Practice Parameter,[3] *food allergy* is defined as an adverse health effect arising from a specific immune response that occurs reproducibly on exposure to a given food. These immune responses may be immunoglobulin E (IgE)-mediated, non–IgE-mediated, or a result of multiple mechanisms. The term *food intolerance* refers to a non–immune-mediated reaction that may include metabolic, pharmacologic, or toxic mechanisms. Another important term is *sensitization,* which refers to having demonstrable IgE antibodies, but this may occur in the absence of clinical symptoms. An immune-mediated food allergy requires both the presence of sensitization and clinical responsiveness when the food is ingested. This chapter focuses on the diagnosis of food allergy. Additional chapters discuss specific disorders (Chapters 33 and 34), prevention (Chapter 36), dietary management (Chapter 35), and immunotherapies (Chapter 37).

Prevalence

Current literature suggests that food allergy may affect up to 10% of the population but probably not more than that percentage.[4–6] Prevalence rates are obtained through numerous methodologies; studies that rely on self-report tend to give the highest prevalence estimates, whereas those applying medically supervised oral food challenges typically give the lowest.[7] There is an impression that food allergy has increased over the past decades and there are

marked geographic differences.[4,8,9] A clinically significant issue is that many more individuals label themselves "food allergic" than are confirmed to have true food allergy.[6,7] This observation underscores the need for a careful medical evaluation to ensure that children are not unnecessarily avoiding foods.

Immunoglobulin E–Mediated Symptoms

IgE-mediated reactions typically have symptom onset within minutes after ingestion of an allergen, but symptoms may begin up to 2 hours after exposure[10] (Box 31.1). An unusual exception is allergy to mammalian meats triggered by a reaction to a sugar moiety, the oligosaccharide galactose-α-1,3-galactose (alphagal).[11] The reaction onset in this disorder is often 4 to 6 hours after ingestion. The following section describes symptoms that are characteristic of IgE-mediated reactions.

Cutaneous Symptoms

Food allergy–induced skin symptoms generally fall into two main categories: atopic dermatitis and urticaria. Urticaria typically begins promptly after the ingestion of a known food allergen, is usually diagnosed early, and the culprit food is determined. Chronic urticaria is rarely caused by a food allergen. Rarely, food additives have been reported to cause chronic urticaria in adults, but there are no systematically confirmed reports in children.

Atopic dermatitis has been shown to be exacerbated by food allergies in numerous carefully controlled studies using double-blind, placebo-controlled food challenges.[12] In some situations, the onset of symptoms is subtle and somewhat delayed, with irritability and then

Immune
IgE Mediated
- Immediate (gastrointestinal, respiratory, cutaneous, ocular, cardiovascular, anaphylactic)
- Oral allergy syndrome or pollen-food allergy syndrome

Mixed IgE and Cell Mediated
- Atopic dermatitis
- Eosinophilic esophagitis and other eosinophilic gastrointestinal diseases

Non–IgE Immune Mediated
- Celiac disease, dermatitis herpetiformis
- Food protein–induced gastrointestinal illnesses
  - Food protein–induced enterocolitis
  - Allergic colitis/proctocolitis
  - Food protein-induced enteropathy (milk, soy, others)
- Food-induced pulmonary hemosiderosis (Heiner's syndrome)

Non–Immune Mediated
- Toxic reactions
- Toxic reactions (food poisoning [e.g., scombroid fish poisoning])
- Nontoxic reactions
- Intolerances
  - Carbohydrate malabsorption (e.g., lactase deficiency, fructose deficiency, sucrase-isomaltase deficiency)
  - Psychological reactions (strongly held beliefs)

itching being the first symptoms to appear, followed by erythema and/or urticaria preceding the more typical erythema and morbilliform eruption that may be most prominent the day after the offending food is consumed. There does not appear to be a single pattern of presentation, but careful observations by families can often make the connection, especially when parents are instructed on the typical presentation. Children with moderate to severe atopic dermatitis are at high risk (~35%) of having food allergies, but this relationship primarily reflects reactions that would result in acute systemic reactions, not isolated eczema flares.[12] The elimination of foods as a treatment for eczema can be considered in a subset of patients but carries risks that include reduced nutrition, impaired quality of life, and possible development of anaphylactic allergy to a previously ingested food. Therefore, this approach requires careful consideration.[12,13] The treatment of atopic dermatitis is addressed in more detail in Chapter 38.

Respiratory Symptoms

Respiratory symptoms of a food allergic reaction include those in the upper respiratory tract: sneezing, nasal pruritus, rhinorrhea, and congestion and periocular pruritus and tearing. In the lower respiratory tract, symptoms and signs include stridor, hoarse voice, cough, dyspnea, and wheezing. It is important to note that a hacking staccato cough may be a sign of impending laryngeal obstruction without other symptoms and may lead to abrupt airway closure. Asthma is infrequently the sole manifestation of an allergic reaction to food. However, when a patient with asthma has symptoms that are not responding in the usual fashion to treatment, a food reaction should be considered and the treatment approach altered to include injected epinephrine. Food allergy in individuals with asthma may predispose them to more severe episodes and may be a risk factor for more severe and fatal asthma.[14–16]

Gastrointestinal Symptoms

Immediate-onset gastrointestinal (GI) symptoms include nausea, abdominal pain and cramps, vomiting, and diarrhea. Nausea and vomiting are often immediate, while the food is being consumed, raising the suspicion of food allergy, especially in an individual with a known food allergy. It should be noted that the GI symptoms may not be accompanied by skin manifestations. Rapid resolution of GI symptoms and return of appetite are frequently noted after a GI food reaction. Diarrhea may occur immediately or be delayed for a few hours.

Several GI symptoms are sometimes attributed to food allergy but remain controversial and are not likely related to IgE-mediated mechanisms. Constipation is not a typical feature of food allergy but a few controlled trials suggest that this is worth considering in toddlers having persistent constipation issues, but this remains controversial.[17] The issue of colic as a GI food allergic reaction in infants remains controversial. With newer feeding guidelines suggesting that delaying food introduction may increase food allergy, it is often difficult to determine whether to try elimination diets.[18] However, when infants and families are under significant distress, a brief trial of dietary elimination may be warranted.[19,20]

Pollen-Food Allergy Syndrome

Pollen-food allergy syndrome (oral allergy syndrome) is a common disorder in which oral symptoms, itching of the throat, and occasionally mild oral edema occur immediately upon the ingestion of certain foods, most commonly raw fruits and vegetables, but also certain nuts (e.g., hazelnuts and peanuts) can trigger these symptoms (see Chapter 35). These complaints are the result of specific IgE antibodies directed to aeroallergens that cross-react with certain food proteins. It is often useful to perform skin tests with fresh fruits and vegetables to confirm the diagnosis, and component protein testing for hazelnut (Cor a 1) and peanut (Ara h 8) will identify IgE to the birch pollen cross-reactive protein, Bet v 1. This constellation of symptoms is often present in children, but it is frequently unrecognized unless patients with pollen allergy (and/or their parents) are specifically queried about the presence of oral symptoms with certain foods.[21]

Cardiovascular Symptoms

Allergic reactions to foods that involve the cardiovascular system in children usually appear as respiratory compromise first and then progress to a drop in blood pressure and shock, as contrasted with adults who may have the sudden onset of cardiovascular symptoms before any other symptoms occur.

Anaphylaxis

The working definition of *anaphylaxis* is "a serious allergic reaction that is rapid in onset and may cause death."[22] The clinical criteria for diagnosing anaphylaxis are outlined in Chapter 44.

Non–Immunoglobulin E Immune-Mediated Reactions to Food

Celiac disease is an autoimmune process that occurs when antibodies directed to gluten cross-react with epithelial cells in the GI tract. When gluten-containing foods are removed from the diet, the GI lesion resolves. An associated but less common condition, dermatitis herpetiformis, is often mistaken for atopic dermatitis. Virtually all individuals with celiac disease exhibit human leukocyte antigen (HLA)-DQ2 or DQ8 genetic haplotypes.[23]

The eosinophilic GI disorders (see Chapter 34), especially eosinophilic esophagitis, appear to be increasing. In the majority of children, food allergy is a significant trigger; however, it is not IgE-mediated, and therefore current diagnostic methods for detection of IgE (skin tests and specific serum antibody measurements) are generally not helpful. A careful and detailed history may be the most important means of raising suspicion of the disease and prompting referral for endoscopy. A pattern of seasonal exacerbation in some individuals raises the possibility of swallowed aeroallergens as triggers. It is often difficult to monitor the effectiveness of food elimination diets because there are no noninvasive tests to examine the esophagus for a response.

Another immunologically mediated GI syndrome is food protein–induced enterocolitis syndrome (FPIES; see Chapter 33). A careful history elicits a pattern of repetitive vomiting that is delayed by about 2 hours after the ingestion of culprit foods. Characteristics of FPIES that distinguish it from IgE-mediated GI reactions are the delayed onset of symptoms; the lack of immediate recovery after the vomiting; and the continuous pattern of vomiting, pallor, and hypotension in about 15% of cases. Food protein–induced proctocolitis is characterized by gross or occult blood in the stools with an otherwise healthy-appearing infant (see Chapter 33).

Nonimmunologic Reactions

Toxic Reactions

A number of toxic reactions have been described that could be confused with allergic reactions to food. Food poisoning resulting from bacterial contamination commonly provokes nausea, abdominal pain, and often profuse diarrhea. Scombroid fish poisoning, which results from histamine in poorly prepared histidine-containing fish, is less common and can more easily mimic an allergic reaction, including triggering skin changes that are not caused by bacterial food poisoning. These skin changes may include flushing, urticaria, and angioedema. Respiratory symptoms may occur because of the large amount of histamine present.

Nontoxic Reactions

Auriculotemporal syndrome (Frey's syndrome) is triggered when foods that increase salivation cause a flushing reflex through the auriculotemporal branch of the trigeminal nerve resulting in a "strap-like" rash on both sides of the face.[24] Gustatory rhinitis occurs when the ingestion of spicy foods triggers rhinorrhea.[25]

Lactose intolerance as a result of lactase deficiency is the most common carbohydrate malabsorption condition. When there is insufficient lactase in the intestinal mucosa, diarrhea and bloating ensue, and the condition may be confused with milk allergy. Depending on the degree of lactase deficiency, some patients may tolerate small quantities of milk products without symptoms. Chronic diarrhea in young children may be due to carbohydrate malabsorption caused by fructose in fruit and especially fruit juice. The diarrhea, which often has an acrid smell, may be accompanied by a scalded skin appearance in the perianal and diaper area in the youngest children.

Psychological Reactions

Families may have concerns that foods trigger various behavioral symptoms in their children. Clinicians must be vigilant to ensure that these beliefs and resulting dietary restrictions do not lead to malnutrition or deficiency in specific nutrients. Occasionally, Munchausen syndrome by proxy must be considered, most often related to behavioral changes or other subjective symptoms.[26]

Evaluation

History

A thorough and detailed history is the most important part of the evaluation and will determine which specific laboratory tests to order, which food challenges and treatments may be required, and the education that will be needed regarding the results and avoidance of food triggers. The details to be ascertained include a detailed description of symptoms that have been observed, including the sequence of those symptoms; timing from onset of symptoms to their resolution; number of events that have occurred for each suspected food; possible ingestion of the food without symptoms; quantity of food eliciting symptoms, including the least amount (threshold) that has triggered symptoms if there has been more than one event; and associated factors such as exercise (in food-dependent exercise-induced anaphylaxis), medication (especially aspirin, other nonsteroidal antiinflammatory medications, and antireflux medication), and alcohol ingestion accompanying the suspected food.[1–3]

A history of anaphylaxis or a severe reaction increases the need for accurate details that include getting the ingredients of a meal from the facility (restaurant, home, or school) where the reaction occurred. This may lead to suspicions about less obvious culprits, especially spices. Emergency department records may be helpful. It is also important in situations in which wheezing has been part of the reaction to inquire if the asthma symptoms responded in the usual manner for that individual. If not, a food might have been the trigger.

Physical Examination

A complete physical examination should be done in children with a history of a food allergic reaction; however, the examination is usually normal unless the reaction is occurring acutely. The major exception is atopic dermatitis, which is a chronic condition that may exacerbate during the acute reaction. Other stigmata to observe include a possible abnormal abdominal examination, signs of malnutrition, or significant failure to thrive in young children placed on a restricted diet.

Laboratory Studies

Skin Testing

Skin testing by the prick/puncture technique is an easy-to-perform, cost-effective method for identifying sensitization to a food and determining the probability that a food challenge is likely to be helpful.[1–3] Food allergens eliciting wheal diameters of at least 3 mm or larger than the negative control are considered positive test results. Negative skin tests have a high negative predictive accuracy, thus usually excluding food allergy to common foods. The negative predictive accuracy for children younger than 3 or 4 years of age tends to be lower than for older children.[1–3]

Food extracts that elicit a positive result in the absence of a strong history of clinical reactivity typically have a positive predictive accuracy of less than 50% and cannot be considered diagnostic of symptomatic food allergy. Some studies suggest that larger skin tests (≥8-mm wheals for some foods) correlate better with symptomatic food allergy, but there is no clear correlation between skin test size and severity of reactions.[28] If there is a history of a convincing allergic reaction to a food and the skin test is positive, the test may be viewed as diagnostic. Skin test outcomes can be variable depending on a few factors: reagents and devices used for testing, experience of the testing personnel, and the interpretation of the test results.[29] A strongly positive history incriminating a specific food in the face of a negative skin test must be evaluated further (e.g., food-specific serum IgE determination and/or physician-supervised oral food challenge [OFC]).

Skin tests must be selected judiciously based on the history rather than performing panels of food skin tests. Selection of numerous foods to be eliminated from the diet based on large numbers of poorly selected skin tests may lead to diets that are difficult for families to follow and may eliminate foods that are clearly tolerated, making adherence to the diet poor.[30]

Commercial skin test extracts vary considerably in allergen content. It is often very useful to use fresh fruits and vegetables for skin testing by the technique referred to as "prick to prick" especially when evaluating patients with pollen-food allergy syndrome. In this technique the fresh food is "pricked with the skin test device and then the skin is pricked immediately."[32,33]

Limitations of skin testing include the following variables: (1) commercially prepared extracts often lack labile proteins responsible for IgE-mediated sensitization to most fruits and vegetables (as noted earlier); (2) skin testing on skin surfaces that have been treated with topical steroids may induce smaller wheals than those measured on untreated skin; (3) negative skin prick tests with commercial extracts that do not confirm convincing histories of food reactions should be repeated with the fresh food before concluding that IgE is absent; and (4) long-term, high-dose systemic steroid therapy may reduce allergen wheal size.

Intradermal skin testing for food is not recommended because of its high false positive rate and its occasional association with systemic reactions. However, intradermal skin tests have been found to be useful in reactions to beef, pork, and lamb because of reactivity to the meat proteins and galactose-α-1,3-galactose.[34]

In Vitro Testing

Numerous studies have shown that specific serum antibody levels correlate well with the outcome of OFCs, especially for peanut, egg, milk, and tree nuts, but there is less information on fish, shellfish, and a few other foods.[1] As with skin testing, detectable antibody in an immunoassay gives probability information on the likelihood of a reaction to a suspected food, but the history and food challenge remain crucial. Numerous studies have correlated clinical outcomes to food-specific IgE antibody levels but values associated with reactivity vary between studies likely because of a number of methodologic factors and characteristics of the patient populations studied.[28,30,35–41] Decision points have also been identified to be used as cut-off values to determine a reasonable level for considering an allergy to be highly likely (e.g., 95% risk, probably resulting in deferring an OFC) or in ranges at which tolerance may have developed (Table 31.1).

TABLE 31.1	Predictive Value of Food-Specific Immunoglobulin E	
Allergen	~95% Reaction Decision Point (kU$_A$/L)	≤50% Reaction Rechallenge Value (kU$_A$/L)
Egg	≥7.0	≤1.5
≤2 years old	≥2.0	
Milk	≥15.0	≤7.0
≤2 years old	≥5.0	
Peanut	≥14.0	≤5.0
Fish	≥20.0	
Tree nuts	≥15.0	≤2.0

Note: Patients with food-specific IgE values less than the listed diagnostic values may experience an allergic reaction after challenge. Unless history strongly suggests tolerance, a physician-supervised food challenge should be performed to determine whether the child can ingest the food safely.

Modified from Sicherer SH, Sampson HA. Food allergy: a review and update on epidemiology, pathogenesis, diagnosis, prevention, and management. J Allergy Clin Immunol 2018;141:41–58.

However, as mentioned earlier, the clinical history is always key in making these decisions.

In vitro measurements are preferred in a number of situations: (1) patients with extensive dermatographism; (2) patients with extensive skin disease (atopic dermatitis or urticaria); (3) patients who cannot discontinue antihistamines; and, more recently, (4) use by nonspecialists who do not perform skin testing to evaluate children for potential food allergy.

There is no consensus on whether skin tests or specific serum antibody levels are most sensitive. However, meta-analysis suggests that skin prick/puncture tests and immunoassays have similar sensitivities and specificities compared with double-blind, placebo-controlled food challenges.[42] At present, most allergists use the two tests together, in concert with the medical history (to ascertain a pretest probability) to decide whether to do food challenges (see later discussion) and the probability of the challenge being positive for a particular food.

Additional diagnostic insight may be obtained by performing IgE antibody tests to specific proteins within foods (components). The benefit of component testing primarily results from the fact that different food proteins may contribute differentially to the allergenic potential of a food. For example, in peanut, the proteins Ara h 2 and Ara h 6 are stable to digestion, and IgE binding to these proteins is particularly correlated with reactions.[35,43] In contrast, Ara h 8 in peanut is a labile pollen-homologous protein, and IgE binding to this protein is often not related to clinical reactivity or only mild symptoms.[44] The following vignette demonstrates the clinical utility of the testing.

A 13-year-old patient with birch pollen allergy had experienced generalized urticaria at age 2 from peanut butter and has not had any known subsequent exposures. Only 20% of children with peanut allergy resolve the allergy, and his peanut-specific IgE increased from 4 kilo units of allergen (kU$_A$)/L at age 2 to 25 kU$_A$/L at age 15, a result typically associated with peanut allergy. However,

TABLE 31.2	Component Tests		
Food	**Component Associated With Significant Reaction**	**Component Not Typically Associated With Significant Reaction**
Peanut	Ara h 2, Ara h 6, Ara h1, Ara h 3, Ara h 9	Ara h 8
Egg	Ovomucoid	Ovalbumin
Walnut	Jug r 1, Jug r 3	
Cashew	Ana o 3	
Brazil	Ber e 1	
Milk	Casein	α Lactalbumin, β lactoglobulin
Hazelnut	Cor a 14, Cor a 9, Cor a 8	Cor a 1

component testing revealed undetectable IgE to all components except Ara h 8, which was 95 kU_A/L. The conclusion is that he likely resolved his early peanut allergy, and the testing was influenced by his new pollen allergy. Table 31.2 shows available food component tests.

It also has been found that patients with antibodies to sequential (linear) epitopes in egg and milk, compared with conformational epitopes to these foods, are more likely to exhibit persistent food allergy. Extensive heating (baking) of milk and egg changes conformational epitopes that are recognized by the majority of youngsters, allowing them to tolerate baked milk- and egg-containing products. Peptide microarray technology is characterizing patient heterogeneity and may more accurately predict clinically significant food allergy as opposed to just allergen sensitization.[45–50]

Serum IgG levels to foods have not been found to have clinical utility. All individuals with a normal immune system will produce some IgG antibodies to many food proteins.[51]

Atopy patch tests have not been found to be consistently useful for detection of clinically significant food allergy, and a number of additional tests, such as applied kinesiology, resistance testing, hair analysis, and others, are considered unproved and experimental and not recommended.[2]

Food Challenges

The best test for food allergy is observing whether a food is tolerated when ingested. This is why the history is so influential in diagnosis. However, when history and skin or serum testing is not sufficient for a diagnosis, a medically supervised gradual feeding, an OFC can be undertaken. The double-blind, placebo-controlled oral food challenge (DBPCFC) is the gold standard for precise diagnosis of allergic reactions to foods and has provided a standard by which to evaluate other tests.[52–54] This format uses both active and placebo foods typically given on two separate days. The DBPCFC is usually reserved for research-related food challenges or when bias is likely, for example, from patient anxiety that could result in a false positive result if the

patient and observer were aware that the potential trigger food was being ingested. However, most OFCs are performed for clinical reasons and are performed without masking (open) or if some bias is a concern the food can be masked for the patient (single blind).

There is no universally accepted regimen for conducting an OFC, although various groups have suggested approaches that are tailored for research or clinical settings.[52–55] Fundamental aspects of the procedure suggest the following: the patient is in good health with a stable baseline before proceeding, the food is given in gradually increasing amounts starting at a dose unlikely to trigger a reaction, dosing is stopped for persistent subjective or objective symptoms, treatments of a reaction are provided promptly, and the procedure is conducted in a setting in which personnel and equipment are available to treat anaphylaxis.

The decision to undertake an OFC for clinical purposes usually begins with an evaluation of the odds of tolerating the food based on history and testing and a discussion of the value of proceeding for the patient (i.e., comfort with the risks and benefits, value of the food to the diet, etc.). For example, an OFC would likely not be undertaken in a 3-year-old patient with a 90% risk of a peanut allergy, but a 17-year-old patient with the same odds may be a good candidate because the patient is embarking on adulthood and because if he or she tolerated peanut, this could be life-changing. Before proceeding, patient and family preparation typically includes reviewing of risk versus benefit, obtaining informed consent, and ensuring the patient is healthy and not taking any medications that could interfere with interpretation of the procedure (e.g., antihistamines), mask an unstable baseline (e.g., recent use of inhaled β agonist), or interfere with treatment of anaphylaxis (e.g., β-blockers). The procedure is undertaken in a location (i.e., medical office, hospital setting) where anaphylaxis can be managed, and the selection of an appropriate setting requires consideration of the risks of a reaction and reaction severity, although emergency management of anaphylaxis always must be possible. Two fatalities have been reported.[56,57] When foods are masked, they may be mixed in other foods such as applesauce, pudding, juices, oatmeal, and so on. The dosing regimen varies, but one approach used for open OFCs is to aim for a typical serving for age and provide the food incrementally 1%, 4%, 10%, 20%, 20%, 20%, and 25%. Another approach based on grams of food protein is to escalate from 1 mg, 3 mg, 10 mg, 100 mg, 300 mg, 600 mg, 1000 mg, 3000 mg, and so on. Dosing intervals are usually 15 to 30 minutes. Various protocols exist, but clinical judgment is crucial regarding when to wait longer between doses or repeat a dose if a reaction may be developing. DBPCFCs often end with less than a full meal size portion of the food for age and are followed with an additional feeding of the food in a typical quantity and preparation for age. Patients are monitored closely throughout an OFC and typically observed 2 hours or longer to ensure the food was tolerated or a reaction, once treated, has fully subsided. Longer observation periods are also needed for alpha-gal allergy.[58] There is a low false negative rate (<2%) for OFC,[59] but a negative or passed challenge is not considered negative until the food is actually in the patient's diet in usual and customary portions on multiple occasions. It is important to counsel families to incorporate the food into the diet.[60,61] Food challenges are associated with improvement in quality of life whether they result in a reaction or identification that a food is tolerated.[62]

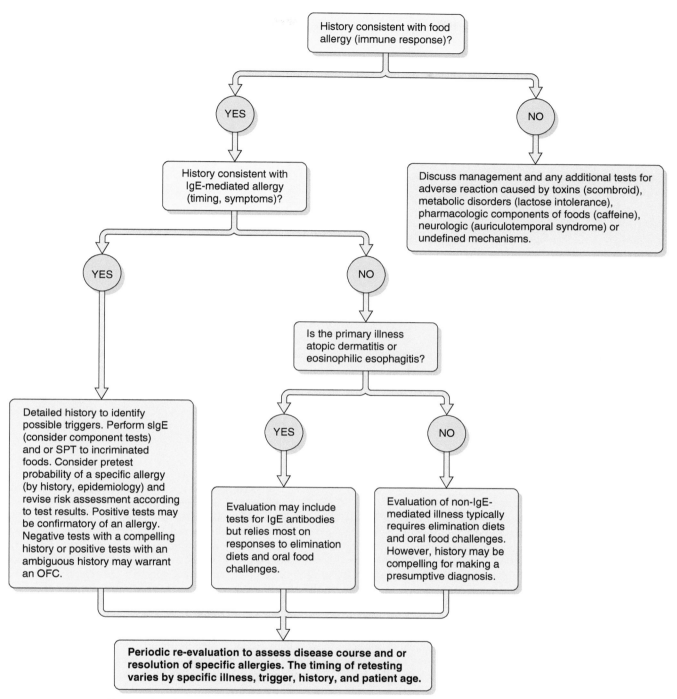

History consistent with food allergy (immune response)?

YES

History consistent with IgE-mediated allergy (timing, symptoms)?

NO

Discuss management and any additional tests for adverse reaction caused by toxins (scombroid), metabolic disorders (lactose intolerance), pharmacologic components of foods (caffeine), neurologic (auriculotemporal syndrome) or undefined mechanisms.

YES

NO

Is the primary illness atopic dermatitis or eosinophilic esophagitis?

YES

NO

Detailed history to identify possible triggers. Perform sIgE (consider component tests) and or SPT to incriminated foods. Consider pretest probability of a specific allergy (by history, epidemiology) and revise risk assessment according to test results. Positive tests may be confirmatory of an allergy. Negative tests with a compelling history or positive tests with an ambiguous history may warrant an OFC.

Evaluation may include tests for IgE antibodies but relies most on responses to elimination diets and oral food challenges.

Evaluation of non-IgE-mediated illness typically requires elimination diets and oral food challenges. However, history may be compelling for making a presumptive diagnosis.

Periodic re-evaluation to assess disease course and or resolution of specific allergies. The timing of retesting varies by specific illness, trigger, history, and patient age.

• **Fig. 31.1** Algorithm diagnosing food hypersensitivity. *IgE,* Immunoglobulin E; *OFC,* oral food challenge; *SPT,* skin prick test. (With permission from Sicherer SH, Sampson HA. Food allergy: a review and update on epidemiology, pathogenesis, diagnosis, prevention, and management. J Allergy Clin Immunol 2018;141:41–58, Fig. 31.1.)

Conclusions

Fig. 31.1 outlines a summary of the approach for the evaluation of children with a history of adverse reactions to food. A detailed history is followed by selection of skin tests and in vitro tests to be performed. The results of these tests allow selection of foods to be challenged under observation or reintroduced at home. Care always must be taken to be certain that any possible food culprit is introduced under observation.

The reference list can be found on the companion Expert Consult website at http://www.expertconsult.inkling.com.

32

Approach to Feeding Problems in the Infant and Young Child

ALEXIA BEAUREGARD, MARION GROETCH

KEY POINTS

- Infants with food allergies are at increased risk of inadequate nutrient intake and poor growth.
- Food allergies and elimination diets may have an impact on feeding skill acquisition.
- Feeding problems may exacerbate poor nutritional intake.
- There are critical windows of opportunity in the oral sensorimotor developmental continuum when specific feeding skills are best acquired.

- Delayed exposure to a variety of flavors and textures in infancy can lead to long-term feeding difficulties and poor variety of foods at 7 years.
- Feeding assessment screenings can be done in the office setting and should be conducted at food allergy diagnosis and follow-up, especially in infants and young children.

Introduction

Food allergies and their associated elimination diets can have a negative impact on nutrient intake and growth, with cow's milk allergy and multiple food allergies having the greatest impact.[1–6] Many factors can influence nutritional intake, including the number of foods eliminated from the diet, the nutritional importance of the eliminated food(s), parental preferences, beliefs, socioeconomic factors, and feeding skills and behaviors.[7] Food allergy, and cow's milk allergy in particular, generally begins in early infancy and may disrupt feeding skill acquisition. Non–immunoglobulin E (IgE)-mediated allergies affecting the gastrointestinal (GI) tract, such as food protein–induced enterocolitis syndrome, eosinophilic esophagitis, and other eosinophilic GI disorders in particular, have been shown to result more commonly in feeding difficulties[8,9] and poor growth.[2,10] Indications for increased nutritional risk can be found in Box 32.1.

Feeding and Developmental Readiness

Feeding is a complex process that requires superb coordination. Developmental skills for feeding tend to be sequential, and each infant develops at his or her own pace. Healthy, full-term infants are born with the innate ability to coordinate sucking, breathing, and swallowing, but other feeding skills are acquired through the presentation of foods. During the first few months of life, the infant learns to master and strengthen these suckling skills and

aims for homeostasis. The infant's achievement of physiologic, oral, and motor developmental milestones for feeding flavors and textures should guide when complementary feeding can begin. Some signs of developmental readiness for complementary feeding, typically emerging around 4 to 6 months of age, include sitting with some support, ability to maintain midline head positioning, diminished protrusion reflex, and anatomic changes that result in the infant having more space for vertical movement of the tongue rather than the in-and-out movement required for suckling.[11] During this early period of complementary feeding the infant is exposed to a variety of flavors (generally through thin purees) and will often accept a new flavor on the first exposure.[12] Minimal exposure with a new food in early infancy enhances not only the infant's acceptance of that food but also of similar foods.[12] Infants gradually gain oral sensorimotor skill and move from thin pureed foods to thicker and lumpier, mashed foods (around 6–9 months), and many infants will begin to self-feed soft and dissolvable textures at this time. From 9 to 12 months, infants will gradually take fewer mashed foods and more finger foods. Through this independent feeding, infants learn about the textures that go along with the previously acquired accepted flavors. By 12 to 15 months of age most children can eat modified (coarsely chopped) foods from the family table.

There appear to be critical windows of opportunity in the oral sensorimotor developmental continuum when specific feeding skills are best acquired.[13] If a lack of experience and exposure to age-appropriate foods during these windows occurs, it becomes

• **BOX 32.1** **Indications for Increased Nutritional Risk in Food Allergy**

- Greater number of eliminated foods
- Greater nutritional value of the eliminated food(s) for the child
- Inappropriate and/or excessive dietary eliminations
- Picky eater
- Feeding delays or feeding difficulties
- Delayed or limited introduction of complementary foods
- Poor variety or volume of foods offered or accepted
- Symptoms affecting dietary intake (abdominal pain, reflux, dysphagia, etc.)

Modified from Groetch M, Henry M, Feuling MB, Kim J. Guidance for the nutrition management of gastrointestinal allergy in pediatrics. J Allergy Clinical Immunol Pract 2013;1:323–31.

more difficult for the child to learn the skill. For example, in contrast to easier flavor and texture acceptance in infancy, 2- to 5-year-old children seem to need multiple exposures to a new food before significant increases in intake are noted.[12,14] Long-term feeding skills and behaviors can be affected with delayed feeding. In a longitudinal, birth cohort study, 7821 mothers of children were surveyed about foods eaten and feeding difficulties in their children at various ages, up to 7 years of age. Children introduced to lumpy solids after the age of 9 months ate less of many of the food groups at 7 years, including fruit and vegetables, than those introduced to lumpy foods between 6 and 9 months (P <.05–.001). In addition, they were reported as having significantly more feeding problems at 7 years (P <.05–.001).[13]

Children with food allergies may have diets that eliminate many foods or entire food groups or symptoms that negatively affect dietary intake and make eating unpleasant. Caregivers of children with food allergy may be anxious to offer new foods that have not been tolerated in the past and thereby limit the provision of a variety of foods. Long-term complications of food acceptance and acquisition of feeding skills are cause for concern, and health professionals can help by encouraging a variety of flavors of tolerated foods from all food groups and the progression from purees when age and developmentally appropriate.

Division of Responsibility and Authoritative Feeding

In addition to what foods are presented, the way foods are presented can have an impact on overall and long-term nutritional intake. We often think of feeding as unidirectional; however, successful feeding in infancy and childhood depends on the reciprocity in the feeding relationship between the caregiver and child. A healthy feeding relationship depends on an appropriate division of responsibility between the caregiver and the child. Caregivers following the Satter Division of Responsibility (sDOR) Model, developed by Ellyn Satter, determine what foods to serve and when and where to serve the food. Children are given autonomy to determine how much food they will eat or whether they will eat any of the food that is served. In other words, the feeding is appetite driven, and the child determines appetite through internal cues of hunger and satiety. In early infancy, the sDOR is even more simple, with the parent choosing what food to serve (breast milk or formula) and the child responsible for everything else (when to eat and how much to eat) because feeding on demand is appropriate in infancy.[15]

In using the sDOR model, caregivers do the following[16,17]:
- Select and prepare developmentally appropriate food that is safe, nutritionally sound, and balanced
- Provide food at regular intervals throughout the day
- Make mealtimes pleasant
- Demonstrate appropriate mealtime behavior
- Trust the child's instincts to know how much to eat and trust that the child will grow in a predictable manner

Additionally, the infant or child has a role and must do the following:
- Signal hunger and satiety through motor actions, facial expressions, or vocalizations
- Learn to trust the caregiver if the response to their signals is appropriate

Another approach to feeding, frequently reported in the literature and similar to sDOR, is responsive feeding. In responsive feeding, feeding styles can be measured along the dimensions of demandingness and responsiveness with demandingness referring to the caregiver's expectations of the child in the feeding relationship and responsiveness relating to the caregiver's sensitivity to the child's individual needs during feeding.[18] Four feeding categories have been described with the authoritative feeding style (high demandingness and high responsiveness) recommended in numerous feeding guidelines and defined as, "reasonable nutritional demands in conjunction with sensitivity toward the child"[18–21] (Table 32.1). Arlinghaus and colleagues reported that an authoritative feeding style as compared to an authoritarian feeding style was associated with higher dietary quality. Additionally, authoritative feeding styles were associated with a higher consumption of fruit and vegetables.[22]

The feeding and eating dynamic can become strained when caregivers provide too little support by not being consistent with food presentation (neglectful feeding style), by allowing the child to make all of the decisions around food (permissive feeding styles), or by applying too much interference by insisting, pressuring, or bribing the child to eat (authoritarian feeding style). Pressure to eat is more common in children with poor growth, but this caretaker behavior is more likely to decrease intake than increase intake.[23] If caregivers are too invested in feeding a certain volume of food, or specific foods, and ignore the child's signals, feeding can go poorly. Additionally, children may not offer signals that the caregivers can read, and caregivers of children with food allergies are more likely to give up (less demandingness) with feeding a food if they misread their child's hesitancy as a sign of a potential allergic symptom.

sDOR and authoritative feeding emphasize normal eating patterns and can help caregivers understand what is developmentally appropriate and what difficulties may be exacerbated by fear and anxiety brought about by food allergy.[24] Caregivers should understand developmentally appropriate feeding and have appropriate expectations of their child but also should be responsive to the child cues.

Picky Eating Versus Problematic Feeding and Eating

Picky eating and problematic feeding appear to afflict boys and girls at equal rates.[25] The terms "picky" and "problematic" feeding are often used interchangeably and have not always been clearly defined. They are, in fact, separate issues that may co-exist

TABLE 32.1	**Parent Feeding Styles**	
	LOW Demandingness FX1	**HIGH Demandingness FX1**
LOW responsiveness to infant/child cues FX2	*Neglectful Feeding* Caregiver does not consistently offer foods in response to child cues and does not attempt to provide support, structure, or boundaries.	*Authoritarian Feeding* Caregiver-centered feeding in which caregiver controls boundaries excessively (insistent on eating or restricting specific foods and specific volumes) and does not respond to infant/child cues.
HIGH responsiveness to infant/child cues FX2	*Indulgent or Permissive Feeding* Child-centered feeding in which child decides what foods to eat, where to eat, when to eat, and how much to eat. Caregiver does not apply appropriate support, structure, or boundaries.	*Authoritative Feeding* Caregiver is consistent in presentation of foods (where, what, and when), applies appropriate support, structure, and boundaries and is responsive to child cues.

Modified from Hughes SO, Power TG, Orlet Fisher J, Mueller S, Nicklas TA. Revisiting a neglected construct: parenting styles in a child-feeding context. Appetite 2005;44:83–92; Hughes SO, Shewchuk RM, Baskin ML, Nicklas TA, Qu H. Indulgent feeding style and children's weight status in preschool. J Dev Behav Pediatr 2008;29:403–10; Arlinghaus KR, Vollrath K, Hernandez DC, et al. Authoritative parent feeding style is associated with better child dietary quality at dinner among low-income minority families. Am J Clin Nutr 2018;108:730–6.

in a child.[25,26] Feeding difficulties also may be transient in some children, which further impedes the ability to clearly define and standardize how these terms are applied outside of literature and in clinic settings. In this text, *picky eating* will refer to children who eat a limited variety of food. The prevalence of picky eating behaviors has been reported in up to 50% of normally developing children, up to 80% of children with developmental delays, and in up to 94% of children with eosinophilic GI disorders.[27] Picky eaters usually behave around the table at meal time and may eat one or two foods offered and simply ignore other food options. They may touch or smell the food that is offered but generally do not demonstrate any fear of or anxiety about the food that is in front of them. A picky eater may simply not be prepared to put some types of foods in their mouth.

Problematic feeding or *feeding difficulties,* in this text, will refer to a wider spectrum of feeding behaviors that include spitting out food; retching at the sight or smell of foods, a spoon, or a bottle; slow eating; increased irritability at meal time; and difficulty swallowing.[26] Problematic feeding behaviors can cause early satiety, excessive fluid intake, and refusal of solid food[28] and may be caused by structural abnormalities, neurologic problems, cardiac or respiratory conditions, gastroenterology abnormalities, or immune system abnormalities such as food allergy. Children with feeding difficulties may have more than one of these problems or abnormalities simultaneously.[28] Problematic feeders may have a very poor quality of life around food, and their family relationships may suffer as a result of this behavior.[24] Research has shown that there is a significant negative correlation between caloric intake and problematic feeding behaviors, which is not seen in children who have been labeled as picky eaters,[29] although the nutritional quality of the diet may be affected in picky eating. Medical conditions that make oral feeding in infancy a challenge can contribute to feeding difficulties later in childhood.[25,30] An infant or a toddler with feeding difficulties may not advance to solid foods, whereas older toddlers and preschool-aged children will begin to self-restrict or may demonstrate an increased fear or anxiety around food, especially new foods. The older child may simply refuse to expand the variety of foods (in terms of flavors and textures), demonstrate anxiety

around food (especially new foods), and begin to have slowed growth. Problematic feeders may cry, throw food, or refuse to come to the table if the food has reached it before they do. They may refuse favorite foods if they are on the same plate as new foods and demonstrate behaviors that are designed to help them avoid all contact with food [25,31]

Food Allergy Impact on Feeding

Children will not eat if they are afraid of allergic reactions or do not feel confident in their self-feeding skills. This fear will override any innate drive to eat to satisfy hunger and may result in malnutrition. The number and severity of allergic symptoms is often correlated with the severity of the feeding difficulty and a worsening number of maladaptive feeding behaviors.[8] Parents of children with food allergies report greater anxiety in feeding, which also may have an impact on the foods offered in the complementary feeding period, and therefore parents require extensive avoidance education and guidance on what foods to feed.[32,33] Children with food protein–induced enterocolitis syndrome (FPIES) may have delayed or slowed introduction of complementary foods affecting feeding skill acquisition and nutritional intake. Blackman and associates[34] reported from their FPIES cohort of 74 children that malnutrition was present in 8% of their population and another 5% were at risk of malnutrition because of restricted food choices and limited knowledge on how to introduce safe foods as documented in the nutrition diagnosis in the electronic medical record.[34] Children with eosinophilic esophagitis coupled with poorly controlled reflux may have poorly developed oral phase skills that will require specialized therapeutic interventions to not only manage the food allergy and reflux but also improve the oral motor feeding skills.[35,36] Common feeding difficulties caused by signs and symptoms of food allergy can be found in Table 32.2.

Why Do Feeding Problems Matter?

Children with very limited diets because of multiple food allergy, picky eating, or severe problematic feeding difficulties are at an

TABLE 32.2	Behaviors and Symptoms Contributing to Feeding Difficulties in Children With Food Allergy	
Food Allergic Disorder	**Behaviors That May Lead to Feeding Difficulties**	
Eosinophilic esophagitis (EoE)	• Fear of eating (i.e., fear of pain with swallowing, dysphagia, worsening reflux, or food impaction) • Selective eating regarding specific foods or textures • Limited appetite, early satiety, and food refusal • Slow eating with frequent beverage intake between bites • Preference for liquids over solids	
Eosinophilic gastrointestinal disorders other than EoE	• Fear of eating (i.e., fear of pain with swallowing, dysphagia, or food impaction) • Selective eating regarding specific foods or textures • Limited appetite and food refusal	
Food protein–induced enterocolitis syndrome	• Fear of feeding new foods • Lack of knowledge of what to feed and when to introduce new foods	
Food protein–induced proctocolitis	• Fear of feeding new foods • Severely limited maternal diet while breastfeeding • Severely limited infant diets	
Anaphylaxis	• Fear of feeding or eating • Fear of offering new foods • Limiting foods to only those tolerated in the past or avoidance skill (label reading)	

Modified from Chehade M, Meyer R, Beauregard A. Feeding difficulties in children with non-IgE mediated food allergic gastrointestinal disorders. Ann Allergy Asthma Immunol 2019;122:603–9.

• **BOX 32.2   Practical Screening Questions for Feeding Difficulties in the Office Setting**

- How long does it take to feed your child a meal? Bottle?
- Do you need to use distraction to get your child to eat?
- Does your child show signs of respiratory distress during or after meals?
- Are mealtimes stressful for the family?
- Does your child eat a variety of foods from each food group?
- Does your child try new foods?
- Does your child eat age-appropriate consistencies?
- Does your child avoid specific textures of foods?
- Is your child growing well?
- Does your child demonstrate anxiety when around food?
- Does your child willingly go to the table at mealtime?
- Do you think you can eat a meal at a restaurant or in someone else's home?

Modified from Chatoor I, Ganiban J, Harrison J, Hirsch R. Observation of feeding in the diagnosis of posttraumatic feeding disorder of infancy. J Am Acad Child Adolesc Psychiatry 2001;40:595–602; Sharp WG, Volkert VM, Scahill L, McCrackern CE, McElhanon BA. Systematic review and meta-analysis of intensive multidisciplinary intervention for pediatric feeding disorders: how standard is the standard of care? J Pediatr 2017;181:116–24; Maslin K, Grundy J, Glasbey G, et al. Cows' milk exclusion diet during infancy: is there a long term-effect on children's eating behavior and food preference. Pediatr Allergy Immunol 2016;27:141–6; Meyer R, Rommel N, Van Oudenhove L, Fleming C, Dzuibak R, Shah N. Feeding difficulties in children with food protein induced gastrointestinal allergies. J Gastroenterol Hepatol 2014;29:1764–9.

Treatment Options

Healthcare providers should screen for any problematic feeding behaviors when the food allergy is diagnosed. There are currently no standardized screening tools available, but common parental concerns can help reveal feeding difficulties.[31,42–44] Providing education on how and what to feed at various developmental stages may help prevent feeding difficulties or minimize their impact (Box 32.3). If a child's nutritional intake has already been affected and feeding difficulties are present, a referral to a multidisciplinary feeding team is warranted.[45] (See the algorithm in Fig. 32.1 for when to refer for feeding intervention.) However, a child must be developmentally ready and medically stable before any therapy can begin. The multidisciplinary approach is necessary to accurately determine the cause of the feeding difficulty, avoid misdiagnosis, and provide the appropriate therapeutic advice.[30] Members of a multidisciplinary healthcare team should include an allergist, a gastroenterologist (if GI allergy is present or if child will require a feeding tube), other specialty physicians to address medical conditions that may be impairing a child's ability to eat by mouth, a dietitian, a behavioral therapist, a speech therapist, and/or occupational therapist.[31] Special therapies may be required to help parents and/or children overcome the fear of new foods and reactions to foods, help older children acquire feeding skills that were missed at younger ages, and assist children in oral-motor skill development. Treatment and management of feeding difficulties must consider parental feeding style and the relationship between the caregiver and the child for it to be successful. In cases of feeding disorders in infants and young children, behavior modification should focus on the parents and not the child because the child is often feeding in response to caregiver behavior. Response to therapy should be measured in terms of diminished anxiety or disappearance of anxiety around food and mealtime by the child, increased variety of accepted foods,

increased risk for long-term health complications. Limited oral intake in childhood can cause slowed growth without realizing catch-up growth, impaired immune systems, and impaired cognitive ability.[27] An elimination diet for a picky eater can have a considerable impact on eating habits and overall food intake,[26] and feeding difficulties can persist long after a food allergy is well-managed and the diet is stable.[37,38] Research has shown that modifying an infant diet can have an impact on overall oral intake that can last between 7 and 10 years.[39] Feeding difficulties may impair a child's psychosocial development and require specialized therapies to help caregivers learn how to feed and children learn how to eat.[40]

Failure to address feeding difficulties that significantly alter overall food intake may necessitate the need for supplemental nutrition provided orally or via a feeding tube, which can dramatically increase the cost of food allergy management and further increase family stress and burden while also impairing social functioning.[41] Children may not be able to meet developmental milestones because of their food allergy and limited diet, parental fear of feeding, or maladaptive feeding behaviors that make progressing to a broader selection of flavors and textures incredibly difficult.[30,35] Practical tips for screening patients and families for feeding difficulties in the office setting are listed in Box 32.2.

• **BOX 32.3**   **Clinical Pearls**
Preventing Feeding Difficulties

In Infancy

- Do not delay complementary feeding beyond 4 to 6 months of age in developmentally ready infants.
- Provide appropriate avoidance education, including foods to avoid and foods to include in the child's diet.
- Encourage the introduction of a wide variety of tolerated foods from all food groups.
- Encourage age- and skill-appropriate progression from puree to greater textures.

Encourage a Division of Responsibility in Feeding and Authoritative Feeding Styles

- Encourage family meals that include the child with allergies so caregivers can provide a role model for eating and enjoying foods.
- Encourage a structured meal and snack scheduled so children can predict when foods will be served and learn how to manage their appetites.
- Encourage the parent to allow children to eat as much or as little as wanted at meal- and snack-time.
- Discourage grazing between meal and snack times on foods and beverages (other than water) to encourage a cycle of hunger and satiety.
- Encourage a diet that is balanced and proportional and meets nutritional needs.

    Screen for feeding skills and feeding dynamics at initial diagnosis and then at least once every 12 months.

Modified from Satter EM. The feeding relationship. J Am Diet Assoc 1986;86:352–6; Satter E. The feeding relationship: problems and interventions. J Pediatr 1990;117:S181–9; Satter E. Eating competence: definition and evidence for the Satter Eating Competence model. J Nutr Educ Behav 2007;39:S142–53.

age-appropriate initiation of feeding by the child, and stabilization of growth curves.[33,41,46,47]

Feeding is a skill that must be learned by caregivers, eating is a skill that must be learned by children, and food allergy can make it harder to develop those skills. Feeding difficulty that develops as a complication of food allergy has been underappreciated, but recognition is gaining momentum across the healthcare spectrum. Eating is essential for survival; feeding and eating are critical for the bonding process between the caregiver and child and is the initial way in which a child explores the outside environment.[30] Caregivers of children with food allergies need a higher level of support in managing all aspects of feeding. Without appropriate tools and education, caregivers can feel incompetent, overwhelmed, and unable to implement feeding management strategies.[48] Once problematic feeding behaviors have been identified, a family should be referred for further assessment and intervention as quickly as possible to minimize the impact the behaviors may have on the nutritional quality of an already limited dietary pattern. Allergists should conduct regular screening assessments of feeding and eating skills and behaviors because feeding difficulties can occur at any age and for a variety of reasons in the food-allergic child. There is no developmental endeavor with greater social or biologic significance than feeding and the gradual acquisition of competence in eating and enjoying nutritious foods, and healthcare professionals should provide support and guidance along the way.[48]

The reference list can be found on the companion Expert Consult website at http://www.expertconsult.inkling.com.

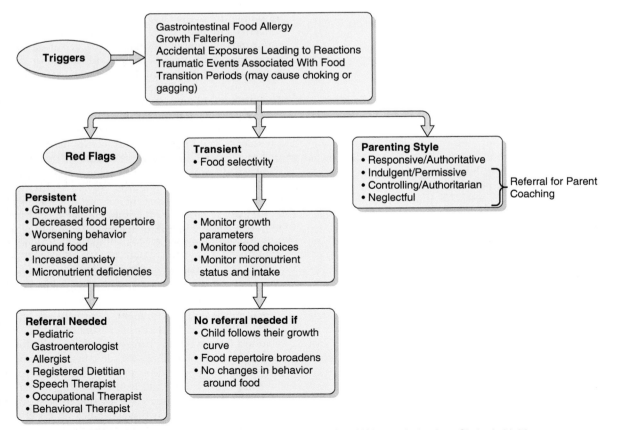

• **Fig. 32.1** Algorithm for when to refer for feeding intervention. (With permission from Chehade M, Meyer R, Beauregard A. Feeding difficulties in children with non-IgE mediated food allergic gastrointestinal disorders. Ann Allergy Asthma Immunol 2019;122:603–9.)

33

Enterocolitis, Proctocolitis, and Enteropathies

SCOTT H. SICHERER, ANNA NOWAK-WĘGRZYN

KEY POINTS

- The differential diagnosis of cell-mediated (non–immunoglobulin E [IgE]-mediated) gastrointestinal food-allergic disorders includes other types of food hypersensitivity (IgE-mediated, eosinophilic gastroenteropathy), nonimmune reactions to foods, and disorders with similar manifestations (infection, anatomic disorders, metabolic disease).
- Diagnosis requires a history, physical examination, exclusion of alternative diagnoses, and selected diagnostic procedures, including dietary elimination and oral challenge, biopsy, and selected laboratory evaluations.
- Food protein–induced allergic proctocolitis occurs in infants and consists of mucous, bloody stools attributed primarily to cow's milk proteins passed in maternal breast milk. However, rectal bleeding in infants is not commonly caused by food allergy.

- Food protein–induced enteropathy occurs in infancy and has symptoms related to protein malabsorption. It is most commonly caused by cow's milk protein and generally resolves by age 1 to 3 years.
- Food protein–induced enterocolitis syndrome occurs in infancy and has symptoms that include prominent vomiting, lethargy, diarrhea, and growth failure with possible progression to a sepsis-like clinical picture. It is usually attributed to cow's milk and/or soy protein and usually resolves by the age of 1 to 5 years.
- Celiac disease often presents at weaning because of an immunologic response to gluten. The disease may present at any age. Classic symptoms include vomiting, anemia, poor growth, and steatorrhea. The diagnosis is assisted through serology for antiendomysial IgA antibodies and is a lifelong disorder requiring elimination of gluten.

Introduction

This chapter focuses on four non–immunoglobulin E (IgE)-mediated food hypersensitivity disorders that affect the gastrointestinal (GI) tract: food protein–induced proctocolitis, enterocolitis, enteropathy, and celiac disease.[1] These disorders have overlapping symptoms but are distinguishable clinically and have distinct patterns of symptoms and clinical course.[2]

Epidemiology

Food Protein–Induced Allergic Proctocolitis

Food protein–induced allergic proctocolitis (FPIAP) is characterized by mucous, bloody stools in an otherwise healthy infant, attributed to an immune response directed against food proteins, usually cow's milk. The mean age at diagnosis is approximately 60 days, with a range of 1 day to 6 months.[3–6] Perirectal fissures are commonly suspected as a culprit; however, bleeding associated with fissures tends to manifest with streaks of blood on hard, formed stool rather than mixed in frothy, mucous stool, which is typical of FPIAP. Failure to thrive is absent. Approximately 60%

of cases occur in breastfed infants in whom the immune response results from maternal food ingestion, usually cow's milk, passed in immunologically recognizable form into the breast milk. In formula-fed infants, the reaction is associated with cow's milk or, less commonly, soy and egg.[4,7] Peripheral blood eosinophilia, hypoalbuminemia, or anemia are uncommon.[4,8,9] Markers of atopy such as atopic dermatitis or a positive family history of atopy are not significantly increased compared with the general population.

Endoscopic examination is not required for diagnostic purposes, but, when performed, shows patchy erythema, friability, and a loss of vascularity generally limited to the rectum.[10] High numbers of eosinophils (5–20 per high-power field) or eosinophilic abscesses are seen in the lamina propria, crypt epithelium, and muscularis mucosa.[8,11] The eosinophils are frequently associated with lymphoid nodules (lymphonodular hyperplasia)[8,12] and rarely with granulomas.[13] However, lymphonodular hyperplasia is not unique to this condition.[8,11] Mucosal infiltration by CD3+ IgA+ lymphocytes has been found.[14] The pathophysiologic process is unknown. Because inflammation is confined to the lower colon and is common in breastfed infants, it has been hypothesized that dietary antigens complexed to breast milk IgA may play a part in the activation of eosinophils and the distribution of the inflammatory process.[3]

The prevalence of FPIAP in the general population is unknown, and the frequency of food allergy causing rectal bleeding in infants has not been extensively studied, with estimates ranging widely between 18% and 64%.[5,15] In a study by Arvola and colleagues,[15] atopic dermatitis and inflammation of the colonic mucosa were associated with persistence of cow's milk allergy to the age of 1 year. This indicates that food allergy is not a common cause of rectal bleeding in infants unless there are additional signs of allergy and that cow's milk (CM)-FPIAP must be differentiated from benign idiopathic neonatal transient eosinophilic colitis.[6,16]

Food Protein–Induced Enterocolitis Syndrome

Food protein–induced enterocolitis syndrome (FPIES) describes a symptom complex of profuse vomiting, lethargy, hypotonia, and diarrhea usually diagnosed in the first year of life and often attributable to cow's milk, soy, rice, and oat[17] (Box 33.1). Adult-onset FPIES also has been reported, most commonly to seafood, but also dairy, egg, and wheat.[18a] Birth cohorts from Israel and Spain estimated a cumulative incidence of infantile FPIES between 0.34% and 0.7%.[18b,18c] A national study of pediatric disease surveillance with use of a strict case definition estimated a cumulative incidence of 0.015% among Australian infants.[18d] Based on population-weighted prevalence estimates from a nationally representative sample, physician-diagnosed FPIES was reported by an overall 0.28% (0.24%–0.33%) of Americans, with 0.51% children and 0.22% adults.[19] Unlike FPIAP, the majority of affected infants are asymptomatic while being exclusively breastfed on an unrestricted maternal diet. When the causal protein remains in the diet (e.g., in the young infants fed with cow's milk or soy-based formula), symptoms of chronic FPIES include watery or bloody diarrhea, intermittent emesis, poor growth, anemia, hypoalbuminemia, and fecal leukocytes; the illness may progress to dehydration and hypotension over the course of days to weeks.[20–22] Removal of the causal food leads to resolution of symptoms but re-exposure results within 1 to 4 hours in repetitive, often projectile vomiting, lethargy, hypotonia, elevation of the peripheral blood neutrophils, reduced core body temperature, thrombocytosis, hypotension, diarrhea, dehydration, acidemia, and methemoglobinemia.[23] The dramatic presentation often results in evaluations for sepsis or surgical diagnoses[24] and a delay in diagnosis until more than one episode occurs.[25]

The pathophysiology process of FIPES remains poorly understood. The limited biopsy data demonstrated the imbalance between tumor necrosis factor-alpha (TNF-α) and transforming growth factor-beta (TGF-β1) in the duodenal mucosa.[26] Serologic studies demonstrated paucity of the humoral responses to cow's milk casein in children with CM-FPIES.[27,28] The evidence for the role of T cells in acute FPIES is inconclusive.[27,29] Studies using peripheral blood have detected massive activation of the innate immune system.[30–35] The available immunologic data are summarized in Table 33.1.

Food Protein–Induced Enteropathy

Food protein–induced enteropathy (FPE) is characterized by protracted diarrhea, vomiting, malabsorption, and failure to thrive. Additional features include abdominal distention, early satiety, edema, hypoproteinemia, and protein-losing enteropathy.[36] Moderate anemia (typically the result of iron deficiency) is present in 20% to 69% of infants with CM-FPE. Bloody stools are typically absent, but occult blood can be found in 5% of patients.

Symptoms usually begin in the first several months of life, depending on the time of exposure to the causal proteins. FPE was described primarily from the 1960s to the 1990s[37–40] and was commonly caused by cow's milk protein. A decrease in prevalence was documented in Finland[41] and Spain[42] and attributed to a rise in breastfeeding and/or the use of adapted infant formula. There have been no clear reports of this diagnosis in the past several years, although early childhood eosinophilic gastroenteritis with protein-losing enteropathy shares many features with previous descriptions of this disorder.[43]

Unlike celiac disease (CD), FPE generally resolves in 1 to 2 years, and there is no increased threat of future malignancy.[44]

Celiac Disease

CD, also termed *celiac sprue* or *gluten-sensitive enteropathy*, estimated to affect 1% of the population, is caused by immune responses to wheat gluten or related rye and barley proteins, resulting in inflammatory injury to the small intestinal mucosa.[45] CD classically manifests in infants after weaning, at the time of cereal introduction into the diet. Early (younger than 4 months of age) or delayed (older than 7 months) introduction of wheat may be a risk factor, and breastfeeding may be protective.[46] Symptoms reflect malabsorption, with patients exhibiting failure to thrive, anemia, and muscle wasting. Additional symptoms include diarrhea, abdominal pain, vomiting, osteoporosis, bone pain, and aphthous stomatitis. Subclinical or minimal disease is possible, delaying diagnosis into adulthood. Chronic ingestion of gluten in patients with celiac is associated with increased risk of T cell lymphoma. CD is associated with autoimmune disorders and IgA deficiency. Another associated disorder is *dermatitis herpetiformis,*[47] a gluten-responsive dermatitis characterized by pruritic, erythematous papules, and/or vesicles distributed symmetrically on the extensor surfaces of the elbows and knees and also on the face, buttocks, neck, and trunk.

Endoscopy of the small bowel in active CD typically reveals total villous atrophy and extensive cellular infiltrate. CD is caused by gliadin-specific T cell responses against deamidated gliadin produced by tissue transglutaminase. Gliadin stimulation of monocytes and macrophages may also contribute to the inflammatory response.[48,49] Antigen presentation appears to be a central issue in immunopathology because about 95% of patients exhibit

TABLE 33.1	Pathophysiologic Pathways in Food Protein–Induced Enterocolitis Syndrome (FPIES)	
Pathway	**Findings in FPIES**
Gastrointestinal factors: defects in the intestinal barrier function[26,27]	• Low expression of TGF-β1 receptor type 1 in duodenal biopsy specimens, leading to reduced gut epithelial barrier function. • Increased TNF-α expression in duodenal biopsy specimens with villous atrophy, resulting in increased intestinal permeability. • Increased IL-9 secretion (measured in supernatants) may contribute to increased intestinal permeability.
Cell-mediated immunity[27,29,30]	• Generally skewed toward T_H2 (measured in supernatants). • High levels of IL-2, suggesting some T_H1 activity. • During reactions, there appears to be pan–T cell activation.
Innate immune system (peripheral blood)*	• Neutrophils: Increased count and activation. • Mast cells: Suspected increased activation or accumulation/density as evidenced by increased baseline serum tryptase; no evidence of degranulation in acute FPIES, because tryptase level does not increase after a reactive challenge. • Lymphocytes: Decreased. • Monocytes: No change in absolute number of circulating monocytes but enrichment of CD14+ monocytes and increased activation. • Natural killer cells: Increased activation. • Increased expression of genes involved in granulocyte adhesion and diapedesis, IL-10 and TREM1 signaling and hub genes reflecting predominance of innate immune activation, including MMP9, IL-1B activation, ICAM, and STAT3. • C-reactive protein: Increased and at levels higher than seen in FPIAP.
Eosinophils[34,74]	• Peripheral blood eosinophilia may be noted at diagnosis and can be marked. • During acute reactions, the peripheral eosinophil count may decrease, although there is evidence of increased circulating eosinophil activation with increased CD69 expression. • An increase in fecal eosinophil-derived neurotoxin has been observed, suggesting possible increases in activated eosinophils in the gastrointestinal tract.
Cytokine profile[27,28,75]	• Patients with active FPIES demonstrate deficient TGF-β response (measured in supernatant from the peripheral blood mononuclear cell culture). • Serum IL-2, IL-8, and IL-10 increase during FPIES reactions. • High serum IL-5 levels correlate with peripheral blood eosinophilia. • Increased serum IL-10 appears to correlate with the development of tolerance although elevated serum IL-10 has been observed in active FPIES.
Serotonin[62,76]	• Emesis and cramping in FPIES responds to ondansetron. • Ondansetron is a serotonin 5-HT3 receptor antagonist; thus, its effectiveness suggests a neurologic component involvement in FPIES.

*References 27, 30, 31, 33, 34, 73.

FPIAP, Food protein–induced allergic proctocolitis; *ICAM*, intercellular adhesion molecule; *IL*, interleukin; *MMP-9*, matrix metallopeptidase 9; *STAT3*, signal transducer and activator of transcription 3; *TGF-β1*, transforming growth factor-beta 1; T_H2, T helper cell type 2 cell; *TNF-α*, tumor necrosis factor-alpha; *TREM1*, triggering receptor expressed on myeloid cells-1.

HLA-DQ2 and the remainder HLA-DQ8 genetic haplotypes. Gliadin is one of the few substrates for tissue transglutaminase, which deamidates specific glutamines within gliadin, creating epitopes that bind efficiently to gut-derived DQ2 T cells.[50] The activation of DQ2- or DQ8-restricted T cells initiates the inflammatory response.[51] Elimination of gliadin from the diet results in down-regulation of the T cell–induced inflammatory process and mucosal healing.

Diagnosis depends on demonstrating villous atrophy and inflammatory infiltrate, resolution of biopsy findings after 6 to 12 weeks of gluten elimination, and recurrence of biopsy changes after a gluten challenge. The revised diagnostic criteria have eliminated the requirement for a gluten challenge and instead place a greater focus on serologic studies. Quantification of antigliadin IgA and antiendomysial IgA antibodies may be used for screening with IgA antitTGase antibodies in patients older than 2 years of age.[45] After the diagnosis of CD is established, lifelong elimination of gluten-containing foods is necessary to control symptoms and reduce the risk of malignancy.

Differential Diagnosis

Because the GI tract has a limited number of responses to inflammatory damage, there is overlap in the symptoms observed with these disorders. Differentiating them from each other requires consideration of key, distinct clinical features and directed laboratory examinations. Moreover, numerous medical disorders must be considered in the evaluation of patients presenting with GI complaints. Some of these disorders include other food hypersensitivities, but food intolerance (nonimmune disorders such as lactase deficiency) and toxic reactions (e.g., bacterial poisoning) are potential considerations.

The differential diagnosis can encompass virtually any cause of abdominal complaint, including the following categories:

infection (e.g., viral, bacterial, parasitic), anatomic (e.g., pyloric stenosis, anal fissures, motility disorders, lymphangiectasia, Hirschsprung's disease, reflux, intussusception), inflammatory bowel disease, metabolic (e.g., disaccharidase deficiencies), malignancy, and immunodeficiency. The differential diagnosis of severe acute FPIES includes anaphylaxis. Depending on the constellation of findings, various diagnostic strategies are used that are beyond the scope of this chapter. However, the presence of a number of clinical elements may underscore the possibility of a food-allergic disorder. The general approach to the diagnosis of food-allergic disorders affecting the gut is outlined in Fig. 33.1. Various features may suggest a differentiation of the disorders described in this chapter from those related to IgE antibody–mediated GI allergies (i.e., oral allergy, GI anaphylaxis) and those that are sometimes associated with IgE antibody (i.e., eosinophilic gastroenteropathies and reflux). The chronicity after ingestion of

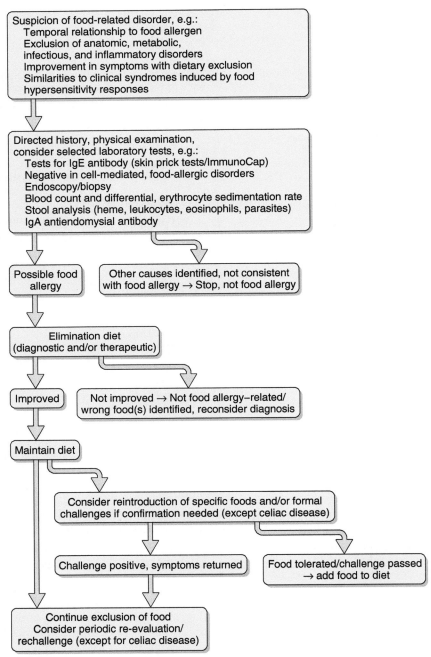

• **Fig. 33.1** The evaluation of food allergy requires a simultaneous consideration for alternative diagnoses (infection, anatomic, metabolic, etc.) and disorders caused by food allergy, including those described in this chapter and others (i.e., oral allergy syndrome, anaphylaxis, eosinophilic gastroenteropathies, food-related reflux disease) and nonimmune adverse reactions to foods (lactose intolerance). Laboratory tests and decisions for elimination and challenge are based on specific elements of the history and an appreciation for the clinical manifestations and course of the various disorders (see text). *IgE,* Immunoglobulin E.

the causal food (acute in IgE antibody–mediated disease), symptoms (e.g., isolated vomiting in gastroesophageal reflux disease), and selected test results (e.g., biopsy revealing an eosinophilic infiltrate in allergic eosinophilic gastroenteropathy) differentiate these food-allergic disorders. The food-related disorders also must

be distinguished from a host of disorders that have similar clinical findings but alternative causes. Table 33.2 delineates the disorders that may most closely overlap the cell-mediated food-allergic disorders.

The distinguishing clinical features of FPIAP, FPIES, FPE, and CD are listed in Table 33.3. Although they may represent a spectrum of disorders with similar causes, the treatment and natural course of the diseases vary, making a specific diagnosis imperative. The causal foods, symptoms, and family history usually indicate the likely disorder. In some cases, the diagnosis requires initial confirmation of reactivity/association determined by resolution of symptoms with an elimination diet and recurrence of symptoms after oral food challenge (OFC). In some cases, specific tests are needed (e.g., serologic tests for IgA endomysial or tissue transglutaminase antibody and small bowel biopsy). The disorders are not IgE antibody mediated, but if there has been immediate onset of symptoms after ingestion or an association of GI allergy with other features of IgE antibody–mediated food allergy (e.g., atopic dermatitis, asthma), screening tests for food-specific IgE antibody (i.e., skin prick tests, serum food-specific IgE antibodies) may be helpful in defining the process causing the reactions. A number of tests are of unproved value for the diagnosis of food allergy and should not be used. These include measurement of IgG_4 antibody, provocation-neutralization (i.e., drops placed under the tongue or injected to diagnose and treat various symptoms), and applied kinesiology (i.e., muscle strength testing).[52]

Evaluation and Management

A diagnosis of FPIAP should be entertained in a well-appearing infant presenting with mucous bloody stools, an absence of symptoms indicating a systemic disease, a coagulation defect, or another source of bleeding. The definitive diagnosis requires withdrawal of the presumed allergen with monitoring for resolution of symptoms; however, additional testing and refeeding of the eliminated protein is advisable after resolution because transient rectal bleeding in infancy is more frequently not related to allergy.[15] A survey of 56 pediatric gastroenterologists showed that 84% prescribe empirical dietary trials.[5] In the absence of biopsy confirmation and especially in the absence of other signs of atopy, refeeding should be considered soon after resolution of symptoms, given the high rate of spontaneous resolution.[6,16] In infants fed cow's milk

TABLE 33.2 Examples of Clinical Disease That May Overlap Symptoms of Cell-Mediated, Food Protein–Induced Disease

Clinical Disease	Symptoms
Food protein–induced allergic proctocolitis	• Anal fissure • Infection (viral, bacterial, fungal, parasitic) • Perianal dermatitis • Transient idiopathic neonatal eosinophilic colitis • Volvulus • Hirschsprung's disease • Intussusception • Coagulation disorders
Food protein–induced enterocolitis syndrome	• Sepsis/infection • Very-early-onset inflammatory bowel disease • Necrotizing enterocolitis • Intussusception • Lymphangiectasia • Volvulus • Ileus • Metabolic disorders
Food protein–induced enteropathy	• Infection • Eosinophilic gastroenteropathy with protein loss • Bowel ischemia • Very-early-onset inflammatory bowel disease • Lymphangiectasia • Autoimmune enteropathy • Immune deficiency • Tropical sprue • Malignancy

TABLE 33.3 Clinical Features Helpful to Distinguish Food Protein–Induced Proctocolitis, Enteropathy, Enterocolitis, and Celiac Disease

	Onset	Vomiting	Diarrhea	Growth	Foods	Other
Food protein–induced allergic proctocolitis (FPIAP)	Days to 6 months	Absent	Minimal, bloody	Normal	Breast/cow's milk/soy/egg	Re-exposure: rectal bleeding within days
Food protein–induced enterocolitis syndrome (FPIES)	Days to 1 year; adult onset to shellfish	Prominent projectile, repetitive	Prominent in chronic FPIES and young infants	Poor	Cow's milk/soy/rice/oat	Re-exposure: severe symptoms within 1–4 hours
Food protein–induced enteropathy (FPE)	2–24 mo	Variable	Moderate	Poor	Cow's milk/soy	Edema resulting from intestinal protein loss
Celiac disease	>4 mo	Variable	Variable	Poor	Gluten	Associated with human leukocyte antigen DQ2 or DQ8

or soy formula, substitution with a protein hydrolysate formula can be undertaken. Few infants who have persistent rectal bleeding when being fed with a hypoallergenic infant formula experience resolution of bleeding with the substitution of an amino acid–based formula (AAF), although follow-up challenges to prove that AAF was required have not been systematically undertaken.[5,53,54] Management in breastfed infants requires maternal restriction of cow's milk or possibly soy, egg, or other foods.[4] In up to 12% of the breastfed infants, bleeding may persist despite extensive eliminations in the maternal diet and requires switching to a hypoallergenic formula. If breastfeeding is continued, chronic bleeding may lead to mild anemia despite iron supplementation and to hypoalbuminemia. Despite persistent symptoms, most children become tolerant to cow's milk by the age of 12 months and have no long-term inflammatory sequelae, although there may be an increased risk for functional GI disorders, including irritable bowel syndrome and functional abdominal pain.[3,55] Progressive bleeding, despite dietary restriction, should prompt re-evaluation

with consideration for proctocolonoscopy and biopsy.[56] Because there is generally no risk of a severe reaction, the foods are gradually reintroduced into the diet at home either as a trial to prove a causal relationship or months afterward to monitor for resolution of FPIAP. However, if there is a suspicion of mild enterocolitis (e.g., vomiting in addition to hematochezia) or history suggests IgE-mediated reactions, repeated testing (e.g., skin or serum tests for specific IgE to the causal food) and medically supervised OFC are warranted.

Food Protein–Induced Enterocolitis Syndrome

The diagnosis of FPIES rests on clinical and OFC criteria (Fig. 33.2).[17,57] Most patients would not undergo a formal OFC during infancy because the diagnosis becomes self-evident after elimination of the causal protein, and frequently patients experience

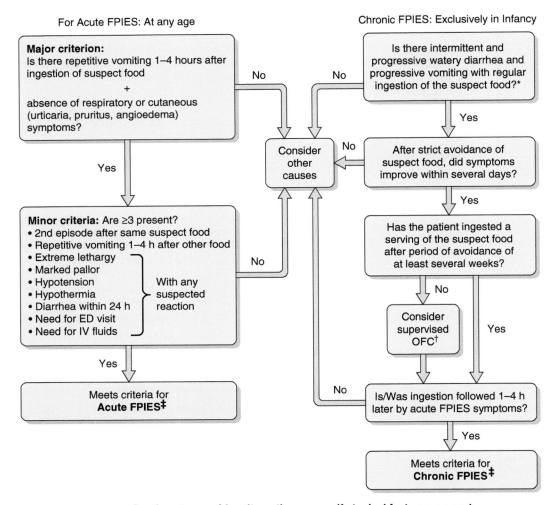

For Acute FPIES: At any age

Major criterion:
Is there repetitive vomiting 1–4 hours after ingestion of suspect food
+
absence of respiratory or cutaneous (urticaria, pruritus, angioedema) symptoms?

Yes ↓

Minor criteria: Are ≥3 present?
- 2nd episode after same suspect food
- Repetitive vomiting 1–4 h after other food
- Extreme lethargy
- Marked pallor
- Hypotension
- Hypothermia — With any suspected reaction
- Diarrhea within 24 h
- Need for ED visit
- Need for IV fluids

Yes ↓

Meets criteria for **Acute FPIES‡**

Chronic FPIES: Exclusively in Infancy

Is there intermittent and progressive watery diarrhea and progressive vomiting with regular ingestion of the suspect food?*

Yes ↓

After strict avoidance of suspect food, did symptoms improve within several days?

Yes ↓

Has the patient ingested a serving of the suspect food after period of avoidance of at least several weeks?

No ↓

Consider supervised OFC†

Is/Was ingestion followed 1–4 h later by acute FPIES symptoms?

Yes ↓

Meets criteria for **Chronic FPIES‡**

Consider other causes

Continue to consider alternative causes if atypical features present

- **Fig. 33.2** Diagnostic Algorithm for Food Protein–Induced Enterocolitis Syndrome. (*ED*, Emergency department; *IV*, intravenous; *OFC*, oral food challenge; *FPIES, food protein–induced enterocolitis syndrome*.) *Chronic FPIES is described almost exclusively with cow's milk or soy in young infants. †Without a confirmatory OFC or other ingestion with emesis onset in 1 to 4 hours, diagnosis of chronic FPIES is presumptive. ‡Based on Nowak-Węgrzyn A, Chehade M, Groetch ME, et al. International consensus guidelines for the diagnosis and management of food protein–induced enterocolitis syndrome: Executive summary—Workgroup Report of the Adverse Reactions to Foods Committee, American Academy of Allergy, Asthma & Immunology. J Allergy Clin Immunol 2017;139:1111–26.

inadvertent re-exposure, proving their sensitivity before a diagnostic OFC.[52] Chronic ingestion, or re-exposure to the causal food, can result in a severe clinical picture that may mimic sepsis and may include acidemia and methemoglobinemia.[17] Approximately half of infants with CM-FPIES also react to soy and among children reacting to cow's milk or soy, about 25% react to additional proteins such as rice or oat. Because there is a high percentage of patients with sensitivity to both cow's milk and soy,

switching directly to a casein hydrolysate is recommended. For the rare patients reactive to hydrolysate, an AAF is appropriate.[58,59] Caution and delay are advised regarding the introduction of common triggers such as rice and oat when cow's milk or soy reactions have already occurred.[17] Follow-up OFCs should be performed to determine tolerance, approximately every 12 to 24 months, depending on the clinical severity and the nutritional and social importance of the food (Fig. 33.3). These OFCs should

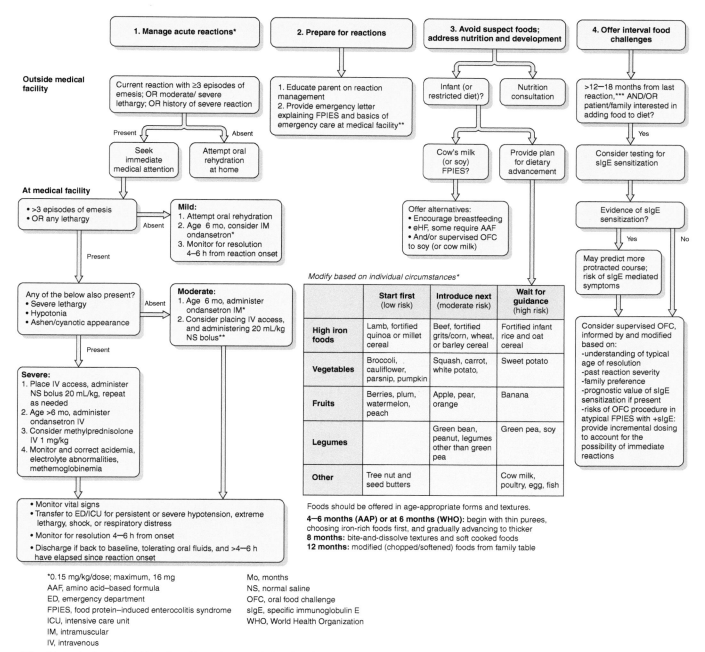

• **Fig. 33.3** Treatment Algorithm for Food Protein–Induced Enterocolitis Syndrome. *Modified from Nowak-Węgrzyn A, Chehade M, Groetch ME, et al. International consensus guidelines for the diagnosis and management of food protein–induced enterocolitis syndrome: Executive summary—Workgroup Report of the Adverse Reactions to Foods Committee, American Academy of Allergy, Asthma & Immunology. J Allergy Clin Immunol 2017;139:1111–26. †Template may be downloaded at https://www.fpies.org/wp-content/uploads/2018/08/IFPIES-ER-Letter-2018.pdf ‡Interval can be modified at the discretion of the treating physician.

TABLE 33.4	Oral Food Challenges for Food Protein-Induced Enterocolitis Syndrome	

Diagnostic Step	Procedures and Assessment
Preparation for challenge	• Verify normal weight gain, no gastrointestinal symptoms while off causal protein • Obtain baseline stool sample and peripheral blood neutrophil count • Consider intravenous access • Medications ready to treat reaction
Administration of challenge	• Administer challenge (typically 0.06–0.6 g food protein/kg body weight) • Observe for symptoms (usual onset of vomiting 1–4 hours) • Repeat neutrophil count 6 hours after ingestion
Evaluation of positive challenge	*Major criterion* Vomiting in the 1- to 4-hour period after ingestion of the suspect food and the absence of classic IgE-mediated allergic skin or respiratory symptoms *Minor criteria* 1. Lethargy 2. Pallor 3. Diarrhea in 5–10 hours after food ingestion 4. Hypotension 5. Hypothermia 6. Increased neutrophil count of ≥1500 cells/mm^3 above the baseline count *Positive oral food challenge* Major criterion and at least two minor criteria are met.

Note: Consider the important caveats to these oral food challenge criteria: (1) With the rapid use of ondansetron, many of the minor criteria, such as repetitive vomiting, pallor, and lethargy may be absent; and (2) not all facilities performing challenges have the ability to perform neutrophil counts in a timely manner. The treating physician may decide that a challenge be considered diagnostic in some instances even if only the major criterion was met. In challenges performed for research purposes, stringent criteria for challenge positivity should be used.

Adapted from Nowak-Wegrzyn A, Chehade M, Groetch ME, et al. International consensus guidelines for the diagnosis and management of food protein-induced enterocolitis syndrome: Executive summary-Workgroup Report of the Adverse Reactions to Foods Committee, American Academy of Allergy, Asthma & Immunology. The Journal of Allergy and Clinical Immunology 2017;139:1111-26.e4.

be performed under physician supervision with intravenous fluids and emergency medications immediately available because dramatic reactions, including shock, can occur. Re-evaluation for the development of food-specific IgE antibody before challenge is helpful because 4% to 30% develop IgE antibodies to the FPIES food (atypical FPIES), and among those with food-specific IgE, one in four converts to IgE-mediated reactions over time.[23,59,60] Patch testing does not provide diagnostic information. About half of positive challenges require treatment (usually intravenous fluids).[61] Considering strong inflammatory responses in FPIES, corticosteroids are administered for severe reactions, although the therapeutic benefit of this practice has not been established. A small case series (n = 5, age older than 3 years) suggested effectiveness of intravenous ondansetron for stopping emesis induced during FPIES-OFC.[62] Intramuscular ondansetron also has been used in five young children (four were under the age of 3 years) with rapid resolution of symptoms during the OFC.[63] A larger retrospective case-control study (n = 66) evaluated ondansetron in acute FPIES reactions and reported a 0.2 relative risk reduction in the onset of vomiting.[64] Almost 20% of patients did not respond to ondansetron; however, those who did respond were less likely to be hospitalized. Ondansetron is usually well tolerated, although special caution may be warranted in children with underlying heart disease because of the potential to prolong the QT interval. More studies are needed to define the role of ondansetron in FPIES management.

The role of epinephrine for treatment is not known, but it should be available for severe cardiovascular reactions. Considering the risk for hypotension, the OFC is best performed under physician supervision with consideration for obtaining intravenous access. FPIES-OFCs are typically performed with 0.06 to 0.6 g/kg of the food protein, with lower doses for those patients with history of severe reactions.[17] The OFC protocol and definition of a positive response are shown in Table 33.4.

The natural history is variable, depending on the population studied. A large birth cohort study from Israel reported resolution of CM-FPIES in 90% by age 3 years.[65] A retrospective study of 35 children from Australia evaluated over a span of 16 years showed rice (14 children), soy (12), and cow's milk (7) to be the most common triggers and sensitivity was lost by the age of 3 years to rice and soy in about 80%.[25] In a cohort of 23 Korean infants with cow's milk or soy FPIES, resolution rates were 64% for cow's milk and 92% for soy by 10 months of age and all were tolerant by 20 months.[66] In a retrospective U.S. study, overall significantly lower rates of FPIES resolution were found, 35% by age 2 years, 70% by age 3 years, and 85% by age 5 years.[60] In a mixed-design U.S. study, overall median age at resolution of CM-FPIES was 13 years, whereas the median age for patients with undetectable cow's milk IgE antibodies was 5 years.[59] These differences reflect differences in study designs and/or selection bias toward more severe and persistent phenotype among children evaluated at referral centers. About 50% of children outgrow rice or oat FPIES by age 4 to 5 years.[60] In addition, some patients maintain FPIES well beyond the age of 6 years, even into adulthood.[67]

Food Protein–Induced Enteropathy and Celiac Disease

There are no specific diagnostic tests for FPE; therefore, the diagnosis depends on exclusion of alternative diagnoses, biopsy evidence of enteropathy, and proof of sensitivity through dietary elimination and re-challenge. Because the symptoms are not as dramatic as those of FPIES, observation during dietary ingestion and exclusion of the causal protein must be undertaken to verify the diagnosis. Unlike FPE, CD can be evaluated with serologic tests. Tests for antiendomysial IgA (using tissue transglutaminase) are sensitive (85%–98%) and specific (94%–100%), with excellent positive (91%–100%) and negative (80%–98%) predictive values.[45] If CD is suspected based on a family history, steatorrhea, anemia, or failure to thrive, serologic tests for antiendomysial IgA and small-bowel biopsy should be undertaken. If there is enteropathy, but negative serology, alternative diagnoses (see Tables 33.1 and 33.2) should be reconsidered. With low suspicion for CD, serologic tests can be undertaken, and, if negative, the diagnosis is generally excluded, but a positive test would warrant confirmation with a biopsy. A gluten-free diet is necessary to treat CD and is maintained indefinitely. However, FPE induced by cow's milk generally resolves in 1 to 2 years, at which time re-challenge is warranted.

Treatment

There are no curative therapies for dietary FPIAP, FPIES, FPE, or CD; treatment is based on dietary elimination. Only patients with FPIES or some individuals with CD and "celiac crisis" experience severe reactions, so these patients also must be instructed on how to proceed in the event of an accidental ingestion. Such patients should report to an emergency department in the event that fluid resuscitation is needed.

Education about the details of avoidance is crucial so that dietary elimination trials and therapeutic interventions are accurately undertaken (reviewed in Chapter 35). Recurrence of symptoms is often caused by poor adherence or insufficient education. Issues of cross-contamination, label reading, restaurant dining, and even the use of medications that may contain causal food proteins make avoidance of major dietary proteins very difficult. Regarding CD, oat does not contain gluten,[51,68] but contamination of oat flour with wheat gluten remains a problem. Support groups and the advice of a knowledgeable dietitian are crucial adjuncts for patients undertaking these nutritionally and socially limiting diets.

Even without performing laboratory tests or OFC to confirm a specific disorder, switching among cow's milk, soy, and casein-hydrolysate formulas is commonly undertaken by pediatricians and families as a test of intolerance or allergy. There are no specific guidelines concerning these formula changes. It is helpful to know that only a small proportion of infants with IgE-mediated cow's milk allergy (14%) will react to soy.[69] In contrast, those with FPIES are more likely (40%–50%) to be reactive to soy. For these infants, hypoallergenic infant formula should be considered. For the few infants with symptoms that persist while taking a casein hydrolysate, AAF may be required.[59,70] Breastfeeding is preferred over commercial formula as the source for infant nutrition, but maternally ingested protein can elicit allergic symptoms in the breastfed infant.[21,71,72] Therefore, maternal dietary manipulation (e.g., avoidance of cow's milk protein) can be undertaken for treatment in breastfed infants, but with infants who have multiple food allergies this may be difficult, so substitution with infant formulas may be needed in some cases.

Except for CD, resolution of the allergy is expected, so a review of the diet, any accidental exposures, and tests as indicated are undertaken on a yearly basis with the expectation that FPIAP will resolve in 1 year and FPE and FPIES would resolve in 1 to 5 years. Although the natural history of adult-onset FPIES is poorly understood, available evidence suggests that it is a long-lasting disorder.

Conclusions

FPIAP, FPIES, FPE, and CD represent cell-mediated hypersensitivity responses to food proteins. These disorders generally manifest in infancy or early childhood and must be differentiated from disorders with similar symptoms and from each other. A careful clinical history, limited laboratory studies, and directed elimination and challenge can readily disclose the type of disorder and causal foods. Knowledge of the course of these disorders assists in long-term planning: either reintroduction of the food to determine whether tolerance has occurred or prolonged dietary elimination. The immunologic mechanisms of these disorders are being elucidated, and these advances are likely to permit improved diagnostic and therapeutic strategies in the future.

The reference list can be found on the companion Expert Consult website at http://www.expertconsult.inkling.com.

34

Eosinophilic Gastrointestinal Diseases

MIRNA CHEHADE, AMANDA B. MUIR, JONATHAN E. MARKOWITZ,
CHRIS A. LIACOURAS, GLENN T. FURUTA

KEY POINTS

- Non–immunoglobulin E (IgE)-mediated food allergies are predominantly T cell mediated. They occur after repetitive ingestion of trigger foods and cause a variety of gastrointestinal (GI) symptoms. These include eosinophilic GI disorders.
- Eosinophilic esophagitis is a chronic eosinophilic disease of the esophagus that causes abdominal pain, vomiting, gastroesophageal reflux symptoms, dysphagia, esophageal food impaction, feeding difficulties, and/or failure to thrive.

- Eosinophilic GI disorders below the esophagus involve eosinophilic infiltration into the stomach, small intestine, and/or colon.
- Eosinophilic proctocolitis is commonly triggered by cow's milk, can cause blood in the stool, and is a disease limited to infancy.

Introduction

Food allergies can affect the gastrointestinal (GI) tract in various ways. Generally, immunoglobulin E (IgE)-mediated food allergies can cause abdominal pain and/or vomiting, which occur almost immediately after ingestion of the culprit food, and at times diarrhea, which can occur either concurrently with the upper GI symptoms or a few hours later.[1] In contrast, non–IgE-mediated food allergic reactions involving the GI tract are generally delayed, causing a chronic inflammation of the GI tract on repetitive exposure to the culprit food(s) and manifesting with a variety of GI symptoms depending on the involved location in the GI tract. These non–IgE-mediated allergic GI disorders include eosinophilic gastrointestinal disorders (EGIDs): eosinophilic esophagitis (EoE), eosinophilic gastritis (EG), eosinophilic gastroenteritis (EGE), eosinophilic colitis (EC), and eosinophilic proctocolitis (EP). Non–IgE-mediated GI allergic disorders also include food protein–induced enterocolitis syndrome (FPIES) and other less well immunologically understood non–IgE-mediated food protein–induced allergic dysmotility disorders affecting various parts of the GI tract and manifesting with gastroesophageal reflux or constipation.[2,3]

The goal of this chapter is to provide an overview of EGIDs, including EoE, summarizing the common food triggers, clinical manifestations, and management approaches.

Food Allergy or Hypersensitivity

Immunoglobulin E–Mediated Allergy and Anaphylaxis

Type I (IgE-mediated) immediate hypersensitivity reactions to foods are most common in young children, with 50% of these reactions developing in the first year of life. The majority are reactions to cow's milk or soy protein from infant formulas.[4] Other food allergies begin to predominate in older children, including egg, fish, peanut, and wheat. Together with milk and soy, these account for more than 90% of food allergy in children.[5] Blinded food challenges have shown that symptoms referable to the GI tract in IgE-mediated allergy typically begin within minutes of the ingestion, although occasionally they may be delayed for up to 2 hours. They tend to be short-lived, lasting 1 to 2 hours.[6,7] Symptoms include nausea, vomiting, abdominal pain, and diarrhea; oral symptoms, skin manifestations, wheezing, or airway edema also may occur.

Eosinophilic Gastrointestinal Disorders

EGIDs are rare but increasingly recognized set of disorders that are defined by location of the GI tract that is infiltrated by large numbers of eosinophils. These include EoE involving the esophagus, EG involving the stomach, EGE involving the stomach and small intestine, and EC limited to the colon. Diagnostically, patients must have symptoms and infiltration of at least one layer of the GI tract with eosinophils in the absence of other known causes for eosinophilia.[8,9] Peripheral eosinophilia is not required for diagnosis, although it is a frequent finding. First reported over 50 years ago, the clinical spectrum of these disorders was defined solely by various case reports. As these reports became more frequent, various aspects of the diseases became better described and stratified. Additional insight into the role of the eosinophil in health and disease has allowed further description of these disorders with respect to the underlying defect that drives the inflammatory response in those afflicted. Perhaps most important to the definition of these disorders has been the understanding of the heterogeneity of the sites affected within the GI tract, resulting in the entities listed previously.

EGIDs arise from interactions between genetic and environmental factors. A family history is noted in 3% to 18% of individuals with one of these disorders.[10,11] In addition, a strong association with atopy has been observed with 75% of patients with EGID having an atopic history,[12,13] and allergen-free diets can reverse disease activity.[12-14] Interestingly, only a minority of individuals with EGIDs have food-induced anaphylaxis,[15] and therefore these disorders exhibit properties that lie between pure IgE-mediated allergy and T cell–mediated hypersensitivity disorders.

Eosinophilic Esophagitis

EoE represents a chronic, immune- and antigen-mediated esophageal disease characterized clinically by symptoms related to esophageal dysfunction and histologically by eosinophil-predominant esophageal inflammation.[16]

Etiology

A number of lines of evidence support the role for atopy and abnormal immunologic responses to specific antigens as an underlying mechanism for EoE.[14,17] In the vast majority of cases the antigens responsible are food antigens, although environmental antigens may contribute in certain individuals.[18] In 1995, Kelly and colleagues[19] reported the seminal finding supporting a role for food allergens in EoE. Ten patients were treated with a strict elimination diet that included an amino acid–based formula (AAF) with two foods (corn and apples/apple juice) for a median of 17 weeks. Symptomatic improvement was observed within an average of 3 weeks after the introduction of the elemental diet (resolution in eight patients, improvement in two), and all patients demonstrated a significant improvement in esophageal eosinophilia. On reintroduction of foods, all patients reverted to previous symptoms. Clinical practice suggests that after ingestion of food allergens, symptoms may be delayed in onset and after elimination of responsible food allergen(s) resolution of the symptoms may not occur for 1 to 2 weeks.

Several authors have suggested that aeroallergens may contribute to the development of EoE. Fogg and associates[20] reported a case of a 21-year-old woman with asthma and allergic rhinoconjunctivitis who also had EoE. The patient's EoE became symptomatic with exacerbations during pollen seasons, followed by resolution during winter months.

T cell–mediated reactions seem to be the predominant mechanism of disease,[21-23] as evidenced by increased numbers of CD4+ and CD8+ T lymphocytes in the esophageal mucosa of patients with EoE.[24,25]

• BOX 34.1 Characteristics of Eosinophilic Esophagitis

Symptoms
- Similar to symptoms of gastroesophageal reflux disease
  - Vomiting, regurgitation
  - Heartburn
  - Epigastric pain
  - Dysphagia
- Symptoms different in infants and adolescents from adults
- Often intermittent symptoms
- Male > female

Comorbidities (>50% patients)
- Asthma
- Atopic dermatitis
- Allergic rhinitis
- Immunoglobulin E–mediated food allergy

Family History (≥50% patients)
- Food allergy
- Atopic diseases

Familial clustering of cases of EoE has led to the assumption that there may be a genetic predisposition to the disease. In recent years, several candidate genes have been identified as risk variants for the development of EoE. Among these are the genes that code for eotaxin-3,[26] thymic stromal lymphoprotein (TSLP),[27] filaggrin,[28] and calpain 14 (CAPN14).[29] More recently, gene and environment interactions were suspected to be at play in causing EoE, with hospitalization in the neonatal intensive care unit and lack of breastfeeding being considered important early life events interacting with susceptibility genes.[30]

Clinical Manifestations

EoE can occur in all age groups, with a male-to-female ratio of about 3:1. The incidence and prevalence of EoE have been increasing, with prevalence estimates currently ranging from 0.5 to 1 case/1000 persons.[31]

Children with EoE typically present with abdominal pain, gastroesophageal symptoms, nausea, vomiting, regurgitation, decreased feeding, and at times failure to thrive.[14,32] Adolescents and adults with EoE typically present with solid food dysphagia and esophageal food impactions, at times necessitating endoscopic removal of the impacted food.[32,33] Symptoms can be frequent and severe in some patients but extremely intermittent and mild in others. It is not unusual for patients to develop coping mechanisms to adapt to their chronic dysphagia, including prolonged chewing of food; drinking excessively during meals to propel food downward; dipping foods in "lubricants" such as ketchup or gravy; and avoiding tough, lumpy, or highly textured foods such as meat, rice, or bread.[34] It is important for the physician to perform a detailed history that will seek to identify these compensatory mechanisms. More than 50% of patients manifest additional allergy-related symptoms such as asthma, eczema, or rhinitis.[11,16] Furthermore, patients often have one or more parents with history of allergy, EoE, food impactions, or esophageal stretching/dilation (Box 34.1).[11] Children with EoE have been studied in comparison to those with gastroesophageal reflux disease.[12,13] Although the symptoms of vomiting and abdominal pain occurred similarly in both groups, some symptoms, especially dysphagia, are predominant in those with EoE (Table 34.1).

	Characteristic	Eosinophilic Esophagitis	Gastroesophageal Reflux Disease
TABLE 34.1	**Contrasting Characteristics of Eosinophilic Esophagitis and Gastroesophageal Reflux Disease**		
	Symptoms	Sometimes intermittent	Persistent
	pH probe	Normal or abnormal	Abnormal
	Number of esophageal eosinophils per high-power field	≥15	1–5

Evaluation and Diagnosis

Patients with chronic refractory symptoms of gastroesophageal reflux disease, dysphagia, or esophageal food impaction should undergo evaluation for EoE. Although laboratory and radiologic assessment may be appropriate, patients will need to undergo an upper endoscopy with biopsy to make the diagnosis.[16,35] According to the most recent consensus guidelines, the threshold of esophageal eosinophilia should be 15 or more eosinophils per high-power field (HPF) on esophageal biopsy samples.[36]

A long-standing clinical observation identified that some children with very high levels of esophageal eosinophilia experienced a symptomatic response and histologic improvement in eosinophilia with the use of proton pump inhibitors (PPIs) alone[37]; this finding led to the development of a now antiquated term, *PPI-responsive esophageal eosinophilia*. As of now, patients with symptoms and endoscopic and histologic findings characteristic of EoE, in whom all findings normalized after treatment with PPIs, are thought to have EoE.[38] A trial of PPIs before endoscopy to establish the diagnosis of EoE is no longer needed, and current criteria state that a diagnostic endoscopy be done on no treatments, including PPIs, topical steroids, or an EoE directed diet.[36]

EoE has been associated with visual findings on endoscopy, including concentric ring formation, called *trachealization;* longitudinal linear furrows; and patches of small, white plaques on the esophageal surface.[39] The white plaques appear to represent the formation of eosinophilic microabscesses (Figs. 34.1 and 34.2). High-resolution probe endosonography in patients with EoE reveals that inflammation may extend past the mucosa into the muscular layers.[40]

Complications

Although failure to thrive is a possible complication of EoE, esophageal food impaction is more common.[41] Food impaction prevalence is increasing in parallel with the incidence of EoE.[42] This may be due to the fact that the esophagus in EoE is both more rigid and dysmotile than a normal esophagus. Up to 37% of patients with EoE have been shown to have abnormal esophageal peristalsis,[43] either weak or absent. In addition, the distensibility of the esophagus in patients with EoE who have a history of food impaction and stricture is decreased.[44]

In addition to esophageal food bolus impactions, esophageal stricture is another significant complication of EoE. Esophageal stricture not only causes esophageal dysfunction and dysphagia but also often requires esophageal dilation for symptom relief. There

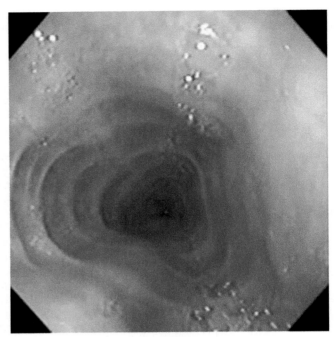

• **Fig. 34.1** "Trachealization" of the midesophagus in a patient with eosinophilic esophagitis. The term arises from the ringed appearance of the esophagus that causes it to resemble a human trachea (which has rings of cartilage).

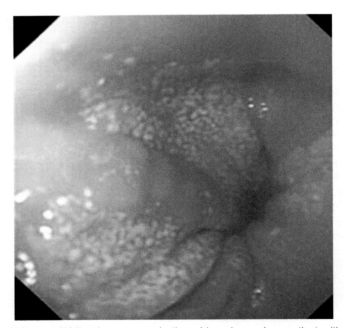

• **Fig. 34.2** White plaques seen in the midesophagus in a patient with eosinophilic esophagitis.

is enhanced collagen deposition in the esophageal lamina propria of patients with EoE[32,45] that can lead to luminal narrowing and stricture. Natural history studies are ongoing and reveal that some patients with long-standing untreated disease are more likely to develop esophageal stricture compared with those with a relatively short duration of disease.[46] Based on this finding, it is postulated that years of unremitting inflammation may lead to excessive esophageal collagen deposition and stricture. Although reversal of collagen deposition has proved to be difficult in successfully treated adults with EoE,[47,48] it may be more readily reversible with successful therapy in children.[49,50] Together, these findings underscore the importance of early diagnosis and treatment of EoE.

Management

Several approaches are available to treat EoE, including dietary exclusion of allergens, topical steroids, and dilation.

Dietary elimination therapies can take several forms, including targeted approach, six-food elimination diet, and use of elemental formula. Comparisons of the two most commonly used dietary therapies, the targeted diet that is directed by history and results of skin prick tests and the empirical elimination of six common food allergens (milk, wheat, egg, soy, nuts, seafood), a diet commonly referred to as the six-food elimination diet (SFED) revealed better outcomes with the SFED.[51] Histologic remission rates in patients with EoE on these diets were 45% versus 72%, respectively.[51] The most effective diet for patients with EoE is the elemental diet, consisting of exclusive feeding with an AAF along with ingestion of only one to two foods that are known to be less common triggers for EoE. The histologic remission rate with this diet was reported to be 91%.[51] Because the empirical SFED demonstrated reasonable efficacy, less restrictive empirical elimination diets also have been trialed, such as the four-food elimination diet consisting of removal of four of the most common six food triggers (milk, wheat, egg, soy/legumes), with histologic remission rates of 54% and 64% in adults and children with EoE, respectively.[52,53] An even more abbreviated diet consisting of elimination of two of the most common four food triggers (milk and wheat/gluten) was tested in a multicenter prospective trial in children and adult patients with EoE. This two-food elimination diet resulted in disease histologic remission in 43% of the patients.[54]

All dietary therapies require the involvement of a dietitian with experience in food allergy to ensure safety and efficacy of the dietary restriction given the multitude of foods removed in some patients, which can lead to caloric insufficiency and imbalance and micronutrient deficiencies, if not properly monitored.[55]

Once EoE remission is achieved with a dietary elimination therapy, foods should be reintroduced in a systematic manner. Because of the possibility of delayed reactions, it is advisable to wait up to 3 weeks before any subsequent food reintroduction. This period is usually sufficient to see a recurrence of symptoms; if symptoms develop, the food should be discontinued. In some cases, however, symptoms do not occur despite recurrence of esophageal eosinophilic infiltration. A repeat endoscopy with biopsy is required to evaluate for EoE histologic relapse. Because clinical symptoms often occur sporadically, obtaining esophageal biopsy samples remains the most important way to accurately determine whether EoE recurred with reintroduction of a food. The goal of food reintroductions is to identify foods that are triggers and foods that are safe to eat, therefore ending up with the minimum number of foods to avoid on a long-term basis.

Another potential problem to watch for with food introduction is that of possible de novo acute allergic reactivity to a food after its reintroduction. This can occur, rarely, despite lack of history of acute reaction or significant allergic sensitization to the food.[56] Therefore, standard allergy tests such as skin prick tests or serum food-specific IgE levels may need to be routinely performed before reintroduction of a food, following a prolonged period of avoidance of that food.

Although removal of the offending food(s) reverses the disease process in patients with EoE, in many cases the identification of these foods can be difficult. Standard allergy tests have shown low positive predictive values for many food triggers,[57] and patients with EoE are typically unable to temporally associate their esophageal symptoms with ingestion of the food triggers. Several days may be required for symptoms to occur on ingestion of a food trigger,[19,58] and it may take days or weeks for symptoms to resolve when the trigger food is eliminated. In addition, most patients with EoE have more than one food trigger for their disease, and the quality of life with the diet can be challenging.

Other management options for patients with EoE include medications. As of 2019, no medications for EoE have been approved by the U.S. Food and Drug Administration (FDA). Although medications can improve the disease and its symptoms, the disease recurs upon their discontinuation. Therefore, chronic therapy is recommended, with close monitoring for potential long-term side effects of these medications.

With the recent change in the consensus recommendations for diagnosing EoE,[36] PPIs are now a treatment option for patients with EoE,[36,59] with approximately a 50% rate of histologic remission in both adults and children.[60] Along with PPIs, corticosteroids are commonly used for patients with EoE. Initial reports identified that systemic corticosteroids improved the symptoms of EoE in adults and children identified with severe EoE.[61,62] In one study, 20 children were treated with oral methylprednisolone (average dose 1.5 mg/kg/day) for 1 month. Symptoms significantly improved in 19 of 20 patients, and esophageal biopsy samples obtained a month after initiation of therapy demonstrated a significant reduction of esophageal eosinophils (from 34 to 1.5 eosinophils per HPF).[63] On discontinuation of corticosteroids, 90% had recurrence of symptoms. A subsequent report of 4 children with EoE reported that swallowing a metered dose of aerosolized corticosteroids was effective in treating the symptoms of EoE in children.[64] Since then, multiple randomized adult and pediatric clinical trials using fluticasone or budesonide in either an aerosolized form to swallow or a liquid form that is thickened have yielded positive results.[65–68] Long-term safety of these medications has not been established. Concerns include growth failure, esophageal and/or oropharyngeal candidal infection, and adrenal suppression. An open-label, single-center prospective study of children with EoE using fluticasone to swallow up to 5.5 years demonstrated continued efficacy of the medication and no evidence of growth failure with the doses used in that trial.[69] More long-term studies are needed to confirm these findings with other topical corticosteroid formulations.

Other forms of medical therapy that have been evaluated previously include the mast cell stabilizing agent cromolyn sodium and the leukotriene antagonist montelukast.[70–74] Although each of these medications may represent an appealing option from a pathophysiologic standpoint, the available data do not support their use, based on either lack of clinical improvement or minimal to no histologic resolution.

Biologic agents have been tested in pediatric patients with EoE, in particular antibodies directed against the cytokine interleukin-5 (IL-5). IL-5 plays in important role in eosinophil recruitment, activation, and proliferation. In the past, two small studies demonstrated the effectiveness of anti–IL-5 in improving both symptoms and esophageal histology.[75,76] The first larger scale multicenter randomized, double-blind, placebo-controlled pediatric trial using an anti–IL-5 monoclonal antibody, reslizumab, had mixed results. Patients receiving active drug showed improvement in esophageal biopsy findings compared with placebo. However, subjects in both active drug and placebo groups showed symptomatic improvement, which resulted in failure to meet one of the study endpoints required to receive FDA approval.[77] Adolescents with EoE were also included in a randomized, double-blind, placebo-controlled trial using omalizumab, an antibody directed against IgE, every 2 to 4 weeks for 16 weeks.[78] No significant reduction in esophageal eosinophilia and no decrease in dysphagia were seen in patients treated with omalizumab compared with placebo.

Eosinophilic Gastrointestinal Disorders Below the Esophagus

EGIDs below the esophagus, which will simply be referred to as EGIDs throughout this section of the chapter, describe a constellation of symptoms attributable to the GI tract, in combination with pathologic infiltration by eosinophils. EGIDs include EG, EGE, and EC. A combination of GI complaints with supportive histologic findings is sufficient to make the diagnosis. These conditions are grouped together under the term EGIDs for the discussion here, though it is likely that they are distinct entities in most patients (Box 34.2).

EGIDs were originally described by Kaijser in 1937.[79] They are characterized by tissue eosinophilia that can affect different layers of the bowel wall, anywhere from the mouth to the anus. The gastric antrum and small intestine are most frequently affected (EG and EGE). In 1970 Klein and colleagues[80] classified EGE into three categories: mucosal, muscular, and serosal forms. Although mucosal disease results in a variety of GI symptoms, such as abdominal pain, vomiting, diarrhea, anorexia, weight loss, and failure to thrive, the muscular disease results in obstructive symptoms such as gastric outlet or bowel obstructive symptoms, and the serosal disease results in ascites.[80,81]

Etiology

EGIDs affect patients of all ages.[81,82] Most commonly, eosinophils infiltrate only the mucosa, leading to one or more GI symptoms, such as abdominal pain, vomiting, melena, failure to thrive, and edema.[81] Mucosal EGIDs may affect any portion of the GI tract. A review of the biopsy findings in 38 children with EGIDs revealed that all patients examined had mucosal eosinophilia of the gastric antrum.[83] Of the patients, 79% also demonstrated eosinophilia of the proximal small intestine, with 60% having esophageal involvement and 52% having involvement of the gastric corpus. Those with colonic involvement tended to be younger than 6 months of age and were ultimately classified as having allergic colitis.

Details of the cause of EGIDs remain unknown. The association between allergy and EGE is supported by disease remission in some patients in response to food allergen removal from the diet and increased likelihood of atopic diseases and IgE-mediated food allergies.[81,84,85] The role of non–IgE-mediated immune dysfunction, in particular the interplay between lymphocyte-produced cytokines and eosinophils, has received attention in EGIDs. IL-5 is a chemoattractant responsible for tissue eosinophilia.[86] Desreumaux and associates[87] found that among patients with EGE, the levels of IL-3, IL-5, and granulocyte-macrophage colony-stimulating factor were significantly increased compared with control patients. Once recruited to the tissue, eosinophils may further recruit similar cells through their own production of IL-3 and IL-5 and leukotrienes.[88] More recently, Caldwell and co-workers[89] demonstrated significantly increased transcripts of the allergic cytokines IL-4, IL-5, and IL-13, as well as increased mast cell–specific transcripts in the gastric tissue of patients with EG.[89]

Clinical Manifestations

The most common symptoms of EGIDs include abdominal pain, bloating, vomiting, diarrhea, weight loss, food aversions, failure to thrive, and edema.[71,81,90] In addition, up to 50% of patients have a personal or family history of atopy.[81,83] Features of severe disease include GI bleeding, iron-deficiency anemia, protein-losing enteropathy, growth failure,[81,90] and, rarely, symptoms of severe GI ulceration and perforation.[91–94] Approximately 75% of affected patients have an elevated blood eosinophilia.[81] Protein-losing enteropathy results in hypoproteinemia, hypoalbuminemia, and loss of IgG but not IgA or IgM.[95]

The muscular involvement by disease in EGID is particularly important to consider in infants, in whom EG involving the gastric muscular layer may manifest in a manner similar to that of hypertrophic pyloric stenosis, with progressive vomiting, dehydration, electrolyte abnormalities, and thickening of the gastric outlet.[81,96,97] When an infant presents with this constellation of symptoms, in addition to atopic symptoms such as atopic dermatitis and reactive airway disease, an elevated eosinophil count, or a strong family history of atopic disease, EG should be considered in the diagnosis before surgical intervention. Serosal infiltration with eosinophils in EGIDs typically results in eosinophilic ascites.[81,98,99]

Evaluation and Diagnosis

EGIDs should be considered in any patient with a history of chronic GI symptoms, including vomiting, abdominal pain, diarrhea, anemia, edema, or poor weight gain, in combination with the presence of eosinophils in the GI tract. Other causes of eosinophilic infiltration of the GI tract include parasitic infection, inflammatory bowel disease, neoplasm, chronic granulomatous disease, collagen vascular disease, and hypereosinophilic syndrome.[100–104]

A number of tests may aid in the diagnosis of EGIDs; however, an endoscopy with biopsy is necessary to make the diagnosis. Eosinophils in the GI tract must be documented before EGIDs can be truly entertained as a diagnosis. This is most readily done with biopsies of either the upper GI tract through esophagogastroduodenoscopy or the lower GI tract through flexible sigmoidoscopy or colonoscopy. Endoscopically, a wide range of findings, including normal mucosa, erosions, ulcerations, and pseudopolyp formation have been described in the gastric mucosa of patients with EG.[81] Ulcers also can be seen in the remainder of the GI tract in some patients with EGIDs. A history of atopy supports the diagnosis but is not a necessary feature. Peripheral eosinophilia occurs in approximately 75% of affected individuals.[81] Radiographic contrast studies may demonstrate mucosal irregularities or edema, wall thickening, ulceration, or luminal narrowing.[105]

Evaluation of other causes of eosinophilia should be undertaken, including stool analysis for ova and parasites and serologic tests for specific parasites in endemic areas. Additional workup for other causes of GI eosinophilia need to be considered, based on the patient's history. Signs of intestinal obstruction warrant abdominal imaging. Allergen-specific IgE testing and skin testing for environmental antigens are rarely useful.

Management

There is as much ambiguity in the treatment of EGIDs as there is in their diagnosis. This is in large part because EGIDs were defined mainly by case series, each of which employed its own mode of treatment. EGIDs are difficult diseases to diagnose and relatively rare in prevalence; thus, randomized trials for its treatment are uncommon, leading to considerable debate as to the optimal treatment.

Food allergy is considered one of the potential underlying causes of EGIDs. The elimination of pathogenic foods, as identified by any form of allergy testing or by random removal of the most likely antigens, should be a first-line consideration. Unfortunately, this approach results in improvement in a limited number of patients, although empirical elimination of common food allergens resulted in a good response in children with EG.[81] In severe cases or when other treatment options have failed, the administration of an elemental diet consisting of exclusive feeding with an AAF has been shown to be successful,[85,106] including in children with concurrent protein-losing enteropathy,[95] with resolution of clinical symptoms and tissue eosinophilia.

When the use of a restricted or elemental diet fails, systemic corticosteroids are often employed because of their high likelihood of success in achieving remission.[71] However, when weaned, the duration of remission is variable and can be short-lived, leading to the need for repeated courses or continuous low doses of corticosteroids. In addition, the chronic use of corticosteroids carries an increased likelihood of undesirable side effects, including cosmetic problems (e.g., cushingoid facies, hirsutism, acne), decreased bone density, impaired growth, and personality changes. A response to these side effects has been to use at times modified oral enteric-coated budesonide regimens in some children with EGE[107] and to look for substitutes that may act as steroid-sparing agents while still allowing for control of symptoms. Orally administered cromolyn sodium has demonstrated only symptomatic relief,[108,109] and montelukast, a selective leukotriene receptor antagonist, has not been effective.[110] No biologic agents have been attempted in children with EGIDs. In adults, omalizumab, a humanized monoclonal antibody targeted against IgE, did not demonstrate efficacy either,[111] but vedolizumab, an antibody targeted against the integrin $\alpha 4\beta 7$, proved to be effective in recent case series reported in 2018 and 2019.[112,113]

Given the limited treatment options for patients with EGIDs, the combination of therapies incorporating the best chance of success with the smallest likelihood of side effects should be employed. When particular food antigens that may be causing disease can be identified, elimination of those antigens should be first-line therapy. Empirical elimination of common food allergens also should be considered. If this approach fails, a total elimination diet using an AAF should be considered. If needed, corticosteroids may be used in conjunction with dietary restriction so that the doses of corticosteroids can be kept minimal while the patient is closely monitored for side effects.

Eosinophilic Proctocolitis

EP, also known as allergic proctocolitis, food protein–induced proctocolitis, or milk protein proctocolitis, has been recognized as one of the most common, benign causes of rectal bleeding in infants.[83,114]

Etiology

Cow's milk protein is the food most frequently implicated in EP. Commercially available infant formulas most commonly use cow's milk as the protein source. There are at least 25 known immunogenic proteins within cow's milk, with β-lactoglobulin and the caseins being the most antigenic.[115] Up to 50% of cases of EP occur in breastfed infants; however, rather than developing an allergy to human milk protein, the infants are manifesting allergy to antigens ingested by the mother and transferred via the breast milk. The transfer of maternal dietary protein via breast milk was first demonstrated in 1921.[116] More recently, the presence of cow's milk antigens in breast milk has been established.[117–119]

Clinical Manifestations

Rectal bleeding, alone or in combination with diarrhea, is typically seen in patients who present with EP.[83] There is a bimodal age distribution, with the majority of patients presenting in infancy, with a mean age reported to be 2 months,[120] and the other group presenting in adolescence and early adulthood.

The typical infant with EP is well appearing, with no constitutional symptoms. Rectal bleeding begins gradually, initially appearing as small flecks of blood. Usually, increased stool frequency occurs, accompanied by water loss or mucous streaks. The development of irritability or straining with stools is also common and can falsely lead to the initial assumption of anal fissuring. Atopic symptoms such as atopic dermatitis and reactive airway disease may be associated. Continued exposure to the inciting antigen causes increased bleeding and may, on rare occasions, cause anemia and poor weight gain. Despite the progression of symptoms, the infants are generally well appearing and rarely appear ill. Other manifestations of GI tract inflammation such as vomiting, abdominal distention, or weight loss almost never occur and would be suggestive of another GI problem.

Evaluation and Diagnosis

EP is primarily a clinical diagnosis, although several laboratory parameters and diagnostic procedures may be useful. Initial assessment should be directed at the overall health of the child. A toxic-appearing infant is not consistent with the diagnosis of EP and should prompt evaluation for other causes of GI bleeding. A complete blood count is at times useful because the majority of infants with EP have a normal or borderline low hemoglobin. An elevated blood eosinophil count may be present. Stool studies for bacterial pathogens such as *Salmonella* and *Shigella* spp. should be considered in the setting of rectal bleeding. A stool specimen may be analyzed for the presence of white blood cells and specifically for eosinophils. The sensitivity of these tests is not well documented, and the absence of a positive finding on these tests does not exclude the diagnosis.[121] Eosinophils can also accumulate in the colon in other conditions such as pinworm and hookworm infections, drug reactions, vasculitis, and inflammatory bowel disease, and it is important to exclude these, especially in older children.

Although not always necessary, flexible sigmoidoscopy may be useful to demonstrate the presence of colitis. Visually, one may find erythema, friability, or frank ulceration of the colonic mucosa. Alternatively, the mucosa may appear normal or show evidence of lymphoid hyperplasia.[122,123] Histologic findings typically include increased eosinophils in focal aggregates within the lamina propria, with generally preserved crypt architecture. Findings may be patchy; therefore, care should be taken to examine many levels of each specimen if necessary.[124,125]

Management

In a well-appearing patient with a history consistent with EP, it is acceptable to make an empirical change in the protein source of the formula. Because of the frequent development of soy protein EP in milk-sensitized individuals, a protein hydrolysate formula is often the best choice.[124] A few infants are sensitive even to that formula and therefore require an AAF for resolution of their symptoms.[126] Symptom resolution begins within a few days of elimination of the problematic food. Although symptoms may linger for several days to weeks, continued improvement is the rule. If symptoms do not quickly improve, or persist beyond 4 to 6 weeks, other antigens and other potential causes of rectal bleeding should be considered. In breastfed infants, dietary restriction of products containing milk and soy from the mother's diet may result in improvement; however, care should be taken to ensure that the mother maintains adequate protein and calcium intake from other sources.

EP in infancy is generally benign, and withdrawing the milk protein trigger resolves the condition. Though gross blood in the stool usually disappears within 72 hours, occult blood loss may persist for longer.[120] The prognosis is excellent, and the majority of patients are able to tolerate the culprit food protein by 1 to 3 years of age. In older individuals, it is more difficult to identify the food triggers, and therefore patients usually require medical management. Though there is a paucity of clinical data regarding therapy for this condition, it appears that glucocorticoids are efficacious.[9] The prognosis for older onset EP is less favorable than the infant presentation and is typically chronic and relapsing.

Conclusions

Eosinophilic disorders of the GI tract are becoming increasingly recognized as distinct clinical entities with specific management strategies. Whereas EG, EGE, and EC are rare and difficult to diagnose, EP and EoE are much more common and more easily diagnosed. EP is a well-accepted entity; however, the diagnosis of EoE has recently been receiving a great deal of attention and the other EGIDs are following suit.

Future research should focus on clarifying the prevalence and natural history of all EGIDs and optimizing their diagnostic approach and treatment options. The particular management challenges posed by these conditions warrant close liaison among gastroenterologists, allergists, and dietitians. In addition, patients and families require particular support, especially when trying to adopt restricted diets. Patient-founded support advocacy groups have been established for this purpose (e.g., American Partnership for Eosinophilic Disorders, http://www.APFED.org).

Awareness of food-induced allergic and eosinophilic disease of the GI tract has increased, but many unanswered questions remain. The variation in geographic distribution of some of the EGIDs such as EoE has yet to be explained. The pathogenesis of EGIDs has to be fully elucidated, in particular the role of environmental agents. Advances need to be made in diagnosing these conditions, especially with the use of less invasive techniques than endoscopy with biopsy, and also in better identifying offending food antigens and allergens. In addition, biochemical studies need to be pursued so we can determine a cause of these disorders. Is the eosinophil dysregulation the result of an immunologic defect or an allergy? These and other research questions reinforce the limitations of our current understanding of EGIDs. We hope that the future will hold promise in answering these questions.

The reference list can be found on the companion Expert Consult website at http://www.expertconsult.inkling.com.

35

Management of Food Allergy

MARION GROETCH, CARINA VENTER

KEY POINTS

- The management of food allergy entails avoidance of the identified allergen to prevent chronic and acute food allergic reactions.
- Allergen elimination diets should not be prescribed lightly because they present challenges to families and come with potential social, psychological, financial, and nutritional burdens.
- Children with food allergies may have inadequate nutrient in-

take and poor growth if the elimination diet is not well designed to substitute for nutrients lost to the elimination diet.
- An individualized avoidance strategy should be developed for each child with food allergy with consideration of cross-sensitization, co-existing allergies, growth status, nutritional deficiencies specific to the food allergy, and tolerance development.

Introduction

The therapeutic management of food allergy entails avoidance of the identified allergen to prevent chronic and acute food allergic reactions. Allergen elimination diets present great challenges to families and come with potential social, psychological, financial, and nutritional burdens.[1–5] Food is an integral part of social gatherings, and without adequate planning the child and family may feel unable to participate fully in daily activities. Going to parties, eating in friends' homes, even going to school or camp requires planning so that these opportunities can be safely enjoyed. Eating competence is also vitally important to the socialization of the child, and children with food allergies may have food aversions and self-limited diets beyond the elimination diet (see Chapter 32). Anxiety issues may even arise about eating and food in general, which will have a further impact on the child's ability to participate fully in activities. Shopping and meal preparation require significantly more time when avoiding allergens, and specialty allergen-free foods can be more expensive. Finally, elimination diets may affect nutrient intake[6–10]; great care must be taken to plan for a diet that continues to provide appropriate nutrition for growth and development and long-term health.

In addition to comprehensive education on how to recognize and treat food allergic reactions, food allergy management entails teaching the family how to avoid the allergen, manage the allergy in all areas of daily living, and provide a nutritionally balanced diet within the context of the allergen avoidance diet. The goal of providing extensive education is to reduce the risk of accidental allergen exposure and empower the family, and eventually the child, to participate in all daily activities while avoiding the food to which the child is allergic. Each child should be evaluated and an

individualized avoidance strategy designed based on patient history, the allergen involved, testing results, and oral food challenge (OFC) outcome.[11] Living with food allergies is a daily challenge, but with planning, activities can be safe and manageable and the allergen avoidance diet nutritionally complete and enjoyable.

Avoidance Diets: General

The elimination of a single allergen from the diet may seem an easy task. If the allergen plays a minor role in our food supply, such as cashew nut, the task may be simple enough. On the other hand, if the allergen is pervasive in our food supply, such as milk or wheat, avoidance issues become much more complex. Avoidance of a single allergen such as cow's milk necessitates avoidance of an entire food group and many common foods of childhood, including not only milk, butter, cheese, yogurt, and ice cream, but also numerous manufactured products, such as crackers, breads, cookies, cereals, cakes, and processed meats and cold cuts, that may also contain milk protein as an ingredient. Allergen avoidance sheets are available (http://www.foodallergy.org or http://www.cofargroup.org—click on Food Allergy Education Program) and are helpful when used as a starting point for allergen avoidance education. It should be noted that avoidance sheets do not provide the extensive education needed for strict dietary elimination.

Label Reading

Food labeling legislation depends on the country or region in which the product is sold. Ingredients considered major allergens based on the labeling laws of a specific country or region are listed in Table 35.1.

TABLE 35.1	Major Allergens by Country or Region			
Country or Countries	**United States, Mexico, Hong Kong, China**	**Australia and New Zealand**	**Canada**	**European Union**
Allergens requiring full disclosure on package labels based on allergy labeling regulation in specified country	Milk	Milk	Milk	Milk
	Egg	Egg	Egg	Egg
	Wheat	Wheat	Wheat	Wheat
	Soy	Soy	Soy	Soy
	Peanut	Peanut	Peanut	Peanut
	Tree nuts	Tree nuts	Tree nuts	Tree nuts
	Fish	Fish	Fish	Fish
	Crustacean shellfish	Crustacean shellfish	Crustacean shellfish	Crustacean shellfish
		Sesame	Mollusks	Mollusks
			Sesame	Mustard
				Celery
				Lupine
				Sesame
				All gluten-containing grains

Note: The specific tree nut, fish, or shellfish species must be identified.

In the United States, the Food Allergen Labeling and Consumer Protection Act (FALCPA) mandates clear, plain language labeling of all ingredients derived from the foods considered major allergens. Those foods considered major allergens in the United States are milk, egg, wheat, soy, peanut, tree nuts, fish, and crustacean shellfish.[12] The plain language stipulation requires the presence of a major food allergen to be listed, using its common FALCPA (e.g., milk) rather than a scientific term (e.g., casein, whey) on the product label in one of the following ways:

- In parentheses, after the food protein derivative, for example: casein (milk)
- In the ingredient list, for example: milk, wheat, peanut
- Immediately below the ingredient list in a "contains" statement, for example: CONTAINS EGG[13,14]

Front of package labeling such as "Dairy-free" or "Peanut-free," is not regulated and should not be used to assess product safety. FALCPA regulations apply only to ingredients derived from the eight foods that are considered the major allergens. An individual with allergy to an ingredient not covered under FALCPA, such as garlic, sesame, or mustard, would still need to call the manufacturer to ascertain if garlic, sesame or sesame oil, or mustard was included in a vague ingredient term such as "spice" or "natural flavoring" of a product. The U.S. Food and Drug Administration is currently considering legislation that may include sesame as a major allergen. (Sesame is considered a major allergen in Canada, Europe, and Australia and must be noted on the label.)

Manufactured food products, including those imported for sale in the United States, dietary supplements, medical foods, and infant formulas are all required to comply with FALCPA.[12] Currently, highly refined vegetable oils derived from major food allergens (including highly refined soy and peanut oils) are not considered allergens by FALCPA because highly refined oils have almost complete removal of allergenic protein and have not been shown to pose a risk to human health.[15,16] In the United States, soy oil is almost always a highly refined oil, meaning it would not be considered an allergenic ingredient. Peanut oil, on the other hand, may or may not be highly refined. Peanut oil also can be present as expeller-pressed, cold-pressed, expelled, or extruded, which may contain enough peanut protein to cause an allergic reaction. Because the ingredient list of a finished food will not tell a consumer how the oil was processed, it will not be possible to tell from a product label if the peanut oil listed is highly refined or otherwise processed. Calling the manufacturer may provide more specific information. However, because peanut oil is infrequently used in manufactured products and the labeling of the oil is not sufficient to determine whether the ingredient is safe, avoidance of peanut oil is frequently recommended. Tree nut oils and sesame oil are typically not highly refined, and unrefined oils may pose a risk to allergic consumers and therefore should be avoided.[13,14]

The presence of ingredients in manufactured foods as a result of cross-contact is not required to be listed on product labels. Cross-contact occurs when an "allergen-safe" food unintentionally comes in contact with an allergen during the use of shared storage, transportation, or production equipment or routine methods of growing and harvesting crops. Cross-contact may lead to significant levels of hidden allergens in a product without identification on the product label. Many manufacturers address the issue of cross-contact with precautionary allergen labeling (PAL), such as "May contain [allergen]," "Manufactured in a facility that also manufactures [allergen]" or "Manufactured on shared equipment with [allergen]." Those with food allergies should be aware that these statements are voluntary and unregulated. A variety of statements are being employed, some of which provide food-allergic consumers with little meaningful information on the potential presence of allergens in prepackaged foods. For instance, in a 2010 study, product labels stating, "Good Manufacturing Practices were used to segregate ingredients in a facility that also processes peanut, tree nuts, milk, shellfish, fish, and soy ingredients," was interpreted to mean that the product was safe for these otherwise undisclosed ingredients; however, milk was detected in two and egg in one of the three products with this PAL.[17] PAL carries a small but real risk to the consumer with food allergies, and no one statement represents a greater or lesser degree of risk than another. In the United States, the National Institutes of Allergy and Infectious Diseases (NIAID) expert panel guidelines for the diagnosis and management of food allergy suggest advising patients to avoid precautionary-labeled products. However, individual guidance based on clinical assessment may be appropriate. For instance, patients with food protein–induced enterocolitis syndrome (FPIES) do not typically require avoidance of products with PAL because infants with FPIES typically have a higher threshold for reactivity.[18]

Although similar legislation exists in many countries, the foods identified as allergens (see Table 35.1)[13] and other slight variations of regulations exist. For instance, in Canada it is recommended that PAL use only the wording, "May Contain –," to prevent misinterpretation of the degree of risk. Unique to the European Union and United Kingdom, food businesses are required to provide allergy information on food sold unpackaged or prepacked for direct sale (e.g., bakeries, delicatessens, and caterers) (https://www.food.gov.uk/business-guidance/allergen-labelling-for-food-manufacturers). In Australia, a voluntary incident trace allergen labeling (VITAL) system may be used by food producers to provide standardized, consistent precautionary advice to consumers with food allergy.

Although label ambiguities continue to exist, the package label provides information to the consumer about the contents of a product and should be read every time a product is purchased. Healthcare professionals must be prepared to offer extensive education to patients with food allergies so safe food selections can be made.

Daily Living With Food Allergies

Once a food item is purchased and brought into the home, that item must continue to be carefully handled to prevent cross-contact with the identified allergen. Storage of ingredients in the home should be planned to prevent cross-contact. A separate shelf in the refrigerator or cupboard may be reserved for the allergen-free foods. Meal preparation to prevent cross-contact in the home is also essential. All food preparation areas, cooking utensils, and cooking equipment should be cleansed with warm soapy water and rinsed. Allergen-free foods and meal items can be prepared first, covered, and removed from the area before the preparation of other foods for the home. Families will also benefit from guidance on how to prepare meals without their allergenic ingredients.

Families living with food allergies report that avoiding eating in restaurants is the leading cause of decreased quality of life because of the food allergy.[19] Those with food allergies may be especially at risk while dining out because restaurants are not required to list ingredients and the wait staff is generally ignorant about the ingredients in a dish. Planning ahead and communication with restaurant staff is the first key step in obtaining a safe restaurant meal. Calling ahead to ask how a food allergy is accommodated and avoiding the restaurant's busiest hours are

often helpful. Families should be taught to inform the staff that their child has a food allergy, not simply to ask if a menu item contains their allergen. "Chef Cards" provide a written list specific allergens and are available free and downloadable from organizations such as Food Allergy Research and Education (FARE; http://www.foodallergy.org). In addition to ingredient inquiries, families must learn to inform restaurant staff about cross-contact risk. For example, the same grill might be used to make a cheeseburger that is used for a plain hamburger, or the French fries may have been cooked in the same deep fat fryer as fried shrimp or egg batter–containing onion rings. The same tongs or mixing bowls may be used to assemble a salad with nuts as are used to assemble a plain green salad. It is important to inform the chef that a clean cooking area, cooking equipment, and utensils must be used. Ordering single-ingredient foods, prepared simply, will decrease the risk for hidden ingredients. When the food arrives at the table, families should confirm with the chef that the meal was prepared correctly and not have their child eat the food if there is any doubt as to the safety of the meal. Finally, as always, emergency medications should be available when eating at home or away from home.

Certain types of eating establishments will present a greater risk of allergen exposure. For example, cafeterias, buffets, and salad bars have inherently greater risk for cross-contact because of spillage and shared serving utensils. Asian and other ethnic restaurants may use more allergenic ingredients (e.g., soy, peanuts, tree nuts, fish, and shellfish) in a wide variety of dishes, and the cooking equipment is generally not washed between each meal prepared. Ice cream parlors use the same scooper for all flavors of ice cream. Asking for a clean scooper may not eliminate the risk because previous servings with a contaminated scooper into the otherwise safe flavor may have already caused cross-contact. For seafood allergies, seafood restaurants may be problematic even if a nonseafood item is ordered because of the greater risk for cross-contact in the kitchen.[20,21]

Children with food allergies will attend schools just like their nonallergic peers, and some planning ahead will help make the environment safer. Management issues in schools involve methods to prevent exposure to allergens and plans to recognize and treat allergic reactions and anaphylaxis.[22] Physicians should provide written, easy-to-follow instructions in the form of an emergency care plan (ECP), which includes direction on recognizing and treating an allergic reaction, including the medication to be given and the appropriate dosing. Parents will need to provide a copy of the ECP to the school staff and inform teachers, nurses, administrators, and food service staff about the food allergy. Families should plan to meet with school personnel before the start of the school year. Communication with the school about topics such as classroom parties, transportation, supervision in the lunch room if needed, substitute teacher notification, field trips, and after-school programs will help plan food allergy management in all areas of the school environment. FARE has developed a variety of resources and products, including a downloadable ECP for physicians to complete and management tips for classrooms and school cafeterias. The Centers for Disease Control and Prevention (CDC) has published a document entitled Voluntary Guidelines for Managing Food Allergies in Schools and Early Care and Education Programs, a PDF that can be downloaded directly from their website (https://www.cdc.gov/healthyschools/foodallergies/pdf/teachers_508_tagged.pdf), and multiple school training programs are available through the FARE website (http://www.foodallergy.org). Parents, physicians, school administrators, teachers, school nurses, food service staff, and childcare and camp staff will find these resources valuable in the planning required to keep children with food allergies safe. Additionally, the Consortium of Food Allergy Research (CoFAR) has developed and validated an extensive food allergy education program that has free and downloadable patient education handouts on specific allergen avoidance diets and fact sheets on specific food allergic disorders, label reading, cross-contact, restaurant meals, cooking without allergens, nutrition, and management issues in schools and camps (http://www.cofargroup. org click on Food Allergy Education Program).[23]

Nutrition

Overview

Children with food allergies may have inadequate nutrient intake if the diet is not well designed to substitute for nutrients lost to the elimination of allergens.[24–26] Additionally, feeding problems such as food aversion and a limited acceptance of a variety of foods are common in children with food allergies and may significantly contribute to poor energy and overall nutrient intake.[27] Certain food allergic disorders, such as eosinophilic gastrointestinal disorders[28–30] and FPIES[31] are commonly accompanied by feeding difficulties and limited diets, which may have an impact on overall nutrient intake. Numerous studies have demonstrated that children with food allergies are at risk for inadequate nutritional intake and poor growth.[7–9,32]

A comprehensive baseline nutrition assessment includes gathering, verifying, and interpreting data from anthropometric measurements, dietary history, medical history, physical examination, and laboratory indices. Key indicators of potential nutritional risk in children with food allergies are a greater number of eliminated foods or greater nutritional value of eliminated foods, picky or self-selective eating, feeding delays or difficulties, poor variety or volume of foods provided or accepted, or an unwillingness of the child to ingest supplemental formula or vitamin or mineral substitutes when required or other substitute foods.[33]

Growth

Several studies have evaluated growth in the pediatric population with food allergy. Isolauri and colleagues[34] found decreased length and weight-for-length indices in a group of 100 infants with food allergy compared with healthy, age-matched controls. Jensen and colleagues[35] found height for age was significantly reduced in a group of patients living with cow's milk allergy for more than 4 years compared with height of parents, siblings, and normal controls. In a 2018 international survey on growth indices in children with food allergies (n = 430),[7] the authors found that children with non–immunoglobulin E (IgE)-mediated allergy and mixed IgE-mediated and non–IgE-mediated food allergy had lowered height-for-age scores than those with IgE-mediated food allergy alone, confirming findings from previous studies that height or length growth may decline before weight. Therefore, it is important that both height/length and weight are routinely assessed. It is also possible that children with food allergies may have decreased growth despite adequate nutritional intake. Flammarion and colleagues[10] conducted a cross-sectional study comparing children with food allergies (N = 96) who had been counseled by a dietitian to paired controls without food allergies (N = 95). Children with food allergies had weights and heights within the normal range; however, they were smaller for their age than the nonallergic controls, even

when they received similar nutrition. Suboptimal nutrition in this population may exacerbate the risk, and decreased growth can more easily become malnutrition. Although there may be other contributing factors associated with decreased growth in children with food allergy (such as subclinical inflammation), in general the primary cause of poor growth likely stems from inadequate substitution in the elimination diet.

The NIAID Food Allergy Guidelines recommend close growth monitoring for all children with food allergies.[36] Review of current and historical growth should be completed according to current standards of care that are based on CDC and World Health Organization (WHO) or other national standards. Measurements, including weight, length or height, and head circumference as age appropriate, should be obtained and plotted on appropriate growth charts (WHO charts for infants and children from birth to 24 months and CDC charts for children ages 2–20 years). Growth typically follows predictable increases in length, weight, and head circumference and significant changes in growth velocity are not expected. Plotting growth measurements on the appropriate standardized growth chart will allow assessment of growth velocity for that particular child and provide a comparison of growth with the reference population.

Dietary Intake Assessment

Dietary intakes can be obtained by 24-hour recall or multiple-day food diary or food frequency questionnaire. A 24-hour recall is generally useful when assessing intake in an infant who is predominantly breastfed or bottle-fed but may provide limited information for older children, because accuracy of a mixed diet may not be reflected with recall. For older infants and children, a food diary will provide a more accurate estimate of intake. A food diary of at least 3 days (including one weekend and two weekdays) should include the amount and types of foods ingested and the timing of meals and snacks. Questions about typical dietary patterns or food frequency questionnaires also may be used and are especially useful in assessing specific nutrient intakes. For example, assessment of calcium and vitamin D intake may be determined by asking about frequency and amounts of dairy or enriched dairy substitutes consumed.

A registered dietitian will be able to compare dietary patterns to recommendations from the Dietary Reference Intakes (DRIs; https://www.nal.usda.gov/fnic/dietary-reference-intakes) or food group guides specified by the U.S. Department of Agriculture (http://www.choosemyplate.gov) or provided by governmental agencies in other countries. The DRIs (https://fnic.nal.usda.gov/fnic/dri-calculator/) and other guidelines may be used as tools to assess nutrient intake, plan interventions, and/or monitor the patient's ongoing nutrient intakes.[37] Even clinicians who are not trained to assess nutrient intake may glean valuable information from a food diary or food frequency questionnaires. For instance, unusual meal or snack patterns such as feeding on demand beyond infancy, or unusual food or beverage intake, such as excessive fruit juice consumption, may become apparent and give clues to potential causes of poor nutritional status in a child. A sample elimination diet menu is provided in Box 35.1.

Eating Competence

Eating competence describes a child's ability to eat and enjoy a wide variety of foods of varying flavors and textures that will support adequate nutrition for growth and development. Eating competence and pediatric nutrition are often discussed side by side because feeding problems are common in childhood, with an

BOX 35.1   Sample Elimination Diet[a]

Breakfast
- Gluten-free oat pancakes[b] or oatmeal with blueberries (or cooked blueberry compote)
- 100% pure maple syrup
- Calcium fortified orange juice—4 ounces

Snack
- Fresh watermelon or applesauce
- Buckwheat or crispy rice crackers with white bean spread (white beans pureed with olive oil)

Lunch
- Homemade chicken fingers[c]
- Baked sweet potato fries or mashed potatoes made with rice milk and milk-free, soy-free margarine or canola oil
- Carrot and red pepper strips with vinaigrette for dipping (or cooked vegetables oven-roasted in olive oil)
- Enriched alternative milk beverage or commercial hypoallergenic formula

Snack
- Enriched alternative milk beverage or commercial hypoallergenic formula
- Homemade Birthday Brownie

Dinner
- Turkey meatballs in tomato sauce (use a fruit puree to bind the meat and a gluten-free breadcrumb or a dry infant oat or rice cereal as a breadcrumb substitute)
- Brown rice or quinoa pasta with olive oil
- Steamed broccoli florets
- Enriched grain "milk" or commercial hypoallergenic formula
- Fresh peach (or canned peaches packed in own juice)

  This sample menu eliminates milk, egg, wheat, soy, peanut, tree nut, fish, and shellfish. For a strict diagnostic elimination diet, you may choose to substitute the cooked fruits and vegetables for the raw versions. Serving size and texture modifications should be individualized and based on the child's nutritional needs and feeding skills.

[a]Furlong-Muñoz A, editor. The food allergy news cookbook. Nashville, TN: Turner Publishing; 1998.

[b]Hendrix E. Sofie safe cooking: a collection of family friendly recipes that are free of milk, eggs, wheat, soy, peanuts, tree nuts, fish and shellfish. Morrisville, NC: Lulu.com; 2006.

[c]Priem MK. Eight degrees of ingredients. St. Paul, MN: Beaver Pond Press; 2008.

estimated 25% to 35% of otherwise healthy children affected.[38] Eating is a complex, learned process involving the acquisition of physical skills, behaviors, acquired tastes, and feelings about eating and about particular food items. Even mild, self-selective or "picky" eating can affect nutrient intake and, in combination with an allergen elimination diet, can have serious nutritional implications. Assessment of eating competencies will provide the information needed to provide an effective nutrition care plan. See Chapter 32 for more information on management of feeding problems.

Common Allergen Elimination Diets of Early Childhood

The prevalence of food allergy in infants and young children is approaching 10%[39] with the major allergens of early childhood being milk, egg, soy, peanut, and wheat.

Cow's Milk Allergy

Cow's milk allergy is the most common and complex presentation of food allergy in early childhood. The prevalence of cow's milk allergy differs according to the population being studied and also the type of cow's milk allergy involved. The most recent data from Gupta and associates[40] indicate that 1.9% of parents in the United States report cow's milk allergy in the child. This is compared with a food challenge–proven prevalence rate of 0.54% in a European cohort of children[41] and 2.4% in a birth cohort from the United Kingdom.[42] The U.S. data did not include data on non–IgE-mediated versus IgE-mediated cow's milk allergy. The European data and the data from the United Kingdom indicated that the majority of infants born in the United Kingdom had non–IgE-mediated cow's milk allergy, whereas no non–IgE-mediated cow's milk allergy was diagnosed in the Netherlands.

Cow's milk allergy affects predominantly the pediatric population, because approximately 80% of children with cow's milk allergy will eventually develop clinical tolerance. The rate at which tolerance develops depends on the population being studied. The EuroPrevall study[41] indicated that almost 70% of children tolerated cow's milk 1 year after diagnosis (around 2 years of age), including children with both IgE-mediated and non–IgE-mediated cow's milk allergy. U.S.-based epidemiologic studies indicate, however, that milk allergy may persist beyond the first few years of life. One large retrospective study from a specialty clinic reported resolution rates in 807 children with cow's milk allergy and found the rates of resolution were 19% at the age of 4 years, 42% by 8 years, 64% by 12 years, and 79% by 16 years.[43] In a 2013 observational U.S. cohort of 244 infants with cow's milk allergy, 52.5% of patients had resolution of milk allergy at a median age of 62 months and a median age of last follow-up at 66 months.[44] These studies indicate that children with cow's milk allergy may be required to eliminate milk, a nutrient-dense food source, for longer durations throughout childhood.

The nutritional impact of cow's milk elimination in the pediatric population is great because milk is not only a good source of fat, protein, calcium, iodine, and vitamin D but is also the primary source for most young children. Milk also provides vitamin B_{12}, vitamin A, pantothenic acid, riboflavin, and phosphorus. Finding a nutritionally dense substitute for cow's milk in the pediatric diet is essential, and parents of children with cow's milk allergy require detailed advice about nutritionally sound food choices.

Numerous cow's milk allergy guidance documents have been published.[45–47] In 2010 the World Allergy Organization (WAO) Diagnosis and Rationale for Action against Cow's Milk Allergy (DRACMA) guidelines provided recommendations for the treatment of cow's milk allergy.[46] Specific guidance was provided on how long an infant should maintain a substitute milk and what kind of substitute milk is appropriate based on the symptom or food allergic disorder. DRACMA recommends a cow's milk substitute of adequate nutritional value for infants and young toddlers until 2 years of age. Adequate substitutes are identified as either breast milk (with maternal milk avoidance when needed) or a substitute formula, which can be either extensively hydrolyzed formula (eHF) or amino acid–based formula (AAF). Soy formula is not recommended for preterm infants or infants before 6 months of age and has no benefit over hypoallergenic formula in cow's milk allergy.[46,48]

The type of substitute formula recommended may vary based on the age and nutritional needs of the patient, the type of food

TABLE 35.2	Pediatric Formula Recommendations Based on DRACMA Guidelines		
Food Allergy Symptom or Disorder	First Formula Recommendation	Second Formula Recommendation	Third Formula Recommendation
IgE-mediated allergy Low-risk anaphylaxis	Extensively hydrolyzed formula	Amino acid–based formula	Soy formula
IgE-mediated allergy High-risk anaphylaxis	Amino acid–based formula	Extensively hydrolyzed formula	Soy formula
Food protein–induced enterocolitis (FPIES) or proctitis/proctocolitis	Extensively hydrolyzed formula	Amino acid–based formula	—
Eosinophilic esophagitis	Amino acid–based formula	—	—
Heiner's syndrome	Amino acid–based formula	Extensively hydrolyzed formula	Soy formula

DRACMA, Diagnosis and Rationale for Action Against Cow's Milk Allergy[46]; IgE, immunoglobulin E.

allergic disorder, and the degree of severity of the presenting symptoms. Meyer and colleagues[49] published a 2018 review indicating that an AAF, opposed to an eHF, may be indicated in the following instances: (1) when symptoms do not fully resolve on eHF; (2) in the case of faltering growth or failure to thrive; (3) in children who need to avoid multiple foods; (4) when suffering from severe complex gastrointestinal food allergies; (5) in children diagnosed with eosinophilic esophagitis (EoE); (6) in children diagnosed with FPIES (although the international consensus guidelines for FPIES indicate that either eHF or AAF can be used[18]); (7) in cases with severe eczema, particularly if not responding to optimal topical treatment; and (8) in infants who are symptomatic while breastfeeding, even though this may occur only in the vast minority of cases. See Table 35.2 for substitute pediatric formula recommendations based on DRACMA guidelines.

Transitioning an infant from a complete formula to cow's milk is typically considered around 1 year of age or, ideally, when at least two-thirds of the total daily caloric intake comes from a varied solid food diet because a wide variety of foods is more likely to contribute to macronutrient and micronutrient adequacy. However, other criteria for the infant with cow's milk allergy must be considered because the milk elimination diet may not be nutritionally equivalent to the diet that is not restricted and the enriched alternative beverage (i.e., soy, tree nut, seed, other legume or grain-based "milks") may not provide comparable nutrition. Alternative mammalian milks, such as goat's or sheep's milk, are also not suitable because homologous proteins and the strong risk for cross-reactivity.[50]

For children with concomitant milk and soy allergy, enriched nut and grain milks may provide a good source of calcium and vitamin D, but they provide essentially no protein and are low in fat. Therefore, protein requirements will need to be met entirely through the solid food diet before switching to these enriched beverages. Fat intake will also need to be assessed, and additional fat in the form of vegetable oils may be required. It is often the case that a 1-year-old child is not capable of meeting protein and fat needs exclusively through the solid food diet; therefore, maintaining the child on a hypoallergenic commercial formula or breast milk, as recommended in DRACMA guidelines, certainly may be warranted. Rice beverage is also very low in protein (1g/8 oz) and fat and has the added risk for higher inorganic arsenic content; therefore, it is not a good substitute for cow's milk in a young child. Soy and pea protein beverages have greater protein

content and may be appropriate if tolerated, but an individualized approach is recommended.

The nutritional impact of milk allergy is great because milk is an excellent source of protein, calcium, vitamin D, phosphorus, vitamin A, vitamin B_{12}, and riboflavin. Possible alternative dietary sources for these nutrients can be found in Table 35.3.

Egg Allergy

Eggs contribute protein, vitamin B_{12}, riboflavin, pantothenic acid, biotin, and selenium in the diet. Many foods supply the nutrients found in eggs. Eggs in the diet do not usually account for a large proportion of daily dietary intake, and therefore the nutrients lost through egg avoidance are not significant if the allergy stands alone and the diet is otherwise varied.

Egg is a common ingredient in many recipes, such as baked goods, casseroles, and meat-based dishes such as meatballs, meatloaf, and breaded meats. Learning to replace egg in the diet will help families continue to enjoy traditional foods. On a practical level, providing egg-free baked products such as cupcakes or muffins may ensure that the child consumes these foods more readily when a baked egg challenge is indicated. Many commercial egg substitutes actually contain egg protein and therefore are not suitable for those with egg allergy, although egg-free replacers for baking are available. A free downloadable cooking handout from the CoFAR food allergy education program (http://www.cofargroup.org) will help families learn how to substitute for egg in their favorite recipes.

Baked Milk and Egg Tolerance

It has been shown that as many as 70% of patients with milk and egg allergy tolerate extensively heated (baked) milk and egg ingredients.[51,52] Heating milk and egg ingredients generally decreases protein allergenicity by destroying conformational epitopes.[53] The introduction of extensively heated milk and egg to the diet of those who tolerate baked milk and egg ingredients can improve the nutritional quality of the diet and decrease the strain and burden of strict avoidance, and extensively heated milk and egg may represent an alternative approach to oral immunomodulation. Kim and colleagues introduced baked milk into the diets of children who were baked milk tolerant yet reactive to unheated milk. Children who incorporated baked milk into the diet were 16 times more likely to become tolerant to

TABLE 35.3	Nutrients Provided by Milk and Milk Products and Alternative Dietary Sources
Nutrients in Cow's Milk	**Alternative Sources**
Macronutrients	
Dietary protein	Commercial formula, meat, fish, poultry, egg, soybean or enriched soy beverage, peanut, other legumes, tree nuts
Dietary fat	Commercial formula, vegetable oils, milk-free margarine, avocado, meats, fish, poultry, peanut, tree nuts, seeds
Micronutrients	
Calcium	Commercial formula, enriched alternative "milk" beverage (soy, rice, almond, coconut, oat, potato), calcium fortified tofu, calcium fortified juice
Vitamin D	Commercial formula, enriched alternative "milk" beverage, fortified milk-free margarine, fortified eggs, liver, fish liver oils, fatty fish (salmon)
Vitamin A	Retinol: Liver, egg yolk, fortified milk-free margarine. Carotene: Dark green leafy vegetables, deep orange fruits and vegetables (broccoli, spinach, carrots, sweet potatoes, pumpkin, apricot, peach, cantaloupe), enriched alternative "milk" beverage
Pantothenic acid	Meats, vegetables (broccoli, sweet potato, potato, tomato products), egg yolk, whole grains, legumes
Riboflavin	Dark green leafy vegetables, enriched and whole grain products
Vitamin B12	Meat, fish, poultry, egg, enriched alternative "milk" beverage, fortified cereals, nutritional yeast

unheated milk compared with a comparison group of children (P <.001) who continued strict avoidance of milk ingredients.[54] Children who incorporated baked egg into the diet were 14.6 times more likely than children in the comparison group (P <.0001) to develop regular egg tolerance, and they developed tolerance earlier (median 50.0 versus 78.7 months; P <.0001).[55] However, a 2017 systematic review (including six studies) could not confirm an accelerated immune tolerance profile with baked milk and egg ingestion.[56]

Although the patients who tolerate baked egg and milk ingredients can have a more liberalized diet, there are additional complexities in avoidance. For instance, a cake may have baked milk or egg ingredients in the cake and unbaked ingredients in the frosting or filling. Flavorings on crackers or chips may be topically applied after the item is baked. Other products such as quiche may have

too much milk or egg protein to be tolerated. A general guideline is to allow only the amount of baked ingredient to which the patient has been shown to be tolerant (based on physician-supervised OFC). Although there are no data to critically evaluate the practice, in the Nowak-Węgrzyn and colleagues' baked milk and egg studies,[51] commercial products were successfully included in the diet that contained baked egg or milk ingredients as long as these ingredients were not listed as the first or second ingredient. Generally, commercial products such as plain cookies or breads that carry a precautionary statement do not need to be avoided but a soy yogurt or vegan cheese for instance may carry the risk for cross-contact with a fresh milk ingredient, so caution is still warranted.

More recently, milk "ladders" have been used to introduce milk in children with mild to moderate non–IgE-mediated cow's milk allergy at home.[57] It is currently unclear if baked milk and egg should be introduced in the diets of children with FPIES or EoE. The practice of using the baked milk and egg ladder approach in children with IgE-mediated CMA[58] and egg allergy[59,60] is gaining acceptance in the United Kingdom but not currently practiced in the United States because of safety concerns.

Wheat Allergy

The child with wheat allergy must avoid all wheat-containing foods, resulting in the elimination of many processed and manufactured products, including bread, cereal, pasta, crackers, cookies, and cakes. Wheat is also commonly used as a minor ingredient in other commercial food products, such as condiments and marinades, cold cuts, soups, imitation seafood, soy sauce, some low or nonfat products, hard candies, licorice, and jelly beans. Wheat contributes carbohydrates as well as many micronutrients such as thiamin, niacin, riboflavin, iron, and folic acid. Whole grain wheat products also contribute fiber to the diet. Alternative dietary sources of these nutrients should be provided. Four servings of wheat-based products, such as whole grain and enriched cereals or breads, generally provide greater than 50% of the Recommended Dietary Allowance/Adequate Intake (RDA)/AI) for carbohydrate, iron, thiamin, riboflavin, and niacin for children 1 year of age and older, as well as a significant source of vitamin B6 and magnesium. Elimination of wheat products from the diet has great nutritional impact when nutrient-dense alternatives are not provided. Alternative sources for the nutrients found in wheat can be found in Table 35.4.

Many alternative flours are available to patients with wheat allergy, including rice, corn, oat, arrowroot, potato, sorghum, soy, barley, buckwheat, rye, amaranth, millet, teff, and quinoa. It has been reported that 20% of individuals with one grain allergy may be clinically reactive to another grain; therefore, use of alternative grains should be individualized and based on tolerance as determined by the patient's allergist.[48] Alternative flours (grain, vegetable, legume, seed, or nut) may improve the nutritional quality, variety, and convenience of the wheat-restricted diet. Many of these flours are commercially available for home use, and there is also a broad array of gluten-free products available that may be suitable for the patient with wheat allergy. Choosing those made from enriched or whole grains will improve the nutritional quality of the diet.

Soybean Allergy

Soybean/soy protein is an ingredient in a surprising variety of manufactured products. Eliminating many manufactured foods

TABLE 35.4	Nutrients Provided by Wheat and Alternative Dietary Sources	
Nutrients Provided by Wheat	**Alternative Dietary Sources**	
Macronutrients		
Carbohydrates	Products made with alternative grains: Amaranth, buckwheat, corn, millet, oat, rice, sorghum, teff, quinoa; fruits, vegetables, legumes	
Fiber	Fruits, vegetables, alternative whole grain products, legumes, nuts seeds	
Micronutrients		
Thiamin	Enriched and whole alternative grain products, nuts, legumes, liver, pork, sunflower seeds	
Riboflavin	Enriched and whole alternative grain products, milk, dark green leafy vegetables	
Niacin	Enriched and whole alternative grain products, meat, fish, poultry, liver, peanuts, sunflower seed, legumes	
Folic acid	Enriched and whole alternative grain products, beef liver, dark green leafy vegetables, legumes, seeds	
Iron	Heme iron: Meat, liver, fish, shellfish, poultry Nonheme iron: Enriched and whole alternative grain products, legumes and dried fruits	

with soy as an ingredient will have an impact on the variety of manufactured products available to those with soy allergy. Highly refined soybean oil is a soy ingredient that is not considered an allergen and does not require labeling as such.[13] Studies show that the vast majority of soy-allergic individuals can tolerate soy lecithin, although soy lecithin must be labeled as an allergen, causing confusion to patients and families.[15] Products containing soy lecithin, with a "Contains soy" statement, may in fact be safe for consumption by most patients with soy allergy if soy lecithin is the only soy ingredient listed and no vague ingredients are listed. However, if a vague ingredient term such as "natural flavoring" is listed, families should not assume that the product is safe without first calling the manufacturer to determine whether any soy ingredient other than soy lecithin is contained in the product. Although soy itself is a nutritionally dense food, it generally is not a major component of the diet, and therefore the nutrients lost because of soy elimination may be easily replaced. However, if a family mainly relies on commercially available foods, this could have a profound effect on food and nutrient intake. If there are other food allergies or dietary patterns such as a vegetarian diet, the child with soy allergy may be at nutritional risk.

Peanut Allergy

Peanut allergy affects approximately 1.4% to 4.5% of children worldwide.[39,61] Avoidance of peanuts in the diet does not necessarily pose any specific nutritional risk when there are no other nutritional risk factors. Approximately 20% of young children with peanut allergy may eventually develop clinical tolerance, and therefore ongoing assessment is recommended. A 2019 review eloquently discusses the issues around peanut avoidance.[62]

Children with peanut allergy are at greater risk for tree nut allergies, and previously patients with peanut allergy were advised to avoid all tree nuts because of the risk of coallergy and the risk for cross–contact with peanuts during processing. However, a study from the United Kingdom indicated that about 30% to 40% of peanut and tree nut allergic individuals are not sensitized to other tree nuts and tolerate them in their diets.[11] In a retrospective case series from the United States, Couch and colleagues[63] found the majority of individuals with a peanut allergy or specific tree nut allergy passed OFCs to other tree nuts even when sensitized. Furthermore, development of tree nut allergy has been reported in sensitized but tolerant individuals after exclusion from the diet.[64] The British Society for Allergy and Clinical Immunology (BSACI) guidelines now recommend active inclusion of "nonallergic" nuts in diets of individuals with tree nut allergy, once tolerance has been ascertained.[65,66] There has been a clear shift toward recommending timely introduction of tolerated nuts with continued intake.[67] There are now many tree nuts and specific tree nut products that are manufactured in dedicated facilities, and therefore inclusion of these nuts in the diet is possible when tolerated.

Cosensitization between peanuts and legumes is very high; however, clinical cross-reactions are rare, with only about 5% of those with a peanut allergy reacting to another legume. However, the legume lupine (lupin) appears to carry a greater risk of cross-reactivity with peanut, in particular Ara h 1, and it also cross-reacts with other legumes, so caution is warranted.[11] In recognition of the risk for cross-reactivity with peanut and the risk for having a primary allergy to lupine, the European Union and the United Kingdom have included lupine as a major allergen, with products containing lupine or its derivatives requiring full disclosure on E.U. and U.K. product labels. Lupine is not, however, considered a major allergen in the United States, Canada, or Australia.[13]

Fruit and Vegetable Allergies

The definitions of oral allergy syndrome (OAS) and pollen-fruit allergy syndrome are distinct in Australia and Europe. OAS describes any oral symptoms after oral exposure to an allergen; pollen-fruit allergy syndrome is the clinical entity in which symptoms, predominantly OAS, occur after exposure to plant foods that contain allergens of structural similarity to pollen, such as grass and trees.[68,69] Pollen-fruit allergy syndrome also has been used broadly to describe cross-reactivity with pollens leading to oral and generalized symptoms.[70]

The terms *oral allergy syndrome* and *pollen-fruit allergy syndrome* are used synonymously in the United States. OAS, also called pollen food allergy syndrome, is a secondary IgE-mediated allergy that is due to cross-reacting, homologous proteins between pollens and raw food proteins in fruits, vegetables, spices, and nuts. These proteins are easily denatured during initial stages of digestion, and therefore the cross-reactive proteins are active mostly in the oral cavity, leading to symptoms primarily localized to the oropharyngeal area. Generalized symptoms have occurred, but this is the exception rather than the rule; symptoms of OAS tend to be mild.[70,71] Additionally, the cross-reactive proteins are heat labile, so cooked versions of trigger foods are typically tolerated without symptoms. For foods that are mostly eaten raw, briefly microwaving to maintain the fruit structure has been reported to be enough to denature trigger proteins; most particularly with Bet v 1 in apple. The increased prevalence of allergic rhinitis and OAS in recent years, along with advances in identification of relevant allergenic proteins, have led to a better understanding of the diverse associations characterizing OAS.

There is no consensus guideline for the management of OAS, and therefore management of OAS is variable among practicing physicians, with some physicians recommending avoidance of entire botanical groups and others recommending avoidance only of those foods triggering symptoms.[72] In one study of 23 individuals with OAS to peach, 63% reported symptoms to more than one Prunoideae fruit,[73] and another study of 26 individuals with fruit allergy reported that 46% had reactions to more than one Rosaceae fruit.[74] As in other areas of food allergy, clinical reactivity to one member of a botanical family does not mean reactivity to all foods in a botanical family, and overrestriction can lead to poor nutritional quality of the diet. Additionally, OAS symptoms can be very specific to one variety of a fruit. For example, Granny Smith apples tend to trigger more OAS symptoms than Fuji apples. The distribution of allergen is also not uniform throughout the fruit. Much higher concentrations are found in the skin (of apples and peaches, for instance) compared with the pulp. In one small study, over 40% of individuals with allergies to apple and pear were able to tolerate the flesh, but had symptoms on ingestion of the whole fruit.[75]

Allergies to fruits and vegetables also can be a primary allergy caused by lipid transfer proteins (LTP), which are more resistant to heat and enzymatic degradation and more likely to present with both oral and systemic symptoms. Allergy to LTP does not require a primary allergy to pollens. LTP allergens are typically to the Rosaceae family and nuts, seeds, and latex. Previous symptoms to a cooked food,[76] positive skin prick test result to commercial extract (which represents a cooked form of the food),[77] lack of pollen sensitization, positive LTP sensitization,[78] and past systemic reactions to the food increase the risk for future systemic reactions in an individual.

Novel Food Allergens

Novel food allergens such as cricket protein powder, which cross-reacts with shellfish, are beginning to appear in common foods such as protein bars. Other novel food allergens such as commercial foods or tilapia caused by cross-reactions to aeroallergens are increasingly being reported and should be considered during the diagnostic workup and food allergy management plan.[11]

Oral Food Challenges

A child with food allergies may undergo an OFC for diagnostic purposes or to determine whether clinical tolerance to a particular food has been acquired. The individual patient history and the results of skin prick tests, food-specific serum IgE values, and in some cases component resolve diagnostics will determine whether an OFC is appropriate. The type of challenge is determined by the history, age of the patient, and likelihood of encountering subjective symptoms. The food challenge requires evaluation of the patient before the procedure and preparation of the office for the organized conduct of the challenge, for a careful assessment of the symptoms and signs and the treatment of reactions.

During the physician-supervised OFC, the challenge food is administered gradually in incremental doses.[79] The patient is observed for symptoms during the procedure and for a period after the full test dose is administered. Challenges can be open, single-blind, or double-blind. Although the utility of the double-blind, placebo-controlled food challenge (DBPCFC) as the gold standard for food allergy testing is acknowledged, the NIAID Food Allergy Guidelines noted that open or single-blind challenges also could be acceptable for food allergy evaluation when the challenge outcome is negative or when objective symptoms are elicited that

recapitulate the reaction history.[36] Regardless of the type of food challenge, emergency medications should be available, and an emergency treatment protocol should be in place.

A number of primary documents are available for the practicing allergist or immunologist to guide the administration of the physician-supervised OFC.[79,80] In 2012 the American Academy of Allergy, Asthma & Immunology (AAAAI) and the European Academy of Allergy and Clinical Immunology (EAACI) jointly published a consensus report on standardizing the DBPCFC, which is part of the PRACTALL initiative.[79] In 2020, AAAAI Adverse Reactions to Foods Committee published a comprehensive guide to conducting physician-supervised oral food challenges, which is an update to the 2009 OFC Workgroup report[80] and an additional document for conducting OFCs to peanut in infants.[81] These documents offer in-depth, practical guidance and should be used by practicing allergists and immunologists to ensure that safe and scientifically sound challenge procedures are conducted.

Conclusions

Current management of food allergy entails dietary avoidance of the identified allergen, requiring extensive education (Box 35.2). Allergen elimination diets should not be prescribed lightly, and

---

the global impact of these diets should be considered. In theory, elimination of dietary allergens may seem an easy enough task, but avoidance issues are complex and accidental ingestions are not uncommon. Thus, food allergy management must also include comprehensive education on how to recognize and treat a food allergic reaction. This topic is discussed fully in Chapter 44.

The reference list can be found on the companion Expert Consult website at http://www.expertconsult.inkling.com.

36

Prevention of Food Allergy

JENNIFER KOPLIN, KATRINA ALLEN

KEY POINTS

- The rise in food allergy is more rapid than genetic deviation would allow, and the current consensus is that environmental factors integrally linked to the modern lifestyle are likely to be key drivers of this phenomenon. The concept that these factors might be modifiable is supported by studies demonstrating that food allergy is more common in developed than developing countries, and the risk appears to be highest in migrants from developing to developed countries.
- There is now strong evidence from randomized controlled trials and a systematic review of randomized trials that delayed introduction of peanut and egg in the infant diet increases the risk of allergy to these foods, with stronger evidence of effect for peanut. In response to this research, updated expert guidelines around the world now call for allergenic foods to be introduced in the first year of life to reduce the risk of developing food allergy.

- There is also emerging evidence that the early immunomodulatory effects of microbial exposure (including through indoor pet ownership and siblings) and nutritional patterns (including breastfeeding and specific nutrient optimization such as vitamin D) are important determinants of the risk of early-onset inflammatory diseases such as allergic disease, including food allergy.
- At present there is no clear evidence that prebiotics, probiotics, or hydrolyzed formula prevent food allergy. Although "breast is best," insufficient data currently exist to support the hypothesis that breastfeeding is protective against food allergy.

Introduction

Allergic diseases have become the most common chronic diseases of childhood as part of a shifting profile of disease in modern societies. An epidemic of food allergy has emerged, particularly in the last 10 to 15 years. For good reason, we have described this as the "second wave" of the allergy epidemic.[1] This phenomenon appears to be still evolving in many regions, and it is unclear why it has occurred decades after the "first wave" of asthma and respiratory allergy reached a peak in industrialized countries.

There is concern that this growing early predisposition for the allergic phenotype may portend a greater burden of later onset allergic diseases such as asthma and allergic rhinitis and contribute to an escalating burden of inflammatory disease in this new generation. The parallel increase in many other immune diseases and inflammatory noncommunicable diseases strongly suggests broader immunologic effects of modern risk factors on human health.[2] In this context, allergy may be regarded as the most common and earliest manifestation of the vulnerability of the immune system to modern environmental change. Strategies to improve early immune health may therefore not only prevent allergic disease but also ultimately reduce the burden of other inflammatory diseases.

Because the rise in food allergy is more rapid than genetic deviation would allow, the current consensus is that environmental

factors integrally linked to the modern lifestyle are likely to be key drivers of this phenomenon. The concept that these factors might be potentially modifiable is supported by studies demonstrating that food allergy is more common in developed than in developing countries, and the risk of food allergy increases with migration to higher risk countries.[3,4]

Factors associated with a modern lifestyle include a myriad of changes to our level of public health, including improved sanitation, secure water supplies (with associated decreased prevalence of *Helicobacter pylori* infection), widespread use of antibiotics and increasing rates of immunization, improved nutrition, decreased helminthic infestation, improved food quality (and presumably less microbial load in the food chain), and generally improved nutrition and associated obesity. These factors might work individually or in concert to effect a failure in the development of oral immune tolerance in the first year of life, when development of immunoglobulin E (IgE)-mediated food allergy is most likely to occur. In addition, there is likely to be at least some component of gene-environment interaction. Thus, lifestyle factors may have a differential effect depending on genetic status of the individual.

Although the exact reasons for the rise in food allergy remain unclear, studies have shown that some food allergy can be prevented. In infants with early eczema or egg allergy, who are at high risk for developing peanut allergy, timely introduction of peanut into the infant diet reduces the risk of peanut allergy.[5] Randomized controlled trials also collectively suggest a reduction in egg allergy with early egg introduction, although the protective effect appears less pronounced compared with early peanut introduction.[6] These interventions are discussed further in the following section.

The Importance and Timing of Early Intervention

This new epidemic of food allergy is most striking in preschool children, particularly in the first year of life. In some high-income countries such as Australia, more than 20% of 1-year-old infants now have evidence of food sensitization and more than 10% now have challenge-proven IgE-mediated food allergy.[7] It is not yet clear whether intervention measures to promote immune health and prevent allergic disease more generally need to be targeted prenatally or will be equally effective if administered postnatally. There is evidence that an atopic predisposition has declared itself by the time of birth in at least some infants; however, food allergy phenotypes cannot be declared until postnatally. Although it is clear that the development of specific food allergies such as peanut allergy can be prevented in some individuals through interventions in the first year of life, the protective effects of these interventions so far appear to be allergen specific.[8]

Antenatal Intervention

During pregnancy there is close immunologic interaction between the mother and her offspring, providing enormous opportunities to influence fetal immune development. The placenta and the fetus are vulnerable to a wide range of exogenous and endogenous maternal influences. Contrary to traditional concepts, human fetal T cells are responsive as early as 22 weeks' gestation.[9] There appear to be emergent differences in immune function at birth in newborns destined to develop allergy,[10–12] indicating that the scene is set to some extent by birth. This highlights the importance of considering a broad range of immunomodulatory factors that may begin to have their effects much earlier in pregnancy than previously suspected. Notably, most of the environmental factors implicated in the development of allergic disease (including microbial exposure, dietary factors, cigarette smoke, and other pollutants) have been shown to influence fetal immune function and contribute to an increased risk of subsequent allergic disease. Moreover, there is also preliminary evidence that each of these has been associated with epigenetic effects, including activation or silencing of immune-related genes through epigenetic modifications.[13,14]

Postnatal Intervention

The early postnatal period also appears to be critical in the development of oral tolerance. Events in the gastrointestinal tract are vitally important for normal immune maturation. After birth we encounter a vast array of new antigenic proteins in relatively high amounts. Most of this foreign antigenic load is derived from colonizing commensal bacteria and food components. We have to learn very quickly to distinguish the harmful ones on a large scale. To prevent inflammatory responses to largely harmless antigens, gastrointestinal-associated lymphoid tissue (GALT) has evolved complex mechanisms to promote tolerance as a default response.[15] The human intestines harbor between 10 and 100 trillion resident microbiota, and this vast and complex ecosystem forms gradually over the first years of life. The collective genetic material of these bacteria (called the *microbiome*) is estimated to contain 150 times more genes than our human genome.[16] Through co-evolution and established "mutualism" the microbiota play an essential role in homeostasis of multiple interconnected host metabolic and immune functions.[17]

The success of oral tolerance appears to depend on a number of oral exposures. Although the best known of these is breast milk, optimal microbial diversity (still an ill-defined concept) and other dietary immunomodulatory factors, including prebiotics (soluble fiber), fat-soluble vitamins (including vitamin D), and polyunsaturated fatty acids (PUFAs), may all have important antiinflammatory effects.[18] There is also some evidence to suggest that both the gastric acid milieu[19] and a window of opportunity of optimal allergenic solids introduction are potential factors for oral tolerance development.

Timing of Exposure to Allergenic Foods

Modifying the age at which allergenic foods such as egg and peanut are introduced into the infant diet is currently the only strategy that has been convincingly shown to prevent food allergy in randomized controlled trials. The first of these trials, the Learning Early About Peanut allergy (LEAP) study was published in 2015 and appropriately hailed as a landmark development in peanut allergy prevention.[5] This study showed that introduction of peanut into an infant's diet from 4 to 11 months of age led to an approximately 80% reduction in peanut allergy compared with peanut avoidance until 5 years of age in a high-risk group of infants. The trial randomized 640 infants with severe eczema or egg allergy, a population at increased risk for developing peanut allergy, to either peanut avoidance for 5 years or regular peanut consumption commencing from 4 to 11 months of age and then evaluated infants for peanut allergy at the age of 5 years. Egg allergy was defined as either a skin prick test (SPT) wheal size of 6 mm or greater with no history of previous egg tolerance or a history of reaction to egg plus an SPT wheal of 3 mm or greater. Severe eczema was defined as either SCORing Atopic Dermatitis (SCORAD) grade of 40 or greater, parental description of very bad rash, or frequent need for topical corticosteroids or calcineurin inhibitors. SPTs to peanut were performed before randomization, and those with a wheal size greater than 4 mm (10.6% of potentially eligible infants) were excluded because of a higher risk of preexisting peanut allergy.

Emerging evidence is showing a potential benefit of earlier introduction of other allergenic foods for food allergy prevention, in particular moderate evidence of a protective effect of early egg introduction at 4 to 6 months of age. This evidence was comprehensively examined in a 2016 systematic review.[6] In response to these findings, updated expert guidelines now recommend that allergenic foods be introduced in the first year of life (from as early as 4–6 months of age) to reduce the risk of developing food allergy. U.S. guidelines specifically targeting peanut allergy prevention recommend introduction of peanut at 4 to 6 months of age for infants with severe eczema, egg allergy, or both.[20] Guidelines published from the peak allergy body in Australia, the Australasian Society for Allergy and Clinical Immunology (ASCIA), recommend that solid foods should be introduced at around 6 months of age, but not before 4 months, and egg and peanut should be included in the first year of life.[21]

Protection from developing food allergy may also depend on the amount and frequency of allergen consumed; however, the evidence base on the amount of allergen exposure required in infancy to prevent the development of food allergy is extremely limited. The dose of peanut recommended by current U.S. guidelines for children at high risk is based on the amount of peanut consumed by 75% of children in the peanut consumption group in the LEAP trial. These recommendations are for 6 to 7 g of peanut per week over three or more feedings[20] and would require three feedings of 2 tsp of peanut butter each per week or similar. It is not clear how long this should continue—in LEAP, this regular peanut consumption continued to 5 years of age for the early peanut introduction group. LEAP achieved good adherence with the protocol through intensive contact with participants that would not be available to parents outside of a trial setting. The proportion of parents of high-risk infants in the United States who meet these specific recommendations has not yet been measured. Currently no evidence indicates whether sporadic peanut consumption throughout infancy is also effective in preventing peanut allergy or whether there is a particular threshold dose and frequency of peanut that needs to be achieved to provide protection. If the latter, additional strategies are likely to be required to ensure that parents, particularly those with infants at high risk, are able to meet these recommendations. Similarly, there is little evidence to guide recommendations around frequency and quantity of exposure for other allergenic foods in infancy.

Finally, although timely introduction of allergenic foods into the infant diet is a promising intervention for food allergy prevention, reversing the "epidemic" of childhood food allergy will require more than earlier introduction of allergenic foods. Some models estimate a maximum population reduction in peanut allergy achievable with timely peanut introduction of around 40% to 60%.[22] Earlier introduction of egg and cow's milk is expected to have a lower impact on the prevalence of allergies to these foods,[6] and currently no evidence exists as to whether and to what degree early introduction of other allergenic foods such as tree nuts will aid in preventing allergies to these foods. Additional prevention strategies are therefore clearly needed, and several trials are currently underway investigating other interventions as described later.

Breastfeeding

It is universally agreed that human milk should be the first and most important source of nutrition for the infant. It contains a vast array of bioactive factors, including hormones, growth factors, neuropeptides, and antiinflammatory and immunomodulatory agents that influence many physiologic systems and promote normal gut colonization for both short-term and long-term benefits.[23]

Allergens are normally secreted in breast milk and appear to be an important early source of exposure.[24,25] This may actually be important in initiating, maintaining, and reinforcing normal tolerance to foods.[26] Although this has been demonstrated in animals, human evidence is limited because randomized controlled trials of breastfeeding versus not breastfeeding are difficult from an ethical point of view. Systematic analysis of observational studies on the protective effect of breastfeeding has shown conflicting results, and many of the studies included were conducted decades ago when food allergy was uncommon and methods of assessment were limited.[27] An early review by Muraro and colleagues,[28] including 15 observational and 14 interventional studies, concluded that breastfeeding for at least 4 months was associated with a reduced cumulative risk of cow's milk allergy in high-risk infants over 18 months of age. None of these studies was either randomized or

prospective, and most systematic reviews since have failed to find a specific beneficial effect on food allergy.[29,30] In this regard, some, albeit limited, evidence exists that continued breastfeeding during the period when complementary foods are initiated may promote tolerance and have protective effects.[31] Even so, some expert bodies recommend that breastfeeding should continue while solids are introduced into the diet, although strong scientific evidence that it plays a role in the prevention of allergic disease is both lacking and unlikely to be available because of the unethical aspects of randomization trials that would need to include a "no breastfeeding" arm.[32]

Formula Feeding

There has been significant interest in the use of modified infant formulas, especially partially hydrolyzed cow's milk formula (PHF) and extensively hydrolyzed cow's milk formula (EHF), for prevention of early childhood allergic disease. Intense expectations from families with a history of allergy seeking readily available primary prevention interventions have been responded to by industry with the development of a range of allergy prevention formulas. Furthermore, expert bodies have felt the need to provide recommendations regarding the use of formula for prevention of allergies.

In the past, infant feeding guidelines in Europe, the United States, and Australia recommended that hydrolyzed formula could be considered as primary prevention therapy for allergic diseases. These guidelines were informed by a Cochrane review in 2006[33] that supported the use of hydrolyzed formula for the prevention of allergy especially in high-risk infants who are unable to be completely breastfed, although the authors themselves recommended further larger trials because of the methodologic concerns and inconsistency of the findings of the studies included in the review. An update of the Cochrane review in 2018 found no evidence to support short-term or prolonged feeding with a hydrolyzed formula compared with exclusive breastfeeding or cow's milk formula for prevention of allergic disease.[34] The review reported very-low-quality evidence suggesting that short-term use of an EHF compared with a cow's milk formula may prevent infant cow's milk allergy, but recommended further trials before implementation of this practice. A 2016 report from the U.S. National Academies of Sciences, Engineering and Medicine also concluded that studies on the effects of partially or extensively hydrolyzed infant formulas for preventing food allergies are inconsistent or have methodologic flaws, and that high-quality randomized clinical studies would be needed before these formulas could be recommended for food allergy prevention.[35]

Timing of First Solids

Along with age at introduction to specific allergenic foods, the association between timing of first introduction of solid foods and food allergy also has been investigated. There have been dramatic changes to timing of solid introduction over time. In the 1960s infants were typically given solid foods in the first 3 months of life, but the 1970s saw the introduction of guidelines recommending delayed introduction of solids until after 4 months of age because of a perceived link between early introduction of gluten and celiac disease.[36] By the late 1990s, expert bodies had begun to recommend delaying solids until after 6 months of age, with further delay in the introduction of allergenic foods such as egg and nuts until at least 2 years of age recommended for infants with a family history of allergy in some guidelines.[37] This did not, however, appear to have the desired effect of reducing the prevalence of food allergy, and in 2008 a lack of evidence of a protective effect led to the removal of advice to delay the introduction of any foods beyond 4 to 6 months of age.

In a large observational cohort study in Melbourne, Australia, we found no relationship between timing of introduction of solid foods and challenge-confirmed egg allergy at 1 year of age.[38] Solid foods in this cohort were predominantly introduced between 4 and 6 months of age, with only 4% introducing solids before age 4 months and 5% after 6 months; thus, an effect of very early or late introduction of solids cannot be ruled out. A 2019 systematic review also found no evidence of an association between age at introduction of complementary solids, defined as before or after 4 months of age, and food allergy.[39]

Vitamin D

The hypothesis that low vitamin D may increase the risk of food allergy[40] is supported by two lines of ecologic inquiry. First, there is a strong latitudinal prevalence gradient, with countries further from the equator (and thus lower ambient ultraviolet radiation) recording more admissions to hospital for food allergy–related events[41] and more prescriptions for epinephrine autoinjectors for the treatment of anaphylaxis.[41,42] These findings appear to be independent of longitude, physician density, or socioeconomic status. Second, season of birth may play a role; children attending emergency departments in Boston with a food-related acute allergic reaction were more likely to be born in autumn or winter, when vitamin D levels reach their nadir, than spring or summer,[43] and there are similar links to birth seasonality in the Southern Hemisphere.[41]

Vitamin D could influence the onset and resolution of food allergy via several plausible mechanisms. The vitamin D receptor is widely expressed in the immune system, including T cells, in particular promoting the expression of interleukin 10–secreting T regulatory cells crucial to maintaining immune tolerance[44] and, potentially, playing a key role in the induction of tolerance in food-allergic individuals.[45] Vitamin D metabolites also contribute to innate epithelial defenses by stimulating production of antimicrobial proteins such as cathelicidins[46,47] and defensins.[48]

We showed that Melbourne, the most southern major city in Australia, has the highest reported prevalence of documented infantile food allergy in the world, with more than 10% of a population sample of 1-year-old infants having challenge-proven IgE-mediated food allergy.[7] In a separate study, we have shown that, compared with the northern states, children residing in Australia's southern states are six times more likely to have peanut allergy at age 6 years and twice as likely to have egg allergy than those in the northern states.[49] Finally, increasing vitamin D insufficiency in Melbourne over the last 20 years,[50] paralleling the rise in food allergy, is supported by data showing that 20% of pregnant women have insufficient vitamin D.[40,51]

Using the Healthnuts population-based study we found that infants of Australian-born parents, but not of parents born overseas, with vitamin D insufficiency (<50 nM/L) were more likely to be peanut (adjusted odds ratio [aOR] 11.51, 95% confidence interval [CI] 2.01, 65.79, P = .006) and/or egg (aOR 3.79, 95% CI 1.19, 12.08, P = .025) allergic than those with adequate vitamin D levels independent of eczema status.[52] Among those with Australian-born parents, infants with vitamin D insufficiency were more likely to have multiple (≥2) than single food allergies (aOR 10.48, 95% CI 1.60, 68.61 versus aOR 1.82, 95% CI 0.38, 8.77, respectively). In contrast, a case-control study (n = 274), also

conducted in Australia, did not find an association between early vitamin D status (at birth or age 6 months) and later food allergy at the age of 1 year.[53] To date there has been only one small trial of maternal vitamin D supplementation for food allergy prevention. No trials have examined vitamin D supplementation in infants.[54] Randomized controlled trials assessing the potential role of infant vitamin D supplementation in the prevention of food allergy are currently underway.[55]

Modulation of the Maternal and Infant Microbiome

The intestinal microbiota plays a critical role in healthy immune development and programming. Early microbial diversity, beginning in utero, is a major driving factor[56] in the normal maturation of both T helper cell type 1 (T_H1) cells[11] and regulatory T (T_{REG}) lymphocyte function[57] and suppressing the propensity for T_H2 allergic responses in early childhood.[12] Alterations in intestinal microbial composition during early life have been associated with an increased risk of food allergy[58,59] and sensitization.[60] Furthermore, these alterations precede the development of food sensitization, suggesting a potential causal role.[61]

Multiple studies have explored whether supplementation with probiotics or prebiotics to modulate the infant intestinal microbiota can prevent allergic diseases; however, few high-quality randomized controlled trials have been conducted specifically looking at food allergy outcomes. The most consistent finding has been protection from eczema. A 2015 systematic review and meta-analysis found that probiotics administered prenatally and/or postnatally reduced the risk of eczema,[62] whereas there were limited studies evaluating probiotics for prevention of food allergy.

There has also been interest in using prebiotic fiber to promote favorable colonization and reduce inflammation. In humans, prebiotic fiber selectively stimulates growth of beneficial gut microbiota, particularly bifidobacteria but also lactobacilli,[63] in a dose-dependent manner. Prebiotic fermentation products, short-chain fatty acids, have direct antiinflammatory effects.[64] This promotes intestinal integrity and reduces systemic endotoxin and antigenic load in experimental models. Acetate, butyrate, and propionate are among the most abundant short-chain fatty acids and play a critical role in local and systemic metabolic function and stimulating regulatory immune responses.[65] A 2017 systematic review reported that prebiotic supplementation to infants reduced the risk of food allergy (relative risk [RR] 0.28, 95% CI 0.08–1.00)[66]; however, the authors caution that the certainty of these estimates is very low because of risk of bias in the trials and imprecision of results. There were no studies evaluating prebiotic supplementation to mothers during pregnancy or breastfeeding that met the inclusion criteria.

In summary, at present there is insufficient evidence to recommend supplementation with probiotics or prebiotics to prevent food allergy.

Skin Barrier and Eczema

A history of eczema in infancy, particularly early infancy, has been consistently recognized as a strong risk factor for developing food allergy. Up to 50% of infants with moderately severe early-onset eczema (within the first 3 months) develop challenge-proven food allergy by the age of 1 year.[67] This population-based observation also has been noted in clinical populations. Eczema genes such as filaggrin (*FLG*) have been suggested to be important determinants of food allergic disease. A multisite study of peanut allergy found that *FLG* null mutations were associated with a significantly increased risk of peanut allergy; however, history of eczema and sensitization status was not available for all infants, so the impact of *FLG* on these outcomes could not be assessed independently of food allergy.[68] In the Healthnuts study, we found that *FLG* null mutations were associated with food sensitization (but not food allergy over and above that risk) independent of eczema status.[69] This suggests that there could be a different pathogenesis for food sensitization and food allergy. That is, the epidermal barrier dysfunction resulting from filaggrin deficiency might lead to food sensitization regardless of clinical eczema status, but filaggrin-induced skin barrier dysfunction might not play a further role in the progression to food allergy from sensitization.

These results are consistent with the dual allergen hypothesis proposed by Gideon Lack.[70] This hypothesis proposes that early cutaneous exposure to food protein through a damaged skin barrier leads to sensitization and allergy and that early oral exposure to food allergen induces tolerance. Expanding on this hypothesis, filaggrin deficiency might provide a mechanism for the development of sensitization, but a second factor (or factors), either environmental or genetic (or both), may be important for converting food-sensitized infants to food allergic status. This two-step hypothesis is also consistent with the findings of the LEAP study, described previously, which show that peanut allergy can be prevented in some peanut-sensitized infants through early peanut introduction.[5] Several studies currently underway aim to prevent the development of food allergy by improving skin barrier and function in early life.[71]

Targeting and Individualizing Prevention Strategies: Considering Phenotypic, Environmental, and Genotypic Risk

The effectiveness of any preventive intervention is likely to vary with both genetic and environmental factors. Just as concepts of individualized precision medicine are being explored for disease treatment, prevention strategies also may ultimately need to be tailored according to the context, conditions, and other factors determining risk. This requires a better understanding of both the genetic and environmental determinants of allergic risk, which are likely to be extremely variable and complex, and raises a series of issues that will become increasingly relevant as technologies evolve, including how to target interventions, how to identify specific groups at risk, and how to refine strategies according to the level of risk.

At present there are no good prenatal markers of genetic risk apart from family history, which remains a common predictor of allergic disease in use. This is crude and imperfect with variable specificity (48%–67%) and sensitivity (22%–72%) and a positive predictive value generally less than 40%.[72–75] Because there are many and diverse genetic determinants of allergy, predicting risk through genotyping is not yet possible.[76] In the meantime there have been attempts to identify early predictive biologic markers; however, currently none of these has any established predictive value.

A better understanding of the genetic predispositions existing to food allergy will lead to the determination of whether a rise in food allergy is occurring asymmetrically between high-risk and

• BOX 36.1   Clinical Pearls

1. Earlier introduction of peanut in the infant diet has been shown to reduce peanut allergy risk in a randomized controlled trial in infants at high risk, and expert guidelines now recommend introduction of peanut into the infant diet in the first year of life, particularly for infants with preexisting risk factors for peanut allergy (eczema or egg allergy).
2. Other current allergy recommendations are that infants should be introduced to solids around the age of 4 to 6 months irrespective of family history risk and that other allergenic solids do not need to be avoided by infants when solids are introduced or by mothers when breastfeeding or lactating.
3. At present the use of prebiotics, probiotics, or hydrolyzed formula cannot be recommended as a food allergy prevention strategy.
4. Although breastfeeding is recommended for the multiple benefits it provides for infants, currently insufficient data exist to support the hypothesis that breastfeeding is protective against food allergy.

low-risk groups. There is evidence that Asian populations may be more susceptible to allergic disease when living in westernized environments. Earlier studies of respiratory disease observed that both allergic symptoms and sensitization were more common in Asian Australians than in non–Asian Australians.[77] Rates were also higher in Australian-born Asians than in Asian immigrants, in whom the prevalence increased with length of stay in Australia. The Healthnuts study found challenge-confirmed food allergy was three times more common in infants with parents born in East Asia compared with those with parents born in Australia.[4] This increased risk appears to have occurred in a single generation, because the prevalence of reported allergic disease was similar or even lower in Asian-born parents compared with Australian-born parents. Furthermore, we showed in a separate study that children born in East Asia who subsequently migrated to Australia in early life were protected against food allergy.[78] These findings suggest a strong genetic propensity that is amplified by a western environment. This is consistent with earlier work indicating evolutionary differences in genetic polymorphisms affecting candidate genes.

Conclusions and Future Directions

Recent years have seen substantial progress in understanding risk factors for food allergy. Although reasons for the rise in food allergy remain incompletely understood, we can now recommend interventions to prevent some children from developing food allergies (Box 36.1). Earlier introduction of allergenic foods, particularly peanut, in the infant diet is currently the most promising intervention for food allergy prevention and has been shown in clinical trials to prevent peanut allergy in some infants at high risk. This is, however, only the first step. Preventing allergy in future generations will require dissemination of advice to introduce peanut early and monitoring of its uptake in the general population. Finally, the impact of earlier peanut introduction on population prevalence of allergy needs to be measured to determine real-world effectiveness. It is also becoming clear that a substantial proportion of childhood food allergy will not be preventable through timely introduction of allergenic foods into the infant diet alone. Additional prevention strategies are needed, and several novel intervention strategies for food allergy prevention, including infant vitamin D supplementation and moisturizing infants to improve skin barrier are currently being tested in rigorous, high-quality clinical trials that will be completed in the next 5 years. There is increasing recognition that cost-effectiveness of new prevention strategies needs to be considered before their implementation, and several of these trials will include a cost-effectiveness analysis. As the results of these trials become available, we hope that strategies that are both efficacious and cost-effective will be revealed and subsequently implemented in the general community. As new prevention strategies are implemented, continuous monitoring at the population level will show whether these strategies are effective in a real-world setting and will allow refinement of these strategies where necessary to optimize food allergy prevention.

The reference list can be found on the companion Expert Consult website at http://www.expertconsult.inkling.com.

37

Immunotherapeutic Approaches to the Treatment of Food Allergy

AMY M. SCURLOCK, WAYNE G. SHREFFLER

KEY POINTS

- Substantial progress in development of active therapies such as oral and epicutaneous immunotherapy has ushered in an exciting new era in food allergy with approval of the first licensed therapy for food allergy and multiple novel approaches in the developmental pipeline.
- Food allergen oral immunotherapy has demonstrated efficacy in promoting immune changes that lead to clinically relevant desensitization in the majority of treated individuals; however, side effects are common and sustained clinical benefits appear to require ongoing antigen exposure.
- Other approaches such as epicutaneous immunotherapy and sublingual immunotherapy have shown generally more moderate clinical and immunologic effects, with typically fewer side effects; further investigation evaluating longer-term outcomes

will inform optimal patient selection and therapeutic application.
- Improved understanding of factors such as biomarkers or patient characteristics that predict successful outcomes after food allergen immunotherapy and the immune mechanisms underlying these outcomes is critical to determining the optimal therapeutic approach for individual patients.
- Enhanced research infrastructure that consistently defines clinical outcomes, regulates data standards, and considers important patient-oriented outcomes will be critical in the coming era of large-scale therapeutic implementation to ensure alignment of therapeutic goals among multiple stakeholders.

Introduction

Food allergy is an immune-mediated disorder with significant medical, psychosocial, and economic impacts on affected individuals and families.[1–4] Food allergy results from immune deviation and a failure to establish oral tolerance to food proteins, resulting in allergic sensitization that leads to clinical allergy.[5] Multiple immune mechanisms have been implicated in development of food allergy, including reductions in regulatory T cell and tolerogenic dendritic cell activity, T helper type 2 (T_H2) cells skewing of the immune response, and T_H2-predominant cytokine production, increased immunoglobulin E (IgE), and elevated mast cell and basophil activation[5,6] (Fig. 37.1).

The standard of care for food allergy is strict dietary avoidance of implicated allergen(s) with ready access to injectable epinephrine and an emergency action plan in case of accidental ingestion.[1,4] Despite its success for other allergic diseases, subcutaneous immunotherapy (SCIT) has not been implemented for the treatment of food allergy because of its unacceptable safety profile in early studies.[7,8] The development of active therapies targeting IgE-mediated food allergy has been the subject of significant clinical and translational research over the past two decades, with

several approaches emerging as promising therapeutic options.[9–12] Presently, oral immunotherapy (OIT) and epicutaneous immunotherapy (EPIT) are the most advanced modalities in the drug-development pipeline, both having completed Phase III clinical trials[9,11,13] (Table 37.1).

Therapeutic outcomes after food allergen immunotherapy have typically been defined using the terms *desensitization* and *sustained unresponsiveness*.[14–17] Desensitization is defined as elimination of clinical reactivity with an increased reaction threshold to a food allergen while on active therapy. Sustained unresponsiveness is defined as elimination of clinical reactivity to a food allergen that persists after a specified period of cessation. Sustained unresponsiveness has been achieved only in a subset of individuals.[18,19] Additional outcomes that have been considered in clinical trials include patient-reported outcomes such as quality of life and reaction severity. Immune tolerance, defined by the U.S. Food and Drug Administration (FDA) as "complete and permanent resolution of clinical response following exposure to any amount of the identified allergenic food" has not been assessed in clinical trials, nor has "field efficacy," defined by the FDA as "the rate and/or severity of reactions to food exposures encountered outside a controlled clinical setting"[17] (Fig. 37.2).

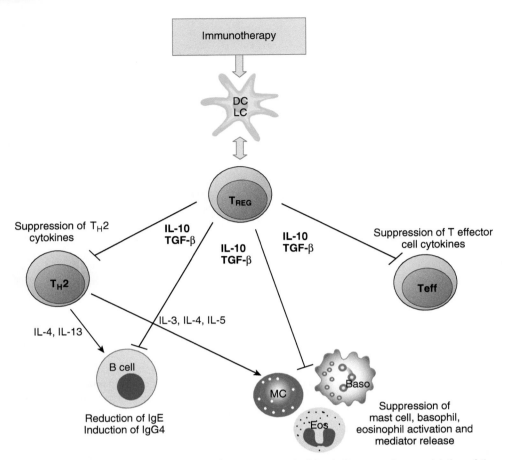

• **Fig. 37.1** Immunotherapeutic approaches for the treatment of food allergy requires modulation of the allergic response to foods through activation of dendritic cells (*DC*), Langerhans cells (*LC*), and regulatory T cells (T_{REG}) with subsequent suppression of a variety of effector cell types. *Baso,* Basophils; *Eos,* eosinophils, *IgG,* immunoglobulin G; *IL,* interleukin; *MC,* mast cells; *Teff,* effector T cell; *TGF-β,* transforming growth factor beta; T_H2, type 2 T helper cells.

TABLE 37.1	Immunologic Changes Immunoglobulin E–Mediated Food Allergy Versus Effective Immunotherapy	
Immune Parameters	**Food Allergy**	**Effective Immunotherapy**
Allergen-specific IgE	Increased	Decreased
Allergen-specific IgG4	Negligible	Increased
Allergen-specific IgA	Negligible	Increased
IgE epitope binding	Variable	Targeted binding
Mast cell and basophil activation	Increased	Decreased
T_H2 cytokines	Increased	Decreased
Regulatory T cell activity	Negligible	Increased

IgE, Immunoglobulin E; T_H2, T helper cell type 2 cell.

This chapter will highlight immunomodulatory approaches to target IgE-mediated food allergy at various stages in the investigative pipeline. To date, no active therapies have achieved the FDA designation for safe use in patients; however, peanut OIT and EPIT have been in Phase III clinical trials and received FDA fast-track designation.[9,11] Refinement of existing approaches to determine optimal dose, duration, age at initiation, and predictors of clinical response and exploration of combination approaches to maximize benefit and minimize side effects are important to continue to advance toward safe and effective therapies for food allergy.

Allergen-Specific Immunotherapy

During the past two decades, clinical trials in food allergy have focused primarily on allergen-specific immunotherapy encompassing three major forms: OIT, SLIT, and EPIT. Each of these forms of immunotherapy is in a different stage of investigation, with similar immunologic targets but with clear differences in the route of administration, antigen dose, and clinical outcomes (Table 37.2).

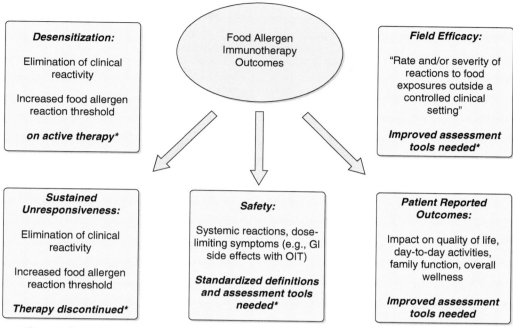

• **Fig. 37.2** Therapeutic outcomes after food immunotherapy have typically been defined in the context of safety and efficacy (desensitization, sustained unresponsiveness); however, standardized assessments of patient-prioritized outcomes and field efficacy will be important as more therapies progress toward broader clinical implementation. *GI,* Gastrointestinal; *OIT,* oral immunotherapy.

TABLE 37.2 Comparison of Allergen-Targeted Immunotherapies in Clinical Trials

Comparison Factors	OIT	SLIT	EPIT
Allergens	Single allergen: Milk, egg, peanut (others: wheat, tree nuts, fish) Multiallergen	Peanut, milk, hazelnut, peach	Milk, peanut
Daily maintenance dose	300–4000 mg	1–10 mg	50–500 mcg
Primary side effects	Oral, gastrointestinal (systemic symptoms associated with infection, exercise, menses)	Oropharyngeal	Skin
Desensitization	Significant effect	Moderate effect	Moderate effect
Sustained unresponsiveness	Effective in subset of patients	Ongoing investigation	Ongoing investigation
Immune modulation	Significant	Present	Present

EPIT, Epicutaneous immunotherapy; *OIT,* oral immunotherapy; *SLIT,* sublingual immunotherapy.

Oral Immunotherapy

OIT is the therapeutic approach with the largest body of evidence in clinical trials for food allergy to date. Early open-label studies demonstrated a beneficial response to OIT for a variety of allergens, such as milk, egg, and fish, with evidence of clinical desensitization in up to 80% of subjects treated.[20,21] Subsequent trials expanded to multicenter, randomized controlled OIT trials that used food proteins as therapies that were bound by FDA regulations for labeling and widespread, safe use in the clinical setting. FDA registered trials are accessible through the National Institutes of Health clinical trials registry (http://www.clinicaltrials.gov).

Randomized, controlled, multicenter clinical trials of OIT have provided valuable efficacy and safety data.[22–28] In a trial of peanut OIT, 28 children (ages 1–16 years) were randomized to receive peanut OIT (maintenance dose = 4000 mg) versus placebo OIT.[28] Peanut OIT treatment was associated with clinical desensitization compared with placebo after 12 months (5000 mg [~20 peanuts] versus 280 mg [~1 peanut], $P < .001$). In another randomized trial, 62% of children (ages 7–16 years) on active OIT could be desensitized to 1400 mg peanut protein (~5 peanuts) after 6 months of OIT at a dose of up to 800 mg compared with none of placebo OIT subjects ($P < .001$).[22] Similar findings were noted during a 6-month milk OIT trial in 20 milk-allergic children (ages 6–21 years) randomized to milk OIT (maintenance dose = 500 mg) compared with placebo OIT when assessing change in reaction threshold at baseline oral food challenge (OFC) compared with 6-month OFC (5100 mg [~160 mL] versus 0 mg, P = .002).[27] Other milk OIT trials in children have shown similar clinical findings.[24–26]

In a study from the Consortium of Food Allergy Research (CoFAR), 55 egg-allergic children (ages 5–18 years) were randomized to egg versus placebo OIT.[23] After 10 months of egg OIT (maintenance dose = 2000 mg), 55% of egg OIT subjects were desensitized to 5 g of egg (~3/4 whole egg) compared with 0% of placebo OIT subjects (5000 mg versus 50 mg; P <.001) and 75% of egg OIT subjects passed a 10 g (~1.5 whole egg) OFC at 22 months. Although further long-term investigation of safety, efficacy, tolerability, and patient-prioritized outcomes is needed, these studies highlight the efficacy of OIT induction of desensitization and treatment-specific immunomodulation.[9,29–32]

Findings from early OIT studies informed the design of larger industry-sponsored trials of a characterized peanut OIT product (AR101) using a standardized dosing protocol. A Phase II clinical trial in eight U.S. centers enrolled 55 peanut-allergic children, adolescents, and adults (with confirmed clinical reactivity during screening peanut double-blind placebo-controlled food challenge at a single maximum dose of 100 mg) to receive peanut OIT using a 300-mg maintenance dose.[10] The primary endpoint was defined as the proportion of subjects who tolerated a cumulative 443-mg exit double-blind placebo-controlled food challenge after 2 weeks of maintenance OIT. Of the peanut-OIT treated participants in the intent-to-treat analysis, 79% tolerated 300 mg posttreatment compared with 19% of the placebo-treated subjects (P <.0001). Study withdrawals were more common in the active treatment group (6/29) versus the placebo group (0/26); one participant in the active treatment group withdrew because of the diagnosis of eosinophilic esophagitis (EoE). In a pivotal Phase III randomized controlled trial of AR101, 554 peanut-allergic subjects ages 4 to 55 years with objective clinical reactivity at a maximum single dose of 100 mg in a screening double-blind placebo-controlled food challenge were randomized 3:1 to active peanut OIT or placebo.[9] The primary endpoint of this Phase III trial was defined as tolerating (with no or mild symptoms) 600 mg or greater single peanut dose in the exit double-blind placebo-controlled food challenge conducted 6 months after reaching the 300-mg maintenance dose; the primary endpoint was met with 67% of the AR101 treated group versus 4% of placebo (P <.0001). Adverse events led to withdrawal in 12.4% of active versus 1.6% of placebo recipients, including one case of documented EoE in the active group.

Several studies have evaluated longer term outcomes of OIT, including sustained unresponsiveness.[19,23,33–35] Many of these studies have been either uncontrolled, open-label studies or open-label extension phases of randomized controlled trials that include years of OIT dosing. In an open-label study of six egg-allergic children (ages 3–13 years), all passed an OFC after 33 months of OIT and introduced egg into their diet.[35] After 5 years of peanut OIT (maintenance dose = 4000 mg), 50% of subjects demonstrated sustained unresponsiveness to 5 g of peanut protein and were considered treatment successes with incorporation of a median of 555 mg/day (range, 0–4000 mg/day) of peanut in their diets approximately 3 days/week.[19] During a 60-week trial of milk OIT compared with milk SLIT, OFCs were performed after 1 and 6 weeks off therapy in subjects demonstrating desensitization at week 60[34]; 10% failed at week 1, and 20% failed at 6 weeks. In the CoFAR egg OIT trial, development of sustained

unresponsiveness increased with extended duration of treatment, with 27.5% noted at 24 months, 47.5% at 36 months, and 55% at 48 months.[23,33] Among subjects on peanut OIT surveyed about duration of treatment effects, none of the treatment successes reported symptoms with peanut consumption after 3 to 4 years.[19] Follow-up of successful milk OIT yielded 22% of subjects reporting limitations with milk consumption because of symptoms, although for various reasons only 20% were ingesting milk on an unlimited basis.[36] Two to three years after completion of egg OIT, 67% of egg OIT subjects, compared with 18.2% of placebo OIT subjects, could consume both baked and concentrated egg.[33] Overall, sustained unresponsiveness is possible in a subset of subjects, but the long-term impact of OIT remains unclear. Varying definitions of the sustained unresponsiveness outcome have been used, and consensus regarding optimal duration off therapy to assess this outcome is lacking. Further, accumulating evidence supports the need for ongoing antigen exposure to maintain therapeutic responses, suggesting OIT should not be considered a "cure" but rather a long-term, continuing therapeutic approach.[13] Indeed, findings from a recently published randomized, double-blind, placebo-controlled, single-center Phase II study of the long-term effects of peanut OIT in children and adults (age 7–55 years) suggested that discontinuation or even reduction in maintenance peanut OIT dose increased the likelihood of regaining clinical reactivity to peanut.[37] Participants were randomized to receive peanut OIT build-up to a maintenance dose of 4000 mg of peanut protein over 104 weeks (2 years) and then discontinue (peanut-0 group, n = 60), decrease to 300 mg peanut protein daily (peanut-300 group, n = 35) or receive placebo dosing (n = 25). When assessing the primary endpoint, the proportion of participants who passed 4000 mg double-blind placebo-controlled food challenge at both 104 and 117 weeks, 21 (35%) of peanut-0 group participants and 1 (4%) placebo group participant passed the 4000 mg challenge (odds ratio [OR] 12 · 7, 95% confidence interval [CI] 1 · 8–554 · 8; P = .0024). When examined at the week 156 double-blind placebo-controlled food challenge, only 8 of 60 (13%) of the peanut-0 group passed the 4000 mg challenge. Sustained unresponsiveness was associated with a higher baseline peanut-specific IgG4/IgE ratio and a lower Arah-2- IgE level and basophil activation response. In the peanut-300 group, the percentage passing the double-blind placebo-controlled food challenge decreased over time, with 13 of 35 (34%) passing the week 156 challenge.

Work from 2017 highlights the potential window of opportunity for early intervention to maximize the therapeutic efficacy of OIT in young children. Investigators evaluated the safety, efficacy, and feasibility of early peanut OIT in 37 children (ages 9–36 months) randomized to either low (300 mg) or high (3000 mg) daily maintenance doses.[38] The primary endpoint, sustained unresponsiveness (SU) 4 weeks after OIT cessation, was achieved in 29 of 37 (78%) in the intent-to-treat analysis (300-mg arm, 17/20 [85%]; 3000 mg, 12/17 [71%]) and 29 of 32 (91%) in the per-protocol analysis, over a median of 29 months. Peanut OIT-treated children were 19 times more likely to successfully incorporate peanut into their diets compared with matched peanut-allergic standard care controls. The Immune Tolerance Network IMPACT trial is evaluating long-term outcomes among peanut-allergic children (ages 1–4 years) in a randomized, controlled 3-year peanut OIT trial; sustained unresponsiveness is evaluated 6 months after cessation of therapy in treated individuals who pass a desensitization challenge on therapy, and analyses are forthcoming. (http://www.clinicaltrials.gov NCT01867671).

To date, the majority of studies have evaluated single-allergen OIT approaches; however, multiallergen OIT has shown promise in initial trials and is the subject of ongoing investigation to address the complex needs of multifood-allergic individuals. Investigators delivered multiallergen OIT to participants (ages 4–25 years) sensitized to up to five foods (N = 25 subjects) compared with those peanut monoallergic (N = 15) and reported that multiallergen OIT could be delivered with safety and efficacy similar to those of single-allergen OIT.[39] Participants received either single-allergen peanut OIT (maximum daily maintenance dose 4000 mg) or multiallergen OIT using up to five allergens (peanut, tree nuts, sesame, milk, and egg; maximum maintenance dose 4000 mg per allergen). Treated subjects demonstrated a 10-fold increase in their reaction threshold; individuals receiving single-allergen peanut OIT achieved this outcome a median of 14 weeks earlier than the multiallergen OIT group. Although the majority of reactions were mild, two severe reactions requiring epinephrine were observed in each group. Successful multifood desensitization was observed in a Phase I trial that paired pretreatment with omalizumab with subsequent rush multiallergen OIT to multiple foods.[40] A subsequent double-blind, single-center, controlled trial randomized 48 participants (age 4–15 years) with multiple OFC-confirmed food allergies to receive multiallergen OIT (two to five foods) paired with omalizumab or placebo; 12 subjects were included as nonrandomized, untreated controls.[41] Participants receiving multiallergen OIT combined with omalizumab passed 36-week OFC at a significantly greater proportion than placebo (30/36, 83% omalizumab treated versus 4/12, 33% placebo) and had fewer OIT-associated adverse events. The sustainability of treatment response after omalizumab-facilitated multiallergen OIT was evaluated in a Phase II randomized controlled, multicenter trial including 70 participants (age 5–22 years) with multiple OFC-confirmed food allergies.[42] After 16 weeks of omalizumab paired with two- to five-allergen OIT during weeks 8 to 30, participants were then randomized to discontinue OIT or to receive 300-mg or 1000-mg maintenance doses followed by a 2-g OFC to at least two foods at week 36. Findings suggested that after omalizumab-facilitated multiallergen OIT, desensitization was best sustained by continued maintenance dosing versus discontinuation.

Immunologic changes associated with clinical findings after successful OIT have been compelling. Single-allergen OIT has been associated with beneficial immunomodulatory effects, including reduced basophil and mast cell activation, down-regulation of T_H2 effector cells and cytokine production, and initial increased T regulatory cell activity and reduced IgE antibodies with increased IgG4 antibodies.[19,23,27,28,34,43–45] Some of these changes after peanut OIT, in particular those related to basophil activation, are antigen specific, but some are also associated with nonspecific stimuli, including evidence of basophil suppression after anti-IgE stimulation or after nonspecific antigen (e.g., egg) stimulation.[45] Peanut OIT also has been shown to increase antigen-induced regulatory T (T_{REG}) lymphocyte function and intracellular interleukin 10 (IL-10) levels and decrease in Foxp3 methylation, an indicator of T_{REG} cell suppressive function.[44] After long-term peanut OIT, treatment successes were associated with reduced peanut specific IgE (sIgE), Ara h 1 and Ara h 2, and skin prick tests (SPTs) compared with treatment failures, parameters that were predictive of outcomes.[19] Low-baseline sIgE levels were predictive of treatment success for desensitization in both milk[46] and egg[47] OIT studies, but not predictive of success in the multicenter CoFAR egg OIT study.[23] Analysis of IgE

and IgG4 binding epitopes before and after milk[48] and peanut[49] OIT identified reduced IgE binding and increased IgG4 binding with overlap of key binding epitopes associated with response to therapy; however, in some individuals, significant discordance indicates that antigen-nonspecific changes may also play a role.[49] Additional mechanisms that are the subject of ongoing investigation include allergen sIgA, component resolved analysis, and elimination of pathogenic versus induction of "anergic" CD4+ T_H2 phenotypes.[50–52]

The potential therapeutic benefits of OIT must be carefully considered in light of the potential for adverse, potentially treatment-limiting events (Box 37.1). Although OIT has demonstrated clinical efficacy, meta-analyses highlight the fact that insufficient data exist for full efficacy assessments and safety concerns persist (Box 37.2).[29,31,32,53–56] Generally, OIT-associated side effects in treatment trials are mild to moderate, predominantly oropharyngeal, and easily treated[23,27,28,57,58]; however, more severe reactions have been reported. Currently, the highest rate of adverse events related to OIT occurs during the first year of therapy, with up to approximately 10% to 15% of subjects withdrawing, often because of gastrointestinal (GI) side effects.[18,19,23] During blinded peanut OIT,[28] symptoms were noted in most active treatment subjects compared with placebo treated subjects. During OIT, approximately 45% of active subjects compared with approximately 10% of placebo subjects experienced dose-associated symptoms, primarily mild and oropharyngeal, but with approximately 1% requiring epinephrine.[27,28] During the first year of blinded egg OIT, 75% of 11,860 OIT doses were symptom free versus 96% of 4018 placebo doses.[23] During years 3 and 4, 95% of OIT doses were symptom free (Box 37.3).[59]

Studies incorporating omalizumab pretreatment for 12 to 16 weeks before milk or peanut OIT demonstrated enhanced safety with reduced side effect profiles, shortened time to maintenance therapy, and higher tolerated OIT dose but no significant change in clinical efficacy outcomes.[60,61] When milk OIT and omalizumab were combined, investigators found that a baseline basophil activity threshold of less than 40% was associated with lower clinical symptoms during OIT, and those with higher basophil reactivity at baseline had fewer symptoms when omalizumab was combined with milk OIT.[62] Further, a combination of lower baseline basophil reactivity and lower sIgE ratios was associated with attainment of SU after treatment, indicating that early biomarkers may predict OIT outcomes. EoE has been associated with peanut OIT despite treatment with omalizumab.[63] To better understand risk factors for peanut OIT-associated side effects, investigators evaluated adverse events in 104 participants in three peanut OIT trials.[64] The authors reported that 80% of participants experienced adverse events, with 42% having systemic symptoms and 49% having GI symptoms; 20% dropped during the study, half because of GI symptoms. Asthma and allergic rhinitis predicted systemic symptoms, and higher SPT wheal size was predictive of GI adverse events. Viral infections, menses, and exercise have been associated with lowering the reaction threshold for patients on stable OIT dosing[65] and often require dose adjustments in the face of acute illness. Additionally, EoE has been reported in association with OIT, adding potential risks for a subset of children (see Box 37.3).[66]

Sublingual Immunotherapy

SLIT employs sublingual delivery of a daily dose of allergen in liquid concentrate or tablet that is held in place for a couple minutes, then spit or swallowed.[67] SLIT involves the use of smaller doses than OIT, typically starting with microgram amounts, advancing incrementally over the course of months to maintenance doses in the 1- to 10-mg range, that are generally continued for multiple years of therapy. Mechanistically, SLIT is thought to take advantage of tolerogenic antigen-presenting cells in the oral mucosa, with further benefit thought to be derived from exposure to the food protein in the intact form before proteins are subjected to gastric digestion.[68] Initial published reports of SLIT for food allergy demonstrated clinical efficacy in individuals with kiwi, hazelnut, and peach allergy.[69–73] SLIT studies have expanded to include both pediatric and adult patients with milk or peanut allergy. In a 6-month, open-label study of eight children (age older than 6 years) with cow's milk allergy, milk SLIT led to an increase in the mean volume of milk that elicited allergy symptoms from 39 to 143 mL.[74] In a study of 30 milk-allergic children (ages 6–17 years), milk SLIT was compared with milk OIT in a two-center study.[34] Participants were randomly assigned to receive SLIT

alone (7 mg) or SLIT followed by OIT at two different doses (1 or 2 g) during 60 weeks of immunotherapy. At the end of the study, 1 of 10 SLIT-only participants achieved desensitization to 8 g of milk protein, and 6 of 10 participants in the lower dose SLIT plus OIT group and 8 of 10 patients in the higher dose SLIT plus OIT group achieved desensitization. Overall, SLIT in combination with OIT was associated with more robust clinical benefits than SLIT alone; however, systemic side effects occurred only in the SLIT plus OIT groups with higher levels of antihistamine and epinephrine usage. Symptoms reported with milk SLIT were limited to the oropharynx.

The first randomized controlled trial of peanut SLIT was performed in a single-center study of 18 children (ages 1–11 years) receiving 12 months of SLIT (maintenance dose = 2 mg daily) with peanut or placebo.[75] At the conclusion of 1 year of treatment, those receiving peanut SLIT were able to safely consume 1710 mg (~8 peanuts) of peanut protein, compared with only 85 mg (<0.5 peanut) in those receiving peanut SLIT (P = .011), representing a 20-fold increase in peanut consumption. During dosing, side effects were minimal and localized to the oropharynx, noted in 11.5% of peanut SLIT subjects compared with 8.6% of placebo SLIT subjects. Symptoms were typically untreated, and no participant required epinephrine during treatment. Immunologic changes were noted in peanut SLIT subjects compared from baseline to OFC at 12 months, including decreased peanut sIgE (P = .003), SPT size (P = .02), basophil activation (P = .009), and IL-5 levels (P = .015), with increase in peanut sIgG4 (P = .014). A subsequent multicenter study from CoFAR of 40 peanut-allergic patients (ages 12–40 years) evaluated the efficacy of peanut SLIT versus placebo SLIT.[76] Treatment success was defined during OFC when 5 g of peanut protein was consumed or when a 10-fold or higher increase in peanut protein consumption was achieved when comparing baseline to follow-up OFC. After 44 weeks of therapy (target maintenance dose = 1386 mcg), 14 (70%) of 20 subjects who received peanut SLIT compared with only three (15%) of 20 subjects who received placebo SLIT demonstrated treatment success—primarily greater than a 10-fold increase in eliciting dose over baseline challenge. The median dose of peanut consumed at the 44-week OFC compared with baseline OFC was significantly higher for peanut SLIT subjects (371 mg [~1 peanut] versus 21 mg, P = .01) compared with placebo SLIT subjects (146 mg versus 71 mg, P = .14). When evaluation took place at week 68 the mean consumed dose rose to 996 mg, which was significantly higher than at week 44 (P = .05). For the 12 of 17 placebo subjects who crossed over to higher dose SLIT (target maintenance dose = 3696 mcg) and completed a 5-g OFC, the median consumed dose was higher than at baseline OFC (603 mg versus 71 mg, P = .02). Although the results were encouraging, none of the subjects treated with low-dose or high-dose SLIT could consume the full 5-g OFC during the desensitization phase. Peanut SLIT was well tolerated, with 95% of subjects on these doses being symptom free when local oropharyngeal symptoms were excluded. Clinical outcomes were associated with modest immunologic changes, including reductions in basophil activation and modest changes in titrated skin tests. No significant changes were noted in peanut sIgE or sIgG4 levels. Both of these trials met inclusion criteria for a 2017 meta-analysis finding a statistically significant effect for desensitization favoring SLIT versus placebo (25/31 active versus 3/27 placebo; relative risk [RR], 7).[77]

A 3-year long-term follow-up study of the CoFAR peanut SLIT cohort reported a "modest level of desensitization" with favorable safety outcomes.[78] However, despite a favorable safety profile, very few subjects in this adolescent and adult cohort continued therapy for the full 3 years. Dose-related symptoms after a year on therapy did not appear to be the primary cause of early study discontinuation; indeed, the most common reasons given for early withdrawal included "participant decision" or nonadherence. Although not formally assessed in this trial, the potential concerns leading to cessation of SLIT included difficulty of maintaining daily therapy, mild oral discomfort, lack of perceived response to therapy, lifestyle issues, and interference with daily activities. Sustained unresponsiveness was observed in a small subset of 4 of 37 subjects (10.8%).

In a small randomized trial directly comparing peanut SLIT to peanut OIT, the median cumulative threshold dose among participants completing treatment increased approximately 20-fold with SLIT and more than 300-fold with OIT.[79] There was no difference between groups in the proportions of subjects who achieved desensitization, defined as minimum 10-fold increase in posttherapy threshold. SLIT-treated individuals had fewer systemic reactions than OIT-treated subjects, and withdrawal rates for SLIT were lower than for OIT. A retrospective comparison study of peanut-allergic children treated with either peanut OIT or SLIT indicated that after 12 months of therapy patients who received SLIT reacted at lower eliciting dose thresholds and were less likely to pass food challenges evaluating desensitization.[80] Thus, available evidence for milk and peanut allergy suggests that SLIT therapy is less effective than OIT for desensitization but has a better safety profile.[34,79,80] In one study, investigators treated children ages 1 to 11 years with peanut SLIT (2 mg peanut/day) observing that 37 of 48 subjects completed 3 to 5 years of treatment, with 67% (32/48) successfully consuming 750 mg or more during double-blind placebo-controlled food challenges and 25% (12/48) passing a 5-g challenge without clinical symptoms.[81] Of the 12 subjects who passed the 5-g challenge, 10 demonstrated sustained unresponsiveness after cessation of therapy for 2 to 4 weeks. Ongoing SLIT studies in younger age groups and using different SLIT delivery systems will help define the best application of SLIT for food allergy in the future.

Epicutaneous Immunotherapy

Epicutaneous immunotherapy uses an allergen-containing patch to deliver antigen for uptake by the epidermal layer of skin activating Langerhans cells that subsequently traffic to regional lymph nodes and promote regulatory immune responses.[82–86] Multiple preclinical studies of EPIT for food allergy in murine models supported effective antigen delivery, beneficial immunomodulation, and treatment outcomes that supported further clinical trials in milk and peanut allergy.[83,84,87]

To date, EPIT clinical trials conducted for food allergy have employed the Viaskin platform developed by DBV Technologies (Paris, France). This technology consists of a small adhesive patch that has been electrostatically coated with allergen and is applied to the upper arm or interscapular space. The first study conducted was a 3-month double-blind, placebo-controlled pilot study in milk-allergic infants and children (3 months to 15 years).[88] Nineteen subjects were randomized to treatment with milk or placebo EPIT applied at 48-hour intervals during 3 months of treatment (using the Diallertest device, a precursor to Viaskin). The cumulative dose of cow's milk consumed during OFC (baseline versus 3 months) trended higher in the milk EPIT group (1.77 ± 2.98 mL versus 23.61 ± 28.61 mL) compared with the placebo group (4.36 ± 5.87 mL versus 5.44 ± 5.88 mL) (P = .13). Adverse events were higher

among milk EPIT-treated subjects compared with placebo treatment and were limited to mild skin reactions at the patch site and increased risk for local eczema (OR 8.20; 2.72–24.5; P <.001).

Since completion of the milk EPIT pilot study in children, the focus of clinical trials has shifted primarily to evaluation of safety and/or efficacy of peanut EPIT. A Phase Ib safety trial conducted at five clinical sites in the United States randomized 100 peanut-allergic participants (ages 6–25 years), categorized as severe and nonsevere based on reaction history to treatment with placebo Viaskin or four different doses of peanut Viaskin patches administered over 2 weeks of therapy.[89] The peanut Viaskin proved safe and convenient up to a dose of 250 mcg for children and up to 500 mcg in adolescents and adults. Overall, 2 of 80 active EPIT and 1 of 20 placebo EPIT subjects dropped out because of adverse events; 90% experienced mild or moderate local symptoms, and systemic symptoms were mostly mild and transient, with no severe reactions and no epinephrine use.

A large randomized controlled Phase IIb trial (the Efficacy and Safety of Several Doses of Viaskin Peanut in Adults and Children With Peanut Allergy [VIPES] trial) enrolled 221 highly peanut-allergic individuals (ages 6–55 years) in 22 centers in the United States and Europe, for a 1-year treatment comparison of placebo versus peanut EPIT.[12] Individuals reacting to an eliciting dose of 300 mg or less of peanut protein at the screening double-blind, placebo-controlled food challenge were randomized 1:1:1:1 to receive placebo or one of three EPIT doses (50, 100, or 250 mg). The primary endpoint was the proportion of treatment responders at the 12-month exit double-blind, placebo-controlled food challenge, defined as either a 10-fold improvement in eliciting dose compared with baseline or an eliciting dose of 1000 mg or greater of peanut protein. The absolute difference in the response rates between the 250-mg patch and the placebo patch was 25% (95% CI, 7.7%–42.3%; P = .01; number needed to treat, 4). In secondary analyses, effects were found to be strongest in the 6- to 11-year-old group, whereas no differences between active and placebo were seen in adolescents or adults. Treatment-related adverse events occurred twice as often with active treatment (95% versus 48%), mostly skin-related, and there were no serious related adverse events, but one moderate episode of anaphylaxis was deemed possibly related.

A multicenter randomized controlled trial was published by COFAR investigators evaluating the safety and efficacy of the Viaskin peanut patch in children and young adults, ages 4 to 25 years.[90] After 52 weeks of treatment, peanut EPIT was associated with modest desensitization and immunologic changes when the 100 mcg and 250 mcg doses were compared with placebo EPIT (P = .003), with the greatest response noted in younger children ages 4 to 11 years compared with those older than 11 years (P = .003). Peanut EPIT was well-tolerated, with an overall favorable safety profile; adherence to therapy approached 97%, with the majority reporting only mild skin irritation at the patch site. In a Phase III double-blind placebo-controlled trial conducted at 31 sites in 5 countries, 356 peanut-allergic children aged 4 to 11 years without a history of severe anaphylaxis and who developed objective symptoms to 300 mg or less of peanut protein during the screening double-blind placebo-controlled food challenge were randomized 2:1 to receive 250 mcg active or placebo patch.[11] The primary endpoint of the study was the proportion of treatment responders at the 12-month exit double-blind placebo-controlled food challenge, defined as either 300 mg or greater eliciting dose in those with baseline eliciting dose of 10 mg or less, or an eliciting dose of 1000 mg or greater in those with baseline eliciting dose of more than 10 mg. Response rates were 35.6% in the active group and 13.6% in the placebo group ($P <.0001$), for a between-group absolute difference of 21.7% (95% CI, 12.4%–29.8%). However, the primary endpoint of the study was not met, because the lower bound of the 95% CI around this between-group difference did not exceed the prespecified minimum of 15%. Ongoing studies evaluating longer term treatment outcomes will provide further insight into the role of EPIT in treatment of food allergy.

Extensively Heated Foods as Oral Immunotherapy

Use of extensively heated (baked) milk and/or egg allergen has been investigated as a potential treatment option that mirrors allergen immunotherapy. Clinical trials performed in milk-allergic[91] and egg-allergic[92] children have demonstrated that approximately 70% to 80% of milk-allergic or egg-allergic children can safely ingest baked milk or egg products because of disruption of conformational epitopes by heating. Daily consumption of one to three servings of baked allergen products was safe and associated with accelerated tolerance development and immunomodulation compared with age-matched controls.[92-94] In patients with IgE-mediated egg allergy who passed physician-supervised OFCs to extensively heated egg (e.g., muffin) and incorporated these foods into their diet, continued consumption of heated egg protein was associated with decreased skin test size, reduced egg allergen specific IgG4 (sIgG4) levels and increased IgG4 levels.[95] Additional questions remain regarding the best way to identify those patients tolerant of baked milk or egg, the effective dose required, the degree of heating needed, the role of the food matrices, and the ability of heated proteins to induce lasting tolerance. In a retrospective study, investigators reported the outcomes of 84 baked milk OFCs performed in a food allergy referral clinic, observing that 72% were baked milk–tolerant and 12% of all individuals challenged (42% of reactors) had mild anaphylaxis that responded to in office medications and did not require prolonged monitoring beyond the 2-hour observation period.[96] Milk sIgE levels were higher in reactive patients, and SPT wheal size was similar in baked milk–tolerant and reactive subjects. To maximize safety and minimize risk, assessment of baked milk or egg tolerance requires supervised challenges in a clinical setting with an allergist who is skilled in the identification and management of food allergic reactions.

"Next-Generation" Therapies for Food Allergy

Several immunomodulatory therapies are under investigation as single agents or adjunctive treatments to synergize with allergen-targeted immunotherapy using novel therapeutic approaches.

Biologic Therapies

Multiple biologic therapies are the subject of investigation for treatment of food allergy either alone or in combination with allergen-specific approaches such as OIT (see Table 37.2). Omalizumab, a recombinant, humanized, monoclonal anti-IgE antibody, is FDA approved for the treatment of allergic asthma and chronic urticaria. The first clinical trial of anti-IgE for peanut allergy used a novel antibody, TNX-901, to demonstrate efficacy in increasing the reaction threshold to peanut during OFC from 178 mg to 2805 mg.[97] However, approximately 25% of subjects were nonresponders. A second multicenter, randomized, controlled trial using omalizumab to treat peanut allergy was initiated in 26 subjects, but was stopped prematurely because of safety issues during baseline OFCs.[98] Fourteen subjects randomized to receive omalizumab or placebo during 20 to 22 weeks of treatment completed OFC assessment before study discontinuation. The dose threshold of peanut flour at 1000 mg or greater was noted in 44% of omalizumab-treated subjects compared with 20% of placebo-treated subjects, but over half of the subjects did not reach the 1000-mg threshold, leaving unanswered questions about efficacy.

Omalizumab treatment before and during OIT has shown benefits in reducing side effects and shortening build-up dosing time to maintenance therapy during a trial of 11 subjects treated with milk OIT[99] and during a trial of 13 children treated with peanut OIT.[100] Both studies report lower overall side effect profiles during build-up and maintenance dosing. Additionally, omalizumab pretreatment in both studies reduced the time interval of OIT build-up phase to maintenance therapy by several months compared with other studies employing OIT alone. In a Phase I study of 25 children and adults with multifood allergy, 16-week pretreatment with omalizumab was used to advance multiallergen OIT over weeks rather than months, with 94% of dosing reactions reported as mild and only one subject reported to have a severe allergic reaction.[40] Investigation using omalizumab pretreatment for 12 to 16 weeks before milk or peanut OIT has demonstrated improved safety, reduced side effects, shortened time to maintenance therapy, and higher tolerated OIT dose but no significant change in clinical efficacy outcomes.[60,61] When milk OIT and omalizumab were combined, investigators found that a baseline basophil activity threshold of less than 40% was associated with lower clinical symptoms during OIT and those with higher basophil reactivity at baseline had fewer symptoms when omalizumab was combined with milk OIT.[62] Further, a combination of lower baseline basophil reactivity and lower sIgE ratios were associated with attainment of SU after treatment, indicating that early biomarkers may predict OIT outcomes. EoE has been associated with peanut OIT despite treatment with omalizumab.[63] New studies are currently assessing the role of omalizumab combined with OIT in randomized, controlled multicenter trials, and FDA Breakthrough Therapy Designation has been granted for omalizumab for the prevention of severe allergic reactions after acute accidental food allergen exposures.

In addition to targeting IgE, there is great interest in studying alternative biologic therapies involving other molecules involved in the allergic response; many of these therapies have been licensed for other allergic disorders. IL-33 is a cytokine that acts upstream of IgE to induce B cell class switching; ANB020 is an experimental monoclonal anti–IL-33 antibody that has been shown to suppress IL-33 function for approximately 3 months after a single dose.[101] A Phase II placebo-controlled trial of ANB020 in adults with peanut allergy is in progress (NCT02920021). Phase II clinical trials with dupilumab (anti–IL-4ra) as either monotherapy (NCT03793608) or an adjunct to peanut OIT (NCT03682770) are currently enrolling. Other molecules such as anti–IL-5 (mepolizumab, reslizumab), IL-5R (benralizumab), tezepelumab (anti-TSLP, AMG157/MEDI-9929), anti–IL-13 (QAX576), and anti–IL-9 (MEDI528) could have potential roles in targeting the relevant immune responses in food allergy; however, further investigation for alternative indications is required (Fig. 37.3 and Table 37.3).

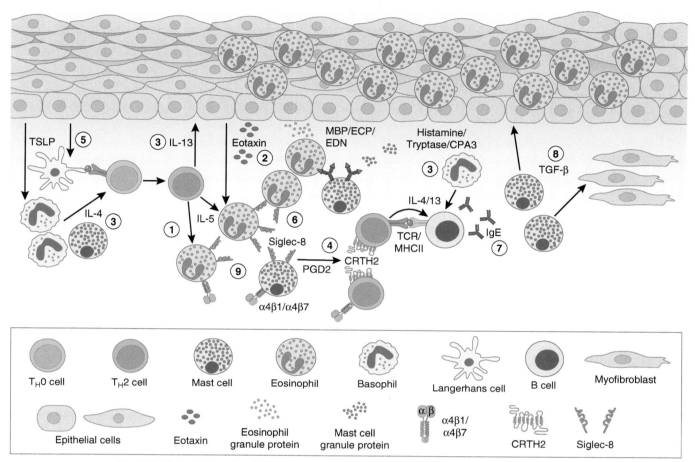

• **Fig. 37.3** Biologic therapies for food allergy have potential to modulate the food-specific immune response through targeting multiple cytokine and cell signaling networks. Some of these potential targets are currently under investigation in food allergy. The numbers in the figure represent potential target immune pathways for biologic immunomodulatory therapies for food allergy. *CPA3*, Carboxypeptidease A3; *CRTH2*, chemoattractant receptor-homologous molecule expressed on T_H2 cells; *ECP*, eosinophil cationic protein; *EDN*, eosinophil-derived neurotoxin; *IgE*, immunoglobulin E; *IL*, interleukin; *MBP*, myelin basic protein; *MHCII*, major histocompatibility complex II; *PGD2*, prostaglandin D2; *Siglic*, sialic acid–binding immunoglobulin-type lectin; *TCR*, T cell receptor; *TGF-β*, transforming growth factor-beta; T_H2, T helper cell type 2 cell; *TSLP*, thymic stromal lymphopoietin.

Modified Proteins

Modified allergen immunotherapy uses recombinant technology to alter the host response to modified allergenic proteins. Based on positive findings from a peanut mouse model using heat-killed *Escherichia coli* (HKE) in combination with modified Ara h 1, Ara h 2, and Ara h 3 proteins (HKE-EMP123),[102,103] a Phase I clinical trial using HKE-EMP123 delivered rectally was conducted in 5 nonallergic adults and 10 peanut-allergic adults.[104] In peanut-allergic subjects, 50% had significant allergic reactions preventing further dosing (30% required epinephrine), whereas healthy controls tolerated the treatment, suggesting that future application of this approach requires further refinement of the allergen modification, dose, or route of administration.

Other approaches using modified allergens are currently under investigation. A Phase I study assessing the safety and tolerability of incremental doses of a chemically modified, aluminum hydroxide–adsorbed peanut extract, aluminum hydroxide adsorbed modified peanut extract (HAL-MPE) administered by subcutaneous injection is in progress in U.S. and Canadian studies of

peanut-allergic adults (NCT02991885). Another approach uses synthetic peptides representing T cell epitope sequences from Ara h 1 and Ara h 2 delivered by intradermal injection (PVX108), with the goal of promoting tolerogenic T cell responses; because this product has minimal IgE binding, these tolerogenic responses are theoretically induced with minimal risk for acute anaphylactic reactions, and further study is ongoing.[105]

DNA Vaccines

DNA vaccines are a novel strategy to target peanut allergy, with a product ASP0892 (http://www.clinicaltrials.gov NCT02851277) currently under investigation in human trials. DNA encoding the peanut allergens Ara h 1 and Ara h 3 is inserted into a single plasmid containing the coding sequence for lysosomal-associated membrane protein (LAMP); after uptake by antigen-presenting cells, a peanut allergen–LAMP fusion protein is synthesized, which is hypothesized to promote T_H1 predominant responses.[106]

| TABLE 37.3 | Current and Potential Biologic and Immunomodulatory Therapies for Food Allergy |

Target	Role in Pathogenesis	Approved Indications	Clinical Trials for IgE-Mediated Food Allergy	Clinical Trials for Other Allergic Indications	Agents	Notes
IgE	FcεRI-crosslinking, "antigen focusing"	Asthma, CIU	Phase II	Allergy prevention trial	Omalizumab	
IL-5	Activation and recruitment of eosinophils	Asthma			Mepolizumab, reslizumab	
IL-5R	Activation and recruitment of eosinophils	Asthma		HES	Benralizumab	
IL13	Epithelial barrier, endothelial permeability, high-affinity IgE?	na		EGID	Tralokinumab, QAX576, RPC4046	
IL-4Ra	IgE class switch and maintenance, T_H2 maintenance/amplification	Atopic dermatitis, Asthma	Phase II monotherapy, in combination with OIT, and head-to-head against omalizumab	EGID, Phase II completed with positive results	Dupilumab	
Siglec-8	Eosinophil apoptosis, mast cell suppression	na		EGID, Phase II	AK002	
TSLPR	Recruitment of T_H2, basophils, conditioning of DCs to promote T_H2	na		Phase III (asthma); Phase II (AD)	Tezepelumab	
alpha4-beta7	Recruitment of T cells, eosinophils and mast cells	IBD			Vedolizumab	Trials in GVHD, a recent retrospective series described improved histopathology in five patients with EGID after therapy with vedolizumab, but exposure to corticosteroids may have affected the responses.
Eotaxin	Recruitment of eosinophils	na		Asthma—negative Phase II	GW766994	
TGF-β	Promote tolerance/pro-fibrotic	na		EGID (losartan)	Fresolimumab, losartan(?)	Trials in sclerosis, oncology, FSGN
TLR4	Induction of T_H1/suppression of T_H2	Vaccine adjuvant (MPL)	Phase I/II		GLA, others	Trial terminated; no results available
IL-9/IL-9R	Promote mast cell proliferation	na		Asthma—negative Phase II	Enokizumab	
IL-33	Drive induction and ? maintenance of T_H2/activate ILC2	na	Phase IIa (POC)—peanut allergy	Phase II (AD and asthma)	Etokimab (MEDI-528)	
IL-31R	Major driver of itch	na			Nemolizumab	Animal models do support clear role in inflammation
Multiple		na	Phase III/IV		AR101, Viaskin	AR101 FDA approved on January 31, 2020
Multiple		na	Phase I/II		Probiotics	
Multiple		na	Phase I complete		PVX108	
Multiple		na	Phase II		ARA-LAMP-VAX	

AD, atopic dermatitis; *CIU*, chronic idiopathic urticaria; *DC*, dendritic cell; *EGID*, eosinophilic gastrointestinal disease; *FcεRI*, high-affinity immunoglobulin E receptor; *FSGN*, focal segmental glomerulonephritis; *GLA*, glucopyranosyl lipid A; *GVHD*, graft-versus-host disease; *HES*, hypereosinophilic syndrome; *IBD*, inflammatory bowel disease; *IgE*, immunoglobulin E; *IL*, interleukin; *ILC2*, type 2 innate lymphoid cell; *MPL*, monophosphoryl lipid A; *OIT*, oral immunotherapy; *POC*, proof of concept; *Siglec*, sialic acid–binding immunoglobulin-type lectin; *TGF-β*, transforming growth factor-beta; T_H1, T helper cell type 1 cell; *TLR4*, Toll-like receptor 4; *TSLPR*, thymic stromal lymphopoietin receptor.

Probiotics

Based on an ever-increasing body of evidence about the role of host microbiome in allergic and inflammatory disease,[107–113] therapeutic intervention with agents that alter the microbiome and affect the immune response are a subject of significant interest and require further investigation. In an Australian study, children with peanut allergy were randomized to receive either peanut OIT combined with *Lactobacillus rhamnosus* or placebo OIT without probiotics once daily for 18 months.[114] When assessed 2 to 5 weeks after the end of the trial, 82.1% of the active group were desensitized to peanut, compared with 3.6% in the placebo group, and a 4-year follow-up study suggested that combination therapy

may be effective in promoting longer term desensitization.[115] Additional study is needed to further evaluate and develop this approach for application in food allergy.

Chinese Herbal Formulas

Traditional Chinese medicine has been used for centuries to treat a variety of disorders, with anecdotal reports of medicinal benefits for allergic disorders. FAHF-2 was developed as a formulation of nine Chinese herbs and studied extensively in preclinical studies. FAHF-2 was shown to block peanut-induced anaphylaxis and induce immunologic changes when comparing peanut-sensitized to sham-sensitized mice, with effects sustained for up to

6 months (25% of the lifespan of a mouse).[116] During a Phase I study, subjects received FAHF-2 tablets or placebo over 1 week.[117] Treatment was well tolerated, with only minor GI symptoms in approximately 10% of participants and with associated reductions in serum IL-5 levels. A Phase II, multicenter clinical trial in multifood-allergic adolescents and adults (ages 12–45 years) reported a favorable safety profile and evidence of in vitro immunomodulation; however, a significant treatment response was not observed, possibly influenced by poor participant adherence to a regimen requiring 10 tablets three times daily over 6 months of treatment.[118] Additional studies of FAHF-2 in combination with multiallergen OIT and omalizumab are ongoing (http://www.clinicaltrials.gov NCT02879006).

Adjuvanted Sublingual Immunotherapy

Conventional SLIT for peanut and milk allergy as described earlier shows moderate efficacy, favorable safety profile, and variable tolerability and is not currently the subject of broad investigation. However, a novel approach using peanut extract combined with glucopyranosyl lipid A (GLA) (SAR439794, http://www.clinicaltrials.gov NCT03463135) is in early-stage development. A Phase I, randomized, double-blind, placebo-controlled study of adolescents and adults with peanut allergy is in progress, including three treatment arms: active peanut extract/active GLA, active peanut allergy/placebo GLA, and placebo peanut allergy/placebo GLA. This trial will evaluate the safety, tolerability, pharmacodynamics, and immunogenicity of daily SLIT over a 12-week treatment period.

Conclusions

Immunotherapeutic approaches for the treatment of food allergy have advanced significantly over the past two decades, with the first licensed therapy for peanut allergy approved and multiple potential therapies in the developmental pipeline. Previously, the standard of care for food allergy has included vigilant dietary avoidance with ready access to emergency medications in the case of accidental exposures; the imminent availability of FDA-approved therapeutic interventions for broader clinical application represents a significant paradigm shift in management of food allergy. However, these therapies are not without risk, and the potential benefits must be carefully considered in the context of safety and efficacy and consideration of outcomes important to patients and caregivers, such as improved quality of life, reduced anxiety about accidental ingestions and unpredicted reactions, and the constant anxiety associated with the need for dietary vigilance to prevent adverse reactions. Continued investigation of novel therapies as well as refinement of existing approaches is critical to address existing knowledge gaps, including optimal duration, age at initiation, maintenance regimen, long-term outcomes, predictors of response, cost-effectiveness, and psychosocial impact that will maximize efficacy, minimize risk, and ultimately allow for development of individualized, patient-centered approaches for future clinical application.

The reference list can be found on the companion Expert Consult website at http://www.expertconsult.inkling.com.

38

Evaluation and Management of Atopic Dermatitis

MARK BOGUNIEWICZ, DONALD Y.M. LEUNG

KEY POINTS

- Proper skin hydration and barrier protection along with identi-fication and elimination of relevant triggers are key to manage-ment of atopic dermatitis (AD).
- Patient and caregiver education is a critical part of caring for patients with AD.

- Topical antiinflammatory therapies include glucocorticoids, calcineurin inhibitors, and phosphodiesterase 4 inhibitor.
- Dupilumab is a systemic biologic therapy approved for patients 12 years and older with moderate to severe AD.

Introduction

Atopic dermatitis (AD) is a common, frequently relapsing inflammatory disease that affects up to 20% of children and has a significant impact on the quality of life of patients and families.[1] Some patients with AD have mutations in the gene encoding filaggrin (*FLG*), a protein essential for normal epi-dermal barrier function.[2] These patients have early-onset, more severe, and persistent disease. Mutations in *FLG* also have been associated with allergic sensitization, food allergy, and asthma, but only in patients with AD. However, most patients with severe AD have lower levels of filaggrin protein in the skin because of type 2 cytokine (interleukin 4 [IL-4] and IL-13) suppression of *FLG*.

Symptoms and Signs

AD has no pathognomonic skin lesions or laboratory param-eters, with diagnosis based on clinical features, including severe pruritus, a chronically relapsing course, and typical morphol-ogy and distribution of the skin lesions (Box 38.1).[1] Acute AD is characterized by erythematous papules with excoria-tions, vesiculations, and serous exudate, whereas chronic AD is characterized by thickened skin with accentuated markings (lichenification). In skin of color, erythema and associated inflammation may be difficult to appreciate. In infants, AD often first manifests on the cheeks, involving face, scalp, and extensor aspects of extremities and typically sparing the diaper region (Fig. 38.1). In older patients, flexural creases of the extremities are the predominant location of lesions, although this distribution can be seen even in infants (Fig. 38.2). Rou-tine skin biopsy does not differentiate AD from other eczema-tous processes but may be helpful in atypical cases. Genetic testing for the most common *FLG* mutations may identify patients who would be at increased risk for more severe, per-sistent AD and be more likely to develop allergic sensitization, food allergy, and asthma; however, *FLG* mutations occur in individuals without AD.

Differential Diagnosis

A number of diseases can present with eczema or pruritic lesions (Box 38.2).[3] Seborrheic dermatitis may be distinguished by a lack of significant pruritus with coarse, yellowish scales and predilec-tion for scalp ("cradle cap"), perinasal, and groin regions. Allergic contact dermatitis may be suggested by specific distribution of lesions and a greater demarcation of the dermatitis compared with AD. However, allergic contact dermatitis can be superimposed on AD and manifest as an acute flare of the underlying disease. Patients with AD who have persistent facial, hand, or foot eczema should be considered for patch test evaluation (see Chapter 40). Nummular eczema is characterized by coin-shaped plaques. Immunodeficiencies that can manifest with eczematous rashes include Wiskott-Aldrich syndrome, severe combined immuno-deficiency disease, hyper–immunoglobulin E (IgE) syndrome, immunodeficiency with dedicator of cytokinesis 8 (DOCK8)

Essential Features

- Pruritus
- Eczema (acute, subacute, chronic)
- Morphology and age-specific patterns
  - Infants and children: facial, neck and extensor involvement
  - Any age group: flexural lesions; sparing of groin
- Chronic or relapsing history

Important Features

- Early age
- Atopy
  - Personal and/or family history of atopic disorders
  - Elevated total serum immunoglobulin E (IgE) or allergen-specific IgE
- Xerosis
- Lichenification

Associated Features

- Atypical vascular responses (e.g., white dermatographism, facial pallor)
- Keratosis pilaris, hyperlinear palms, ichthyosis
- Ocular, periorbital changes
- Other regional findings (perioral, periauricular)
- Perifollicular accentuation, prurigo lesions

Congenital Disorders

- Netherton's syndrome
- Familial keratosis pilaris

Chronic Dermatoses

- Seborrheic dermatitis
- Contact dermatitis (allergic or irritant)
- Nummular eczema
- Psoriasis
- Ichthyoses

Infections and Infestations

- Scabies
- Human immunodeficiency virus–associated dermatitis
- Dermatophytosis

Malignancies

- Cutaneous T cell lymphoma (mycosis fungoides/Sézary syndrome)
- Letterer-Siwe disease

Autoimmune Disorders

- Dermatitis herpetiformis
- Pemphigus foliaceus
- Graft-versus-host disease
- Dermatomyositis

Immunodeficiencies

- Wiskott-Aldrich syndrome
- Severe combined immunodeficiency syndrome
- Hyper–immunoglobulin E syndrome
- Dedicator of cytokinesis 8 (DOCK8)-associated immunodeficiency
- X-linked immune dysregulation, polyendocrinopathy, enteropathy (IPEX) syndrome

Metabolic Disorders

- Zinc deficiency
- Pyridoxine (vitamin B_6) and niacin
- Multiple carboxylase deficiency
- Phenylketonuria

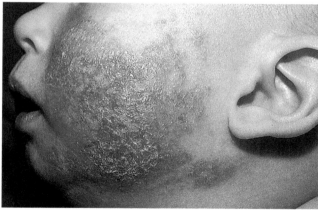

• **Fig. 38.1** Infant with acute atopic dermatitis. Note the oozing and crusting skin lesions. (Reproduced with permission from Weston WL, Morelli JG, Lane A, editors. Color textbook of pediatric dermatology. 3rd ed. St. Louis: Mosby; 2002.)

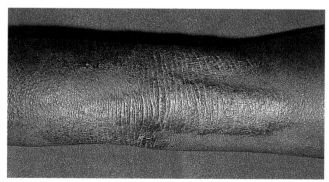

• **Fig. 38.2** Adolescent with lichenification of the popliteal fossa from chronic atopic dermatitis. (Reproduced with permission from Weston WL, Morelli JG, Lane A, editors. Color textbook of pediatric dermatology. 3rd ed. St. Louis: Mosby; 2002.)

mutations, and X-linked immunodeficiency with polyendocrinopathy and enteropathy (IPEX) (see Chapter 6). Scabies can manifest with intensely pruritic lesions, although their distribution in the axillary and groin regions and presence of linear lesions should differentiate it from AD. In addition, skin scrapings should establish a definitive diagnosis. Cutaneous T cell lymphoma (most commonly mycosis fungoides), although rare, has been described in children and is diagnosed by skin biopsy. Eczematous rash has been reported in patients with human immunodeficiency virus (HIV) infection. Other disorders that may resemble AD include zinc deficiency, phenylketonuria, and Letterer-Siwe disease.

Complications

Patients with AD have increased susceptibility to infection or colonization with a variety of organisms.[4] These include viral infections with herpes simplex, molluscum contagiosum, and human papillomavirus. Superimposed dermatophytosis may cause AD to flare. *Staphylococcus aureus* can be cultured from the skin of the majority of patients with AD. *S. aureus* toxins can

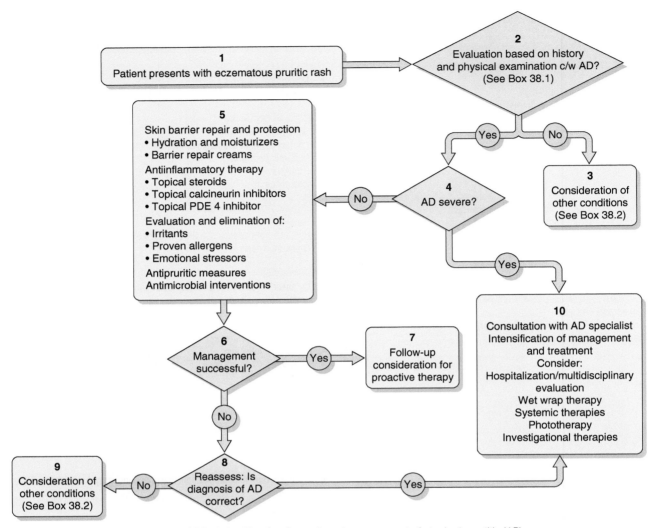

• **Fig. 38.3** Clinical algorithm for diagnosis and management of atopic dermatitis (*AD*).

act as superantigens contributing to persistent inflammation or exacerbations of AD. Community-acquired methicillin-resistant *S. aureus* (MRSA) has become an increasing problem, especially in patients treated with frequent antibiotics. Although recurrent staphylococcal pustulosis can be a significant problem in AD, invasive *S. aureus* infections occur rarely and should raise the possibility of an immunodeficiency.

Ocular complications associated with AD include atopic keratoconjunctivitis, which is always bilateral with intense itching, burning, tearing, and copious mucoid discharge. It is frequently associated with eyelid dermatitis and chronic blepharitis and may result in visual impairment from corneal scarring (see Chapter 41). Keratoconus in AD may result from persistent rubbing of the eyes. Anterior subcapsular cataracts may develop during adolescence or early adult life.

Patients with AD can develop nonspecific hand dermatitis. This is frequently irritant in nature and aggravated by repeated wetting.

Management

Management approaches in AD have evolved with increasing understanding of the mechanisms underlying this

skin disease. Although AD is the most common chronic skin disease of children, it is important to bear in mind the differential diagnosis of a pruritic rash when starting therapy, especially if there are atypical features or the response to treatment is suboptimal (see "Differential Diagnosis" section, earlier). Given the complex nature of AD and its chronic, relapsing course, it will often require a multipronged approach directed at healing or protecting the skin barrier and addressing the immune dysregulation to improve the likelihood of successful outcomes. This includes proper skin hydration and identification and elimination of flare factors, such as irritants, allergens, infectious agents, emotional stressors, and pharmacologic therapy (Fig. 38.3).[1,3]

Hydration and Skin Barrier Protective Measures

As discussed previously, patients with AD have genetic or immune-mediated abnormalities in skin barrier function.[2] Of note, filaggrin contributes not only to barrier integrity but also to hydration through generation of hygroscopic amino acids that are a key component of natural moisturizing factor, which is also involved in the maintenance of skin pH and regulation of key biochemical events, including protease activity, barrier permeability, and cutaneous antimicrobial defense. Filaggrin may also contribute to the acid mantle through acid degradation products. Children with AD have dry skin (xerosis) with microfissures and epidermal defects that serve as portals of entry for irritants, allergens, and skin pathogens. Transepidermal water loss occurs even through normal appearing skin.

Hydration of the skin can be accomplished through warm (note that lukewarm and tepid are not comfortable temperatures for bathing) soaking baths for approximately 10 minutes, followed by immediate application of a moisturizer or medication to prevent evaporation and promote healing. Bathing also removes irritants, allergens, and skin pathogens and provides symptomatic relief. It is important that areas involved by eczema are immersed, not just wet. Wet towels can be used to hydrate the head and neck regions, with masks created to make the experience both therapeutic and enjoyable. Young children need to be supervised. Baths can be taken several times per day during eczema flares, and showers may be substituted in milder disease. Cleansers with minimal defatting activity and a neutral pH can be used as necessary. Preparations formulated for sensitive skin that are dye and fragrance free are generally well tolerated. Antibacterial cleansers may be helpful for patients with folliculitis or recurrent skin infections. Patients should be instructed not to scrub with a washcloth while using cleansers. Addition of bleach (sodium hypochlorite) to bath water, especially for patients with MRSA, has been advocated. However, the amount of bleach per volume of water (e.g., an eighth to a half cup per tub of water) and the frequency of such treatments (e.g., one to three times weekly) have not been well studied and bleach baths can cause skin irritation. A 2017 meta-analysis found that dilute bleach baths are no more effective in decreasing eczema severity than plain water baths,[5] although they may still be useful in patients requiring frequent courses of topical or systemic antibiotics to treat infectious complications of AD.

Use of an effective moisturizer combined with hydration therapy will help restore and preserve the stratum corneum barrier.[6] Moisturizers can also improve skin barrier function, reduce susceptibility to irritants, improve clinical parameters of AD, and decrease the need for topical corticosteroids.[7] Ingredients that contribute to effective moisturizers include humectants to attract and hold water in the skin, such as glycerol; occlusive, such as petrolatum, to retard evaporation; and emollients, such as lanolin, to lubricate the stratum corneum.[8]

Moisturizers are available as ointments, creams, lotions, and oils. Although ointments have the fewest additives and are the most occlusive, in a hot, humid environment they may trap sweat, causing associated irritation of the skin. Lotions and creams may be irritating as a result of added preservatives, solubilizers, and fragrances. Lotions contain more water than creams and may be drying because of an evaporative effect. Moisturizers should be obtained in the largest size available because they may need to be applied several times each day on a chronic basis. Vegetable shortening (Crisco) can be used as an inexpensive moisturizer. Of note, patients and caregivers should understand that petroleum jelly (Vaseline) is an occlusive, not a moisturizer, and thus needs to be applied on damp, not dry, skin. Even young children can be taught to apply their moisturizer, allowing them to participate in their skin care.

Patients and caregivers need to be instructed to apply moisturizers routinely but not over or immediately before topical medications to avoid dilution or interference with medication on skin.

A number of studies suggest that AD is associated with decreased levels of ceramides, contributing not only to a damaged permeability barrier but also making the stratum corneum susceptible to colonization by *S. aureus*.[9] A ceramide-dominant emollient added to standard therapy in place of moisturizer in children with "stubborn-to-recalcitrant" AD was shown to result in clinical improvement.[10] Ceramide-containing creams are available, including Epiceram, which is registered as a medical device and thus available only by prescription. These "barrier repair" creams are not regulated by the U.S. Food and Drug Administration (FDA) and have no restrictions on age or length of use. They may be especially attractive to parents who have concerns about using topical corticosteroids and calcineurin inhibitors. However, their place in the treatment algorithm for AD has not been definitively established.

Topical Antiinflammatory Therapy

Topical Glucocorticoids

Glucocorticoids have been the cornerstone of antiinflammatory treatment for over 50 years. Because of potential side effects, topical glucocorticoids are used primarily to control acute exacerbations of AD.[1]

Patients should be carefully instructed in the use of topical glucocorticoids to avoid potential side effects. The potent fluorinated glucocorticoids should be avoided on the face, the genitalia, and the intertriginous areas. Failure of a patient to respond to topical glucocorticoids is often due to an inadequate amount applied. It is important to remember that it takes approximately 30 g of cream or ointment to cover the entire skin surface of an adult-sized patient for one application. The fingertip unit (FTU) has been proposed as a measure for applying topical corticosteroids and has been studied in children with AD.[11,12] This is the amount of topical medication that extends from the tip to the first joint on the palmar aspect of the index finger. It takes approximately 1 FTU to cover the hand or groin, 2 FTUs for the face or foot, 3 FTUs for an arm, 6 FTUs for a leg, and 14 FTUs for the trunk. Of note, adequate application of topical corticosteroids has been shown to correlate with clinical improvement.[13] Obtaining medications in larger quantities can result in significant savings for patients.

There are seven classes of topical glucocorticoids, ranked according to their potency based on vasoconstrictor assays from superpotent (class I) to low potent (class VII). Because of their potential side effects, the superpotent and high-potent glucocorticoids should be used for only short periods and in areas that are lichenified, but not on the face or intertriginous areas. The goal is to use moisturizers to enhance skin hydration and lower potency glucocorticoids or nonsteroidal agents for long-term therapy, if needed. Side effects from topical glucocorticoids are related to the potency ranking of the compound, the length of use, and the area of the body to which the drug is applied, so it is incumbent on the clinician to balance the need for a more potent steroid with the potential for side effects. In general, ointments have a greater potential to occlude the epidermis, resulting in enhanced systemic absorption compared with creams. Side effects from topical glucocorticoids can be divided into local and systemic. Local side effects include the development of striae and skin atrophy.[14] Systemic side effects in AD are uncommon unless high-potency steroids are used under occlusion, but adrenal suppression and cataracts have been reported.[15–17] However, disease activity, rather than the use of topical corticosteroids, was shown to be responsible for low basal cortisol values in patients with severe AD.[18] Of note, patients and caregivers continue to use topical corticosteroids suboptimally, primarily because of concerns about their use.[19] This may include delaying application of the medication for a number of days after the start of a flare, which contributes to suboptimal outcomes. An expert consensus from the Dermatology Working Group pointed out that "in an ideal world, dermatologists, dermatology nurses, . . . practitioners, . . . pharmacists would work together to advise and reinforce information about the correct way to apply topical corticosteroids, and to address concerns about the safety of these highly effective agents. But in the real world, expert advice, even when given, is soon forgotten."[12] Patients and caregivers need to have a basic understanding of topical corticosteroids, including their risks and benefits. Patients may erroneously assume that the potency of a topical corticosteroid is defined by the percent stated after the compound name (as discussed under "Education of Patients and Caregivers" later in this chapter). At times, patients may be prescribed a high-potency corticosteroid with instructions to discontinue it within 7 to 14 days without a plan to step down, resulting in rebound flaring of their AD. Of note, only a few topical corticosteroids have been approved for use in very young children. These include desonide and fluticasone cream down to 3 months of age, alclometasone down to 1 year of age, and mometasone down to 2 years of age. Indications are typically for up to 3 to 4 weeks.

Patients with AD are often labeled as topical corticosteroid treatment failures. Reasons for this may include inadequate potency of the preparation or insufficient amount dispensed or applied, *S. aureus* superinfection, steroid allergy, and possibly corticosteroid insensitivity. A much more common reason for therapeutic failure is nonadherence to the treatment regimen. As with any chronic disease, patients or caregivers often expect quick and lasting benefits and become frustrated with the relapsing nature of AD.[20] These factors need to be considered when faced with a patient not responding to therapy before considering alternative therapy, especially systemic treatment.

Topical Calcineurin Inhibitors

Since their approval by the FDA in 2000 and 2001, respectively, the topical calcineurin inhibitors (TCIs)—tacrolimus ointment (Protopic 0.03% and 0.1%) and pimecrolimus cream (Elidel 1%)—have become well-established, effective, and safe nonsteroidal treatments for pediatric AD.[21] They are currently indicated as second-line treatment for intermittent, noncontinuous use in children aged 2 years and older with moderate to severe AD (i.e., tacrolimus ointment 0.03%) and mild to moderate AD (i.e., pimecrolimus cream 1%). Tacrolimus ointment 0.1% is indicated for patients 16 years and older. Nevertheless, patients and caregivers frequently misunderstand their place in the treatment algorithm and have concerns about the boxed warning for these drugs. A Joint Task Force of the American College of Allergy, Asthma and Immunology and the American Academy of Allergy, Asthma & Immunology (AAAAI) reviewed the available data and concluded that the risk-to-benefit ratios of tacrolimus

ointment and pimecrolimus cream are similar to those of most conventional therapies for the treatment of chronic relapsing eczema.[22] In addition, a case-control study of a large database that identified a cohort of 293,253 patients with AD found no increased risk of lymphoma with the use of TCIs.[23] Children may be prescribed TCIs to replace topical corticosteroids when they are not doing well or during a flare of AD, with unrealistic expectations for this class of drugs. Patients and caregivers may not be instructed about potential side effects, a common reason for TCIs being discontinued, and patients labeled as treatment failures. Although several studies have explored the use of TCIs in children under 2 years of age[24] and as early intervention to reduce the incidence of flare and need for topical corticosteroid rescue,[25] they would currently be considered to be off-label therapy.

Topical Phosphodiesterase 4 Inhibitor

Phosphodiesterase 4 (PDE4) is a key regulator of inflammatory cytokine production in AD, with PDE4 activity increased in circulating inflammatory cells of patients with AD.[26] Crisaborole, a topical PDE4 inhibitor, has been shown to be safe and effective in children and adults with AD[27] and has been approved in the United States for patients 2 years and older with mild to moderate AD. Stinging or burning at the site of application has been a commonly reported adverse event.

Proactive Therapy

Nonlesional skin in AD can have skin barrier and immune abnormalities and *S. aureus* colonization.[28] In patients whose eczema tends to relapse in the same location, proactive therapy is an approach that has gained increased attention. After a period of stabilization, topical antiinflammatory therapy is instituted in areas of previously involved but normal-appearing skin, rather than waiting for a flare of eczema in a traditional reactive approach. Studies with topical corticosteroids and TCIs,[29] including in pediatric patients,[30,31] have shown clinical benefit with this approach. Of note, it is important to recognize that eczema first needs to be brought under control before a 2- to 3-times weekly, long-term regimen can be instituted. This approach would currently be considered off-label in the United States, but it has been approved in E.U. countries for children 2 years and older for up to 12 months with tacrolimus ointment and shown to be a cost-effective approach by the National Health Service of the United Kingdom.[32]

Identification and Elimination of Triggering Factors

Patients with AD have hyperreactive skin, and a number of different triggers, including irritants, allergens, infectious agents, and emotional stressors, can contribute to cutaneous inflammation and flare of eczema.

Irritants

Patients with AD are more susceptible to irritants than are normal individuals. Thus, it is important to identify and eliminate or minimize exposure to irritants such as soaps or detergents, chemicals, smoke, abrasive clothing, and extremes of temperature and humidity. Alcohol and astringents found in toiletries can be drying. Cleansers, ideally formulated for sensitive skin, should be used in place of soaps, especially fragranced ones. Using a liquid rather than powder detergent and adding a second rinse cycle will facilitate removal of the detergent. Recommendations regarding environmental conditions should include temperature and humidity control to avoid problems related to heat, humidity, and perspiration. Every attempt should be made to allow children to be as normally active as possible. Certain sports such as swimming may be better tolerated than others that involve intense perspiration, physical contact, or heavy clothing and equipment, but chlorine should be rinsed off after swimming with the aid of a cleanser and the skin lubricated. Although ultraviolet light may be beneficial to some patients with AD, sunscreens should be used to avoid sunburn. Sunscreens formulated for the face are often better tolerated.

Specific Allergens

Potential allergens can be identified by taking a careful history and performing selective allergy tests. Negative skin tests or serum tests for allergen-specific IgE have a high predictive value for ruling out suspected allergens. Positive skin or in vitro tests, particularly to foods, often do not correlate with clinical symptoms and should be confirmed with controlled food challenges and, if indicated, trials of specific elimination diets.[33] Avoidance of foods implicated in controlled challenges has been shown to result in clinical improvement. Infants who do not improve on formulas containing hydrolyzed proteins can be tried on amino acid formulas. However, these can add a significant financial burden for the family. Extensive elimination diets, which in some cases can be nutritionally deficient, are rarely if ever required, because even with multiple positive allergy tests, the majority of children will react to three or fewer foods on controlled challenge. Unfortunately, patients with multiple positive allergy tests are often labeled as multifood-allergic, with no attempts to prove clinical relevance. Food challenges after getting the eczema under control and establishing a baseline for immediate and, less frequently, delayed reactions can be of immense value in managing the patient and helping the family with this stressful issue. It is noteworthy that in one retrospective study, 325 (89%) of 364 supervised oral food challenges were reported as negative.[34] In addition, consultation with a dietitian familiar with food allergies can be extremely helpful to ensure a nutritionally sound diet for the child and suggest practical advice to caregivers.[35] The Food Allergy Research & Education website (http://www.foodallergy.org) is a useful resource for patients and families with food allergy (see Chapter 31).

In patients allergic to dust mites, prolonged avoidance of dust mites has been found to result in improvement of AD.[36–39] Avoidance measures include using dust mite–proof casings on pillows, mattresses, and box springs; washing bedding in hot water weekly; removing bedroom carpeting; and decreasing indoor humidity levels with air conditioning. Because there are many triggers that can contribute to the flare of AD, attention should be focused on identifying and controlling the flare factors that are important to the individual patient. In addition, allergic contact dermatitis may be overlooked in children and patch testing should be considered in children with AD (see Chapter 40).[40,41] In a study to determine the frequency of positive and relevant patch tests in children referred for patch testing in North America, of the children with a relevant positive reaction, 34% had a diagnosis of AD.[42]

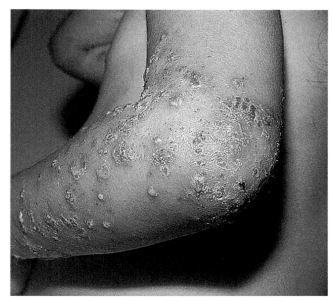

• **Fig. 38.4** Patient with atopic dermatitis who is secondarily infected with *Staphylococcus aureus*. Note multiple pustules and areas of crusting. (Reproduced with permission from Weston WL, Morelli JG, Lane A, editors. Color textbook of pediatric dermatology. 3rd ed. St. Louis: Mosby; 2002.)

Emotional Stressors

Patients with AD often respond to frustration, embarrassment, and other stressful events with increased pruritus and scratching. In some instances, scratching is simply habitual; less commonly it is associated with secondary gain. Psychological evaluation or counseling should be considered in patients who have difficulty with emotional triggers or psychological problems contributing to difficulty in managing their disease. Relaxation, behavioral modification, or biofeedback may be helpful in patients who habitually scratch.[43]

Infectious Agents

Children with AD often are colonized or infected with various microbial organisms, including bacteria, especially *S. aureus* (Fig. 38.4); viruses, including herpes simplex virus; and occasionally yeast or fungi. MRSA has become an increasingly important pathogen in patients with AD. Antistaphylococcal antibiotics are helpful in the treatment of patients who are heavily colonized or infected with *S. aureus*.[44] Cephalosporins or penicillinase-resistant penicillins are usually beneficial for patients who are not colonized with resistant *S. aureus* strains. Erythromycin and other macrolide antibiotics are usually of limited utility because of increasing frequency of erythromycin-resistant *S. aureus*. Topical mupirocin is useful for the treatment of localized impetiginized lesions; however, in patients with extensive skin infection, a course of systemic antibiotics is more practical. Retapamulin ointment 1%, used twice daily for 5 days, was shown to be as effective as oral cephalexin twice daily for 10 days in the treatment of patients with secondarily infected dermatitis and was well tolerated.[45] Use of topical neomycin can result in development of allergic contact dermatitis because neomycin is among the more common allergens causing contact dermatitis.[42] Treatment for nasal carriage with an intranasal antibiotic may lead to clinical improvement of AD.[46] MRSA may require culture and sensitivity testing to assist

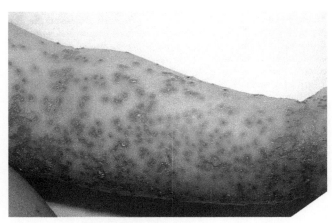

• **Fig. 38.5** Eczema herpeticum, the primary skin manifestation of herpes simplex in atopic dermatitis. (From Fireman P, Slavin R, editors. Atlas of allergies. 2nd ed. London: Mosby-Wolfe; 1996.)

in appropriate antibiotic selection. However, patients and caregivers need to be instructed that the best defense against microbes is an intact skin barrier, and basic skin care principles, as discussed previously, should be emphasized. Of note, antiinflammatory therapy alone, with either a topical corticosteroid or a TCI, has been shown to improve AD and reduce *S. aureus* colonization of the skin.[47]

Although antibacterial cleansers have been shown to be effective in reducing bacterial skin flora,[48] they may be too irritating to use on inflamed skin in AD. Baths with dilute sodium hypochlorite (bleach) may benefit patients with AD, especially those with recurrent MRSA, as discussed earlier, although they can be irritating. An approach to recurrent MRSA infections in patients with AD has been reviewed in detail.[49]

AD can be complicated by disseminated herpes simplex virus infection, resulting in Kaposi's varicelliform eruption or eczema herpeticum (Fig. 38.5). Vesicular lesions are umbilicated, tend to crop, and often become hemorrhagic and crusted. These lesions may coalesce to large denuded and bleeding areas that can extend over the entire body. Herpes simplex can provoke recurrent dermatitis and may be misdiagnosed as impetigo, although herpetic lesions can become superinfected by *S. aureus*.[50] The presence of punched-out erosions, vesicles, and/or infected skin lesions that fail to respond to oral antibiotics should initiate a search for herpes simplex. This can be diagnosed by a Giemsa-stained Tzanck smear of cells scraped from the vesicle base or by viral culture or polymerase chain reaction. Test results may be falsely negative if the samples are inadequate. Ideally, vesicle fluid should be obtained by unroofing one or more intact vesicles. Ophthalmology consultation should be obtained for patients with periocular or suspected eye involvement. Treatment may be with oral acyclovir for less severe infections or intravenous acyclovir for widely disseminated disease or toxic-appearing patients at 30 mg/kg/day divided every 8 hours (for patients younger than 1 year) or 1500 mg/m^2/day divided every 8 hours (for patients older than 1 year) for 7 to 21 days, depending on the clinical course.[51] Valacyclovir is indicated in pediatric patients 12 years or older for treatment of herpes labialis (2 g every 12 hours for 1 day) and patients 2 to younger than 18 years of age for treatment of chickenpox (20 mg/kg three times daily for 5 days) up to a maximum dose of 1 g three times daily. Detailed instructions on preparing a liquid suspension (including shelf life) are available under "Extemporaneous Preparation of Oral Suspension" in the manufacturer's package insert. Of note,

the suspension needs to be used within 4 weeks of being prepared. Acyclovir prophylaxis may be necessary for patients with recurrent eczema herpeticum.

In patients with AD, smallpox vaccination, or even exposure to vaccinated individuals, may cause a severe widespread skin rash called *eczema vaccinatum* that is similar in appearance to eczema herpeticum.[52] An increased risk of fatalities resulting from eczema vaccinatum has been reported in AD. Even if not fatal, eczema vaccinatum is often associated with severe scarring and lifelong complications after recovery from this illness.

Fungi may play a role in chronic inflammation of AD. *Malassezia sympodialis* is a lipophilic yeast commonly present in the seborrheic areas of the skin. IgE antibodies against *M. sympodialis* are found in patients with AD, most frequently in patients with a head and neck distribution of dermatitis. The potential importance of *M. sympodialis* and other dermatophyte infections is further supported by the reduction of AD skin severity in patients treated with antifungal agents.[53] However, even patients with IgE antibodies to *M. sympodialis* often respond better to topical steroids than to topical antifungal therapy, and systemic antifungal therapy may benefit patients with AD through antiinflammatory properties.[54]

Control of Pruritus and Sleep Disturbance

The treatment of pruritus in AD should be directed primarily at the underlying causes.[55] Reduction of skin inflammation and dryness with topical glucocorticoids and skin hydration, respectively, will often symptomatically reduce pruritus. Inhaled and ingested allergens should be eliminated if documented to contribute to eczema. Systemic antihistamines act primarily by blocking the histamine 1 (H$_1$) receptors in the dermis and thereby ameliorating histamine-induced pruritus. However, histamine is only one of many mediators that can induce pruritus of the skin, minimizing benefit from antihistamine therapy. Studies of nonsedating antihistamines have shown variable results in the effectiveness of controlling pruritus in patients with AD, although they may be useful in the subset of patients with AD with concomitant urticaria. Because pruritus is usually worse at night, sedating antihistamines such as hydroxyzine or diphenhydramine may offer an advantage with their soporific side effects when used at bedtime. Doxepin hydrochloride has both tricyclic antidepressant and H$_1$- and H$_2$-histamine receptor blocking effects. Thus, it may be useful in treating children and adolescents who do not respond to H$_1$ sedating antihistamines. If nocturnal pruritus remains severe, short-term use of a sedative to allow adequate rest may be appropriate. Treatment of AD with topical antihistamines or topical anesthetics is not recommended because of potential cutaneous sensitization. Other treatment options for sleep disturbance used by the behavioral health clinicians in the AD program at National Jewish Health include clonidine and melatonin.

Tar Preparations

Coal tar preparations may have antipruritic and antiinflammatory effects on the skin.[56] They also may have a beneficial effect on the skin barrier by increasing filaggrin protein in the skin.[57] Tar shampoos can be beneficial for scalp dermatitis. Tar preparations should not be used on acutely inflamed skin because this can result in skin irritation. Side effects associated with tars include folliculitis and photosensitivity.

Systemic Therapy

Children who are considered candidates for systemic therapy should be evaluated by specialists in AD.[3] Patients with refractory AD often will respond to conventional therapy with appropriate education regarding the relapsing nature of AD and proper skin care.[58] In addition, other diseases with eczematous rash may need to be considered (see Box 38.2).

Biologic Therapy

Dupilumab is a fully human monoclonal antibody directed at the IL-4 receptor alpha subunit.[59] It has been approved in patients 12 years or older with moderate to severe AD who have failed to respond to topical prescription medications or when such medications are not advised. In patients 12 to 17 years, dosing is weight based, with patients less than 60 kg receiving an initial dose of 400 mg, then 200 mg every 2 weeks by subcutaneous injection, and patients 60 kg or more receiving a 600-mg initial dose, then 300 mg every 2 weeks. Injections can be self-administered at home, and at present there is no requirement for any laboratory monitoring. Injection site reactions and conjunctivitis have been the most commonly reported adverse events.

Systemic Glucocorticoids

The use of systemic glucocorticoids, such as oral prednisone, is rarely indicated in the treatment of chronic AD.[1,60] The dramatic clinical improvement that may occur with systemic glucocorticoids is frequently associated with a severe rebound flare of AD after the discontinuation of systemic glucocorticoids. Short courses of oral glucocorticoids may be appropriate for an acute exacerbation of AD while other treatment measures are being instituted. If a short course of oral glucocorticoids is given, it is important to taper the dosage and begin intensified skin care, particularly with topical glucocorticoids and frequent bathing followed by application of emollients, to prevent rebound flaring of AD. Patients with oral steroid-dependent AD or who are treated with frequent courses of systemic steroids need to be evaluated for corticosteroid side effects, including adrenal suppression, osteoporosis, cataracts, and muscle weakness, and switched to other therapy.

Nonapproved Systemic Immunosuppressives

Cyclosporine A (CsA) is a potent immunosuppressive drug not approved for use in children with AD, but it has been used off-label. Studies in children have demonstrated that patients with severe AD refractory to conventional treatment can benefit from short-term CsA treatment, with reduced skin disease and improved quality of life.[61] A 1-year study of CsA (5 mg/kg/day) in a pediatric population using either intermittent or continuous treatment showed no significant differences between these two approaches with respect to efficacy or safety parameters, and a subset of patients remained in remission after treatment was stopped.[62] In addition, children as young as 22 months of age were shown to respond to low-dose (2.5 mg/kg/day) CsA.[63] Nevertheless, risks must be weighed against benefits and laboratory parameters, especially serum creatinine and blood pressure, monitored.[3,60]

Methotrexate (MTX) is a folic acid antagonist that affects T cell activities and is used routinely in treating psoriasis in adults and children. In AD, time to maximum effect averages 10 weeks, with minimal to no further efficacy after 12 to 16 weeks with further dose escalation.[60] In a study of children with severe AD, MTX and CsA had similar efficacy over 12 weeks of treatment.[64]

Dosing of MTX in AD is derived from the dosing used in psoriasis. The medication is generally given once weekly and can be titrated upward until effect is reached. In adults, dosing ranges from 7.5 to 25 mg/wk, and in children it is weight based at 0.2 to 0.7 mg/kg/wk.[48] Folic acid supplementation is recommended and may be protective against hematologic and gastrointestinal toxicity. Common side effects include nausea, vomiting, and stomatitis, which can be minimized by administering medication in three divided doses given 12 hours apart.[3,60] Patients should be monitored for rare, but severe and potentially irreversible side effects, such as bone marrow suppression and pulmonary fibrosis.

Azathioprine is a purine analog with antiinflammatory and antiproliferative effects. It has been used for severe AD, including in children, although no controlled trials have been reported, and it is not approved for use in AD.[65] Myelosuppression is a significant adverse effect, although thiopurine methyltransferase levels may predict individuals at risk.[3,60]

Mycophenolate mofetil (MMF), a purine biosynthesis inhibitor used as an immunosuppressant in organ transplantation, has been used for treatment of refractory inflammatory skin disorders.[3,60] The drug has generally been well tolerated, although herpes retinitis and dose-related bone marrow suppression have been reported. A retrospective analysis of children treated with MMF off-label as systemic monotherapy for severe, recalcitrant AD found that of 14 patients, 4 achieved complete clearance, 4 had more than 90% improvement, 5 had 60% to 90% improvement, and 1 failed to respond.[66] Initial responses occurred within 8 weeks (mean 4 weeks), and maximal effects were attained after 8 to 12 weeks at MMF doses of 40 to 50 mg/kg/day in younger children and 30 to 40 mg kg/day in adolescents. MMF was well tolerated in all patients, with no infectious complications or significant laboratory abnormalities.

Phototherapy

Broad-band ultraviolet B, broad-band ultraviolet A, narrow-band ultraviolet B (NB-UVB) (311 nm), UVA-1 (340–400 nm), and combined UVAB phototherapy can be useful adjuncts in the treatment of AD.[1,60] Of note, UVB therapy was shown to increase skin barrier proteins, including filaggrin, in AD.[67] Studies in children are limited, and, in general, UV therapy should be restricted to adolescents, except in exceptional cases.[1] Short-term adverse effects with phototherapy may include erythema, pain, pruritus, and pigmentation; long-term adverse effects include premature skin aging and cutaneous malignancies.

Education of Patients and Caregivers

Education is a critical component of AD management, especially when the disease is severe or relapsing. Important components include teaching about the chronic or relapsing nature of AD, exacerbating factors, and therapeutic options, with risks versus benefits and prognosis. Strategies include one-on-one communication, direct demonstration with reinforcement, group discussions, classroom teaching, and written materials, including an AD home care or action plan. Observing the patient's or caregiver's method of treatment will often reveal fundamental errors that may explain why a patient is not experiencing the expected therapeutic response. Patients or caregivers are often observed applying inadequate amounts of topical medications; layering therapy, thus diluting or blocking specific drugs; and misunderstanding the potency of topical corticosteroids based on the misperception that corticosteroid potency is based on the percent value (e.g., 2.5% versus 0.05%), rather than on the specific corticosteroid preparation (e.g., mometasone versus hydrocortisone). AD home care and action plans are integral to the management of children with AD; without them, patients or caregivers may forget or confuse skin care recommendations.[43] These plans should fit the child's and family's needs and should be reviewed and modified at all follow-up visits.

Providing patients and caregivers with appropriate educational resources is an important component of management. Educational brochures and videos can be obtained from the National Eczema Association (800-818-7546 or http://www.nationaleczema.org). Information, instruction sheets, and brochures, including the comprehensive booklet, *Understanding Atopic Dermatitis*, are available from National Jewish Health Lung Line (800-222-LUNG or http://www.nationaljewish.org) and from national organizations such as the AAAAI (http://www.aaaai.org) or the American Academy of Dermatology (http://www.aad.org).

Wet Wrap Therapy

Wet wrap therapy has been used successfully as part of a step-up therapy regimen for treating severe or recalcitrant AD for over two decades.[68] This therapeutic intervention can improve penetration of topical medications, reduce pruritus and inflammation, and act as a barrier against trauma from scratching.[43] A study of wet wraps demonstrated recovery of the epidermal barrier, with clinical improvement associated with release of lamellar body and restoration of intercellular lipid lamellar structure.[69] Of note, 1 week after discontinuation of wet wraps, increased water content and decreased transepidermal water loss were still maintained. Wet wrap therapy has been shown to benefit patients during acute flares of AD.[70] This study points to the usefulness of this intervention in acute AD flares and suggests that the time for topical corticosteroid application may be shortened. A technique used successfully at National Jewish Health in Denver employs clothing such as long underwear and cotton socks selectively wetted based on distribution of the patient's eczema, applied over an undiluted layer of topical corticosteroids with a dry layer of clothing on top.[43] Treating facial eczema requires nursing skills with wet, followed by dry, gauze expertly applied with spaces for eyes and mouth carefully cut out and secured with a dressing such as surgical Spandage (Fig. 38.6). Wraps may be removed when they dry out (after ~2 hours); however, it is often practical to apply

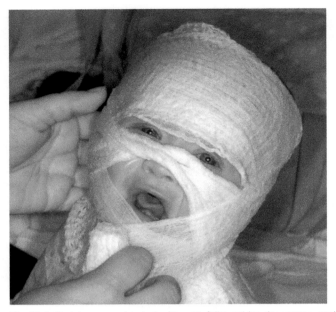

• **Fig. 38.6** Facial eczema treated with wet, followed by dry, gauze, and secured with a dressing such as surgical Spandage. (Reprinted from Boguniewicz M, Nicol N, Kelsay K, et al. A multidisciplinary approach to evaluation and treatment of atopic dermatitis. Semin Cutan Med Surg 2008;27:115–27, with permission from Elsevier.)

them at bedtime and most children are able to sleep while wearing them. Overuse of wet wraps may result in chilling or maceration of the skin and may be complicated by secondary infection. However, a controlled study of wet wrap therapy with topical corticosteroids found that *S. aureus* colonization was decreased with this intervention.[71] Use of wet wrap therapy over TCIs is not indicated per current package labeling. Wet wrap therapy should be thought of as an acute crisis intervention, not as part of maintenance therapy, although occasionally it can be used on a more chronic basis to select areas of resistant dermatitis with appropriate monitoring. An evidence-based critical review of wet wrap therapy in children concluded, with a grade C recommendation, that (1) wet wrap therapy using cream or ointment and a double layer of cotton bandages, with a moist first layer and a dry second layer, is an efficacious short-term intervention treatment in children with severe and/or refractory AD; (2) the use of wet wrap dressings with diluted topical corticosteroids is a more efficacious short-term intervention treatment in children with severe and/or refractory AD than wet wrap dressings with emollients only; (3) the use of wet wrap dressings with diluted topical corticosteroids for up to 14 days is a safe intervention treatment in children with severe and/or refractory AD, with temporary systemic bioactivity of the corticosteroids as the only reported serious side effect; and (4) lowering the absolute amount of applied topical corticosteroid to once-daily application and further dilution of the product can reduce the risk of systemic bioactivity.[72] The largest controlled study of wet wrap therapy in children using a validated scoring tool and patient questionnaire showed that in patients with moderate to severe AD, SCORing Atopic Dermatitis (SCORAD) improved significantly. Importantly, the benefit of this intervention could be demonstrated 1 month after discharge from the program, even though the treatment itself was discontinued before discharge (used for an average of 4 days).[68] In addition, none of these patients required treatment with a systemic immunosuppressive agent.

Multidisciplinary Approach to Atopic Dermatitis

Given the complex nature of AD, its relapsing course, and its incompletely understood pathogenesis, a significant number of patients have suboptimal outcomes with their prescribed treatment regimens. In addition, there is a significant impact on the quality of life of patients and families that leads to frustration and often a search for alternative therapies, which may not be in the best interest of the child. Although children with AD of all severities could benefit from a multidisciplinary approach, those who especially should be considered candidates include those failing conventional therapy, those with recurrent skin infections, those diagnosed with multiple food allergies, those whose disease is having a significant impact on their or their family's quality of life, those with concerns about medication side effects, and those with need for in-depth education. The significant and sustained clinical improvement often seen in patients treated with a multidisciplinary approach may be due, in large part, to in-depth, hands-on education, along with changes in environmental exposures, reduction in stressors and ensuring adherence to therapy. Of note, a high percentage of these patients experience significant improvement, even when treated with medications that previously were thought to be ineffective, when the treatment is integrated into a comprehensive and individualized management program.

The Atopic Dermatitis Program (ADP) at National Jewish Health in Denver, Colorado, consists of a team of pediatric allergist-immunologists with extensive experience in basic and clinical research in AD, a nurse practitioner/dermatology clinical specialist, pediatric psychiatrist, child psychologists, allergy-immunology fellows-in-training, physician assistants, nurse educators, child life specialists, creative art therapist, social workers, dietitians, and rehabilitation therapists.[3,43] Dermatologists are available for consultation if the diagnosis of AD is in question or phototherapy is being considered. Patients undergo comprehensive evaluation and treatment that is tailored to their needs and the goals of the family. Our ADP provides single-day consultations; multiday outpatient clinic visits; rarely, inpatient hospitalization; and a day program for more extensive evaluation, education, and treatment, typically over 5 to 14 days. In the controlled environment of the day program, patients and caregivers interact with members of the multidisciplinary team and, importantly, with other patients and families in group meetings and informal settings. In addition, sleep disturbance and response to interventions can be evaluated with overnight observation.[73]

Allergen Immunotherapy

Allergen-specific immunotherapy (AIT) has been added as a therapeutic consideration in the most recent AD Practice Parameter Update for selected patients with AD with environmental allergies, based on studies with house dust mite immunotherapy.[55] Most of the studies have been done in adult patients, and, anecdotally, patients on AIT may have flares of their eczema with allergen injections. Well-controlled studies in children with AD are still required to determine the role for AIT in this disease. In addition, preliminary studies with sublingual immunotherapy suggest a role for a subset of children with AD sensitized to dust mite allergen,[74] but again these data need to be reproduced in a larger pediatric population, especially in light of the natural history of AD for different subsets of patients.

Investigational or Unproven Therapy

Intravenous Immunoglobulin

High-dose intravenous immunoglobulin (IVIG) could have immunomodulatory effects in AD. In addition, IVIG could interact directly with microbes or toxins involved in the pathogenesis of AD. IVIG has been shown to contain high concentrations of staphylococcal toxin–specific antibodies that inhibit the in vitro activation of T cells by staphylococcal toxins.[75]

Treatment of severe refractory AD with IVIG has yielded conflicting results. Studies have not been controlled and have involved small numbers of patients.[76,77] Children appear to have a better response than adults, including to IVIG as monotherapy, and the duration of response was also shown to be more prolonged in children. However, additional controlled studies are needed to establish efficacy in a more definitive manner.

Interferon-Gamma

Interferon-gamma (IFN-γ) is known to suppress IgE responses and down-regulate T_H2 cell proliferation and function. Several studies of patients with AD, including a multicenter, double-blinded, placebo-controlled trial, have demonstrated that treatment with recombinant IFN-γ results in clinical improvement.[78] Reduction in clinical severity of AD was correlated with the ability of IFN-γ to decrease total circulating eosinophil counts. Influenza-like symptoms are commonly observed side effects seen early in the treatment course.

Probiotics

Data from one meta-analysis suggest a modest role for probiotics in children with moderately severe disease in reducing the Scoring of Atopic Dermatitis Severity Index score (mean change from baseline, –3.01; 95% confidence interval, –5.36 to –0.66; P = .01).[79] Duration of probiotic administration, age, and type of probiotic used did not affect outcome. Another meta-analysis found that current evidence is more convincing for probiotic efficacy in prevention rather than treatment of pediatric AD.[80] On the other hand, supplementation with *Lactobacillus* GG during pregnancy and early infancy neither reduced the incidence of AD nor altered the severity of AD in affected children, but it was associated with an increased rate of recurrent episodes of wheezing bronchitis.[81] A Cochrane review concluded that probiotics are not an effective treatment for eczema in children and that probiotic treatment carries a small risk of adverse events.[82] In contrast, a subsequent meta-analysis of randomized controlled trials through 2011 that attempted to overcome some of the limitations of earlier reviews found a reduction of approximately 20% in the incidence of AD and IgE-associated AD in infants and children with probiotic use.[83] To add to the continued uncertainty, a study in pregnant women and infants up to age 6 months given a multistrain probiotic did not show any difference in diagnosis of eczema at 2 years compared with placebo.[84] However, the frequency of allergic sensitization and allergic eczema (defined as eczema with one or more positive allergy skin tests) was significantly reduced.

Vitamin D

Vitamin D deficiency is being increasingly recognized in the U.S. population and may play a role in various allergic illnesses.[85] Of interest, vitamin D may play an important role in regulation of antimicrobial peptides in keratinocytes.[86] A trial with oral vitamin D supports this hypothesis.[87] In one small pediatric study, children with AD were treated with oral vitamin D in a randomized controlled trial. Investigator Global Assessment (IGA) score improved by 1 IGA category in four of five subjects treated with vitamin D versus one of six on placebo. Similar improvements were seen for change in the Eczema Area and Severity Index (EASI) score.[88] The updated practice parameter states that patients with AD may benefit from supplementation with vitamin D, particularly if they have low vitamin D levels or low dietary intake.[55]

Omalizumab

Anecdotal reports suggest clinical benefit in some patients with AD, including children treated for their asthma with monoclonal anti-IgE (omalizumab) subcutaneous injections.[89] Adult patients with severe AD and significantly elevated serum IgE levels did not show benefit when omalizumab was used as monotherapy.[90] In contrast, significant improvement in three adolescent patients was observed when omalizumab was added to the usual therapy.[91] In addition, in an open study of seven patients (aged 6–19 years) with severe AD treated with omalizumab, baseline SCORAD was 75.4 (53–96.2) with a mean serum IgE of 16,007 IU/L (7520–35,790 IU/L).[92] After 12 months of treatment, mean SCORAD was 30.0 (16.2–43), a mean improvement of 45.6 (31.6–59.6; P <.0005). Specific markers have not been found to identify potential responders, although a 2014 study suggested that adult patients with AD who respond are wild type for filaggrin mutations.[93] At present, omalizumab remains an investigational therapy in AD.

Conclusions

AD is a common, genetically transmitted inflammatory skin disease frequently found in association with respiratory allergy. Key management concepts include protection of the skin barrier, skin hydration, avoidance of irritants and proven allergic triggers, and effective use of topical antiinflammatory agents and appropriate use of systemic therapy (Box 38.3). Education of patients and caregivers is an essential part of treating patients with AD of all levels of severity, and a multidisciplinary approach to management may be the best approach for some patients. Better understanding of the complex genetic and immunoregulatory abnormalities underlying AD may allow for development of more specific treatments and suggest new paradigms for managing this disease.

Helpful Websites

National Jewish Health (http://www.nationaljewish.org)
The National Eczema Association (http://www.nationaleczema.org)
The American Academy of Allergy, Asthma & Immunology (http://www.aaaai.org)
The American Academy of Dermatology (http://www.aad.org)

The reference list can be found on the companion Expert Consult website at http://www.expertconsult.inkling.com.

39

Urticaria and Angioedema

SHYAM R. JOSHI, DAVID A. KHAN

KEY POINTS

- The distinction between acute and chronic urticaria and angioedema has important diagnostic and therapeutic implications. Recurrent angioedema without urticaria suggests the possibility of hereditary angioedema.
- The most common type of swelling in children is acute urticaria and angioedema. The cause of acute urticaria often can be determined and is most likely to involve viral infections, immunoglobulin E–mediated reactions, or stings.
- Chronic urticaria and angioedema are typically idiopathic; however, physical stimuli, including cold, heat, and pressure, often

contribute to the symptoms. Extensive diagnostic evaluation of chronic urticaria is not usually warranted.
- First-line treatment of urticaria and angioedema is nonsedating antihistamines with dosing up to four times the approved dose.
- Omalizumab is recommended for patients with chronic urticaria who do not respond to high-dose antihistamines.

Introduction

Urticaria (hives or wheals) typically presents as a pruritic generalized eruption with erythematous circumscribed borders and pale, slightly elevated centers (Fig. 39.1A). Angioedema is characterized by an asymmetric, nondependent swelling that is generally not pruritic (see Fig. 39.1B). The pathophysiologic processes of urticaria and angioedema are similar and the result of increased vascular permeability. However, the underlying mechanisms can be very distinct: mast cells are often implicated in urticaria, but angioedema may be caused by histamine or bradykinin.

Affected patients may manifest symptoms that range from transient and mildly bothersome hives to severe and potentially fatal angioedema. Quality of life has been reported to be moderately to severely impaired in patients with chronic urticaria,[1–4] and children with chronic urticaria exhibit significantly greater psychiatric morbidity than controls.[5] An efficient and cost-effective approach to the management of both acute and chronic urticaria and angioedema depends on a careful assessment of the characteristics and likely cause of the swelling. This chapter provides a framework to differentiate the various types of urticaria and angioedema and then outlines a directed evaluation and treatment plan based on the cause (Box 39.1).

Classification of Urticaria and Angioedema

Urticaria and angioedema are conventionally classified as either acute or chronic, the latter being defined as the continuous or frequent occurrence of lesions for longer than 6 weeks.[6] Although arbitrary, this distinction has significant implications regarding the cause, course, and treatment of the swelling. Most cases of urticaria and angioedema are acute, particularly in children. Acute

urticaria and angioedema can occur during anaphylaxis, and this possibility needs to be considered when urticaria or angioedema is associated with respiratory, gastrointestinal (GI), cardiovascular, or nervous system involvement.

Epidemiology

Approximately 50% of affected patients experience both urticaria and angioedema, 40% only urticaria, and 10% only angioedema.[7] Surveys have indicated that 15% to 23% of the population experience urticaria at least once during their lifetime,[8] and the prevalence of chronic urticaria is estimated to be 0.5% to 5%, with females overrepresented.[9,10] Chronic urticaria is less common in children than in adults. Atopic individuals are at increased risk for acute urticaria or angioedema and some forms of physical urticaria; however, most patients with chronic urticaria or angioedema do not have atopy.

The prevalence of hereditary angioedema (HAE) resulting from C1 inhibitor (C1INH) deficiency (HAE-C1INH) is approximately 1:50,000.[11] The prevalence of HAE with normal C1INH (HAE-nlC1INH) is less than HAE-C1INH. Acquired C1INH deficiency occurs predominantly in adults and has an estimated prevalence of 1:500,000.[12] Bradykinin-mediated angioedema also can be associated with use of angiotensin-converting enzyme (ACE) inhibitors and possibly with recurrent idiopathic angioedema.

Pathophysiology

Most urticaria and angioedema is caused by mast cell degranulation with released mediators leading to activation of sensory nerves, vasodilation, plasma extravasation, up-regulation of

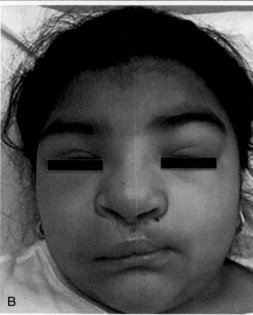

• **Fig. 39.1** Typical examples of urticaria and angioedema. (A) Urticarial lesions with areas of central pallor and confluence. (B) Angioedema of the eyelids, nose, and lips.

• **BOX 39.1   Key Concepts**
Urticaria and Angioedema

- The distinction between acute and chronic urticaria and angioedema has important diagnostic and therapeutic implications.
- The most common types of swelling in children are acute urticaria and angioedema.
- The cause of acute urticaria often can be determined and is most likely to involve infections (mainly viral), immunoglobulin E–mediated reactions, or bites and stings.
- The cause of chronic urticaria and angioedema is typically idiopathic; however, physical stimuli often contribute to the symptoms.
- Chronic urticaria and angioedema should be distinguished from urticarial vasculitis.
- Recurrent angioedema without urticaria suggests the possibility of hereditary angioedema.
- Most cases of chronic urticaria or angioedema resolve within 3 to 4 years.

endothelial cell adhesion molecules, and recruitment of inflammatory cells.[13–15] Basophils may also play an important role.[16] The causes of mast cell degranulation in urticaria and angioedema are variable. Immunoglobulin E (IgE)-mediated mast cell degranulation is responsible for many cases of acute urticaria and angioedema in children, most commonly from drugs and foods. Many acute and most chronic urticaria and angioedema cases involve mast cell activation as a result of immune or nonimmunologic processes not involving IgE, such as direct mast cell degranulators, viral infections, anaphylatoxins, various peptides and proteins, and several types of physical stimuli. Viral infections are the most common cause of acute urticaria in children.[17,18]

The underlying cause of mast cell degranulation in chronic urticaria and angioedema usually cannot be determined. Lesions demonstrate a nonnecrotizing mononuclear cell infiltrate around small venules, with increased numbers of eosinophils, basophils, and T helper cells.[13,19] Filaggrin is overexpressed in urticarial lesions, the level correlating with urticaria severity.[20] Activation of thrombin with subsequent generation of complement component 5a (C5a) also has been suggested as a potential underlying mechanism in chronic urticaria.[21] Some children with celiac disease and severe chronic urticaria showed improvement of the urticaria after institution of a gluten-free diet.[22] A number of IgE autoantibodies have been implicated in the pathogenesis of chronic urticaria. At least 40% of patients with chronic urticaria have circulating autoantibodies with specificity for IgE or the high-affinity Fc epsilon receptor 1(FcεRI). [23–25] Skin testing with autologous serum or plasma may detect these antibodies.[26] Approximately 30% of children with chronic urticaria have positive autologous serum skin tests.[27,28] Recently, elevated IgE anti–interleukin 24 (IL-24) autoantibodies have been found in a majority of patients with chronic urticaria and correlate with disease severity.[29] The functional and prognostic significance of these autoantibodies remains unclear, and routine testing for these autoantibodies is not recommended.

An increased prevalence of thyroid antimicrosomal and antithyroglobulin antibodies has been described in urticaria and angioedema, with about half of these patients having goiters or abnormal thyroid function[30–33]; however, no causal relationship has been demonstrated.[34] Conversely, an increased cumulative prevalence of urticaria and angioedema has been found in patients with thyroid disease with antimicrosomal and antithyroglobulin antibodies (primarily Hashimoto's thyroiditis) but not in patients with other types of thyroid disease.[35] Activation of complement by the complement controller domain of thyroperoxidase has been suggested to be an important contributor to development of urticaria and angioedema in patients with thyroid autoimmunity.[36] An association between urticaria and a variety of other autoimmune diseases has also been described, although the nature of the relationship remains uncertain.[37,38] Evaluation of underlying autoimmunity, including thyroid disease, is not routinely performed unless the history is suggestive.

HAE-C1INH is an autosomal dominant disease caused by a functional deficiency of the plasma protein C1INH. Two major types of HAE-C1INH have been described: type 1 HAE comprises 85% of cases and is characterized by low C1INH antigenic and functional levels; type 2 HAE comprises the other 15% of cases and is characterized by normal C1INH antigenic levels with low C1INH functional activity resulting from secretion of a dysfunctional protein.[39] Types 1 and 2 HAE are caused by mutations in the C1INH gene (*SERPING1*), resulting in increased plasma kallikrein activity and generation of the vasoactive mediator

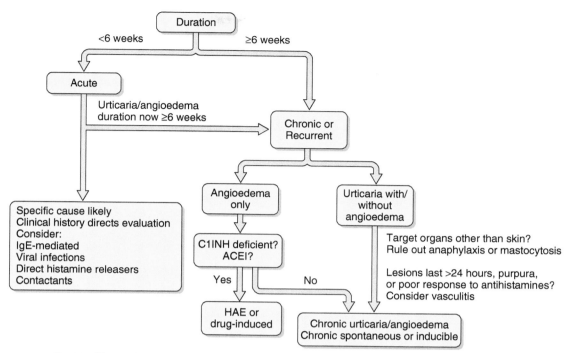

• **Fig. 39.2** Diagnostic algorithm for urticaria and angioedema. *ACEI*, Angiotensin-converting enzyme inhibitor; *AE*, angioedema; *C1INH*, C1 inhibitor; *HAE*, hereditary angioedema; *IgE*, immunoglobulin E.

bradykinin.[39] Familial recurrent angioedema with normal C1INH gene and protein was originally called type 3 HAE,[40,41] but has now been renamed HAE-nlC1INH.[42] Coagulation factor XII gene mutations were the first mutations discovered; subsequently, several other mutations have been reported associated with HAE-nlC1INH, including mutations in genes for plasminogen and angiopoietin-1.[43,44] Nevertheless, the underlying cause of the disease remains unclear in most patients, although mechanisms have been proposed.[45] C1INH deficiency also may be acquired; however, this occurs primarily in older adults and has not been reported in children.

Cryopyrin-associated autoinflammatory syndromes (CAPS) are associated with mutations in a gene that encodes cryopyrin and are referred to as cryopyrinopathies.[46,47] Familial cold auto-inflammatory syndrome (FCAS) is the mildest form, and Muckle-Wells syndrome (MWS) is a more severe subtype associated with hearing impairment and amyloidosis. Neonatal-onset multisystem inflammatory disease (NOMID) is a particularly devastating cryopyrinopathy. Cutaneous lesions associated with CAPS are referred to as *pseudourticaria* and often are not pruritic but may be associated with a burning sensation. Antagonists of the IL-1 pathway, including anakinra and canakinumab have been used successfully to prevent attacks.[48,49] *PLCG2*-associated antibody deficiency and immune dysregulation (PLAID) syndrome is due to a gain of phospholipase Cγ2 function that is characterized by cold urticaria, antibody deficiency, increased susceptibility to infection, autoimmunity, and skin granuloma formation.[50,51]

Differential Diagnosis

Recognition of urticaria and angioedema on examination is generally straightforward. The single most important step in the differential diagnosis is to visualize acute lesions. Individual urticarial lesions

---

• BOX 39.2 Common Causes for Acute Urticaria and Angioedema in Children

Infections
- Viral, bacterial, fungal, parasitic

Mast Cell–Mediated
- Drugs
  - Nonsteroidal antiinflammatory drugs, antibiotics
- Foods
  - Cow's milk, egg, wheat, soy, peanut, tree nuts, fish, shellfish
- Insect bites/stings
  - Mosquitos, spiders, chiggers, hymenoptera, (fire) ants, bed bugs, fleas, mites

Contact allergens
- Poison ivy, foods, animals, latex

---

seldom last for more than a few hours (up to 24 hours), which distinguishes urticaria from almost all other skin diseases. In addition, urticarial lesions blanch with pressure, and new hives frequently develop as the older ones fade. If the lesions do not itch or last longer than 24 hours, the diagnosis should be reconsidered. Angioedema is not a dependent edema and is typically not symmetric. Fig. 39.2 presents an algorithm for the approach to the differential diagnosis.

Acute Urticaria and Angioedema

Etiology

Acute urticaria and angioedema by definition lasts less than 6 weeks and is most commonly caused by infections or exposure to allergens, toxins, or sensitizers. A cause for acute urticaria or angioedema frequently can be determined by history and testing (if appropriate). Most cases in children will be secondary to infection (up to 50%), but other causes also should be considered, including IgE-mediated reactions to drugs and foods.[17,18] Box 39.2 lists many common triggers in children.

The most common foods associated with IgE-mediated urticaria and angioedema vary with the age of the patient. In younger children, egg, milk, soy, peanut, and wheat are the most common allergens, whereas fish, seafood, tree nuts, and peanuts are common offenders in older children.[52] Acute urticaria also can be triggered by ingestion of dark-fleshed fish containing high levels of bioactive amines in the absence of specific IgE (scombroid poisoning).[53] Urticaria and angioedema are the most common manifestations of anaphylactic reactions to insect stings. Immunologic reactions to the saliva of bedbugs, fleas, or mites can cause papular urticaria, especially on the legs of children. Papular urticaria lesions typically last longer than 24 hours. Acute urticaria or angioedema occurring 3 to 6 hours after the ingestion of beef, pork, lamb, or venison has been described in patients with IgE against galactose-α-1,3-galactose.[54]

Urticaria multiforme (or acute annular urticarial hypersensitivity) is distinguished by transient annular, arcuate, and polycyclic urticarial lesions, which are often accompanied by angioedema.[55] It is frequently triggered by an underlying infection or medications (e.g., nonsteroidal antiinflammatory drugs [NSAIDs], antibiotics).

Urticaria and angioedema also can result from exposure to direct mast cell degranulators (e.g., opiates, fluoroquinolones, vancomycin, or dextran volume expanders), penetrating substances (e.g., nettles, Portuguese man-of-war, other forms of sea life), or substances that can produce urticaria on contact with intact skin (e.g., latex, industrial chemicals, benzoic acid, sorbic acid, and numerous other agents).[56] Aspirin and other NSAIDs can provoke acute urticaria or angioedema in children and adults.[57,58]

Idiopathic anaphylaxis often includes a prominent component of urticaria or angioedema and can be difficult to distinguish from severe urticaria or angioedema.[59]

Clinical History

A discerning history is the most important diagnostic procedure in the evaluation of urticaria and angioedema. One should determine whether the urticaria or angioedema is acute or chronic, the duration of the individual lesions, the presence of pruritus (a defining symptom for urticaria), *when* lesions occur, *where* the patient is when lesions occur, *what* the patient suspects is the cause, and the response to prior treatment. Specific inquiry should be made about recent infections, drugs (including over-the-counter products), foreign sera, foods, herbal or homeopathic treatments, stings, direct contact of skin with various agents, connective tissue diseases, and exposure to physical stimuli. Associated respiratory, GI, or cardiovascular symptoms should be inquired about to determine whether the cutaneous lesions are part of an anaphylactic-type reaction.

Physical Examination

Most importantly, close examination of active lesions or pictures of previous lesions should be performed to ensure they are consistent with urticaria.[60] Urticarial rashes typically are generalized and may involve any part of the body. Individual lesions often coalesce

- Avoidance of known provoking stimuli can greatly improve treatment outcomes.
- Histamine 1 (H1) antihistamines are the mainstay of treatment, and second-generation H1 antihistamines are preferred because they have fewer side effects.
- Difficult cases may require treatment with various combinations of second-generation H1 antihistamines, first-generation H1 antihistamines, H2 antihistamines, and leukotriene receptor antagonists.
- Omalizumab is effective for antihistamine-resistant chronic urticaria.
- Delayed-pressure urticaria does not generally respond well to antihistamines.
- Corticosteroids should be avoided for long-term therapy.
- The angioedema of hereditary angioedema does not respond to antihistamines, corticosteroids, or epinephrine; oropharyngeal attacks of hereditary angioedema must be treated as a medical emergency.

into large lesions. If the lesions are localized, the location may provide a clue to the cause. For example, urticarial lesions around the mouth of infants may be secondary to a contact reaction with foods, or lesions isolated to the lower legs of toddlers may be associated with insect bites.

Diagnostic Procedures

The laboratory evaluation of patients with urticaria and/or angioedema must be tailored to the clinical situation. Biopsies or imaging studies are rarely required to confirm urticaria or angioedema and should not be routinely performed. If the history or examination provides clues to the cause of the urticaria or angioedema, the evaluation should be pursued using the appropriate tests. Most commonly, skin testing and in vitro specific IgE testing can be used to confirm IgE-mediated food, drug, or venom allergy. In the absence of a specific probable cause, the laboratory evaluation should be minimal. Routine testing for food or inhalant allergy is not recommended.[6]

Treatment

Guidelines for treating patients with urticaria and angioedema are summarized in Box 39.3. For obvious reasons, the preferred treatment is avoidance of causative agents when these can be identified through history and diagnostic testing. One should avoid generating undue anxiety about laryngeal edema because the only known fatalities from this cause have been in patients with HAE or anaphylactic reactions. True laryngeal edema is very rare in patients with idiopathic urticaria.

Antihistamines are the mainstay of treatment for acute or chronic urticaria or angioedema.[6] Used at a sufficient dose, they alleviate pruritus and suppress hive formation. Most first-generation histamine 1 (H1) antihistamines are effective in urticaria; however, common side effects (particularly drowsiness and anticholinergic effects) may be a significant issue, and thus they are typically considered after second-generation antihistamines have been tried.[61] In addition, children may experience either sedation or a paradoxical agitation response to first-generation H1 antihistamines.[62]

Second-generation H1 antagonists cross the blood-brain barrier poorly, producing much less central drowsiness or agitation,

TABLE 39.1	Dosing of Second-Generation Histamine 1 Antihistamines in the Pediatric Population		
Drug	**Supplied As**	**Usual Dosage**	**Earliest Approved Age**
Cetirizine	Tablets: 5, 10 mg Oral suspension: 1 mg/mL	6 mo–1 yr: 2.5 mg/day 1–2 yr: 2.5 mg bid 2–5 yr: 2.5 mg bid or 5 mg daily 6–11 yr: 5–10 mg/day ≥12 yr: 10 mg/day	6 mo
Loratadine	Tablets/Reditabs: 10 mg Oral suspension: 1 mg/mL	2–6 yr: 5 mg/day ≥6 yr: 10 mg/day	2 y
Fexofenadine	Tablets: 30, 60, 180 mg Oral suspension: 6 mg/mL	6 mo–2 yr; 15 mg/day 2–11 yr: 30 mg bid ≥12 yr: 60 mg bid or 180 mg/day	6 mo
Desloratadine	Tablets/Reditabs: 5 mg Oral suspension: 0.5 mg/mL	6 mo–1 yr: 1 mg/day 1–5 yr: 1.25 mg/day 6–11 yr: 2.5 mg/day ≥12 yr: 5 mg/day	6 mo
Levocetirizine	Tablets: 5 mg Oral suspension: 2.5 mg/5 mL	6 mo–6 yr: 1.25 mg/day 6–11 yr: 2.5 mg/day ≥12 yr: 5 mg/day	6 mo

and have much less anticholinergic effect. Second-generation H1 antagonists have thus become the preferred drugs for the first-line treatment of urticaria and angioedema, including for infants as young as 6 months.[6,63] The most commonly used second-generation H1 antihistamines in the United States are cetirizine, loratadine, desloratadine, fexofenadine, and levocetirizine. Each of these has been shown to be well tolerated and effective for the treatment of urticaria and angioedema.[64] The recommended doses for the pediatric population are shown in Table 39.1.

Because the cutaneous vasculature expresses H2 and the more abundant H1 receptors, the addition of an H2 antihistamine may provide significant benefit for patients who are refractory to H1 antihistamines alone, although the evidence for their efficacy is weak.[6] Leukotriene receptor antagonists have shown some promise in the treatment of urticaria and angioedema, particularly in combination with an antihistamine regimen[65]; however, evidence of benefit from randomized, double-blinded studies is mixed.[66] Although many patients will respond to antihistamine therapy, some patients may have partial or even no response to even high-dose antihistamines.

In cases of severe antihistamine-resistant urticaria or angioedema, a brief course of corticosteroids may be used, but long-term use of corticosteroids is not recommended.[6,67] The potential side effects from chronic use of corticosteroids mandate that they be used at the lowest possible dose for the shortest period.[68,69]

For situations in which other systemic symptoms are present consistent with anaphylaxis, epinephrine should be used. This topic is discussed in more detail in Chapter 46.

Chronic Urticaria and Angioedema

Etiology

Urticaria and angioedema are considered chronic when symptoms occur continuously or frequently for a period of 6 weeks or more. The vast majority of cases are idiopathic, and the diagnosis is one of exclusion based on history, examination, and carefully selected testing (although testing is often not indicated). No clear relationship has been found between chronic urticaria and food allergy, ingestion of food additives, or focal infections.[70] Viral, parasitic, and *Helicobacter pylori* infections have been suggested as having a link to chronic urticaria, although causation has not been established.[71–73] Patients with chronic urticaria may have autoimmune features (see on "Pathophysiology" section).

Severe urticaria or angioedema associated with marked weight gain, pronounced leukocytosis, and striking eosinophilia (Gleich syndrome) has been shown to involve increased serum levels of cytokines (including IL-5) during attacks.[74,75] Other cases of urticaria or angioedema have been reported in association with parathyroid disease, polycythemia vera, hemolytic uremic syndrome, lymphoproliferative diseases, Schnitzler syndrome (chronic urticaria, monoclonal IgM, arthralgia, fever, and adenopathy), and pregnancy.[6] Cyclical urticaria occurring before menses may be a hypersensitivity to progesterone.[76,77] Genetic causes of urticaria and angioedema include HAE, CAPS, PLAID syndrome, vibratory angioedema, familial localized heat urticaria of delayed type, erythropoietic protoporphyria with solar urticaria, C3 inactivator deficiency with urticaria, and serum carboxypeptidase N deficiency with angioedema.

Chronic urticaria is further subdivided into chronic spontaneous urticaria (CSU, previously referred to as chronic idiopathic urticaria) or inducible urticaria (previously known as physical urticaria) based on whether there is a precipitating stimulus.[6] CSU has no identifiable cause and is the most common form of chronic urticaria, with up to 40% of cases involving angioedema. Inducible urticaria involves mast cell degranulation precipitated by discrete physical stimuli (Table 39.2). Inducible urticaria is often but not always encountered in the setting of co-existing CSU. The percentage of children in whom chronic urticaria also has a physical component ranges from 1% to more than 10% based on data from multiple studies.[78] Patients may urticate in response to one or several physical stimuli, including mechanical pressure or stroking, heat, cold, sunlight, or water. Specific physical challenges can be performed to confirm inducible urticaria

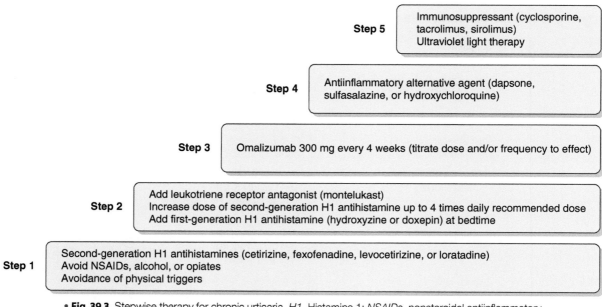

Step 5	Immunosuppressant (cyclosporine, tacrolimus, sirolimus) Ultraviolet light therapy
Step 4	Antiinflammatory alternative agent (dapsone, sulfasalazine, or hydroxychloroquine)
Step 3	Omalizumab 300 mg every 4 weeks (titrate dose and/or frequency to effect)
Step 2	Add leukotriene receptor antagonist (montelukast) Increase dose of second-generation H1 antihistamine up to 4 times daily recommended dose Add first-generation H1 antihistamine (hydroxyzine or doxepin) at bedtime
Step 1	Second-generation H1 antihistamines (cetirizine, fexofenadine, levocetirizine, or loratadine) Avoid NSAIDs, alcohol, or opiates Avoidance of physical triggers

• **Fig. 39.3** Stepwise therapy for chronic urticaria. *H1,* Histamine 1; *NSAIDs,* nonsteroidal antiinflammatory drugs.

or angioedema (see Table 39.2). Dermographism may occur in up to 5% of the general population (Fig. 39.4A) and can account for the majority of urticaria in some patients.[8] Delayed pressure urticaria is more angioedematous than urticarial and causes significant morbidity.[2]

Primary and secondary acquired forms of cold urticaria have been described.[79] Primary acquired cold urticaria is often seen in children and is frequently associated with asthma and allergic rhinitis and may progress to anaphylaxis.[80] In rare cases, patients with acquired cold urticaria have drowned when exposed to cold water as a result of hypotension and should be warned to avoid swimming in cold water and never to swim alone. Cold urticaria should be distinguished from FCAS, which is marked by cold-induced erythematous rash, fever, arthralgias, leukocytosis, and conjunctivitis.[46]

Cholinergic urticaria (see Fig. 39.4B) is relatively common in children, may be confused with exercise-induced anaphylaxis (EIAn), and can be associated with angioedema, wheezing, or even syncope.[81] Cholinergic urticaria can be differentiated from EIAn by passively warming the patient. Patients with EIAn will not display symptoms in this setting, whereas those with cholinergic urticaria will. Persistent cholinergic erythema, a variant of cholinergic urticaria, can be mistaken for a drug eruption or cutaneous mastocytosis.[82] Many patients have combinations of different physical urticarias, such as cold and cholinergic urticaria, cold and localized heat urticaria, or dermographism with cold urticaria.

Clinical History

Chronic urticaria is a clinical diagnosis; therefore, a careful history and physical examination are required to rule out any potential underlying conditions or external factors. A detailed history should be taken to evaluate for possible autoimmunity, malignancy, and infections. In many patients, chronic urticaria can be aggravated by vasodilating stimuli such as heat, exercise, emotional stress, alcoholic drinks, fever, and hyperthyroidism. Premenstrual exacerbations also are common. Aspirin and other cyclooxygenase 1 (COX-1) inhibiting NSAIDs can cause exacerbations in up to

30% of patients. COX-2 inhibitors and acetaminophen do not typically trigger urticaria or angioedema.[57,83]

For chronic inducible urticaria, an understanding of all physical triggers is helpful because avoidance can lead to significant symptom improvement but is not always feasible (see Table 39.2).

Urticarial vasculitis may be distinguished from chronic idiopathic urticaria or angioedema by lack of pruritus, persistence of individual urticarial lesions for more than 24 hours, bruising, hyperpigmentation, or a poor response to antihistamine therapy. Urticarial vasculitis ranges from relatively benign cutaneous hypersensitivity vasculitis to the hypocomplementemic urticarial vasculitis syndrome.[84,85] In children, most cases of cutaneous vasculitis represent Henoch-Schönlein purpura or hypersensitivity vasculitis.[86] Hypocomplementemic urticarial vasculitis syndrome is rarely seen in children.[87]

Physical Examination

Urticaria and angioedema should be confirmed by a detailed physical examination. Occasionally, the appearance of the lesions gives a clue as to the type of urticaria being encountered: linear wheals suggest dermographism; small wheals surrounded by large areas of erythema suggest cholinergic urticaria; wheals limited to exposed areas suggest solar or cold urticaria; and wheals mainly on the lower extremities suggest papular urticaria or urticarial vasculitis. In addition, signs of cutaneous bruising may help favor the diagnosis of urticarial vasculitis, and signs of autoimmunity, including joint swelling or presence of a goiter, may warrant additional laboratory testing.

Diagnostic Procedures

In most cases of chronic urticaria and angioedema, no specific cause can be established, and the diagnostic approach should therefore be carefully selected and cost effective. For most cases, no workup is indicated. Box 39.4 summarizes a limited laboratory evaluation that can be performed in patients with chronic urticaria or angioedema if features are present that are suggestive of an underlying disease process. Because the cause of chronic urticaria

TABLE 39.2   Major Physical Urticaria Syndromes

Type	Provoking Stimuli	Diagnostic Test	Comment
Mechanically Provoked			
Dermographism (urticaria factitia)	Rubbing or scratching of skin causes linear wheals.	Stroking the skin (especially the back) elicits a linear wheal.	Primary (idiopathic or allergic) or secondary (urticaria pigmentosa or transient after virus or drug reaction).
Delayed dermographism	Same.	Same.	Rare.
Delayed-pressure urticaria	At least 2 hr after pressure is applied to the skin, deep, painful swelling develops, especially involving the palms, soles, and buttocks.	Attach two sandbags or jugs of fluid (5–15 lb) to either end of a strap and apply over the shoulder or thigh for 10–15 min. A positive test exhibits linear wheals or swelling after several hours.	Can be disabling and may be associated with constitutional symptoms such as malaise, fever, arthralgia, headache, and leukocytosis.
Immediate-pressure urticaria	Hives develop within 1–2 min of pressure.	Several minutes of pressure elicit hives.	Rare; seen in conjunction with hypereosinophilic syndrome.
Thermally Provoked			
Acquired cold urticaria	Change in skin temperature rapidly provokes urticaria.	Place ice cube on extremity for 3–5 min, then observe for pruritic welt and surrounding erythema as the skin rewarms over subsequent 5–15 min.	Relatively common, may occur transiently with exposure to drugs or with infections; other rare cases may be associated with cryoproteins or may be transferable by serum.
Familial cold autoinflammatory syndrome	Intermittent episodes of rash, arthralgia, fever, and conjunctivitis occur after generalized exposure to cold.	Genetic testing for *C1AS1* mutation.	Autosomal dominant inflammatory disorder previously called familial cold "urticaria"; results from mutation of *CIAS1* gene, coding for cryopyrin.
Cholinergic urticaria	Heat, exertion, or emotional upset causes small punctate wheals with prominent erythematous flare. May be related more to sweating than to heat per se.	Exercise for 30 minutes or bathe in 42° C for 15 minutes. Urticaria appear after body temperature increases by 1° C.	Differs from exercise-induced anaphylaxis in that it features smaller wheals and is induced by heat and exercise but does not generally cause patients to collapse. Relatively common in patients with chronic urticaria; can be passively transferred by plasma in some patients.
Localized heat urticaria	Urtication occurs at sites of contact with a warm stimulus.	Hold a test tube containing water 44° C against the skin for 5 min.	Rare.
Miscellaneous Provoked			
Solar urticaria	Urticaria develops in areas of skin exposed to sunlight.	Controlled exposure to light; can be divided depending on the wavelength of light eliciting the lesions.	Types include genetic abnormality in protoporphyrin IX metabolism and types that can be passively transferred by immunoglobulin E in serum.
Aquagenic urticaria	Tiny perifollicular urticarial lesions develop after contact with water of any temperature.	Apply towel soaked in 37° C water to the skin for 30 min.	Rare; systemic symptoms can occur; females affected more than males; familial form has been described.

or angioedema is not related to extrinsic allergen exposure in the vast majority of cases, routine skin testing is not recommended.[6] Patients with a history suggestive of physical urticaria may be challenged to confirm the diagnosis (see Table 39.2).

Testing to detect IgG autoantibodies against the high-affinity immunoglobulin E receptor (FcεRI) or IgE, thyroid antibodies, or autologous serum or plasma skin testing is not recommended.[6] This is due to the lack of data supporting abnormal test results having prognostic value or providing any meaningful changes in management.

Treatment

Reassurance is an important aspect of therapy for urticaria and angioedema. Skin lesions are often more frightening in appearance than the generally favorable prognosis warrants and are self-limited. Most urticaria and angioedema spontaneously remits without any irreversible damage.

An explanation of the disease process and its triggers is also helpful for patients with physical urticaria such as dermographism,

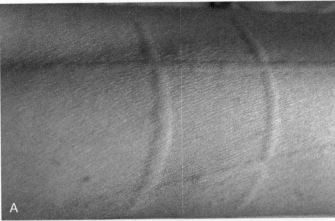

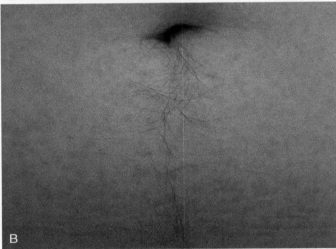

• **Fig. 39.4** Examples of physical urticaria. (A) Dermographism. (B) Cholinergic urticaria.

cholinergic urticaria, and delayed-pressure urticaria (Table 39.2). Treatment of any discovered underlying disease is imperative, and genetic counseling is helpful to families with hereditary forms of these conditions. In addition, patients should avoid, to the extent feasible, potentiating factors such as alcoholic drinks, heat, exertion, and NSAIDs when these are found to be triggers.

Antihistamines remain the first-line therapy for chronic urticaria and angioedema (Fig. 39.3). A detailed explanation of the types of antihistamines, dosing, and side effects is described earlier in this chapter. Lack of response to antihistamines may indicate the possibility of an underlying urticarial vasculitis, particularly when individual hives last for longer than 24 hours. Patients should be treated with second-generation H1 antihistamines for at least 1 week before a given dose is considered ineffective and dose escalation may be considered. Furthermore, it is often helpful to counsel the patient and patient's family that the goal of therapy is not necessarily to suppress urticaria totally, but rather to minimize the urticaria or angioedema to the point that it is not adversely affecting their quality of life. Addition of a potent first-generation antihistamine (hydroxyzine or doxepin) titrated to tolerance may help in patients who are not fully responsive to high-dose second-generation antihistamines.[88] As previously mentioned, H2 blockers and leukotriene antagonists may be considered, with some guidelines recommending their use and others against their

use.[89] Avoidance of dietary "pseudoallergens" (i.e., substances that induce hypersensitivity or intolerance reactions such as food additives, vasoactive substances such as histamine, and some natural substances in fruits, vegetables, and spices) has been reported to improve CSU in a minority of patients and is controversial.[90]

In patients whose symptoms remain inadequately controlled despite aggressive antihistamine therapy, omalizumab is the next recommended therapy per international guidelines.[67] Omalizumab has been shown in randomized placebo-controlled trials to be highly effective in antihistamine-resistant urticaria in adults and children.[91–95] It is approved in the United States for children 12 years of age and older but is often used in younger children because of its proven safety in asthma trials.[96] Omalizumab has also been shown to be safe and effective in meta-analyses.[97,98] Additionally, it is helpful in many types of inducible urticaria and angioedema.[99,100] The most effective approved dose of omalizumab is 300 mg every 4 weeks, yet some reports suggest splitting the dose (150 mg every 2 weeks) may be effective in nonresponders.[101,102] Most patients respond within weeks to omalizumab, but delayed responses occur in approximately one-third of patients. A trial of 4 to 6 months at 300 mg every 4 weeks is generally considered an adequate trial. If omalizumab 300 mg is not effective, some observational studies suggest higher doses may increase the number of patients whose symptoms are able to be controlled.[103] In patients whose symptoms are not adequately controlled with omalizumab, several alternative agents have been used.[104] Evidence for the majority of alternative agents is generally of low quality. Cyclosporine has been studied in refractory urticaria, and although two randomized placebo-controlled studies have demonstrated efficacy, a review of the evidence suggests it is of low quality with a weak recommendation.[105–107] The safety of cyclosporine in children is less well established than in adults; however, it has also been shown to be efficacious in children with chronic urticaria.[108,109] Other alternative therapies for refractory chronic urticaria include dapsone, mycophenolate, tacrolimus, colchicine, hydroxychloroquine, methotrexate, and sulfasalazine among others. The safety of these alternative agents has been demonstrated in adults treated with chronic urticaria.[110]

Isolated Angioedema

Etiology

Angioedema is usually associated with urticaria that is nondependent, asymmetric, and nonpruritic. When it occurs with urticaria, the diagnosis and treatment of angioedema mirrors the parameters described for urticaria. Recurrent angioedema without urticaria (including recurrent unexplained abdominal pain) should suggest a possible diagnosis of HAE. Accurate diagnosis of HAE is essential to avoid morbidity and mortality; however, delays in HAE diagnosis are unfortunately very common. Repeated surveys have shown a 10- to 20-year interval between onset of symptoms and establishment of the correct diagnosis.[111] Half of all patients with HAE begin swelling during the first decade of life, with almost all patients manifesting symptoms by age 18.[112] HAE has been categorized in three distinct types, which are described in detail earlier in this chapter.

The most common form of angioedema without urticaria in children is idiopathic.[113] Idiopathic angioedema can be further categorized into histaminergic and nonhistaminergic. The underlying pathophysiology is not well understood but bradykinin appears to play a role in idiopathic nonhistaminergic angioedema.[114] Infections, IgE-mediated allergies, and autoimmunity have also been associated with angioedema without urticaria.

Angioedema may occur during the treatment of hypertension with ACE inhibitors.[115] ACE is a peptidase that degrades bradykinin (among other peptides), and the mechanism of ACE inhibitor–associated angioedema is suspected to be due to diminished catabolism of bradykinin.[116] In addition, a retrospective review of 1007 charts of children with atopy revealed that 41 (4.07%) had experienced NSAID-induced facial angioedema.[117] Intermittent use of NSAIDs was associated with a higher rate of angioedema than chronic regular use.[118]

There are also several forms of facial edema that can be confused with angioedema, including the granulomatous cheilitis accompanying Crohn's disease and Melkersson-Rosenthal syndrome (a rare syndrome including recurrent orofacial swelling, relapsing facial paralysis, and fissured tongue).

Clinical History

A detailed personal and family history is imperative to help narrow the proper diagnosis. Establishing the lack of urticarial lesions during the angioedema episodes will guide diagnostic workup and therapeutic options. Important factors to consider include the age of onset, severity and frequency of symptoms, duration of swelling, location on the body, and association with other signs or symptoms. Questioning should lead to an understanding of all prescription and over-the-counter medications taken (specifically ACE inhibitors and NSAIDs), autoimmune history, and effectiveness of treatments during previous episodes.

Angioedema attacks in HAE-C1INH have distinct manifestations, including prolonged duration (typically ≥48 hours); frequently triggered by minor trauma or stress; often preceded by a prodromal syndrome; displaying periodicity with attacks of angioedema interspersed by periods of remission (daily episodes suggest an alternative diagnosis); swelling most commonly affecting the extremities, face, GI tract, or upper airway; and a history of lack of response to prior treatment with antihistamines, corticosteroids, or epinephrine.[111] Virtually all patients with HAE-C1INH experience extremity and GI attacks during their lifetime. Recurrent school absences because of abdominal pain may be a presenting symptom. It is not unusual to obtain a history of a normal exploratory laparotomy for presumed appendicitis. Laryngeal attacks are considerably less common, although over 50% of patients with HAE-C1INH will experience a laryngeal attack at some point in their life. Angioedema of the larynx in HAE-C1INH can result in closure of the airway and asphyxiation. In the past, over 30% of patients with HAE-C1INH died from airway attacks, but fatal laryngeal edema is rarer now.[111] A positive family history of angioedema can usually be elicited, although up to 25% of patients with HAE-C1INH have de novo *SERPING1* mutations.[119]

HAE-nlC1INH is also characterized by recurrent prolonged attacks of angioedema that can cause asphyxiation.[40,41,120] Attack frequency varies considerably among affected individuals, from carriers who are asymptomatic to patients with multiple attacks per year. There is a striking female preponderance of patients, and affected women tend to have more severe symptoms than affected men.[121,122] Like that of HAE-C1INH, the inheritance pattern of HAE-nlC1INH is autosomal dominant; however, the penetrance is often much lower, with evidence of obligate asymptomatic carriers, particularly men. Patients with HAE-nlC1INH appear to manifest symptoms at a somewhat older age than those with HAE-C1INH.[123] They are also less likely to have abdominal attacks and have more frequent orofacial swelling.

Physical Examination

Angioedema is usually asymmetric and typically involves loose connective tissue such as the face or mucous membranes such as the lips or tongue. For HAE, extremities are the most frequently affected areas, and abdominal attacks can resemble a surgical abdomen in severe cases. A full skin examination is warranted to ensure urticarial lesions are not present, because the differential would be considerably different in that situation.

Diagnostic Procedures

Patients with recurrent angioedema without urticaria should be evaluated for HAE with complement testing, which can readily establish the diagnosis of type 1 or type 2 HAE (Table 39.3). Patients with HAE-nlC1INH have a normal C4 and normal C1INH antigenic and functional levels. Consensus criteria for making a diagnosis of HAE-nlC1INH have been published.[42] A minority of patients with HAE-nlC1INH may have a mutation in the *F12* gene, and testing for these mutations is warranted in suspected cases.

Treatment

For patients with allergic or idiopathic angioedema, management should mirror that of urticaria in that H1 antihistamines should be trialed first. In severe cases, systemic corticosteroids and intramuscular epinephrine may be considered.

The treatment of HAE is distinct from that of allergic or idiopathic angioedema. Treatment of HAE is best considered as three separate goals: treatment of acute attacks, short-term prophylaxis, and long-term prophylaxis.[124] It is crucial to recognize that standard angioedema treatment modalities, such as epinephrine,

TABLE 39.3   Complement Evaluation of Patients With Recurrent Angioedema

	C4	C1INH Level	C1INH Function	C1q
Idiopathic angioedema	Normal	Normal	Normal	Normal
Type 1 HAE	Low	Low	Low	Normal
Type 2 HAE	Low	Normal	Low	Normal
HAE-nIC1INH	Normal	Normal	Normal	Normal
Acquired C1INH deficiency	Low	Low	Low	Low
Urticarial vasculitis	Low or normal	Normal	Normal	Low or normal

C1INH, C1 inhibitor; *HAE-nIC1INH*, hereditary angioedema with normal C1INH; *nl*, normal.

TABLE 39.4   Drugs Used for Treatment of Acute Hereditary Angioedema Attacks in Children

Drug Class and Name	Dose	Side Effects
C1INH Concentrates		
Berinert	≥5 yr: 20 units/kg, IV	*Common:* Bruising and pain at site of injection
Cinryze	≥6 yr: 20 units/kg, IV (approved only in Europe for acute attacks)	*Uncommon:* Thrombosis, allergic reaction
Ruconest	≥13 yr: 50 units/kg, IV (maximum dose of 4200 units)	
Plasma Kallikrein Inhibitor		
Ecallantide	≥12 yr: 30 mg, subcut	*Common:* Bruising and pain at site of injection *Uncommon:* Anaphylaxis
Bradykinin B$_2$ Receptor Antagonist		
Icatibant	≥18 yr: 30 mg, subcut	*Common:* Wheal and pain at injection site *Uncommon:* None

C1INH, C1 inhibitor; *IV*, intravenous; *subcut*, subcutaneous.

corticosteroids, or antihistamines, do not have a significant impact on the swelling in HAE. Because of the complexity of treatment of HAE, involvement of an expert physician and extensive patient education are recommended.[124]

Acute HAE attacks should be treated with drugs that specifically and effectively target the pathophysiology of the disease (Table 39.4). Published guidelines concur that all patients with HAE should have ready access to these drugs, that attacks at all sites are eligible for treatment, and that treatment is most effective when administered early in an attack.[12,124,125] Two different C1INH concentrates have been approved in the United States for treatment of HAE attacks: plasma-derived C1INH (Berinert) and recombinant human C1INH (Ruconest). Both are administered by intravenous injection and have been approved for use in adolescent and adult patients with HAE. Home therapy with intravenous C1INH was also shown to be safe and effective in children.[126] Two other drugs that antagonize bradykinin generation or action have been approved for treatment of acute HAE attacks: a plasma kallikrein inhibitor (ecallantide) and a bradykinin B$_2$ receptor antagonist (icatibant). Ecallantide and icatibant have been approved for use in the United States for treatment of acute attacks in patients with HAE patients age 12 and older, and 18 and older, respectively.

Prophylactic treatment of HAE is used to reduce the likelihood of swelling in a patient undergoing a stressor or procedure likely to precipitate an attack (short-term prophylaxis) or to decrease the number and severity of angioedema attacks (long-term prophylaxis). The extent of the local trauma may influence the decision on whether to treat the patient prophylactically. C1INH replacement given for short-term prophylaxis should be administered as soon as possible before the stressor (e.g., tooth extraction). In the past, high-dose anabolic androgens have been used for short-term prophylaxis in adults when started 5 to 10 days before the stressor, but this treatment is rarely used anymore.[125] It is critically important that effective on-demand treatment also be available regardless of whether the patient is given short-term prophylaxis.

There is little consensus regarding which patients should receive long-term prophylactic treatment. In general, the decision to start a patient on long-term prophylaxis should be individualized, taking into account attack frequency, attack severity, comorbid conditions, access to emergent treatment, and patient experience and preference.[125] The most commonly used medications for long-term prophylaxis of HAE are plasma-derived C1INH concentrate (Cinryze, HAEGARDA) and monoclonal antibody–inhibiting plasma kallikrein (lanadelumab) (Table 39.5). Both subcutaneous C1INH concentrate and lanadelumab have been shown to be able

TABLE 39.5	Drugs Used for Long-Term Prophylaxis of Hereditary Angioedema in Children	
Drug Class and Name	**Usual Pediatric Dose (Typical Range of Doses)**	**Side Effects**
Antifibrinolytic Agents[a]		
Epsilon aminocaproic acid	0.05 g/kg bid (0.025 g/kg bid–0.1 g/kg bid)	*Common:* Nausea, vertigo, diarrhea, postural hypotension, fatigue, muscle cramps with increased muscle enzymes
Tranexamic acid	20 mg/kg bid (10 mg/kg bid–25 mg/kg tid)	*Uncommon:* Thrombosis
17α-Alkylated Androgens		
Danazol	50 mg/day (50 mg/wk–200 mg/day)	*Common:* Weight gain, virilization, acne, altered libido, muscle pain/cramps, headache, depression, fatigue, nausea, constipation, menstrual abnormalities, increase in liver enzymes, hypertension, altered lipid profile
Stanozolol	≤6 yr: 0.5–1 mg/day ≥6 yr: 1–2 mg/day	
Oxandrolone	0.1 mg/kg/day	*Uncommon:* Decreased rate of growth in children, masculinization of female fetus, cholestatic jaundice, peliosis hepatis, hepatocellular adenoma
C1INH Concentrate		
Cinryze	6–11 yr: 500 units every 3–4 days ≥12 yr: 1000 units every 3–4 days	*Common:* Bruising and pain at injection site *Uncommon:* Thrombosis, allergic reaction
HAEGARDA	≥12 yr: 60 units/kg subcut every 3–4 days	
Plasma Kallikrein Inhibition		
Lanadelumab	≥12 yr: 300 mg every 2 wk	*Common:* Bruising and pain at injection site, headaches *Uncommon:* Allergic reaction

[a]Not approved in the United States.
subcut, Subcutaneous.

to eliminate attacks in up to 40% of patients. Anabolic androgens, however, are relatively contraindicated in children under the age of 16.[127,128] Antifibrinolytic drugs, epsilon aminocaproic acid, or tranexamic acid also can be used for long-term prophylaxis but are typically less effective. Treatment for HAE-nlC1INH is varied, and no controlled trials have determined efficacy of any specific agent.

Conclusion

Urticaria and angioedema are common clinical problems whose manifestations range from trivial and intermittent to life threatening. To minimize unnecessary time and money spent on complicated workups, while simultaneously not overlooking important diagnoses, the clinician must be able to characterize urticaria and angioedema by chronicity, type, and, increasingly, pathogenesis. The cause of acute urticaria and angioedema often can be determined and appropriate interventions taken that should lead to prompt resolution of the problem. A discrete cause of chronic urticaria, by contrast, is rarely established, forcing the clinician

into the role of controlling symptoms but not curing the problem. Although frequently frustrating for both the patient and the physician, the treatment of chronic urticaria can almost always achieve adequate results until the swelling disorder spontaneously remits. HAE is a rare but important cause of recurrent angioedema, and timely screening for HAE is the key to protecting these patients from potentially severe morbidity and mortality.

Helpful Websites

The American Academy of Dermatology (http://www.aad.org/)
The American Academy of Allergy, Asthma & Immunology (http://www.aaaai.org)
The American College of Allergy, Asthma & Immunology (http://www.acaai.org)
The Hereditary Angioedema Association (http://www.hereditary-angioedema.com)

The reference list can be found on the companion Expert Consult website at http://www.expertconsult.inkling.com.

40

Contact Dermatitis

LUZ FONACIER, ERIN BANTA

KEY POINTS

- Allergic contact dermatitis is recognized as the prototypic cutaneous type 4 cell-mediated hypersensitivity reaction.
- Allergic contact dermatitis (ACD) in children is not uncommon and should be suspected in patients with chronic dermatitis.
- Patch testing is the gold standard for diagnosis of ACD even in children and should be considered for children with chronic or recurrent eczematous dermatitis, including those with atopic dermatitis (AD) who fail to improve with standard treatment. The greatest abuse of patch testing is lack of use.

- Identify the causative allergen if possible and counsel the patient and/or family by providing a list of the chemicals the patient is sensitive to, giving synonyms and sources, and providing a list of safe products to use, alternatives, and substitutions.
- Patients with a suggestive history or physical findings but negative results on the thin-layer rapid-use epicutaneous test (T.R.U.E. TEST) should be considered for further evaluation in a patch testing clinic with an expanded panel of allergens.

Introduction

Contact dermatitis (CD) is a spectrum of inflammatory skin reactions induced by exposure to external agents. Clinically, CD most commonly manifests as a dermatitis or eczema, but it can manifest as urticaria, erythroderma, phototoxic or photoallergic reactions, hypopigmentation or hyperpigmentation, and even as an acneiform eruption.

CD is traditionally divided into irritant contact dermatitis (ICD), accounting for 80%, and allergic contact dermatitis (ACD), accounting for 20% of these reactions. The more common type of CD results from tissue damage caused by contact with irritants (ICD), whereas contact with allergens causes ACD. The former is seen commonly in infants as diaper dermatitis, whereas nickel and poison ivy are more frequent causes of ACD in the pediatric population.[1]

However, there are other diseases that are caused by an external inciting factor such as contact urticaria (CU) and protein contact dermatitis (PCD).[2]

CU, a type 1 immediate hypersensitivity reaction, manifests as pruritic wheals after contact with the triggering substance. CU can be nonimmunologic or immunologic; the latter requires a prior sensitization phase and can spread beyond the localized contact point.[3]

PCD manifests as chronic or recurrent eczematous dermatitis on to which develops vesicular, urticarial or edematous papules on exposure to specific proteins such as shrimp, fish, meat, or latex[4,5] and is thought to be caused by a combination of type 1 and type 4 reactions.[4] Both CU and PCD can be caused by contact with external allergens and can respond to antihistamines and topical corticosteroids.

An estimated 85,000 chemicals exist in the world, and approximately 2800 substances have been identified as contact allergens.[6] The majority of these agents, when applied to the skin, can induce an ICD.[7]

Epidemiology

It was previously thought that ACD occurs less frequently in children, possibly because of reduced exposure to contact allergens or because the immune system in children may be less susceptible to contact allergens. Moreover, in clinical practice, ACD is often misdiagnosed as AD or ICD, thus leading to an underestimation of its incidence and prevalence. International published data in the healthy pediatric population indicate that the point prevalence of contact allergy documented with positive patch test reaction ranges between 13.3% and 24.5%.[8–11] Despite the existing data, the true incidence of ACD in children and adolescents remains largely unknown because not all patients with suspected ACD are confirmed by patch testing.

In patients suspected of having ACD and referred for patch testing, the positive patch test rates ranged from 14% to 70%. Current relevance was reported at 56% to 93%. Very young children (0–5 years old) showed a high rate of relevant positive patch test reactions to common haptens.[12] In a study by Seidenari and associates[13] in Italian children, the highest percentage of positive responses was found in children younger than 3 years of age. Bruckner and colleagues[14] found that 24.5% of asymptomatic children aged 6 months to 5 years were sensitized to one or more contact allergens, with approximately half of the sensitized children younger than 18 months. In the adolescent age group, females have significantly higher rates of ACD on the face, likely to be explained by increased exposure to nickel in piercing and to preservative and fragrance in cosmetic products. A U.S.-based study showed nickel, fragrance, cobalt, thimerosal, balsam of Peru, potassium dichromate, neomycin, lanolin, thiuram mix, and p-phenylenediamine (PPD) to be common allergens in children.[15] Less common, but emerging allergens include cocamidopropyl betaine (CAPB) in "no tears" shampoos, baby washes, cleansers, and disperse dyes in clothing materials.

Pathogenesis

Innate Immunity

The innate immune system offers multiple layers of protection starting with the physical barrier of the stratum corneum and also including antimicrobial peptides, complement, Toll-like receptors (TLRs), and the inflammasome. Penetration of the stratum corneum by small compounds (<500 Da) acting either as direct irritants (in ICD) or as haptens (in ACD) leads to activation of these systems and resultant inflammation.

In ACD, most environmentally encountered contact sensitizers are small organic molecules (<500 Da) that require chemical interaction with self-protein to be recognized as a neoantigen and elicit an adaptive immune response. This process is known as *haptenization*. The chemical sensitizer is referred to as the *hapten*.[16,17] Once the hapten has penetrated the stratum corneum barrier, it encounters keratinocytes and Langerhans cells (LCs) within the epidermis. There, haptens induce the production of reactive oxygen species, which leads to the release of adenosine triphosphate (ATP) and can induce the breakdown of high molecular weight hyaluronic acid. The resultant low molecular weight hyaluronic acid can activate TLR2 and TLR4, resulting in increased expression of pro–interleukin 1 beta (IL-1β) and pro–IL-18. TLRs then work in coordination with the inflammasome to further inflammation. Activation of the inflammasome by ATP with resultant caspase 1 activity is able to cleave pro–IL-1β and pro–IL-18 products into their active forms, IL-1β and IL-18.[16] Interestingly, nickel has been shown to directly bind human TLR4. This process requires the presence of two nonconserved histidines that are absent in mouse TLR4, which has explained the absence of development of CD to nickel in mice.[18]

Another innate immune cell, the natural killer (NK) T cell may be important. Absence of this cell impairs contact hypersensitivity in animal models[19] and concentration of NK T cells is found to be significantly increased in the skin in human patients with ACD.[20] These cells likely play a role in the inflammatory reaction in the epidermis, where they mediate cytotoxicity against keratinocytes. Both ICD and ACD begin with activation of the innate immune system.

Irritant Contact Dermatitis

ICD results from contact with agents that directly irritate the skin. Irritation is usually a cytotoxic event produced by a wide variety of chemicals, detergents, solvents, alcohol, creams, lotions, ointments, and powders and by environmental factors such as wetting, drying, perspiration, and temperature extremes. This interaction leads to the release of cytokines, chemokines, and recruitment of inflammatory cells, all of which activate the innate immune response.[21] ICD, unlike ACD, does not require prior sensitization, and immunologic memory is not involved in the clinical manifestation. ICD typically develops more quickly than with ACD, and epidermal necrosis can be seen within 24 hours of exposure to a moderately strong irritant.[22]

A number of studies have identified the epidermal keratinocyte as a key effector cell in the initiation and propagation of contact irritancy. Keratinocytes can release both preformed and newly synthesized cytokines and up-regulate major histocompatibility complex class II (MHCII) molecules and adhesion molecules in response to irritants.[23] In experimental models, the application of sodium lauryl sulfate to the epidermis leads to direct toxic effects on keratinocytes, epidermal barrier disruption, and lamellar body lipid extrusion.[24,25] These epidermal changes lead to the release of innate immune mediators IL-1α, IL-1β, IL-6, IL-8, and TNF-α, which[26] activate LCs, dermal dendritic cells (DCs) and endothelial cells leading to further inflammatory cell infiltration with neutrophils, lymphocytes, macrophages, and mast cells. Irritants can also function as "danger signals," activating the inflammasome and nuclear factor kappa-light-chain-enhancer of activated B cells (NF-κB) pathways through TLRs and Nod-like receptors, which also leads to release of cytokines and chemokines[21,23] (Fig. 40.1). These inflammatory mediators can cause direct tissue damage and further activation of the inflammatory cascade, leading to the release of additional inflammatory mediators from activated nonsensitized T cells.

The inflammatory response is dose and time dependent. Any impairment to the epidermal barrier layer (e.g., fissuring, overhydration) renders the skin more susceptible to an irritant effect. The presence of ICD itself increases susceptibility to the development of contact sensitization to allergens, and this has been demonstrated in both mouse models and human studies.[26–28] The activation of the innate immune system by irritants appears to prime the skin for development of ACD, and a decreased elicitation threshold for cobalt and nickel has been demonstrated after skin priming with sodium lauryl sulfate.[29,30]

Allergic Contact Dermatitis

ACD is recognized as the prototypic cutaneous cell–mediated hypersensitivity reaction, in which the epidermal LCs play a pivotal role.[23] The hapten initiates the immunologic reaction at the site of contact with the skin and enlists both an innate response similar to the early steps of ICD and an adaptive immune response.

ACD reactions have both a sensitization (afferent) phase and elicitation (efferent) phase. During the sensitization phase, the hapten gains entrance to the epidermis, where it binds to a self-protein and activates keratinocytes, leading to release of TNF-α, granulocyte-macrophage colony-stimulating factor (GM-CSF), IL-1β, and IL-10. These inflammatory molecules activate LCs, dermal DCs, and endothelial cells, leading to an accumulation of even more DCs at the site of hapten contact. In addition, the release of IL-1β by epidermal LCs promotes their egress from the epidermis. After the uptake of hapten, LCs process it while migrating to regional lymph nodes, where they present the processed peptide to hapten-specific T cells. An important property of LCs and DCs is their ability to present exogenous antigens on both MHCI and MHCII molecules. This cross-priming leads to the activation of both CD4+ and CD8+ hapten-specific T cells.[31] Hapten-specific T cells have been shown to include T helper cell type 1 (T$_H$1), T$_H$2, T$_H$17, and T regulatory subsets, and it is thought that each hapten may have its own propensity to induce a specific T cell subset.[23,32,33] These effector T cells proliferate, enter circulation and move to the site of initial epidermal exposure.

The elicitation (efferent) phase then occurs on skin re-exposure to a hapten. On diffusion through the skin, hapten is taken up by other antigen-presenting cells (APCs), including macrophages and dermal DCs. These cells then stimulate hapten-specific memory T cells.[21] The sensitized hapten-specific T cells home in on the hapten-provoked skin site, releasing their inflammatory mediators, which results in epidermal spongiosis (eczema) through their

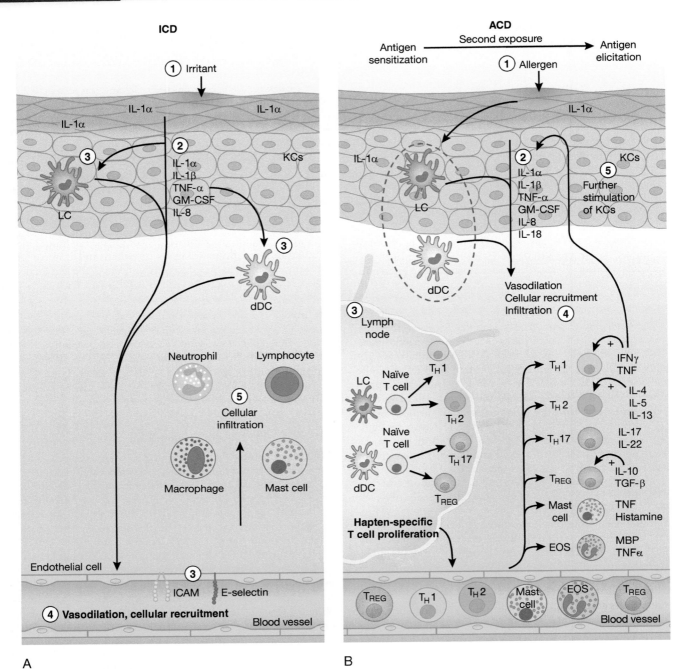

• **Fig. 40.1** Pathogenesis. Immune mechanism in the pathogenesis of irritant contact dermatitis (*ICD*) and allergic contact dermatitis (*ACD*). (A) In patients with ICD, exposure to an irritant exerts toxic effects on keratinocytes, activating innate immunity with release of interleukin 1 alpha (*IL-1α*), *IL-1β*, tumor necrosis factor alpha (*TNF-α*), granulocyte-macrophage colony-stimulating factor (*GM-CSF*), and *IL-8* from epidermal keratinocytes. In turn, these cytokines activate Langerhans cells (*LCs*), dermal dendritic cells (*dDCs*), and endothelial cells, all of which contribute to cellular recruitment to the site of keratinocyte damage. Infiltrating cells include neutrophils, lymphocytes, macrophages, and mast cells, which further promote an inflammatory cascade. (B) In the sensitization phase of ACD, similar to ICD, allergens activate innate immunity through keratinocyte release of IL-1α, IL-1β, TNF-α, GM-CSF, *IL-8*, and *IL-18*, inducing vasodilation, cellular recruitment, and infiltration. LCs and dermal DCs encounter the allergen and migrate to the draining lymph nodes, where they activate hapten-specific T cells, which include T helper cell type 1 (*TH1*), *TH2*, *TH17*, and regulatory T (*TREG*) cells. These T cells proliferate and enter the circulation and site of initial exposure, along with mast cells and eosinophils (*EOS*). On re-encountering the allergen, the elicitation phase occurs, in which the hapten-specific T cells, along with other inflammatory cells, enter the site of exposure and, through release of cytokines and consequent stimulation of keratinocytes, induce an inflammatory cascade. Circled numbers represent sequence of events. *IFN-γ*, Interferon gamma; *IL-22*, interleukin 22; *KCs*, keratinocytes; *MBP*, major basic protein. (With permission from: Gittler JK, Krueger JG, Guttman-Yassky E. Atopic dermatitis results in intrinsic barrier and immune abnormalities: implications for contact dermatitis. J Allergy Clin Immunol 2013;131(2):300–13. © Elsevier.)

effects on keratinocytes. Secondary or subsequent hapten exposure may have a shorter period of latency from contact to appearance of the rash.

Initial evidence from mouse studies with strong skin sensitizers suggested a T_H1/T_H17 (interferon-γ [IFN-γ]) polarized T cell profile for ACD.[32,34,35] Multiple studies have demonstrated that hapten-specific CD8 T cells are predominant in effector mechanisms of tissue damage.[35–38] Roles for T_H2/T_H22 (IL-4) involvement also have been defined in both animal and human studies.[39–41] The immunologic mechanism of ACD appears to be hapten-specific with allergens such as nickel inducing T_H1/T_H17 polarization, and fragrance induces T_H2/T_H22 polarization.[43] The concept that ACD may differ mechanistically according to allergen is likely to have significant therapeutic relevance as a consideration in the choice of future targeted therapy.[34]

Evaluation and Management

Differential Diagnosis

A number of both eczematous and noneczematous dermatoses should be considered in the evaluation of a child with suspected CD. Eczematous dermatoses such as seborrheic and atopic dermatitis occur commonly, whereas psoriasis and zinc deficiency are less common. Nummular eczema, neurodermatitis (lichen simplex chronicus), and adverse drug reaction also should be considered. Noneczematous dermatoses such as dermatophytosis, bullous impetigo, vesicular viral eruptions, urticarial vasculitis, mycosis fungoides, and Sézary syndrome may mimic CD.

Allergic Contact Dermatitis and Atopic Dermatitis

The relationship between ACD and AD is complex. The skin in AD has a defective skin barrier, bacterial colonization, and chronic immune dysregulation. The dysfunctional skin barrier in patients with AD allows for increased penetration of chemicals, which may increase the risk of contact sensitization and ACD. This increased penetration of irritants through AD skin makes patients with AD more prone to ICD even when their AD is quiescent,[44] resulting in further compromise of the skin barrier. Also patients with AD apply emollients and topical antiinflammatory therapy frequently and liberally for treatment and maintenance. A large proportion of these so-called hypoallergenic pediatric cosmetic products contained potent contact allergens such as fragrances and preservatives.[45] Bacterial colonization that is prominent in AD has been shown to activate cells in the inflammatory milieu that are also involved in potentiating contact sensitization and ACD.[46–48]

Differentiating AD from ACD in some patients, especially those with widespread eczematous lesions, can be challenging. Thus, patient misdiagnosis or underdiagnosis can commonly occur. Both ACD and AD can manifest as a flexural dermatitis, localized and systemic dermatitis with predominantly flexural involvement.

The incidence of ACD in AD is controversial. Earlier literature suggested that patients with AD, especially severe AD, had a depressed T_H1 immune system and therefore were less likely to become sensitized to allergens and develop ACD.[49,50] However, conflicting data suggest that development of ACD may be enhanced in patients with chronic moderate to severe AD.[51–53] Other clinical studies have suggested that contact sensitization and ACD could be decreased in patients with severe AD but elevated in patients with mild AD.[54–56]

In 2010, Jacob and colleagues[57] reported that 95.6% of 69 children with suspected ACD had at least one positive patch test reaction, and of these 76.7% had a history of AD.[57] Other studies have identified AD as a risk factor for polysensitization (i.e., the presence of contact sensitization to multiple [three or more] allergens).[58,59]

Although many of the common allergens seen in AD, such as fragrances and lanolin, are similar to those seen in the general population, certain topical agents are especially relevant in AD.

Increased prevalence of ACD in AD to these specific allergens include metals, fragrances, preservatives, plants (e.g., Compositae), antiseptics (e.g., chlorhexidine), emollients (e.g., lanolin), topical medicaments (e.g., neomycin, corticosteroids), surfactants (e.g., CAPB), and rubber accelerators.[56,60–66]

Patch testing remains the criterion standard for diagnosing ACD, even in patients with AD. A consensus recommendation by allergists and dermatologists on when and how to patch test individuals with AD was published in 2016.[55] Patch testing should be considered in patients with AD with dermatitis that fails to improve with topical therapy, with an atypical or changing distribution of dermatitis, with a pattern suggestive of ACD, with therapy-resistant hand eczema in the working population, with adult- or adolescent-onset AD, and/or before initiating systemic immunosuppressants for the treatment of dermatitis. Failure to patch test when appropriate may result in overlooking an important and potentially curable complicating comorbidity.

When patch testing the patient with AD, it should be remembered that irritant reactions, especially to metals, fragrances, formaldehyde, lanolin, and personal rinse-off products, are common and may be misinterpreted as allergic reactions. Between patch readings, the typical "crescendo" pattern is not observed to the same degree in patients with AD.[67] Patch testing should be avoided at the time of an AD flare because it may lead to false negative results and/or increased irritancy. Concomitant systemic immunosuppressive therapy may result in false negative results and should be avoided whenever possible or reduced to the minimum necessary to clear the back.

Diagnosis of Contact Dermatitis

History

A careful, comprehensive, and age-appropriate history should include possible contact exposure of the child such as to diapers, hygiene products, perfume-containing products, moisturizers, cosmetics, sun blocks, tattoos, body piercing, textiles with dyes and fire retardant, medications, pets and pet products, school projects, recreational exposure, sports, work, and so on. ICD may be the cause of the dermatitis or an aggravating factor. Frequent handwashing and use of water and soaps, detergents, and cleansers should be noted. The evolution of the skin reaction is influenced by many factors, including the patient's skin, age, and color; ambient conditions; use of topical or other oral medication; and response to all prior treatment. Because the majority of contact reactions manifest as eczematous eruptions, it is essential to note clinical evolution from acute vesiculation to chronic lichenification.

Unfortunately, although history can strongly suggest the cause of CD, relying solely on the history, other than with obvious nickel reactions and a few other allergens, may confirm sensitization in only 10% to 20% of patients with ACD.

Physical Examination

The diagnosis of ACD is suspected from the clinical presentation of the rash and the possible exposure to a contact allergen. CD can be described as acute, subacute, or chronic. Acute dermatitis can manifest with erythematous papules, vesicles, and even bullae. Chronic CD is generally pruritic and erythematous and may be associated with crusting, scaling, fissuring, excoriations, and lichenification. ICD usually manifests as well-demarcated, erythematous macules, papules, and plaques confined to the area of the skin in direct contact with the offending agents, with little or no extension beyond the site of contact (Fig. 40.2). ICD generally spares "protected" areas such as the inguinal folds in diaper dermatitis. In ACD the dermatitis can spread beyond the areas of contact and even cause an activation of dermatitis at distant sites of prior dermatitis, as in systemic CD.

Although the geographic location of dermatitis can aid in the determination of the suspected allergen, other factors may influence the location of the dermatitis. In connubial dermatitis, the product may be transferred to the child by the parent/caregiver or to the patient by a partner. Clinically, it is difficult to differentiate CD from AD, especially in the common areas of involvement such as the eyelids, lips, hands, flexural areas of the neck, and even dermatitis with scattered generalized distribution.

Regional Considerations in Children

Hand Dermatitis

Hand dermatitis in children is extremely common. Its differential diagnosis can be challenging, and it is not often studied with patch testing. Hand dermatitis may be due to ICD, ACD, AD, dyshidrosis, or psoriasis. ICD commonly manifests as a localized dermatitis without vesicles over webs of fingers extending onto the dorsal and ventral surfaces ("apron" pattern), dorsum of the hands, palms, and ball of the thumb. Because the skin on the palm is much thicker than that on the dorsum of the hands, ACD is often associated with vesicles, occurring most often on the thinner skin on the dorsum of the hands, the fingertips, nail folds, and less commonly the palms (Fig. 40.3). In a study by Toledo and associates,[68] 36% of the children with hand eczema had ACD, supporting the recommendation of patch testing of children with chronic hand eczema, independently of age, sex, personal history of atopic dermatitis, or distribution of the eczema.

Patch tests in patients with hand eczema showed that relevant allergens included nickel sulfate (17.6%); potassium dichromate (7.2%); rubber elements, including thiuram mix, carba mix, PPD, and mercaptobenzothiazole (MBT) (19.6%); and cobalt chloride (6.4%).[69,70]

The prevalence of hand eczema in patients with AD is 2- to 10-fold higher than in individuals without atopy. Involvement of the dorsal aspect of the hand and fingers, combined with volar wrist involvement, suggests AD as a contributing etiologic factor. Because of the significant overlap it is often difficult to distinguish the cause of hand dermatitis. Because ICD of the hands can precede ACD, pattern changes such as increasing dermatitis from web spaces to fingertips or from palms to dorsal surfaces should prompt patch testing.[71]

Face and Eyelid Dermatitis

Eyelid dermatitis may be due to ACD (55%–63.5%), ICD (15%), AD (<10%), and seborrheic dermatitis (4%).[72] The eyelid is susceptible to ACD because of higher exposure to allergens, greater sensitivity to allergens, including aeroallergens, and easy accessibility to touch, facilitating the transfer of chemicals from other areas of the body (e.g., nails, scalp) to the eyelid. Although CD is considered the most common cause of eyelid dermatitis, it is thought that 25% of patients with AD may have chronic eyelid dermatitis.

Pure eyelid dermatitis may be distinct from dermatitis with other areas of involvement.[73] Common allergens causing eyelid dermatitis are fragrances (e.g., facial tissues, cosmetics), preservatives, nickel (e.g., eyelash curlers), thiuram (e.g., rubber sponges, masks, balloons, toys), tosylamide formaldehyde resin (e.g., nail polish), and gold.[74] CAPB, found in shampoos, is a common source of eyelid dermatitis in children.[75] Facial tissues may contain fragrances, formaldehyde, or benzalkonium chloride. PPD and ammonium persulfate can cause urticaria and or eyelid edema.

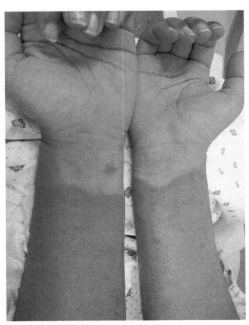

• **Fig. 40.2** Irritant contact dermatitis of the arms.

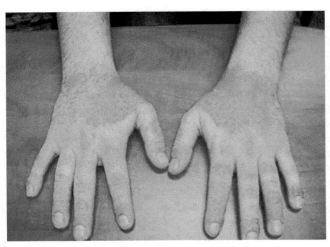

• **Fig. 40.3** Allergic contact dermatitis of the hand.

Facial dermatitis may also occur secondary to allergens transferred to the face from other regions of the body. Facial presentation of dermatitis was seen in 19.7% of children examined by the North American Contact Dermatitis Group (NACDG), making it second only to generalized presentation in frequency by location in this pediatric-specific study. It ranks third by location in the results from the NACDG in their results from 2015 to 2016.[76] Distribution patterns can help determine clinically relevant products. Symmetric, central or patchy distribution tends to be seen with cosmetics and personal products (e.g., moisturizers, sunscreens, foundations, and powders) whereas peripheral face (i.e., preauricular, submental and jawline areas) involvement can be due to shampoos, conditioners, and facial cleansers. ACD that affects the lateral neck is most likely secondary to perfumes/colognes and nail cosmetics. Unilateral facial dermatitis in an infant or toddler may be due to connubial CD resulting from PPD in recently dyed hair or fragranced products used by a caregiver.[77] In an adolescent, unilateral facial dermatitis may result from nickel or chromate used in cell phones or from headsets.[78]

The scalp skin is relatively resistant to allergens. Shampoos, conditioners, hair sprays, gels, and mousses may cause eyelid or facial dermatitis without causing scalp or forehead lesions. Severe burns of the scalp and hair can be caused by the misuse of hair straighteners and relaxers. The manufacturers of hair dyes recommend patch testing with the product before each application.

Oral Mucous Membranes, Perioral Dermatitis, and Cheilitis

Perioral dermatitis and cheilitis are common in children and are associated with lip licking, lip chewing, thumb sucking, or excessive drooling. Objectively, changes may be barely visible or may vary from a mild erythema to a fiery red color, with or without edema. Juices of foods and even chewing gum may contribute to skin irritation of these areas. Cinnamon flavorings and peppermint are the most common causes of allergic cheilitis from toothpastes.[79]

Contact allergy of the mucous membrane is rare, and use of patch testing to evaluate patients with mucosal involvement is controversial. In a series of 331 patients with different oral diseases (i.e., burning mouth syndrome, cheilitis, gingivitis, orofacial granulomatosis, perioral dermatitis, lichenoid tissue reaction, and recurrent aphthous stomatitis), metals (i.e., nickel and gold) were most frequently positive on patch testing.[80] Metals, including mercury, chromate, nickel, gold, cobalt, beryllium, and palladium, have been used in orthodontic materials and are important allergens in patients with dental implants or orthodontic devices presenting with oral lichenoid lesions. Other allergens with a high percentage of positive reactions on patch testing include flavorings and preservatives. "Fragrances" are used as flavoring in food products, skin care products, and dentifrices. Balsam of Peru is found in dentifrice, mouthwash, lipstick, and food. Dodecyl gallate is a preservative used to extend the shelf life of oil-based foods such as peanut butter, soups, and pastries. Toothpaste, fluoride mouth washes, chewing gum, and other foods may contain cinnamic aldehyde, flavorings, and peppermint, which are common causes of allergic cheilitis. Thus, an oral antigen screening series in patients with cheilitis should include not only metals but also an even more comprehensive panel of flavorings, preservatives, medications, and dental acrylates. The usefulness of patch testing in the evaluation of orofacial granulomatosis and recurrent aphthous stomatitis is questionable.[80]

Flexural Areas of Neck and Axillary Dermatitis

The thin intertriginous skin of the neck is vulnerable to irritant reactions from "perms," hair dyes, shampoos, and conditioners. Berloque dermatitis from certain perfumes or nail polish presents as localized areas of eczema. Nickel-sensitive individuals may react to wearing a necklace or to zippers.

ACD can be caused by deodorants but is rarely caused by antiperspirants, which usually cause ICD. These agents generally cause a dermatitis involving the entire axillary vault, whereas textile ACD spares the apex of the vault. However, sweat and perspiration may cause increased deodorant allergen in the periphery, giving a dermatitis that is less intense in the apex of the axillae. ACD resulting from disperse dyes such as disperse orange 1, disperse blue 106, and disperse blue 124 in clothing can elicit eczematous eruptions in the axillae, arms, and groin.[81–83]

Diaper Dermatitis

Children are especially susceptible to dermatitis in the diaper region because of their dependency on diapers and their extended toilet seat exposure during transition out of diapers. Eruptions in the diaper area are the most common dermatologic disorder of infancy.[84] Friction, occlusion, maceration, and increased exposure to water, moisture, urine, and feces[85] contribute to ICD. The prevalence of diaper dermatitis, an ICD, in infants has been estimated to be 7% to 35%, with a peak incidence between the ages of 9 and 12 months.[86] However, a large-scale study in the United Kingdom demonstrated an incidence of 25% in the first 4 weeks of life alone.[87] During the transition to toileting, ICD can be seen with the harsh detergents used in disinfection.[88]

Common allergens in diaper dermatitis include mercaptobenzothiazole, fragrance mix, cyclohexylthiopthalimide, p-tert-butylphenol resin, sorbitan sesquioleate, and historically disperse dyes.[89] Early disposable diapers were coated with antileak rubber material, resulting in a characteristic pattern of dermatitis on the outer buttocks and hips, termed the "Lucky Luke" or "gun holster" pattern.[90] In these cases, mercaptobenzothiazole and p-tert-butylphenol–formaldehyde resin were the clinically relevant allergens.[91] Changes in diaper design led to reports of ACD resulting from dyes concentrated in the inner thighs, hips, and waistband region.[92]

Medication, douches, spermicides, sprays, and cleaners can cause CD in the genital area. Fragrances found in liners, toilet paper, soap, and bubble baths can cause a reaction in sensitized patients. Contraceptive devices can affect rubber- and latex-sensitive individuals. Ammonia and/or the acidity of urine may cause ICD, especially in incontinent patients. The ingestion of spices, antibiotics, or laxatives may cause anal itching.

Leg and Foot Dermatitis

Shaving agents, moisturizers, and rubber in the elastic of socks can cause allergic reactions in children. Irritant dermatitis of the feet may occur in children because of excessive perspiration or the use of synthetic footwear. More common than ICD, ACD can be the cause of dermatitis of the feet, and "shoe dermatitis" accounts for around 10% of all cases presenting for patch testing.[93] The increased maceration and enhanced absorption of chemicals within the shoe is thought to aid in the development of ACD and rubber accelerators (i.e., MBT mix, thiuram mix, carba mix, and PPD mix), dichromates (Fig. 40.4), or glues used in manufacturing have been noted to be causative. Chrome used in the tanning

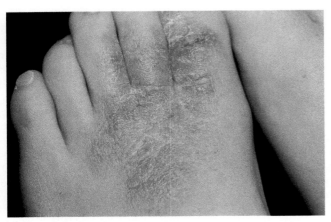

• **Fig. 40.4** Chronic dermatitis on dorsa of feet and toes caused by potassium dichromate allergy from chronic exposure to leather tennis shoes. (From Weston WL, Lane AT, Morelli JG. Dermatitis. In: Color textbook of pediatric dermatology. 4th ed. St. Louis, MO: Mosby; 2007.)

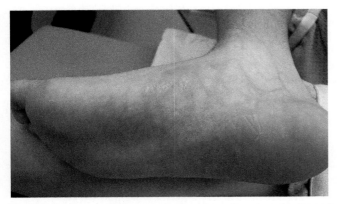

• **Fig. 40.5** Foot dermatitis from insoles involving sole and sparing the arch.

and dyeing processes of leather and colophony used in glues in soles and insoles may be sensitizing. Other chemicals in footwear (e.g., leather, adhesives, glues, and dyes) or in topical medications (e.g., creams, ointments, and antiperspirants) can cause ACD. Reactions to nickel sulfate were also frequent with metal in footwear buckles, eyelets, and ornaments.[94] Regional differences in causative agents can be seen and likely relate to climate, varied footwear styles, and differences in manufacturing practices (i.e., additives and chemicals). In ACD the involvement of the dorsal aspect of the foot and toes, especially the hallux, and sparing of the interdigital areas is characteristic. For ACD caused by rubber, insoles can lead to rash on the sole of the foot, often with sparing of the arch (Fig. 40.5). Advising patients to avoid the causative allergen by switching shoes, changing insoles, or wearing cotton socks is recommended. Treatment of hyperhidrosis also can be considered.[93]

Generalized Dermatitis

Dermatitis with scattered generalized distribution is a difficult diagnostic and therapeutic challenge because it lacks the characteristic distribution that gives a clue as to the possible diagnosis of ACD. Interestingly, the most common body location of dermatitis in the pediatric-specific NACDG in 2015 was the scattered

generalized pattern, followed by the face and then arm.[95] This differs from the more recent NACDG data in children and adults, which found generalized dermatitis second to hand dermatitis as the most common body locations.[76] Zug and colleagues[96] reported that approximately half (49%) of patients with scattered generalized distribution referred for patch testing had a positive patch test deemed at least possibly relevant to their dermatitis, the prevalence being higher in patients with a history of AD. The two allergens most commonly identified were nickel and balsam of Peru. Hjorth[5] reported two children who had positive patch test results for balsam of Peru whose eczema flared after oral intake of naturally occurring balsams. Other relevant positive patch test reactions included preservatives (formaldehyde, quaternium 15, methyldibromo glutaronitrile/phenoxyethanol, diazolidinyl urea, 2-bromo-2-nitropropane-1, 3-diol, imidazolidinyl urea, and DMDM hydantoin) and propylene glycol. Dyes such as disperse blue 106 in synthetic fibers in children's garments also have been implicated.[13]

Advising patients to use skin care products without the most frequent, relevant allergens (i.e., formaldehyde-releasing preservatives, fragrances, and propylene glycol) is one strategy that may be helpful while awaiting definitive patch testing results. However, 8% to 10% of patients with scattered generalized distribution remain in the unclassified eczema category.[96]

Systemic CD should be considered a possible cause of dermatitis with scattered generalized distribution. It manifests as a localized or generalized inflammatory skin disease that occurs in sensitized individuals when they are exposed to the specific allergen orally, transcutaneously, intravenously, or by inhalation. There is a variety of manifestations of systemic CD reactions, including a reactivation of a previous dermatitis, reactivation of a previously positive patch test (localized "recall reactions"), a systemic inflammatory skin disease such as the "baboon syndrome,"[97–101] and/or oral lichenoid reactions. Patients allergic to ethylenediamine may react to systemic aminophylline and antihistamines of the piperazine or ethanolamine families. Similar reactions have been reported to glucocorticoids, diphenhydramine, neomycin, penicillin, sulfonamides, thiuram, colophony, balsam of Peru, fragrance mix, and nickel (Table 40.1).

Patch Testing

Unfortunately, even with an extensive history and physical examination, only about 10% to 20% of patients with ACD can be diagnosed accurately without patch testing. Patch testing is needed to identify the responsible allergens, is helpful in young children suspected of ACD, and remains the gold standard for confirming ACD. Although the application of antigens for patch testing is rather simple, antigen selection and patch test interpretation require an experienced clinician.

Selection of Appropriate Subjects to Test

The higher the index of suspicion, the more frequent is the diagnosis of ACD. Patch testing should be considered for children with a chronic, pruritic, or recurrent eczematous dermatitis, especially those with eyelid or hand involvement,[102] those with uncontrollable or worsening chronic dermatitis of greater than 2 months duration, and those who fail to improve after standard treatment protocols, including a preliminary avoidance regimen of formaldehyde and fragrance. Indeed, the observation that the greatest abuse of patch

TABLE 40.1 Reported Causes of Systemic Allergic Contact Dermatitis

Contact Sensitizer	Systemic Reaction to:
Glucocorticoids	Oral hydrocortisone
Benadryl cream	Oral diphenhydramine
Neomycin	Oral neomycin
Penicillin	Oral penicillin
Sulfonamide	p-Amino sulfonamide hypoglycemics (tolbutamide, chlorpropamide)
Thiuram	Antabuse
Colophony, balsam of Peru, fragrance mix	Spices: Clove, nutmeg, cinnamon, cayenne pepper Citrus fruits: Oranges, lemon, tangerines Tomatoes
Ethylenediamine	Aminophylline (Alternative: Oral theophylline, intravenous theophylline) Piperazine and ethanolamine (Atarax, Antivert) (alternatives: diphenhydramine, chlorpheniramine, fexofenadine)
Nickel	Nickel in tap water, utensils and food high in nickel content such as soy, chocolate, lentils, cashews
Chromate	Inhaled chromium: Oral potassium dichromate

TABLE 40.2 Pediatric Baseline Series

Pediatric (≥6 years) baseline series: American Contact Dermatitis Society Pediatric Contact Dermatitis Workgroup minimum recommended allergens

1	Nickel sulfate	20	Carba mix
2	Quaternium 15	21	Imidazolidinyl urea
3	Neomycin	22	Amerchol L101
4	Balsam of Peru	23	Compositae mix
5	Fragrance mix 1	24	Cinnamic aldehyde
6	MCI/MI	25	Paraben mix
7	Bacitracin	26	Thiuram mix
8	Propylene glycol	27	Bronopol
9	Methylchloroisothiazolinone	28	Sesquiterpene lactones (SQL)
10	Fragrance mix II	29	Colophony
11	Cocamidopropyl betaine (CAPB)	30	p-tert-Butylphenol formaldehyde resin
12	Cobalt chloride	31	Clobetasol-17-propionate
13	Formaldehyde	32	Decyl glucoside
14	Propolis	33	Iodopropynyl butylcarbamate
15	Tixocortol-21-pivalate	34	Benzophenone-3
16	Hydrocortisone-17-butyrate	35	Amidoamine
17	Diazolidinyl urea	36	Tea tree oil (TTO)
18	1,3-Dimethylol-5,5-dimethyl (DMDM) hydantoin	37	Carmine
19	Budesonide	38	Dimethylaminopropylamine

MCI, Methylchloroisothiazolinone; MI, methylisothiazolinone.

testing is its lack of use holds true even for the pediatric population. Immunocompromised patients, including those on oral steroids or those on cancer chemotherapy or immunosuppressive drugs, are not appropriate candidates for patch testing. Ideally, the patient's dermatitis should be quiescent, because flare-up reactions may be elicited during patch testing. The patch test site should have had no potent topical immune modulators or steroid applied for 5 to 7 days before testing. Patients should avoid sun or ultraviolet light exposure for 5-7 days. Systemic antihistamines have no effect on patch test results. However, not all children with suspected ACD can have patch testing. Given the smaller surface area for patch testing, especially in young children, if comprehensive patch testing cannot be done, a detailed exposure history may guide the choice of potential allergens to test based on the history of exposures and the patient's own personal care products.

Sources of Allergens

Commercially available standardized patch testing allergens have been calibrated with respect to nonirritant concentrations and compatibility with the test vehicle. Test systems currently available in the United States are the T.R.U.E. TEST and the standardized allergens are loaded in patch test chambers. Certain screening panels such as the NACDG recommended series or the American Contact Dermatitis Society Core Allergen Series, with a range from 65 to 70 allergens are not approved by the U.S. Food and Drug Administration (FDA) but conform to standards of care recommended by CD experts. The T.R.U.E. TEST is a ready-to-use patch test panel that is FDA approved for pediatric patients as young as 6 years of age.

Allergens

The ACDS pediatric CD workgroup published their recommended allergens to be included in the pediatric patch test panel of children 6 years and older.[103] The 38 allergens reflected in Table 40.2 are a minimum number the group recommended be studied in this population. As a side note, the workgroup experience was that the back of a child aged 6 years can fit 40 to 60 allergens, allowing for expanded testing.

The German Contact Dermatitis Group (GCDG)[104] recommends that children under 6 should only be subjected to patch testing if there is a high degree of clinical suspicion and that only the suspected allergens should be used. Some authors suggest dose adjustment in younger children for allergens such as nickel, formaldehyde, formaldehyde releasers, mercaptobenzothiazole, thiuram, and potassium dichromate to avoid irritant false-positive reactions.[105] Jacob and colleagues[106] recommend a reduced concentration of nickel, formaldehyde, and rubber additives in children under 5, especially in those who also have AD. Children over the age of 12 can be tested in the same manner as adults, and most studies to date suggest that the same test concentrations as in adults can be used.[9]

The ideal number of patch tests to be applied depends on the patient. The usefulness of patch testing is enhanced with the number of allergens tested. Allergens not found on commercially available screening series in the United States frequently give relevant reactions, and personal products are a useful supplement, especially in facial or periorbital dermatitis.

Further study suggested that false-negative results may occur with the T.R.U.E. TEST, particularly with fragrance mix and rubber additives (thiuram and carba mix)[107] and with neomycin, cobalt, and lanolin.

Other standardized allergens can be tested individually with a loading chamber such as the Finn Chamber, but clinicians need to be aware of the limitations of each system of patch testing for individual allergens.[108] Caution should be exercised when testing for nonstandardized antigens to avoid adverse effects and false-positive or false-negative responses. "Leave-on" cosmetics (i.e., makeup, perfume, moisturizer, nail polish), clothing, and most foods are tested "as is," whereas "wash-off" cosmetics (e.g., soap, shampoo) are tested at 1:10 to 1:100 dilution.

Patch testing should never be performed with an unknown substance. Photopatch tests should be performed by physicians with expertise in ultraviolet radiation if photocontact dermatitis is suspected. Additional guidelines for patch testing, including strength of recommendations and quality of evidence, have been published by the British Association of Dermatologists' Therapy Guidelines and Audit Subcommittee.[109] The T.R.U.E. TEST may serve as triage or a screening tool in an allergist's practice, but occupational exposures may benefit from early referral for supplemental testing.

Patch Testing Procedure

Standardized criteria for patch testing have been set by the Task Force on Contact Dermatitis of the American Academy of Dermatology. All results depend on the recommended protocol for application, removal, and interpretation of results.

Patch tests are typically applied to the upper back or midback areas (2.5 cm lateral to a midspinal reference point), which must be free of dermatitis and hair and are kept in place for 48 hours. Patients are instructed to keep the area dry and avoid activities that will cause excessive sweating or excessive movement that may cause displacement of the patches. In infants and small children, the patch test can be covered with fabric adhesive tape or a stockinette vest. Patch tests are removed after 48 hours and read 30 minutes after to allow resolution of erythema and irritative effect from the tape and/or chamber if present. A second reading should be done 3 to 5 days after the initial application. Thirty percent of relevant allergens negative at the 48-hour reading become positive in 96 hours. Irritant reactions tend to disappear by 96 hours. Metals (e.g., gold, potassium dichromate, nickel, cobalt), topical antibiotics (e.g., neomycin, bacitracin), topical corticosteroids, and PPD may become positive after 7 days. More than 50% of positive patch testing to gold was delayed for about 1 week.

The International Contact Dermatitis Research Group has developed a grading system that is almost universally recognized and continues to be widely used (Table 40.3).

TABLE 40.3 Patch Test Interpretation Based on the Recommendation of the International Contact Dermatitis Research Group

Grade	Patch Test Grading
(−)	Negative reaction
(?+)	Doubtful reaction with faint erythema only
1+	Weak positive reaction with nonvesicular erythema, infiltration, possible papules
2+	Strong positive reaction with vesicular erythema, infiltration, and papules
3+	Extreme positive reaction with intense erythema and infiltration coalescing vesicles, bullous reaction
IR	Irritant reaction

TABLE 40.4 Relevance

Definite	If a use test with the putative item containing the suspected allergen is positive or positive patch to object/product
Probable	If the substance identified by patch testing can be verified as present in the known skin contactants of the patient
Possible	If the patient is exposed to circumstances in which skin contact with materials known to contain the putative allergen will likely occur
Past	If the patient had previous exposure but is currently not exposed
Unknown	

Determining Clinical Relevance

The relevance of positive reactions to clinical ACD can be established only by carefully correlating the history, including exposure to the allergen. A positive patch test reaction may be relevant to present or previous dermatitis, multiple true-positive results can occur, and mild responses may still represent allergic reaction. Conversely, patients with negative results may need to be referred for more complete testing to a patch testing clinic. Thus, understanding the sources of antigen in the patient's environment is required to be able to advise the patient adequately regarding avoidance and alternatives in ACD. A positive patch test is considered to be a "definite" reaction of ACD if the result of a "use test" with the suspected item was positive or the reaction of the patch test with the object or product was positive. It would be "probable" if the antigen could be verified as present in known skin contactants and the clinical presentation was consistent, and it would be "possible" if the patient is exposed to circumstances in which skin contact with materials known to contain allergen was likely (Table 40.4). Multiple sensitivities are possible if different allergens are present in different products used simultaneously or concomitant sensitization occurs if allergens are present in the same products and both induce sensitization.

The repeat open application test (ROAT) or exaggerated use test may be done to confirm the presence or absence of ACD. The suspected allergen (for "leave-on" but not "wash-off" products) is applied to the antecubital fossa twice daily for 7 days and observed for dermatitis. The absence of a reaction makes CD unlikely. If eyelid dermatitis is considered, ROAT can be carried out on the back of the ear.

Additional tests used less frequently in the diagnosis of CD include skin biopsy to differentiate from other diseases. Prick or intradermal testing may be helpful, especially in the evaluation of CU. CU also can be evaluated with an "open" patch test. Potassium hydroxide preparation for fungal hyphae or cultures may be needed to identify fungal disease.

Allergens of Particular Importance in Children

Nickel

Nickel is a more common cause of ACD than all other metals combined, even in children. Of 391 children aged 18 years or younger who were patch tested by the NACDG, 28% had a positive patch test to nickel and 26% were deemed to have a nickel allergy of either current or past relevance.[110] Nickel allergy is more common in adolescents, girls more than boys, and ear piercing is the most important predisposing factor. Ear piercing at a young age and greater number of piercings both appear to increase risk of nickel sensitization.[111–114] Thus, some authors recommend that ear piercing be delayed until after 10 years of age, presumably to allow for the development of immune tolerance.[115] The Danish Ministry of the Environment and the European Union have both introduced legislation to decrease exposure to prolonged contact with nickel-containing products. These measures are thought to have contributed to a reduction in nickel sensitization.[116,117]

Nearly 5 million people per year in the United States and Canada undergo orthodontic treatment. In patients with contact allergy to orthodontics, nickel is the most common allergen. Nickel is commonly used in orthodontics; stainless steel, which contains about 8% nickel that is not normally biologically available, is generally considered safe in patients who are allergic to nickel. Orthodontics before ear piercing have been associated with decreased rates of nickel hypersensitivity.[114,118] The mechanism responsible was suggested to be oral tolerance,[119] and in vitro studies support this hypothesis.[120,121] Certain flexible titanium-nickel arch wires used in orthodontics release increased amounts of nickel compared with stainless steel and may need to be avoided in patients with known nickel sensitivity.[122]

The presence of releasable nickel from the surface of any object can be detected using the dimethylglyoxime spot test; a pink color indicates the presence of releasable nickel. In children, instrument mouthpieces with worn coatings are potential sources of nickel exposure[123] as are cell phones.[124] Nickel is also found in foods, though despite some studies suggesting benefit,[125,126] the evidence for dietary avoidance of nickel is not strong (quality of evidence IV, strength of recommendation C).[109]

Chromate

Potassium dichromate is used in manufacturing and construction, and chromates are commonly found in products made of chrome and stainless steel, cement, and leather. They are found in shoes and gloves, in which chromium salts are used in the tanning process. Chromate sensitivity can be associated with hand or foot dermatitis, which can persist even after chromate avoidance. In chromate-sensitive individuals, chromium-free tanned leather shoes should be selected when available; when they are not available, discarding leather shoes after a few months can decrease chromium exposure because it leaches out during prolonged use. In pediatric patients, potassium dichromate sensitization also likely occurs through its use as a pigment in tattoo ink, green felt fabric, cosmetics, radiator coolants, and dental and orthopedic implants.[127]

Cobalt

Cobalt is another metal that often causes a positive result on patch testing in pediatric patients. Sensitization to cobalt may occur independently of nickel sensitization.[95,128,129] Although chromium typically has been considered the cause of dermatitis related to leather goods, cobalt may be another source. Additional cobalt exposures come from jewelry and orthopedic and other implanted devices.[129]

Thimerosal

Thimerosal is a mercuric derivative of thiosalicylic acid used as a preservative in vaccines, cosmetics, tattoo inks, eye drops, contact lens solutions, and a disinfectant (i.e., merthiolate).[130,131] Past reporting of thimerosal-positive patch testing found little to no significant clinical relevance,[132,133] earning it the title of the American Contact Dermatitis Society's "(non)allergen of the year" in 2002.[134] Sensitization to thimerosal is likely associated with routine vaccination, and this sensitization is lifelong. Thimerosal was removed from the NACDG screening allergen series for the 2003 to 2004 assessment.[133] However, thimerosal still can be found in ophthalmic solutions and some eye makeup and may have relevance in eyelid dermatitis. Because of its potential toxicity and allergenicity in children, precautionary measures are underway to remove thimerosal from vaccines.[135] Notably, sensitization to thimerosal is not a contraindication to vaccination,[136–138] and the only vaccine for children under 6 years of age that still contains thimerosal is the inactivated influenza vaccine in the multidose units; the single-dose units do not contain thimerosal.[139]

Aside from thimerosal, reactions to adjuvants (e.g., aluminum hydroxide), stabilizers (e.g., gelatin), preservatives, and antibiotics (e.g., neomycin) in vaccines have been reported.

Methylisothiazolinone and Methylchloroisothiazolinone

Both methylisothiazolinone (MI) and methylchloroisothiazolinone (MCI) are common preservatives used in personal products.

MI is a highly relevant cause of preservative contact allergy and dermatitis.[140,141] Its use as a preservative in a wide array of products has been increasing, and it can be found in baby products (lotions and wipes), bath products (soaps and detergents), cosmetics (makeup and makeup removers), hair care products (shampoo, conditioner, color products, and straighteners), nail care products, deodorants, shaving products, and skin care products. For the second consecutive 2-year reporting cycle, MI has held the top rank in the significance-prevalence index number rating, a weighted calculation of relevance combined with prevalence. MI contained in the MCI/MI patch test mix is only 25 ppm. Testing MI alone at a higher concentration increases detection of contact allergy to this allergen and should be considered.[142] Because of its widespread use, avoidance is difficult and high relapse rates have been reported.[143]

Aluminum

Aluminum may cause cutaneous granulomas in response to vaccines containing aluminum hydroxide. These tend to resolve spontaneously, although children subsequently have positive patch test results to metallic aluminum or its salts.[144] The aluminum sensitivity appears to be lost with time, because it occurs rarely in adults.

Rubber Chemicals

Rubber chemicals (i.e., thiuram mix, mercaptobenzothiazole, mercapto mix) are used in the manufacturing of both dipped (e.g., balloons, gloves) and molded (e.g., pacifiers, handle bars) rubber products. Mixed dialkyl thioureas, a mixture of two thiourea chemicals, is used for rubber acceleration and as an antioxidant in the manufacturing of neoprene. Large quantities of thioureas have been shown to leach from neoprene compounds, and the levels were sufficient to elicit ACD.[145a] ACD from neoprene includes cases caused by orthopedic braces, prostheses, splints and foot supports; athletic shoes; rubber masks, swim goggles and wet suits; computer wrist rests; neoprene gloves; and rubber-based materials in automobiles.

Special Considerations

Plant Dermatitis (Phytodermatoses)

Plants of the *Toxicodendron* group, including poison ivy and poison oak, are the most common causes of allergic plant dermatitis in children in the United States. Even newborns can be sensitized to the oleoresin (urushiol). The clinical reaction is typically vesicles and bullae, often with a characteristic linear appearance (Fig. 40.6) Although the fluid content of vesicles is not antigenic, the oleoresin can be transferred by handling exposed pet dander,

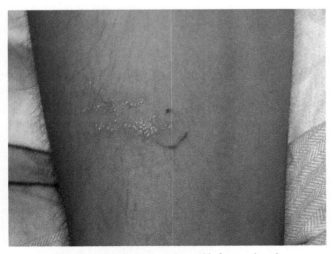

• **Fig. 40.6** Allergic contact dermatitis from poison ivy.

clothing, or sports equipment. Soap and water inactivate the antigen. Urushiol is also found in cashew nut trees, Japanese lacquer, *Ginkgo biloba,* and mango skin, and the ingestion of cashews or contact with mango skin can cause a similar rash. Rhus patch testing is not recommended because it has a significant sensitizing capacity.

The Compositae family (Asteraceae), the second largest plant family, represents approximately 10% of the world's flowering plants. ACD to Compositae may manifest as acute or chronic dermatitis of exposed sites. Although ACD to Compositae is typically seen in florists, farmers, and professional gardeners, studies by Fortina et al[145b] indicate that it may be more common in children than previously thought. The dermatitis has an airborne contact pattern distribution in the exposed areas of the hands and face with symptoms worse in late spring or summer and worse after picking daisies or dandelions or playing outdoors. ACD to Compositae should be suspected in children with a family or personal history of atopy, summer-related or summer-exacerbated dermatitis, and a history of plant exposure.

Ambrosia spp., which include ragweed, can cause allergic plant dermatitis when pollinating, in individuals both with and without atopy. Repeated contact with ornamental cut flowers, including *Alstroemeria* (the lily and tulip family of plants), can result in an ACD that manifests with a fissured dermatitis of the fingertips. Plants that contain furocoumarins (psoralens), including parsley, parsnips, and wild carrots, can cause phototoxic reactions, especially in summer when psoralens are most abundant in the plants where children are playing. These reactions occur when the skin, contaminated with psoralens, is exposed to ultraviolet A light.

Dermatitis From Topical Medications

The topical application of anesthetics, antihistamines, antibiotics, and even antiinflammatory drugs, along with preservatives or fragrances, has been implicated in sensitization and contact reactions. Neomycin, found over the counter in medicated adhesive bandages, and topical diphenhydramine are frequent and potent sensitizers in children (ranked third most common allergen yielding positive patch testing in children).[95] Contact allergy to topical corticosteroids can be difficult to diagnose[146] and should be suspected in patients (especially those with AD) whose dermatitis worsens with the application of a corticosteroid. There have been reports of contact allergy in the nasal mucosa to budesonide nasal spray and stomatitis with budesonide for oral inhalation.[147] Patch testing to some corticosteroids is commercially available, but, because of concurrent antiinflammatory action, delayed readings beyond 72 hours have to be done. Corticosteroids representative of different structural groups A to D with cross-reactivity based on two immune recognition sites—C 6/9 and C16/17 substitutions—are typically used in patch testing[148] (Box 40.1). Cross-reactivity within a group is higher than between agents in different groups.

Contact Dermatitis to Cosmetics

An average adult applies 12 personal hygiene products daily and, in the course of using these products, is exposed to 168 discrete chemicals. Children, especially adolescents, may be exposed to similar numbers. Cosmetics for children are sold in toy stores and are not regulated. Exposure to multiple potential allergens occurs repeatedly with the use of cosmetics, and it is not unusual for these

BOX 40.1 Structural Groups of Corticosteroids
Cross-Reactivity Based on Two Immune Recognition Sites: C 6/9 and C16/17 Substitutions

- *Class A:* Hydrocortisone and tixocortol pivalate—has C17 or C21 short-chain ester
  - Hydrocortisone, -acetate, tixocortol, prednisone, prednisolone, -acetate, cloprednol, cortisone, -acetate, fludrocortisone, methylprednisolone-acetate
- *Class B:* Acetonides—has C16 C17 *cis*-ketal or -diol additions
  - Triamcinolone acetonide, -alcohol, budesonide, desonide, fluocinonide, fluocinolone acetonide, amcinonide, halcinonide
- *Class C:* Nonesterified betamethasone; C16 methyl group
  - Betamethasone sodium phosphate, dexamethasone, dexamethasone sodium phosphate, fluocortolone
- *Class D1:* C16 methyl group and halogenated B ring
  - Clobetasone 17-butyrate, -17-propionate, betamethasone-valerate, dipropionate, alclometasone dipropionate, fluocortolone caproate, -pivalate, mometasone furoate
- *Class D2:* Labile esters without C16 methyl or B ring halogen substitution
  - Hydrocortisone 17-butyrate, -17-valerate, -17-aceponate, -17-buteprate, methylprednisolone aceponate

Wilkinson, SM. Corticosteroids cross reactions: an alternative view. Contact Derm 2000;42:59–63.

TABLE 40.5 Cosmetic Preservatives

Formaldehyde Releaser	Nonformaldehyde Releaser
Quaternium 15	MCI/MI
Diazolidinyl urea	Parabens
Imidazolidinyl urea	Chloroxylenol
Bromo nitropropane DMDM hydantoin	Iodopropynyl butylcarbamate Benzalkonium chloride Thimerosal

Note: Paraben, quaternium 15, and formaldehyde preservatives are frequently combined and co-sensitize.

MCI, Methylchloroisothiazolinone; *MI,* methylisothiazolinone.

products to manifest as contact allergy distant from the sites of application (termed *ectopic contact dermatitis*).

Fragrance is the most common cause of ACD from cosmetics in the United States. Fragrances can be found in cosmetics, personal hygiene products, diapers, and even scented toys, either overtly to add an appealing scent or to mask unpleasant odors.

The term *unscented* can erroneously suggest that a product does not contain fragrance when, in fact, a masking fragrance can be present. *Fragrance-free* products are typically free of classic fragrance ingredients and generally acceptable for the patient with allergy. However, if a fragrance-based chemical (such as the preservative benzyl alcohol) is added for a purpose other than to act as a fragrance, the product can still claim it is fragrance free. The addition of botanical and natural chemicals also can alter the smell of the product. Fragrance Mix II is one of the top 10 most frequently positive allergens of the NACD patch test but is not included in the current T.R.U.E. TEST and may therefore be missed.

Preservatives, present in most aqueous-based cosmetics and personal hygiene products to prevent rancidity, are grouped into two broad categories: formaldehyde releasers and nonformaldehyde releasers (Table 40.5). Individuals who are allergic to formaldehyde cannot use any of the formaldehyde releasers. Paraben is the most commonly used preservative in cosmetic, pharmaceutical, and industrial products because of its broad spectrum of activity against yeasts, molds, and bacteria.

Excipients, including propylene glycol, ethylenediamine, and lanolin, serve to solubilize, sequester, thicken, foam, or lubricate the active component in a product. They can cause ACD or, in higher concentrations, can act as irritants. Lanolin is a common component of consumer products whose composition has not been fully characterized. Medicaments containing lanolin are more sensitizing than lanolin-containing cosmetics. Lanolin is a weak sensitizer when applied on normal skin but a stronger sensitizer on damaged skin.

Hair products are second only to skin care products as the most common cause of cosmetic allergy. Allergy to routine hair care products is usually due to fragrance and CAPB, an amphoteric surfactant often found in shampoos, bath products, eye and facial cleaners, roll-on deodorants, and other skin and hair care products. CAPB is less irritating than the older polar surfactants such as sodium lauryl sulfate,[149] but is more allergenic.

New trends in permanent and temporary tattoos have emerged in our adolescent population. Black henna mixtures, containing indigo, henna, PPD, and/or diaminotoluenes, to temporarily paint the skin are used in some cultures, primarily before major events. There is increasing use of PPD to give henna (auburn to red color) a darker shade of brown to black for body painting, and the need for a policy for use in children has been suggested.[150] Adolescents working in hair salons may be exposed to PPD, the most common allergen affecting hairdressers. A number of chemicals may cross-react with PPD[151] such as PABA in sunscreens, sulfonamides, *p*-aminosalicylic acid, benzocaine and related "caines" anesthetics, azo dyes, and black rubber mix.

Glycerol thioglycolate, the active ingredient in permanent wave solutions, is a more common cause of occupational ACD in hairdressers than consumers. Unlike PPD, thioglycolates may remain allergenic in the hair long after it has been rinsed out; thus, allergic individuals may continue to have skin eruptions weeks after application of the perm, and allergic hairdressers may be unable to cut permanent waved hair.

Nail cosmetics have become increasingly popular and fashionable, and ACD to acrylics can manifest locally at the distal digit or ectopically on the eyelids and face. The currently marketed products contain various methacrylate ester monomers, dimethacrylates and trimethacrylates, and cyanoacrylate-based glues.

Sunscreens are frequently present in cosmetics such as moisturizers, lip preparations, and foundations. As a group they are the most common cause of photoallergic CD. Chemical-free sun blocks use physical blocking agents instead of photoactive chemicals and include titanium dioxide and zinc oxide, which are rarely sensitizers.

Contact Dermatitis in Children Athletes

The skin of athletes is exposed to repeated trauma, heat, moisture, and numerous allergens and chemicals and is predisposed to ICD or ACD. Early recognition can facilitate appropriate therapy and prevention.[152]

In swimmers, chemicals such as chlorine used to disinfect swimming pools can cause both ICD and ACD. The dermatitis may spare the area under the swimwear. However, swimwear and equipment, including goggles, nose plugs, nose clips, ear plugs, fins, and swim caps, also may cause CD. Although ACD from swimming goggles usually manifests with well-demarcated, bilateral periorbital edema and erythema with varying degrees of pruritus, exudate, and scaling, conjunctival injection and hypopigmentation have been reported.[153,154] Allergens include rubber and chemicals used in manufacturing (neoprene, benzoyl peroxide, phenol-formaldehyde resin, thioureas, and antioxidants).

"Jogger's nipples" are painful, erythematous, and crusted erosions representing an ICD caused by friction from the running shirt.[155] Other skin and nail problems are associated with ICD and ACD from shoes, shirts, and topical medications. Contact allergens include components of rubber, leather, glues, or dyes used in the manufacture of running shoes. Sweat helps leach out the chemicals from the shoes. Rubber insoles containing mercaptobenzothiazole and dibenzothiazyl disulfide have been reported to cause recurrent eczematous eruptions of the feet, which can be prevented by switching to new insoles made of materials such as polyurethane.[156] In a large case series of student athletes, benzocaine and lanolin (found in topical anesthetics and massage creams) were the most prevalent allergens responsible for CD in runners.[157]

CD in soccer or football players is usually caused by equipment or chemicals used on the field. "Cement burns" presenting as erythematous, edematous plaques, bullae, and erosions on the upper inner thighs are due to the lime component used in field markings. The characteristic rash, a history of exposure to wet field lines, and worsening of symptoms after taking a hot shower point to the diagnosis. Treatment includes removing contaminated clothing, cleaning the areas with water, and applying topical antibiotics or petroleum jelly.

Like runners, soccer players may develop ACD from topical anesthetic creams, epoxy resins, nickel in certain athletic shoes, and tincture of benzoin used in conjunction with athletic tape.[152] Urea-formaldehyde resin in shin pads has caused ACD in soccer players.

Ball handling in baseball and basketball can cause both ICD and ACD. "Basketball pebble fingers," manifesting as small petechiae and abrasions on a shiny denuded surface of the fingertips and pads, is an ICD resulting from mechanical irritation from the ball's pebbled surface. An eczematous rash on both palms, the palmar fingertips and base of the thumbs may be due to rubber allergy.[158] Protective knee padding and adhesives in athletic tape contain rubber accelerators and formaldehyde resins.

Tennis players can develop ICD as a result of friction of the medial thighs. This manifests as erythematous eruptions over the opposing areas. ACD can be caused by isophorone diamine and epoxy resin used in the manufacture of tennis rackets, neoprene splints for tennis elbow, squash balls with N-isopropyl-N′-phenyl-p-phenylenediamine, rubber, and anesthetic sprays with ethyl chloride.

Fiberglass in hockey sticks, epoxy resin adhesives in a facemask, and dyes used in the manufacture of hockey gloves have caused ACD.[159] Weightlifters have developed ACD to the nickel and palladium in weights or bars[160] and the chalk used to achieve a better grip.[161]

In summary, the young athlete is constantly exposed to allergens in clothing, equipment, environment, and medications. The unique presentation of the rash, a careful sports-directed history, and allergen-directed patch testing enhances the ability to diagnose and care for the young athlete with dermatitis.

Treatment and Prevention

Identification of the allergen to improve avoidance of contact to the allergen and education of patients and/or families is the mainstay of treatment for ACD. All other measures are palliative and temporary.

The deceptively simple application of the patch test is actually complicated by barriers, including interpretation of the patch test and assigning relevance, patient education, and patient compliance. Once the offending agent is identified, patients and/or caregivers must be educated regarding the nature of the dermatitis, triggering agents, and irritant factors.

This process includes the following:

1. *Providing the patient/caregiver the information:* Patient/caregiver understanding improves with visual material such a simple written instruction and/or video-based education.[162–164] A list of potential exposure alternatives and substitutes should be offered to the patient to increase compliance.[165,166] There are two U.S. databases of products free of allergens: the Contact Allergen Management Program (CAMP) of the American Contact Dermatitis Society (http://www.contactderm.org) and the Contact Allergen Replacement Database (CARD) of the Mayo Clinic (http://www.AllergyFreeSkin.com). There are also online sources of allergen handouts and videos (http://www.contactderm.org, http://www.allergeaze.com, http://www.dormer.com, http://www.contactdermatitisinstitute.com).

2. *Ensuring retention and recall of information:* Information overload is a state of confusion and uncertainty when the amount of information provided exceeds the person's capacity to process the information. The names of the allergens are long, complex, and confusing. There are also numerous synonyms and cross-reactions. Reducing the amount of information, limiting the information per visit, and addressing conflicting information at every visit can substantially reduce this risk. Physician time factors into this process, and providing written or online information may improve this process. The written information must be easy to read, composed at a 5th- or 6th-grade reading level. This can be combined with a personalized, verbal review and reinforcement.

Topical corticosteroids are the first-line treatment for ACD and are most effective when treating localized dermatitis. Low-potency corticosteroids (class 4 or 5) are recommended for the thinner skin of the face and flexural areas, and high-potency corticosteroids (class 1) are indicated for thickened, lichenified lesions and areas such as the palms and soles. Ointments are generally more potent, more occlusive, and contain fewer sensitizing preservatives than creams and lotions. Patients with sensitivity to preservatives can use preservative-free corticosteroids. Of note, ACD to the topical corticosteroid molecule and preservatives in corticosteroids has been reported. Cool compresses with aluminum subacetate (Burow's solution), calamine, or colloidal oatmeal may help acute, oozing lesions. Excessive handwashing should be discouraged in patients with hand dermatitis, and nonirritating or sensitizing moisturizers must be used after washing. Soaps and nonalkaline cleansers should be avoided.

For extensive and severe CD, such as in extensive poison ivy, systemic corticosteroids may offer relief within 12 to 24 hours. Because of its high side effect profile of systemic corticosteroids, their use for chronic ACD is not recommended.

Topical calcineurin inhibitors, approved for children with AD, have been used in both animal models and patients with ACD.[167–177] These agents do not induce skin atrophy and may be especially valuable in treating facial or eyelid dermatitis, although use in CD would be off-label at the present time.

Antihistamines may offer some benefit in CU and some relief from pruritus. Oral diphenhydramine should not be used in patients with ACD to diphenhydramine in a calamine base (Caladryl) or hydroxyzine hydrochloride (Atarax) in ethylenediamine-sensitive patients.

Phototherapy (ultraviolet B [UVB]) may be effective in the treatment of ACD, especially in chronic ACD of the hands.[165]

Other immunomodulating agents such as cyclosporine, methotrexate, azathioprine, and mycophenolate mofetil have been used especially in patients who could not avoid their allergens. There are conflicting reports on whether dupilumab is effective or exacerbates some cases.[178]

Mechanical barriers such as protective gloves and clothing and barrier creams are helpful in some cases. For nickel-allergic patients, barriers such as gloves, covers for metal buttons, and identification of nickel by the dimethylglyoxime test can be prescribed, but results can be disappointing.[166]

Frequency of diaper changes using improved product design features, such as superabsorbent disposable diapers, is thought to explain the decline in diaper dermatitis among infants.[179] Low-potency corticosteroids and barrier ointments or creams can be used for a limited period.[180] A topical antifungal agent should be used in secondary *Candida albicans* infection. A gentle cleansing routine, frequent diaper changes, and a thick barrier cream help control this condition.[181]

Patient education regarding the nature of the dermatitis, triggering, agents, and irritant factors plus instruction for avoidance and appropriate substitutes will not only aid in clearing the dermatitis but will also prevent or minimize recurrences. At present, hyposensitization of patients with ACD is not a viable therapy.[182]

Conclusions

CD includes irritant and allergic forms and can affect patients of any age. Identification, patient education, and avoidance of the relevant allergen are key to the successful treatment of ACD. Patch testing remains the gold standard for diagnosis of ACD even in children, and negative results in the face of a convincing clinical presentation should prompt further evaluation by a specialist in CD.[183] A limited number of interventions effectively prevent or treat ICD and ACD, but well-controlled, outcome-blinded studies, particularly in the area of ACD prevention, are needed.[184] New insights into the immune mechanisms involved may lead to better treatment strategies, including induction of tolerance, especially with difficult-to-avoid allergens.[185]

Helpful Websites

American Contact Dermatitis Society website includes "Find a Physician" for patch testing (http://www.contactderm.org)
The American Academy of Dermatology website (http://www.aad.org)
T.R.U.E. TEST website (http://www.truetest.com)

The reference list can be found on the companion Expert Consult website at http://www.expertconsult.inkling.com.

41

Allergic and Immunologic Eye Disease

LEONARD BIELORY, BRETT P. BIELORY

KEY POINTS

- The hallmark of allergic conjunctivitis is itching. Bacterial and viral conjunctivitis commonly manifest with pain or the feeling of a foreign body rather than pruritus.
- Bacterial and viral conjunctivitis generally have a self-limited course ranging from 5 to 14 days. Signs and symptoms of acute allergic conjunctivitis wax and wane over longer periods (weeks to months) coinciding with the circulating allergen (e.g., seasonal pollens).
- Chronic conjunctival vascular injection, "red eye" or "pink eye," may occur in children with dry eye disease related to intense viewing of computers and other mobile devices.

- Disorders of the tear film as in meibomian gland disease can result in chronic blepharoconjunctivitis.
- Topical ophthalmic corticosteroids should be used with caution in treating pediatric forms of ocular surface disease because of their intrinsic potential to raise the intraocular pressure (glaucoma) or exacerbate herpes simplex virus keratoconjunctivitis.
- Oral antihistamines are associated with anticholinergic receptor binding and are associated with ocular surface drying and associated symptoms that confound the diagnosis of allergic conjunctivitis.

Introduction

Ocular allergy symptoms have increased over the past several decades, with specific assessments noting a doubling in the continental United States and up to 40% of the population reporting ocular symptoms in the National Health and Nutrition Examination Survey (NHANES) study compared with earlier reporting of 32% of the pediatric population.[1,2] These increases coincide with the international market growth in the treatment of anterior ocular inflammatory disorders with antiallergics occupying 25% of the market.[3]

Eye Anatomy, Histology, and Immune Function

Because of its considerable vascularization and vessel sensitivity, the eye is a common target of local and systemic inflammatory disorders that have the potential to induce visual loss, potentially causing a tremendous impact on a patient's quality of life.

The eye is essentially constructed of two immunologically active portions, as follows (Fig. 41.1):

1. Externally the eyelids, conjunctiva (palpebral and bulbar), and tear fluid layer provide the primary barrier against environmental aeroallergens, pollutants, and infectious agents; the conjunctiva are contiguous with the collagenous sclera, which is involved in systemic autoimmune disorders.

2. Internally the highly vascular uvea is involved in systemic immune complex and cell-mediated inflammatory disorders. The retina is an extension of the central nervous system.

Ocular immunologic hypersensitivity reactions incorporate the spectrum of the classic Gell and Coombs classification (Table 41.1).[4,5]

Eyelids

The eyelids provide the first line of defense as a mechanical barrier lubricating and cleaning the anterior ocular surface. The palpebral skin is extremely thin (0.55 mm thick compared with the 2 mm integument of the face) and commonly involved in delayed hypersensitivity reactions and fluid retention (e.g., periorbital edema and anasarca).

Conjunctiva

The conjunctiva, a thin mucous membrane that extends from the eyelid margin to the limbus of the eye consists of (1) the palpebral conjunctiva lining the inner surface of the eyelids, (2) the bulbar conjunctiva covering the sclera, and (3) the fornix or conjunctival sac at the junction between the bulbar and palpebral conjunctiva. Histologically, the conjunctiva consists of two distinct histologic layers: the epithelium, which is composed of two to five layers of stratified columnar cells, with interspersed mucin-producing goblet cells, and the substantia propria, which is composed of connective tissue.

Inflammatory cells such as mast cells, eosinophils, and basophils normally do not reside in the ocular epithelium. In the substantia propria, mast cells (~6000/mm³) are present, predominantly (>95%) of the connective tissue mast cell type (MC_{TC}).[6,7] In the more chronic forms of allergic conjunctivitis, mucosal type mast cells (MC_T) increase in the epithelial layer. Tear fluid demonstrated an extensive proinflammatory capability bathing the ocular surface that includes tumor necrosis factor alpha (TNF-α), interleukin 4 (IL-4), IL-6, IL-10, IL12, IL-33, TGF-β, eotaxin, and intracellular adhesion molecules (ICAM-1).[7–13] Additional

arms of the anterior surface immune response in the epithelium include various mononuclear cells, antigen-presenting Langerhans cells, CD3+ lymphocytes, and CD4+/CD8+ lymphocytes. The primary lymphoid organ for intraocular reactions is the spleen, and the external lymphatics drain the lateral conjunctiva to the preauricular nodes (e.g., parotid node) and the nasal conjunctival lymphatics drain to the submandibular nodes. Activated conjunctival lymphocytes travel first to regional lymph nodes, then to the spleen, and traffic back to the conjunctiva.

Tear Film

The conjunctival surface is bathed in a thin layer of tear film that appears approximately 2 to 4 weeks after birth. Tear film includes an aqueous layer with a gradient of mucin that decreases from the ocular surface to the overlying lipid layer.[14,15] Mucin produced by conjunctival surface goblet cells decreases the surface tension of the tear film. The lipid component of the tear film floats on the aqueous layer and decreases the evaporation rate of the aqueous tears. The aqueous portion of the tear film contains a soup of immunologically active proteins, including immunoglobulin A (IgA), IgG, IgM, IgE, tryptase, histamine, lysozyme, lactoferrin, ceruloplasmin, vitronectin, and cytokines.

Uveal Tract

The uveal tract is highly vascular and comprises the pigmented iris, ciliary body, and choroid. The ciliary body produces the aqueous humor, a common site for the deposition of immune complexes and involved in autoimmune conditions. Disturbances in the production or outflow of aqueous humor may lead to increased intraocular pressure (IOP; i.e., glaucoma) that may be immune mediated, but nonimmunologic congenital forms of glaucoma must be considered in the differential diagnosis of pediatric conjunctivitis (pink eye or red eye).

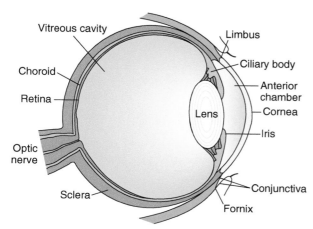

• **Fig. 41.1** Sagittal cross-sectional view of the human eye revealing the parts commonly involved in immunologic reactions: eyelids (blepharitis and dermatitis), conjunctiva (conjunctivitis), cornea (keratitis), sclera (episcleritis and scleritis), optic nerve (neuritis), iris (iritis), vitreous (vitreitis), choroid (choroiditis), and retina (retinitis). The last four parts constitute the inner portion of the eye (the uveal tract) and are classified as forms of uveitis.

TABLE 41.1 Categories of Pediatric Ocular Inflammation

Category	Recognition Component	Soluble Mediators	Time Course	Cellular Response	Clinical Example
IgE/mast cell	IgE	Leukotrienes Arachidonates Histamine	Seconds Minutes	Eosinophils Neutrophils Basophils	Allergic conjunctivitis Anaphylaxis Vernal keratoconjunctivitis
Cytotoxic antibody	IgG IgM	Complement	Hours Days	Neutrophils Macrophages	Mooren's ulcer Pemphigus Pemphigoid
Immune complex	IgG IgM	Complement	Hours Days	Neutrophils Eosinophils Lymphocytes	Serum sickness uveitis Corneal immune rings Lens-induced uveitis Behçet's syndrome Kawasaki's disease Vasculitis
Delayed hypersensitivity	Lymphocytes Monocytes	Lymphokines Monokines	Days Weeks	Lymphocytes Monocytes Eosinophils Basophils	Corneal allograft rejection Sympathetic ophthalmia Sarcoid-induced uveitis

IgE, Immunoglobulin E.

Differential Diagnosis

The differential diagnosis of the pediatric red eye can be broadly divided into four categories: allergic, infectious, immunologic, and nonspecific, with distinct signs and symptoms (Fig. 41.2 and Table 41.2).[16]

History

A well-performed anamnesis and external ocular examination provides a better understanding of the cause of the conjunctivitis: immune-mediated versus other causes of pediatric red eye. The medical history should include all ocular symptoms (i.e., itching, burning, photophobia, discharge, visual changes, pain) associated with the red eye; unilateral or bilateral; duration; presence of allergies or systemic diseases; prior treatments; family history; seasonal, environmental, and occupational exposures; contact lens use; ocular medication use and prior surgery.

Newborn assessment includes a prenatal history, maternal infections (e.g., herpes simplex virus, *Chlamydia*, or human immunodeficiency virus) and developmental delays. Ocular trauma from forceps or vacuum delivery has been known to occur. The ophthalmic application of silver nitrate and erythromycin applied at birth may cause chemical irritation. Recent exposure within the family or at school to individuals with conjunctivitis or upper respiratory tract infection may suggest adenovirus infection in an endemic area. Family history is particularly important when inherited disorders are suspected. Trauma resulting in corneal abrasions or ocular foreign bodies may occur in the curious and mobile toddler, but with increased frequency or with other physical features child abuse also must be considered. In teenagers, a sexual history may

suggest a chlamydial or neisserial infection. The overuse of over-the-counter (OTC) topical medications (e.g., vasoconstrictors, artificial tears, cosmetics, or contact lens wear) may be associated with conjunctivitis medicamentosa or toxic keratopathy. Environmental factors and temporal relationships that include to outdoor (e.g., pollen seasons) or indoor (e.g., tobacco smoke, cleaning supplies, pets) sources of allergens and irritants are to be considered.

Many of the signs and symptoms of allergic conjunctivitis are nonspecific because they involve the four classic signs of inflammation (calor, dolor, rubor, and tumor) and include heat, pain, redness, swelling, tearing, stinging, and burning, with photophobia with itching being the most prominent symptom, which may last from hours to days. A stringy or ropy discharge characteristic of a persistent ocular allergy may range from serous to purulent. A purulent discharge present in the morning with crusting and difficulty opening the lids is more characteristic of bacterial causes (e.g., gram-negative organisms, *Neisseria*, and *Haemophilus* spp.). Ocular effects of environmental allergen exposure are bilateral, although a unilateral reaction may occur from direct hand transfer. Ocular pain is not typically associated with allergic conjunctivitis and suggests an extraocular process such as a corneal abrasion, scleritis or foreign body, or an intraocular process such as uveitis.

Eye Examination

The eye should be examined for external evidence of eyelid involvement (e.g., blepharitis, dermatitis, swelling, discoloration, ptosis, or blepharospasm) (Table 41.3). Conjunctival involvement may include chemosis, hyperemia, cicatrization, or formation of papillae on the palpebral and bulbar membranes.

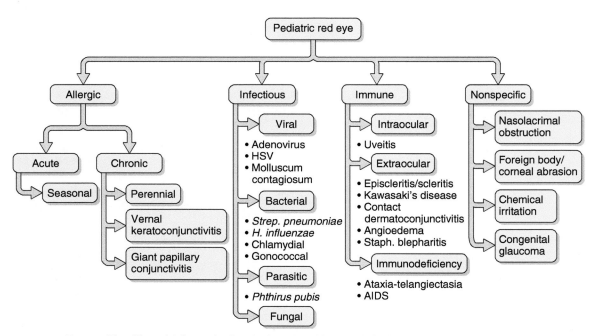

• **Fig. 41.2** The differential diagnosis of pediatric "red eye" includes infectious agents (e.g., chlamydial disease, adenovirus), allergic conditions (e.g., seasonal allergic conjunctivitis, perennial allergic conjunctivitis, giant papillary conjunctivitis, vernal keratoconjunctivitis), immunologic disorders (e.g., Kawasaki's disease, uveitis, ataxia-telangiectasia) and nonspecific causes (e.g., foreign body, chemical irritation, nasolacrimal obstruction). *AIDS,* Acquired immunodeficiency syndrome; *H. influenzae, Haemophilus influenzae; HSV,* herpes simplex virus; *Staph., Staphylococcus; Strep., Streptococcus.*

TABLE 41.2 Differential Diagnosis of Pediatric Conjunctivitis[a]

	Predominant Cell Type	Chemosis	Lymph Node	Cobblestoning	Discharge	Lid Involvement	Pruritus	Gritty Sensation	Pain	Seasonal Variation
Allergic										
AC	Mast cell EOS	+	-	-	Clear mucoid	-	+	+/-	-	+
VKC	Lymph EOS	+/-	-	++	Stringy mucoid	+	++	+/-	+/- if cornea is involved	+
GPC	Lymph EOS	+/-	-	++	Clear white	-	++	+	-	+/-
Infectious										
Bacterial: *Streptococcus, Staphylococcus, Haemophilus*	PMN	+/-	+	-	++ Mucopurulent	-	-	+	+/-	+/-
Viral	PMN Monolymph	+/-	++	+/-	Clear mucoid	-	-	+	+/-	+/-
Chlamydial	Monolymph	+/-	+/-	+	++ Mucopurulent	-	-	+	+/-	+/-
Immunologic										
Kawasaki's disease	PMN, lymph	+/-	++	-	Serous mucoid	-	-	+/-	+/-	-
Uveitis	Lymph	-	-	-		-	-	-	++	-
Sarcoidosis	Lymph	-	-	-		Gray flat papules	-	-	+/-	-
JIA	Lymph	-	-	-		-	-	-	+/-	-
Episcleritis	Lymph	-	-	-		-	+	-	++	-
Contact dermatoconjunctivitis	Lymph	+/-	-	-	+/-	++	+	-	+/- if cornea is involved	-
Angioedema	Mast cell	++	-	-		+++	+/-	-	-	-
Ataxia-telangiectasia	-	-	-	-		-	-	-	-	-
Staphylococcal blepharitis	Monolymph	+/-	-	-	++ Mucopurulent	++	+	++	+/- if cornea is involved	-
Nonspecific										
Congenital entropion epiblepharon	-	-	-	-	Serous watery	++	-	+	+++	-
Congenital glaucoma	-	-	-	-	Serous	+/-	-	+/-	+++	-
Corneal abrasion	-	-	-	-	Serous watery	+	-	+/-	+++	-
Chemical	-	-	-	-	Serous mucoid	++	-	+/-	+++	-
Nasolacrimal obstruction	PMN if secondary infection	-	-	-	Mucopurulent	+	-	+/-	+/-	-

[a]These indicators can be used as a guide to delineate pediatric red eye.

AC, Allergic conjunctivitis; *EOS,* eosinophils; *VKC,* vernal keratoconjunctivitis; *GPC,* giant papillary conjunctivitis; *PMN,* polymorphonuclear leukocytes; *JIA,* juvenile idiopathic arthritis.

TABLE 41.3	Ocular Clinical Signs
Disorder	**Description**
Blepharitis	Inflammation of the eyelids; sometimes associated with the loss of eyelashes (madarosis)
Chalazion	A chronic, granulomatous inflammation of the meibomian gland
Chemosis	Edema of the conjunctiva because of transudate leaking through fenestrated conjunctival capillaries
Epiphora	Excessive tearing; may be the result of increased tear production or more commonly congenital obstruction of the nasolacrimal drainage system. This may occur in as many as 20% of infants, but resolves spontaneously in most cases before 1 year of age. Children with chronic sinusitis and/or rhinitis may have intermittent nasolacrimal duct obstruction because the distal nasolacrimal duct drains below the inferior meatus. Congenital glaucoma may also present with epiphora but has other characteristic findings (e.g., corneal enlargement, photophobia, and eventually corneal edema manifesting as a corneal haze) usually within the first year of life.[a]
Hordeolum	Synonymous with a stye
Keratitis	Inflammation and infection of the corneal surface, stroma, and endothelium, with numerous causes
Leukocoria	A white pupil; seen in patients with Chédiak-Higashi syndrome (a neutrophil defect), retinoblastoma, cataracts, and retrolental fibroplasia
Papillae	Large, hard, polygonal, flat-topped excrescences of the conjunctiva seen in many inflammatory and allergic ocular conditions
Phlyctenule	The formation of a small, gray, circumscribed lesion at the corneal limbus that has been associated with staphylococcal sensitivity, tuberculosis, and malnutrition
Proptosis	Forward protrusion of the eye or eyes
Ptosis	Drooping of the eyelid, which may have neurogenic, muscular, or congenital causes. Conditions specific to the eyelid that may cause a ptotic lid include chalazia, tumors, and preseptal cellulitis
Scleritis	Inflammation of the tunic that surrounds the ocular globe. Episcleritis presents as a red, somewhat painful eye in which the inflammatory reaction is located below the conjunctiva and only over the globe of the eye. The presence of scleritis should prompt a search for other systemic immune-mediated disorders
Trichiasis	In-turned eyelashes; usually results from softening of the tarsal plate within the eyelid
Trantas' dots	Pale, grayish-red, uneven nodules made up of eosinophils with a gelatinous composition seen at the limbal conjunctiva in vernal conjunctivitis

[a]Data from Seidman DJ, Nelson LB, Calhoun JH, et al. Signs and symptoms in the presentation of primary infantile glaucoma. Pediatrics 1986;77:399–404.

The presence of increased or abnormal secretions also should be noted. A fundoscopic examination should be performed to detect such conditions as uveitis (associated with autoimmune disorders), cataracts, and lack of the red reflex (associated with atopic disorders and chronic corticosteroid use).

Allergic shiners are dark circles beneath the eyes thought to result from impaired subcutaneous venous return from congestion beneath the skin (Fig. 41.3). Angioedema commonly affects the conjunctiva with chemosis and the periorbital tissue with increased prominence around the lower lids secondary to gravity. Eyelid or nasal vesicular eruptions are often seen in ophthalmic zoster and in recurrent bacterial infection–associated staphylococcal blepharoconjunctivitis secondary to constant eyelid rubbing. Examination of the bulbar and palpebral conjunctiva is noted for its "milky" appearance that is characteristic of allergy and is the result of the obscuring of blood vessels by conjunctival edema (Fig. 41.4). In contrast, a velvety, beefy-red conjunctiva with purulent discharge suggests a viral or bacterial cause, whereas follicular or papillary hyperplasia of the conjunctival surface reflects a more persistent or chronic inflammatory condition. Follicles appear as grayish, clear, or yellow bumps 1 to 2 mm in diameter, with conjunctival vessels on their surface; papillae contain a centrally located tuft of vessels. Papillae are generally not seen in active viral or bacterial conjunctivitis, and the presence of follicles represents a lymphocytic conjunctival

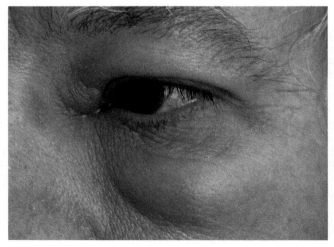

• **Fig. 41.3** Patient with periorbital swelling.

infiltration that commonly occurs in viral and chlamydial infections but are also seen in chronic and persistent forms of ocular allergy.

The cornea is best examined with a slit lamp biomicroscope, although many important clinical features can be seen with the

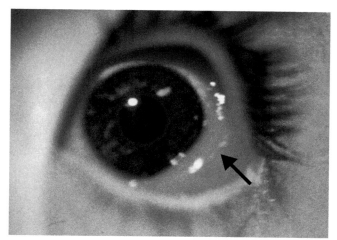

• **Fig. 41.4** Conjunctival edema or chemosis with milky appearance obscuring conjunctival vessels in an acute allergic reaction.

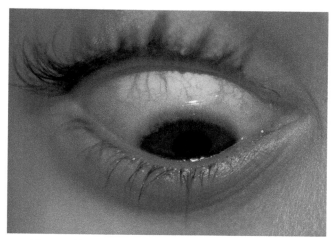

• **Fig. 41.6** Limbal conjunctivitis (a form of vernal conjunctivitis).

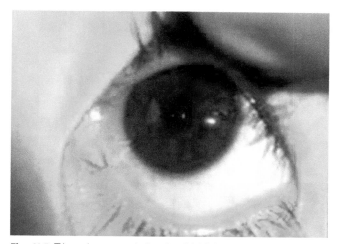

• **Fig. 41.5** Triangular corneal abrasion highlighted with fluorescein dye. The end of the fluorescein strip is touched to the marginal tear meniscus. When the patient blinks, the dye is dispersed throughout the ocular surface and stains wherever an epithelial defect exists, as in a corneal or conjunctival abrasion. A light using a cobalt filter, found on most modern ophthalmoscopes, will best demonstrate abnormal accumulations of the dye.

naked eye or with the use of an ophthalmoscope. The cornea should be perfectly smooth and transparent. Dusting of the cornea may indicate punctate epithelial keratitis. A localized corneal defect may suggest erosion or a larger ulcer that could be related to major basic protein deposition. Surface lesions can be best demonstrated by applying fluorescein dye to the eye, preferably after the instillation of a topical anesthetic drop (Fig. 41.5). Mucus adhering to the corneal or conjunctival surfaces is considered pathologic.

The ciliary body underlying the limbus at the juncture of the cornea and sclera becoming intensely inflamed with a deep pink coloration ("ciliary flush") is pathognomonic for anterior uveitis or iritis. Discrete limbal swellings are indicative of degenerating cellular debris, which is commonly seen in vernal conjunctivitis (Fig. 41.6). The anterior chamber provides a window into the aqueous humor for the presence of blood (i.e., hyphema) or pus (i.e., hypopyon). A shallow anterior chamber suggests narrow-angle

glaucoma that can be estimated by illuminating it from the side with a pen light; if the iris creates a shadow on the far side from the light, there is a high index of suspicion for increased IOP (i.e., glaucoma).

Allergic Disorders

Conjunctivitis caused by immunoglobulin E (IgE) mast cell–mediated reactions is the most common hypersensitivity response of the eye. Direct exposure of the ocular mucosal surface to the environment stimulates these mast cells, clinically producing the acute and late phase signs and symptoms of allergic conjunctivitis.[7,17] In addition, the conjunctiva is infiltrated with inflammatory cells such as neutrophils, eosinophils, lymphocytes, and macrophages. Interestingly, acute forms of allergic conjunctivitis lack an eosinophilic predominance, as seen in asthma. However, eosinophils and other immunologically active cells are prevalent in the more chronic forms.

Seasonal Allergic Conjunctivitis

Seasonal allergic conjunctivitis (SAC) is the most common allergic conjunctivitis, representing over half of all cases. As its name implies, SAC is characterized by symptoms that are seasonal and related to specific aeroallergens. Symptoms predominate in the spring and in some areas during the fall (Indian summer). Grass pollen is thought to produce the most ocular symptoms. Patients report itchy eyes and/or a burning sensation with watery discharge, commonly associated with nasal or pharyngeal symptoms. A white exudate may be present that turns stringy in the chronic form of the condition. The conjunctiva appears milky or pale pink and is accompanied by vascular congestion that may progress to conjunctival swelling (chemosis). Symptoms are usually bilateral but not always symmetric in degree of involvement. SAC rarely results in permanent visual impairment but can interfere greatly with daily activities.

Perennial Allergic Conjunctivitis

Perennial allergic conjunctivitis (PAC) is considered a variant of SAC that persists throughout the year. Dust mites, animal dander, and feathers are the most common allergens. Symptoms are analogous to those of SAC, and 79% of PAC patients have seasonal exacerbations. In addition, both PAC and SAC are similar in distribution of age, sex, and associated symptoms of asthma or eczema. The prevalence of PAC has been reported to be lower than that of SAC (3.5:10,000). It is subjectively more severe,[18] but with the increasing prevalence of allergies as reported in the International Study of Asthma and Allergies in Childhood this may be underrepresented; in fact, perennial forms of ocular allergy may be more common than pure seasonal forms.

Vernal Keratoconjunctivitis

Vernal keratoconjunctivitis (VKC) is a severe, bilateral, recurrent, chronic inflammatory process of the upper tarsal conjunctival surface. It has a marked seasonal incidence, and its frequent onset in the spring has led to use of the term *vernal catarrh*. It occurs most frequently in children and young adults who have a history of seasonal allergy, asthma, and eczema. The age of onset for VKC is usually before puberty, with boys being affected twice as often as girls. After puberty it becomes equally distributed between the sexes and "burns out" by the third decade of life (about 4–10 years after onset). VKC may threaten sight if the cornea is involved and is more common in persons of Asian or African origin.

Symptoms of VKC include intense pruritus exacerbated by time and exposure to wind, dust, bright light, hot weather, or physical exertion associated with sweating. Associated symptoms involving the cornea include photophobia, foreign body sensation, and lacrimation. Signs include conjunctival hyperemia with papillary hypertrophy ("cobblestoning") reaching 7 to 8 mm in diameter in the upper tarsal plate; a thin, copious, milk-white fibrinous secretion composed of eosinophils, epithelial cells, and Charcot-Leyden granules; limbal or conjunctival "yellowish-white points" (Horner's points and Trantas' dots) lasting 2 to 7 days; an extra lower eyelid crease (Dennie's line); corneal ulcers infiltrated with Charcot-Leyden crystals; or pseudomembrane formation of the upper lid when everted and exposed to heat (Maxwell-Lyon's sign; Fig. 41.7). Although VKC is a bilateral disease, it may affect one eye more than the other.

VKC is characterized by conjunctival infiltration by eosinophils, degranulated mast cells, basophils, plasma cells, lymphocytes, and macrophages. Degranulated eosinophils and their toxic enzymes (e.g., major basic proteins) have been found in the conjunctiva and in the periphery of corneal ulcers, a fact that may suggest their etiopathogenic role in many of the problems associated with VKC.[19] MC$_T$ cells are increased in the conjunctiva of these patients. Tears from patients with VKC have been found to contain higher levels of leukotrienes and histamine (16 ng/mL) compared with controls (5 ng/mL).[20] Tears from patients with VKC also contain major basic protein, Charcot-Leyden crystals, basophils, IgE and IgG specific for aeroallergens (e.g., ragweed pollen), and eosinophils (in 90% of cases).[21] The tear-specific IgE does not correlate with the positive immediate skin tests that patients with VKC may have; thus, it represents more than a chronic allergic response as reflected in a study that suggested that exposure to house dust mite allergen aggravates VKC symptoms.[22]

Giant Papillary Conjunctivitis

Giant papillary conjunctivitis (GPC) is associated with the infiltration of basophils, eosinophils, plasma cells, and lymphocytes. GPC has been directly linked to the continued use of contact lenses with a seasonal increase of symptoms during the spring

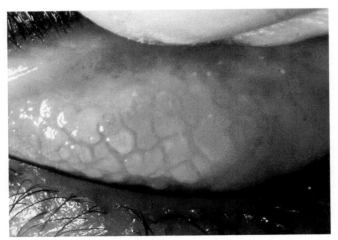

• **Fig. 41.7** Conjunctival hyperemia with papillary hypertrophy (cobblestoning) on the everted palpebral conjunctiva of the upper eyelid in a patient with vernal conjunctivitis.

pollen season, including itching. Signs include a white or clear exudate on awakening that chronically becomes thick and stringy. Patients may develop Trantas' dots, limbal infiltration, and bulbar conjunctival hyperemia and edema. Upper tarsal papillary hypertrophy ("cobblestoning") has been described in 5% to 10% of soft and 3% to 4% of hard contact lens wearers. The contact lens polymer, the preservative (thimerosal), and the proteinaceous deposits on the surface of the lens have been implicated in GPC, but this remains controversial. Analysis of disposable soft contact lenses has revealed that the higher the water content, the higher the protein integration (lysozyme, tear-specific prealbumin, and the heavy chain components of IgG) into the lens.[23,24]

Immunologic Disorders

Kawasaki's Disease

Kawasaki's disease (KD) (mucocutaneous lymph node syndrome) is the most common systemic vasculitis after Henoch-Schönlein purpura and the most common cause of acquired heart disease in the pediatric population. KD is an acute exanthematous illness that almost exclusively affects children: 50% of cases occur in males younger than 2 years of age, with an increased prevalence in individuals of Japanese ancestry. Five of the following six criteria must be present for diagnosis: (1) fever, (2) bilateral conjunctival injection, (3) changes in upper respiratory tract mucous membrane, (4) changes in skin and nails, (5) maculopapular cutaneous eruptions, and (6) cervical lymphadenopathy. The cutaneous eruption characteristically involves the extremities and desquamates in the later stages. The disease may occur in cyclic epidemics, supporting an infectious hypothesis, but an increased odds ratio has been reported with the number of concurrent allergic disorders including urticaria and atopic dermatitis.[25] It was originally associated with toxin-producing *Staphylococcus aureus*,[26a] but more recently *Rickettsia*-like organisms have been demonstrated by electron microscopy. A similar presentation has been reported in children with Coronavirus 2019 infection.[26b] KD is usually benign and self-limited, although 2% of Japanese KD cases (nearly all males) experience sudden cardiac death as a result of an acute thrombosis of aneurysmally dilated coronary arteries secondary to direct vasculitic involvement.[27]

The most typical ocular finding is bilateral nonexudative conjunctival vasodilation, typically involving the bulbar conjunctiva, with medium to large blood vessels being tortuous and engorged. No ocular discharge or pretragal lymph nodes are noted. However, there appears to be an increase in neutrophilic infiltration in conjunctival epithelial cells.[28] Anterior uveitis is seen in up to 80% of patients and is usually mild, bilateral, and symmetric without ciliary injection (most common in children older than 2 years of age); superficial punctate keratitis is seen in 12% of patients. Vitreous opacifications and papilledema have been reported. Choroiditis has been reported in a case of infantile periarteritis nodosa, which may be indistinguishable from KD.

Uveitis

Uveitis may be anatomically classified as anterior, intermediate, posterior, or diffuse. Patients typically complain of diminished or hazy vision accompanied by black floating spots. Severe pain, photophobia, and blurred vision occur in cases of acute iritis or iridocyclitis. The major signs of anterior uveitis are pupillary miosis and ciliary/perilimbal flush (a peculiar injection seen adjacent to the limbus) that can be easily confused with conjunctivitis. Vitreous cells and cellular aggregates are characteristic of intermediate uveitis and can be seen with the direct ophthalmoscope. Cells, flare, keratic precipitates on the corneal endothelium, and exudates with membranes covering the ciliary body can be visualized with the slit lamp and indirect ophthalmoscopy.

Anterior uveitis may be confused with conjunctivitis because its primary manifestations are a red eye and tearing; ocular pain and photophobia are also present. Anterior uveitis may be an isolated phenomenon that presents to an ophthalmologist or may be associated with a systemic autoimmune disorder that presents to a general practitioner. The inflammatory response in the anterior chamber of the eye results in an increased concentration of proteins (flare [i.e., Tyndall effect]), a constricted pupil (miosis) with afferent pupillary defect (a poor response to illumination), or cells in the aqueous humor. White cells can pool in the anterior chamber, forming a hypopyon, or stick to the endothelial surface of the cornea, forming keratic precipitates. The sequelae of anterior uveitis may be acute, resulting in synechia (adhesions of the posterior iris to the anterior capsule of the lens), angle-closure glaucoma (blockage of the drainage of the aqueous humor), and cataract formation.

Posterior uveitis commonly manifests with inflammatory cells in the vitreous, retinal vasculitis, and macular edema, which threatens vision. Posterior uveitis caused by toxoplasmosis occurs as a result of congenital transmission. Serologic assays for toxoplasmosis (enzyme-linked immunosorbent assay or immunofluorescent antibody) assist in the diagnosis.[29]

Panuveitis is the involvement of all three portions of the uveal tract, including the anterior, intermediate (pars plana), and posterior sections. In an Israeli study it was clearly linked (>95% of cases) to a systemic autoimmune disorder, such as Behçet's disease.[30] Although sarcoidosis is rare in children, 50% to 80% have ocular involvement associated with anterior, intermediate, posterior, or diffuse nongranulomatous uveitis with classic noncaseating granulomas appearing as "mutton fat precipitates" on the endothelial surface of the cornea, obstructive glaucoma, Koeppe's nodules at the pupillary margin, or sheathing of retinal blood vessels ("candle wax drippings").

Blepharitis

Inflammation of the eyelid margin, blepharitis, is a common cause of a pediatric red eye that may involve the anterior lash line or posterior, involving the meibomian glands; these conditions commonly occur together and are strongly associated with atopic dermatitis (76% of blepharitis cases) and rosacea (Table 41.4). Ulcerative blepharitis is almost exclusively associated with atopic dermatitis.

A specific form of anterior blepharitis involves colonization of the lid margin by *S. aureus,* although coagulase-negative staphylococci normally colonize the normal lid without causing blepharitis (6%–15% of normal eyelids). Staphylococci enterotoxin may directly cause a form of noninfectious conjunctivitis.[31]

Blepharitis is typically associated with persistent burning, itching, tearing, and a feeling of "dryness" being more severe in the morning. An exudative crust may be present, leading to a child's eye becoming "glued shut." Staphylococcal blepharitis is associated with conjunctival injection, dilated blood vessels, scales, collarettes of exudative material around the eyelash bases, crusting, foamy exudates, telangiectasias, chronic papillary formation, lid ulceration, and folliculitis, leading to the loss of eyelashes (madarosis). In addition, corneal immune deposits may cause severe photophobia. Treatment is directed toward eyelid hygiene with detergents (baby shampoo) and corticosteroid ointments.

Posterior blepharitis is primarily manifested by meibomian gland obstruction that may result in an acute infection (internal hordeolum or stye) or a localized painless granulomatous inflammation caused by an accumulation of lipids and waxes within the meibomian gland (chalazion).

Phthirus pubis, the pubic or crab louse, has a predilection for eyelash infestation and may also cause blepharitis, as can *Demodex* spp.[32,33] Often the lice may be visualized with direct inspection.

Ocular rosacea is a rare cause of blepharitis in children and is underdiagnosed because of its typically mild symptoms.[34–37] The majority of cases are unilateral and manifest with a chronic red eye or recurrent chalazia with a female-to-male ratio of 3:1. Conjunctival phlyctenules that appear as clear vesicles are pathognomonic because of inflammation directed against the bacterial flora of the eyelids. Treatment with lid hygiene, antibiotics, topical corticosteroids, and topical cyclosporine may prevent serious complications, including corneal involvement.

Episcleritis

Inflammation of the scleral surface, *episcleritis,* occurs mainly in adolescents and young adults, manifesting as a localized injection of the conjunctiva around the lateral rectus muscle insertion (Fig. 41.8). Typically, the inflammation is bilateral and accompanied by ocular pain. The presence of pain and absence of pruritus distinguishes episcleritis from allergic conjunctivitis. Episcleritis is self-limited and usually not associated with systemic disease.

Contact Dermatoconjunctivitis

The thin eyelid skin has an increased susceptibility to contact dermatitis with acute development of erythema and edema and thickening and crusting in cases of longer standing. In the pediatric population, ophthalmic medications or preservatives are the cause of contact dermatoconjunctivitis, rather than cosmetics as seen in adults. Ophthalmic lubricants such as thimerosal, which are found in contact lens cleaning solutions and other topical agents, have been shown by patch tests to be among the culprits. Because

TABLE 41.4	Blepharoconjunctivitis: Inflammation of the Eyelid Can Involve Different Portions of the Anterior and Posterior Eyelid (Either Alone or in Combination)			
	ANTERIOR		Posterior Meibomian Gland Dysfunction	Anterior and Posterior Blepharo-keratoconjunctivitis
	Staphylococcal	Seborrheic		
Lashes	Soft scales around roots	Soft greasy scales in between eyelashes	Unremarkable	Crusty
Lid margin	Ulceration Notching microabscesses	Shiny	Posterior oil capping with occlusion of meibomian glands	Chronic anterior and posterior involvement
Tear film	Dry	Dry	Dry and frothy	Dry
Conjunctiva	Papilla Phlyctenules	Unremarkable	Unremarkable	Follicular and papillary hypertrophy
Cornea	Punctate erosions Marginal infiltrates	Punctate erosions Peripheral infiltrates	Punctate erosions	Punctate erosion, vascularizations
Associated dermatitis	Atopic dermatitis	Seborrheic dermatitis	Acne rosacea	None
Cysts	Hordeolum		Meibomian	Styes (often multiple) and meibomian gland blockage

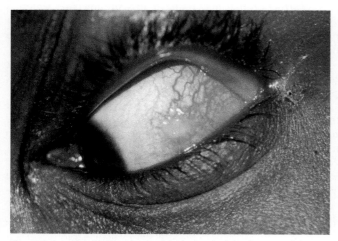

• **Fig. 41.8** Localized bulbar conjunctival vascular injection in a patient with nodular episcleritis.

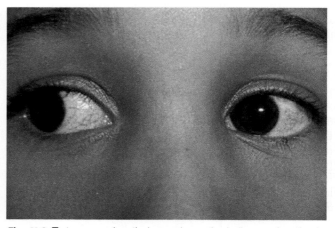

• **Fig. 41.9** Tortuous conjunctival vessels on the bulbar conjunctiva in a patient with ataxia-telangiectasia.

of the high incidence of irritant false-positive reactions, patch testing is generally used only as a confirmatory tool.

Angioedema

The periocular dermal tissue and the conjunctiva are one of the most commonly involved sites in angioedema from systemic hypersensitivity reactions because of the eyelid consisting of loose epidermal tissue providing an extensive reservoir for edema. Localized IgE-mast cell sensitization against papain enzyme in contact lens cleaning solution has been associated with chemosis and angioedema.[38]

Ataxia-Telangiectasia

Louis-Bar Syndrome

Ataxia-telangiectasia initially presents with large bulbar conjunctival tortuous vessels in the exposed canthal regions[34,35] (Fig. 41.9)

that typically become evident and progress between ages 1 and 6 years as they eventually develop ataxia, hypogammaglobulinemia (with absent or deficient IgA), and recurrent sinopulmonary infections. There are no other signs or symptoms of conjunctivitis.

Infections

Conjunctivitis

Contact lens use is associated with several forms of bacterial and parasitic conjunctivitis requiring vigilance with eyelid hygiene and contact lens procedures.

Cellulitis

Orbital cellulitis is an infectious process that manifests with "pain" and lid edema mimicking angioedema and when involving the extraocular muscles leads to proptosis and diplopia. A majority of cases are due to extension of sinusitis. Preseptal cellulitis may resemble orbital cellulitis with lid swelling, except that ocular movement is normal and there is no inflammation of the globe.

TABLE 41.5	Clinical Staging of Conjunctival Acute Graft-Versus-Host Disease
Stage 1	Hyperemia
Stage 2[a]	Hyperemia, chemosis, serosanguineous exudate
Stage 3	Pseudomembranous conjunctivitis
Stage 4	Pseudomembranous conjunctivitis with corneal epithelial sloughing

[a]Occurs in 12% of patients and is associated with increased mortality rate of approximately 90%.

However, delay in diagnosis may lead to extension of infection into the orbit. The orbital and septal infectious agents are commonly *Streptococcus pyogenes, S. aureus,* and *Haemophilus influenzae.* Necrotizing fasciitis of the eyelid, caused by β-hemolytic *S. pyogenes* Lancefield groups A, C, and G and *S. aureus,* is associated with septic thrombophlebitis that can lead to septicemia and is considered a medical emergency.

Transplantation

Corneal transplantation, one of the most frequently performed transplant procedures, does not require histocompatibility testing because the cornea is avascular. The primary indication for corneal allografts is maintaining optical integrity, as noted in patients with keratoconus, but they are also performed for other keratopathies (e.g., interstitial keratitis, corneal scars or ulcers, herpetic keratitis) and endothelial dystrophies.

Ocular complications involving the conjunctiva and the lacrimal system are noted in patients undergoing bone marrow versus heart/lung organ transplantation. In acute graft-versus-host disease (GVHD), conjunctival involvement progresses from erythema to chemosis, to serosanguineous exudate, and ultimately to the sloughing of the conjunctiva and potentially the cornea (pseudomembranous conjunctivitis) (Table 41.5).[39–41] In chronic forms of GVHD there is increased scarring of the conjunctiva and lacrimal inflammation, with over 50% of patients developing a Sjögren's-like dry eye syndrome.

Treatment

Once an allergic cause is identified, treatment is approached in a stepwise fashion. Treatment can be divided into primary, secondary, and tertiary interventions (Table 41.6) and acute (seasonal) versus chronic (persistent).

Current treatment of allergic inflammation of the anterior surface of the eye is primarily aimed at restoring the patient's quality of life and may require at least 2 weeks of therapy.[42–44]

Primary Intervention

Nonpharmacologic interventions are commonly the first line of treatment to be considered. Interventions include minimizing or avoiding contact with environmental allergens, application of cool compresses to the eye, lubrication and use of disposable contact lenses, and use of preservative-free lubricants.[45]

Environmental Control

Avoidance of allergens remains the first option in the management of any ocular disorder.

Cold Compresses

Cold compresses and refrigeration of ophthalmic medications provide considerable symptomatic relief, especially from ocular pruritus. In general, all ocular medications provide additional subjective relief when refrigerated and immediately applied in a cold state.

Lubrication

Many conditions require the use of lubricants that are based on various cellulose formulations that provide hydration for either temporary relief (e.g., seasonal ocular allergy, corneal abrasion) or for more long-term complications (e.g., keratoconjunctivitis sicca in patients undergoing bone marrow transplantation).[46] Tear substitutes consist of a viscosity agent in three formulations to increase the length of action while decreasing the length of time vision is blurred after instillation: aqueous (seconds), gel (a few minutes), and ointment (~30 minutes). Ointments are best tolerated overnight. Most are buffered to pH 7.7 to 7.8 and contain a preservative. Artificial tears can be applied topically 2 to 4 times daily as necessary. If drops are used more than four times a day, a preservative-free preparation should be considered. Lubrication primarily assists in the direct removal and dilution of allergens that may come in contact with the ocular surface. Ocular lubricants vary by class, osmolarity, and electrolyte composition; no product has yet emerged as a clear favorite. Parents should be given the name of one or two brands from each class of lubricant to try until a suitable product or combination of products is found. A tip for the application of eye drops in a recalcitrant child is to have the child tilt the head back (or supine) and close the eyes. The parent then places the drops in the inner canthi of both eyes; the child then opens the eyes, and the eye drops fall onto the ocular surface.

Contact Lenses

In general, patients with seasonal allergies should use daily disposable lenses because long-term lenses accumulate allergenic deposits as 67% of patients reported that the 1-day disposable lenses provided improved comfort compared to the lenses they wore before the study.[15,47]

Overall, the newer soft silicone lenses with increased gas permeability have had a higher comfort satisfaction rate (56%) than the rigid gas-permeable lens (14%); 63% of subjects without atopy and only 47% of those with atopy described their lenses as very comfortable to wear.[48,49]

Secondary Intervention: A Step Approach[50]

The development of therapeutic agents to specifically address the various signs and symptoms of allergic inflammation of the conjunctival surface is ongoing. In the search for more effective medications for ocular allergy, the conjunctival allergen challenge (CAC), also known as the conjunctival provocation test (CPT), has been critical as a standardized model for the assessment of efficacy and duration of effect that new agents have on the allergy signs and symptoms of erythema (redness), pruritus (itching), epiphora (tearing), lid swelling, and conjunctival swelling (chemosis). Many of the newer agents are also being evaluated for potential treatment of the more chronic ocular allergy-associated disorders, such as atopic keratoconjunctivitis, or the potential to treat both ocular and nasal symptoms as the medication drains down the nasolacrimal duct onto the nasal mucosa.

TABLE 41.6	Overview of the Treatment of Pediatric Ocular Allergic Disorders in a Stepwise Format			
Therapeutic Intervention	**Clinical Rationale**	**Pharmaceutical Agents**	**Comments**
Primary			
Avoidance	Effective, simple in theory, typically difficult in practice		>30% symptom improvement
Cold compresses	Decrease nerve C-fiber stimulation, reduce superficial vasodilation		Effective for mild to moderate symptoms
Preservative-free tears	Lavage, dilutional effect	Artificial tears	Extremely soothing, recommend refrigeration to improve symptomatic relief, inexpensive OTC, safe for all ages, comfortable, use as needed
Secondary			
Topical antihistamine and decongestants	Antihistamine relieves pruritus, vasoconstrictor relieves injection	Antazoline naphazoline, pheniramine naphazoline	No prescription required, quick onset, more effective than systemic antihistamines, limited duration of action, frequent dosing required
Topical antihistamine and mast cell stabilizer (plus other mechanisms)	Single agent with multiple actions, has immediate and prophylactic activity, eliminates need for two-drug therapy, comfort enhances patient compliance	Olopatadine (Patanol), ketotifen (Zaditor), azelastine (Optivar), bepotastine (Bepreve), cetirizine (Zerviate)	Twice-daily dosing, dual-acting agents, antihistamine, mast cell stabilizer, inhibitor of inflammatory mediators, more effective at relieving symptoms than other classes of agents, longer duration of action, safe and effective for 3 years and older
Topical mast cell stabilizers	Safe and effective for allergic diseases, especially those associated with corneal changes	Cromolyn (Crolom), lodoxamide (Alomide), nedocromil (Alocril), pemirolast (Alamast)	Cromolyn relieves mild to moderate symptoms of vernal keratoconjunctivitis, vernal conjunctivitis, vernal keratitis. Lodoxamide is highly potent
Topical antihistamines	Relieves signs and symptoms of pruritus and erythema	Levocabastine (Livostin), emedastine (Emadine)	Dosing 1–4 times daily, safe and effective for 3 years and older
Topical NSAIDs	Relieves pruritus	Ketorolac (Acular)	Stinging and/or burning on instillation experienced up to 40% of patients
Tertiary			
Topical corticosteroids	Relieves all facets of the inflammatory response, including erythema, edema, and pruritus	Loteprednol (Lotemax, Alrex), rimexolone (Vexol), fluorometholone (FML)	Appropriate for short-term use only, contraindicated in patients with viral infections
Immunotherapy SCIT SLIT	Identify and modulate allergen sensitivity		Adjunctive, although may be considered in secondary treatment in conjunction with allergic rhinitis
Ancillary			
Oral antihistamines	Mildly effective for pruritus	Loratadine, fexofenadine, cetirizine	May cause dry eyes, worsening allergy symptoms; may not effectively resolve the ocular signs and symptoms of allergy

NSAID, Nonsteroidal antiinflammatory drug; *OTC,* over the counter; *SCIT,* subcutaneous immunotherapy; *SLIT,* sublingual immunotherapy.

Decongestants

Topical decongestants act primarily as vasoconstrictors that are highly effective in reducing erythema and are widely used in combination with topical antihistamines. The decongestants are applied topically two to four times daily as necessary. They have no effect in diminishing the allergic inflammatory response. The primary contraindication is narrow-angle glaucoma. Excessive use of these agents has been associated with an increased conjunctival hyperemia known as the *rebound phenomenon* (a form of conjunctivitis medicamentosa) that is reportedly less when using brimonidine.[45,51,52]

Antihistamines

Initially, oral antihistamines were extensively employed to systemically control the symptoms of allergic rhinoconjunctivitis, although with an obvious delayed onset of action on the ocular domain compared with topical antihistamine agents. However, oral antihistamine appears to have a longer biologic half-life and can have a longer lasting effect. Information on oral antihistamine use in the treatment of allergic conjunctivitis is commonly buried within studies on allergic rhinitis instead of *rhinoconjunctivitis.* Oral antihistamines, especially the older generation (e.g., chlorpheniramine), appear to have an effect on excessive

TABLE 41.7 Topical Multiple Action Agents for Treatment of Ocular Allergy						
	Azelastine HCl 0.05% (Optivar)	Epinastine HCl 0.05% (Elestat)	Ketotifen Fumarate 0.25% (Zaditor)*	Olopatadine HCl 0.2% (Pataday)	Bepotastine Besilate 1.5% (Bepreve)	Alcaftadine 0.25% (Lastacaft)	Cetirizine 0.24% (Zerviate)
Indication	Relief of itching associated with allergic conjunctivitis	Relief of itching associated with allergic conjunctivitis	Temporary prevention of itching of the eye caused by allergies	Relief of itching associated with allergic conjunctivitis	Treatment of itching associated with allergic conjunctivitis	Prevention of itching associated with allergic conjunctivitis	Relief of itching associated with allergic conjunctivitis
Dosage	1 drop in each affected eye twice a day	1 drop in each affected eye twice a day (age 3 yr and older)	1 drop in each affected eye bid to tid	1 drop in each affected eye once a day	1 drop in each affected eye twice a day (age 2 yr and older)	1 drop in each eye daily (2 yr or older)	1 drop in each eye twice a day (2 yr or older)
Adverse event	Transient sting (≈30%) Headache (≈15%) Bitter taste (≈10%)	Cold symptoms (≈10%) Upper respiratory infection (≈10%)	Headache (≈10%–25%) Conjunctival injection (≈10%–25%) Rhinitis (≈10%–25%)	Cold syndrome (≈10%) Pharyngitis (≈10%)	Taste (≈25%)	Eye irritation, burning and/or stinging upon instillation (<4%)	Instillation site pain 3.6%

ªKetotifen (Zaditor) is now available over the counter in the United States.

tearing (lacrimation and epiphora) and may aggravate tear film disorders.[45,50,53–55] Oral antihistamines can offer relief from the symptoms of ocular allergy but have a delayed onset of action, but ophthalmic agents treat ocular allergic symptoms more effectively.

In general, the older topical antihistamines are known to be irritating to the eye, especially with prolonged use, and may be associated with ciliary muscle paralysis, mydriasis, angle-closure glaucoma, and photophobia, especially those that are nonselective and block muscarinic receptors. Interestingly, this effect is more pronounced in patients with lighter irides and has not been reported with the newer topical agents.

The newer topical antihistamines have also been found to have other potential antiinflammatory actions, such as mast cell stabilization, cytokine expression, or interleukin release.

Antihistamines With Multiple Antiinflammatory Activities (Table 41.7)

Olopatadine. Olopatadine 0.01% (Patanol, Pataday, Pazeo) possesses antihistaminic activity and mast cell stabilizing effects. Olopatadine was approximately 10 times more potent as an inhibitor of cytokine secretion. Olopatadine was originally approved for controlling the ocular itch and subsequently for relieving itching and redness for up to 8 hours. In a reformulated form it has been approved for once-daily treatment of ocular allergy (Pataday) and longer duration with the formulation with a cyclodextrin (Pazeo) for the control of ocular itching.[43,56–58]

Epinastine. Epinastine 0.05% (Elestat) is another topical antihistamine with other antiinflammatory properties that include histamine 2 (H2)-receptor antagonism, mast cell stabilization, and inhibition of cytokine production. Pretreatment by epinastine differentially reduced histamine, TNF-α, TNF-β, IL-5, IL-8, and IL-10. In vivo, epinastine and olopatadine pretreatment significantly reduced clinical scores and eosinophil numbers and epinastine also reduced neutrophils, reflecting that there are different patterns of inhibition of

inflammation.[59] In CAC placebo trials, multiple signs and symptoms (i.e., ocular itching, eyelid swelling, conjunctival and episcleral hyperemia, and chemosis) of allergic conjunctivitis were significantly reduced by instillation of epinastine compared with vehicle.[60]

Bepotastine. Bepotastine 1.5% (Bepreve) is ophthalmic antihistamines having multiple antiinflammatory properties that include H1-receptor antagonism, mast cell stabilization and inhibition of cytokine production, including IL-5.[61–63] Because bepotastine relieves antihistamine-resistant pruritus, it is possible that mechanisms of action other than H1-receptor antagonism are also responsible for the antipruritic effects of this agent. In CAC placebo trials, multiple signs and symptoms (ocular itching, eyelid swelling, tearing, total nonocular symptoms score, nasal congestion, and rhinorrhea) of allergic conjunctivitis were significantly reduced by instillation of bepotastine compared with vehicle.[64]

Ketotifen. Ketotifen 0.025% (Zaditor) is a benzocycloheptathiophene that has been shown to display several antimediator properties, including strong H1-receptor antagonism and inhibition of leukotriene formation.[65] Ketotifen has also been shown to have pronounced antihistaminic properties that result in moderate to marked symptom improvement in the majority of patients with allergic conjunctivitis. Ketotifen is distinguished from sodium cromolyn and nedocromil by a conjoint mast cell stabilizer with several antimediator effects, including strong H1-receptor antagonism and inhibition of leukotriene formation.[66,67] It is now available as an OTC therapy for ocular allergy.

Azelastine. Azelastine 0.05% (Optivar) is a second-generation H1-receptor antagonist. It was demonstrated in a pediatric SAC study that the response rate in the azelastine eye drops group (74%) was significantly higher than that in the placebo group (39%) and comparable with that in the levocabastine group[68]; it has been shown to down-regulate ICAM-1 expression during the early and late phase components of ocular allergic response, probably leading to a reduction of inflammatory cell adhesion to epithelial cells.[69] It is safe to use in children 3 years and older.

Alcaftadine. Alcaftadine 0.25% (Lastacaft) is an antihistamine with affinity to H1, H2, and less to H4 receptors that is superior to placebo and as effective as olopatadine 0.1% in preventing ocular itching and conjunctival redness at 15 minutes and 16 hours after administration.[70] Interestingly, in an animal model for allergic conjunctivitis, alcaftadine demonstrated a decrease of eosinophil infiltration compared with controls and olopatadine.[71] In one of the few head-to-head studies, alcaftadine was found not to be inferior to olopatadine.[72a] It is approved for children 2 years and older.

Cetirizine. Cetirizine 0.24% (Zerviate), is the first new prescription topical ophthalmic histamine H1 – receptor antagonist (an inverse agonist), that has been approved by the US Food and Drug Administration in the past 10 years (US NDA approved May 30, 2017) for the treatment of ocular itching associated with allergic conjunctivitis, in adults and children more than 2 years old. Cetirizine is the carboxylated piperazine major metabolite of hydroxyzine in humans, cetirizine has high affinity for peripheral H1-receptors. Overall, the analyses demonstrated that a significant reduction of ocular itch compared to vehicle, even in severe itch patients within 3 minutes of application. Of special interest was that there was a statistically significant effect seen with eyelid swelling, chemosis, rhinorrhea and nasal congestion. The most common treatment adverse events of ophthalmic cetirizine included ocular hyperemia (6.7% vs 6.7%), instillation site pain, (3.6% vs 0.9%) and reduced visual acuity (0.5% vs 2.1%) (cetirizine vs vehicle). Of 551 patients exposed to cetirizine, only one complained of dry eye. It is approved for children 2 years and older.[72b]

Mast Cell Stabilizers

Cromolyn. Cromolyn 4% (Crolom) is the prototypic mast cell stabilizer. The efficacy of this medication appears to depend on the concentration of the solution used (i.e., 1% = no effect, 2% = possible effect, and 4% solution = probable effect).[65,73] Sodium cromolyn was originally approved for more severe forms of conjunctivitis with corneal involvement (e.g., GPC, VKC), but many physicians have used it for the treatment of SAC and PAC. Cromolyn sodium 4% ophthalmic solution requires application four to six times daily for effectiveness. It is approved for children 3 years and older. The major adverse effect is burning and stinging, which has been reported in 13% to 77% of patients treated.

Lodoxamide. Lodoxamide 0.1% (Alomide) is a mast cell stabilizer that is approximately 2500 times more potent than cromolyn in the prevention of histamine release in several animal models. Lodoxamide is effective in reducing tryptase and histamine levels, the recruitment of inflammatory cells in the tear fluid after allergen challenge, and tear eosinophil cationic protein and leukotrienes (BLT and CysLT$_1$) compared with cromolyn.[74–76] In early clinical trials, lodoxamide (0.1%) was shown to deliver greater and earlier relief in patients with more chronic forms, such as VKC, including upper tarsal papillae, limbal signs (i.e., papillae, hyperemia, and Trantas dots), and conjunctival discharge and to improve epithelial defects seen in the chronic forms of conjunctivitis (VKC, GPC) than cromolyn.[19,53,74–77] In patients with allergic conjunctivitis, it is approved for the treatment of VKC at a concentration of 0.1% four times daily. Lodoxamide may be used continuously for 3 months in children older than 2 years of age.

Pemirolast. Pemirolast potassium 0.1% (Alamast) is a mast cell stabilizer for the prevention and relief of ocular manifestations of allergic conjunctivitis. It was originally marketed for the treatment of bronchial asthma and allergic rhinitis and then registered in Japan as an ophthalmic formulation for the treatment of allergic and vernal conjunctivitis.[78] It has been studied in children as young as 2 years of age, with no reports of serious adverse events. In various animal and in vitro studies it was found to be superior and, in others, equivalent to cromolyn.[79–81] The usual regimen is 1 to 2 drops four times daily for each eye.

Nedocromil. Nedocromil 2% (Alocril) is a pyranoquinoline derivative of cromolyn that inhibits various activities on multiple cells involved in allergic inflammation, including eosinophils, neutrophils, macrophages, mast cells, monocytes, and platelets. Nedocromil inhibits activation and release of inflammatory mediators (e.g., histamine, prostaglandin D$_2$, and leukotriene C4 from eosinophils) that may be partly the result of inhibition of neuropeptide release (substance P, neurokinin A, and calcitonin gene-related peptides). Nedocromil does not possess any antihistamine or corticosteroid activity.[82] Nedocromil has been shown to improve clinical symptoms in the control of ocular pruritus and irritation in the treatment of SAC.[83–87] Its safety profile is similar to that of sodium cromolyn, but it is more potent and can be given just twice daily.

Nonsteroidal Antiinflammatory Drugs

Topically applied inhibitors of the cyclooxygenase system (1% suprofen[88]) have been used in the treatment of VKC.[89] Ocufen (diclofenac) is one of three topical nonsteroidal antiinflammatory drugs (NSAIDs) approved for the treatment of intraocular inflammatory disorders.[90] Another topically applied NSAID (0.03% flurbiprofen) has been examined for the treatment of allergic conjunctivitis and was found to decrease conjunctival, ciliary, and episcleral hyperemia and ocular pruritus compared with the control (vehicle-treated eyes). Pruritus is associated with prostaglandin release. It has been shown that prostaglandins can lower the threshold of human skin to histamine-induced pruritus, which also may be the primary benefit of these medications in the eye.

Ketorolac Tromethamine. Ketorolac tromethamine (Acular, Allergan) was approved for the treatment of SAC with a primary mechanism of action on the inhibition of cyclooxygenase, thus blocking the production of prostaglandins but not the formation of leukotrienes. Clinical studies have shown that prostanoids are associated with ocular itching and conjunctival hyperemia, and thus inhibitors can interfere with ocular itch and hyperemia produced by antigen-induced and seasonal allergic conjunctivitis. NSAIDs (e.g., ketorolac) do not mask ocular infections, affect wound healing, increase IOP, or contribute to cataract formation, unlike topical corticosteroids. One study compared diclofenac sodium with ketorolac tromethamine, and the results for both agents were similar.[91] Treatment group differences were observed for the pain/soreness score, with an advantage observed for the diclofenac sodium group over the ketorolac tromethamine group. In another head-to-head study, ketorolac in combination with olopatadine was not as good as combining olopadatine with a corticosteroid for the control of mucus production and chemosis.[92]

Tertiary Intervention

Topical Corticosteroids

In the algorithm of treatment for ocular allergy, mild topical corticosteroids are considered for moderate to severe involvement of the ocular surface and are even required for control of some of the more severe variants of conjunctivitis, including VKC and GPC. Topical administration can be associated with increased IOP (e.g., in glaucoma), viral infections, and cataract formation. Topical agents that are absorbed or systemically administered corticosteroids will produce a transient rise in IOP in genetically susceptible individuals. Unlike efficacy, which varies among the corticosteroid esters, IOP effects are consistent among the different esters of the same corticosteroid base.

Loteprednol. Loteprednol 0.2% (Alrex) is a site-specific corticosteroid (i.e., the active drug resides at the target tissue long enough to render a therapeutic effect with limited secondary effects such as increased IOP and posterior subcapsular cataract) approved for the treatment of ocular allergy. The higher dose loteprednol (0.5%) formulation has demonstrated decreased signs and symptoms of GPC, acute anterior uveitis, and inflammation after cataract extraction with intraocular lens implantation and as prophylactic treatment for SAC when administered 6 weeks before the onset of individual seasonal allergic conjunctivitis.[54,93–97]

In patients with more chronic forms of allergic conjunctivitis the routine use of topical corticosteroids for more than 2 weeks should be done in consultation with an ophthalmologist to assess for cataract formation or increased IOP.

Immunotherapy

The efficacy of allergen immunotherapy is well established, with nasal symptom improvement greater than the ocular symptoms of allergic conjunctivitis, but has been reported to be underused.[50,98] Most of the studies on subcutaneous immunotherapy have demonstrated a clinical effect[99] as well as with conjunctival provocation testing,[100,101] and more recently sublingual immunotherapy has also demonstrated an effect.[102–104] In patients with allergic asthma who are allergic to cat dander (Fel d-I allergen), immunotherapy clearly improved the overall symptoms of rhinoconjunctivitis, decreased the use of allergy medications, and required a 10-fold increase in the dose of allergen to induce a positive ocular challenge test (OCT) reaction after 1 year of immunotherapy with the specific cat allergen.[105] Specific ragweed immunotherapy over a 2-year period generated improvement in nasal more than ocular symptoms.[99]

New Directions and Future Developments[45]

The immunophilins, a group of agents that includes cyclosporine, tacrolimus, and sirolimus, have been used for the more severe form of ocular surface disorders, including VKC and AKC.[106–111] Cyclosporine as a suspension has been approved for tear film dysfunction in patients under 16 years of age, and treatment of VKC has demonstrated marked and lasting improvement in symptoms with an ophthalmic solution or ointment, with results occurring in as little as 1 week.[19,107,112] These agents also have been used in the treatment of corneal graft rejection, keratitis, scleritis, and ocular pemphigoid.

Studies have demonstrated the potential of the positive impact of intranasal treatment (intranasal corticosteroids and possibly intranasal antihistamines) on allergic rhinitis and its associated ocular allergy symptoms.[113–115] It appears that this treatment would be best for mild to moderate cases, such as in seasonal allergic conjunctivitis (more than in perennial allergic conjunctivitis). Such patients would still benefit the most from topical allergy medications.

Although there is some evidence of the potential use of several herbal remedies (e.g., butterbur, *Urtica dioica,* citrus unshiu

powder), dietary products (e.g., *Spirulina,* cellulose powder), Indian Ayurvedic medicine, and traditional Chinese medicine allergic in treatment of rhinoconjunctivitis. Additional studies specifically addressing the pediatric population are required.[116,117]

Conclusions

Ocular disorders in children seen in the clinical subspecialty of allergy and immunology are increasing as our basic understanding of underlying mechanisms of the eye's immune response coupled with a stepwise diagnostic approach facilitates proper diagnosis and treatment, especially for allergic disorders (Boxes 41.1 and 41.2). As we develop a greater understanding of the biomolecular mechanisms of these disease states, treatment will continue to progress from symptomatic relief to more directed therapeutic interventions.

The reference list can be found on the companion Expert Consult website at http://www.expertconsult.inkling.com.

• BOX 41.1   Key Concepts Allergic Eye Disease

- Conjunctivitis caused by immunoglobulin E mast cell–mediated reactions is the most common hypersensitivity response of the eye.
- Seasonal allergic conjunctivitis is the most common allergic conjunctivitis, representing over half of all cases.
- Grass pollen, dust mites, animal dander, and feathers are the most common allergens.
- Most environmental allergens affect both eyes at once.
- The hallmark of allergic conjunctivitis is pruritus.
- A stringy or ropy discharge also may be characteristic of allergy.
- A detailed history is the cornerstone of proper diagnosis.
- Eye examination: Simple observation alone may be diagnostic.
- Ocular inflammation caused by systemic immunologic diseases is frequently observed in children.
- Immunologic disorders of the eye commonly affect the interior portion of the visual tract and are associated with visual disturbances.

• BOX 41.2   Therapeutic Principles of Allergic Eye Disease

- Approached in a stepwise fashion:
  - *Primary:* Avoidance, cold compresses, artificial tears
  - *Secondary:* Topical antihistamines, decongestants, mast cell stabilizers, nonsteroidal antiinflammatory drugs, multiple action agents
  - *Tertiary:* Topical corticosteroids, immunotherapy (immunotherapy may be considered in the secondary category for some cases)
- Novel approaches: Cyclosporine, tacrolimus, liposomal drug delivery systems, cytokine antagonists, anti–immunoglobulin E therapy, complementary and alternative medicine
- Ophthalmology consultation is merited for any persistent ocular complaint or if the use of strong topical corticosteroids or systemic corticosteroids is being considered

42

Drug Allergy

ANCA M. CHIRIAC, PASCAL DEMOLY

KEY POINTS

- True drug hypersensitivity is relatively uncommon; however, many children are labeled as being "allergic" to various medications, particularly antibiotics. They end up carrying this label into adulthood and are likely to be treated with alternative antibiotics that may be less effective, more toxic, and more expensive and lead to the development and spread of certain types of drug-resistant bacteria.
- In children, the drugs most frequently involved in suspected drug hypersensitivity reactions (DHRs) are similar to those in the adult population: antibiotics (especially β-lactams), nonsteroidal antiinflammatory drugs, acetaminophen/paracetamol, and others.

- The entire spectrum of DHRs can be seen in children, even the most severe cutaneous and organ-specific types.
- Most of the lessons learned from DHRs in adults can be and have been extrapolated and applied to the pediatric population. However, some peculiarities arise in children in terms of prevalence, involved classes, and practical aspects of the drug allergy workup.
- Certain approaches such as simplifying and reducing the protocol steps in highly selected pediatric populations seem increasingly attractive. It remains to be seen whether they will be accepted as a general rule in drug allergy workup in children.

Introduction

Drug hypersensitivity reactions (DHRs) are adverse effects of pharmaceutical formulations (including active drugs and excipients) that clinically resemble allergy.[1] Iatrogenic by nature, drug allergy goes against the ultimate purpose of prescribing a drug, which is to alleviate, and not to induce, a disease. DHRs represent a public health problem whose burden arises from the following:

- *Misdiagnosis:* Both underdiagnosis (as a result of underreporting[2,3]) and overdiagnosis (because of overuse of the term "allergy" [e.g., in the presence of symptoms from co-existing factors such as infections[2,4]]).
- *Prevalence:* Affecting more than 7% of the general population.[2]
- *Misbeliefs:* Not only is the suspicion of DHRs long-lasting, with patients carrying the "allergy" label into adulthood but also the field of DHRs must be one of the very few in medicine in which the suspicion of a condition may persist even after the diagnosis has been discarded with the best available means.[5,6]

The work of numerous groups dealing with DHR management has provided a growing body of evidence leading to guidelines and/or consensus documents to support medical decision making on several aspects of DHR. These documents vary in scope and methodology in that they (1) are national,[7,8] regional, or international[9–22]; (2) concern one specific drug class[8,14-16,18,20,21,23,24]; (3) focus

specifically on evaluation tools and management[9,11-13,17,19,24,25]; or (4) are more general.[7,10,23,26,27] Recently, the International Collaboration in Asthma, Allergy and Immunology (iCAALL) contributed to the issue of an International Consensus (ICON) on drug allergy,[28] a comprehensive reference aimed at highlighting the key messages that are common to the existing guidelines and critically reviewing and commenting on any differences. Unmet needs, research, and guideline update recommendations were generated.

Most of the lessons learned from DHR in adults have been extrapolated and applied to the pediatric population. However, some peculiarities arise in terms of prevalence, involved classes, and practical aspects of the drug allergy workup. A growing body of evidence allows us to propose shorter algorithms for drug allergy workup in some cases.

Clinicians and researchers working in the field of DHR are aware that there is a risk of iatrogenesis in individuals with histories that suggest, but do not always confirm, DHR. Proper identification of a DHR, and all the steps leading to it, upholds the principle of *"primum non nocere."*

Because of space limitation, the entire spectrum of DHRs cannot be addressed, and, for this, the reader is referred to the previously mentioned guidelines. This chapter will focus on the most clinically relevant reactions to antibiotics, aspirin (acetylsalicylic acid [ASA]), other nonsteroidal antiinflammatory drugs (NSAIDs), and vaccines. There is an emphasis on novel approaches in drug allergy workup in children.

TABLE 42.1	Classification of Drug Allergies			
Type	Type of Immune Response	Pathophysiology	Clinical Symptoms	Typical Chronology of the Reaction
1	IgE	Mast cell and basophil degranulation	Anaphylactic shock Angioedema Urticaria Bronchospasm	Within 1–6 h after the last intake of the drug
2	IgG and complement	IgG and complement-dependent cytotoxicity	Cytopenia	5–15 days after the start of the eliciting drug
3	IgM or IgG and complement or FcR	Deposition of immune complexes	Serum sickness Urticaria Vasculitis	7–8 days for serum sickness/urticaria 7–21 days after the start of the eliciting drug for vasculitis
4a	T_H1 (IFNγ)	Monocytic inflammation	Eczema	1–21 days after the start of the eliciting drug
4b	T_H2 (IL-4 and IL-5)	Eosinophilic inflammation	Maculopapular exanthem, DRESS	1 to several days after the start of the eliciting drug for MPE 2–6 weeks after the start of the eliciting drug for DRESS
4c	Cytotoxic T cells (perforin, granzyme B, FASL)	Keratinocyte death mediated by CD4 or CD8	Maculopapular exanthem, SJS/TEN, pustular exanthem	1–2 days after the start of the eliciting drug for fixed drug eruption 4–28 days after the start of the eliciting drug for SJS/TEN
4d	T cells (IL-8/CXCL8)	Neutrophilic inflammation	Acute generalized exanthematous pustulosis	Typically 1–2 days after the start of the eliciting drug (but could be longer)

CXCL8, C-X-C motif chemokine ligand 8; *DRESS*, drug reaction with eosinophilia and systemic symptoms; *FASL*, FAS ligand; *FcR*, Fc receptor; *IFN-γ*, interferon gamma; *IgE*, immunoglobulin E; *IL*, interleukin; *SJS*, Stevens-Johnson syndrome; *TEN*, toxic epidermal necrolysis; T_H1, T helper cell type 1.
With permission from Demoly P, Adkinson NF, Brockow K, et al. International Consensus on drug allergy. Allergy 2014;69(4):420–37.

Epidemiology: Prevalence, Manifestations, and Culprit Drugs

DHRs are classified artificially into two types, according to the delay in onset of the reaction after the last administration of the drug: (1) immediate reaction, occurring less than 1 hour after the last drug intake, and (2) nonimmediate reaction, with variable cutaneous symptoms occurring after more than 1 hour and up to several days after the last drug intake.

The entire spectrum of DHRs (Table 42.1) can be seen in children, even the most severe cutaneous and organ-specific types.[29,30]

Patients and physicians commonly refer to all adverse drug reactions (ADRs) as being "allergic." This causes confusion and misconception with regard to DHRs. Drugs can indeed induce several different types of immunologic reactions that, together with nonallergic DHRs, account for 15% of all ADRs.[28] Nonallergic DHRs resemble allergy but have no proven immunologic mechanism. It is assumed that in children most skin reactions are attributable to infectious diseases or interactions between drugs and infectious agents rather than to the drugs themselves.[31–33]

In a 2017 systematic review and meta-analysis of prevalence studies aiming to assess the frequency of self-reported drug allergy,[34] its frequency was lower in studies performed only in children (5.1%; range, 1%–10.2%) than in studies performed only in adults (10.0%; range, 1.5%–38.5%), and it varied according to the target pediatric population (4.8% in the general population versus 7.1% in inpatients and outpatients). Cutaneous manifestations were the most frequently reported (72%), as published elsewhere,[35] whereas anaphylaxis was less frequent in studies performed in children (7.6%; range, 2.1%–10.0%). In a subgroup of children who underwent a confirmatory allergy workup, the frequency of suspected (i.e., after drug allergy questionnaire, 169 patients) DHR was merely 17% (of the initially alleged self-reported DHR, 995 patients), and the confirmed prevalence was 7.7% (13 patients; i.e., 1.3% of the self-reported group). These numbers clearly show the danger of overdiagnosis by self-reporting and the importance of delabeling, as soon as possible. Not surprisingly, antibiotics (especially β-lactams) and NSAIDs are the drug classes for which participants more often reported allergies.

Lovegrove and colleagues[35] used nationally representative public health surveillance data (extracted from a sample of hospitals in the United States and its territories) to identify the antibiotics that result in the highest frequencies and rates of emergency department (ED) visits for ADR in the pediatric population (age up to 19 years). ED visits for antibiotic ADRs accounted for 46.2% of all ED visits for ADRs from a systemic medication. Most ADRs (86.1%) were deemed allergic, with mild allergic (cutaneous) reactions being the most common manifestation. Oral penicillins (55.7%), oral cephalosporins (11.9%), and sulfonamides (11.1%) were the most common culprits, but the number needed to harm (NNH) for ED visits that involved a presumed allergic reaction depended on the severity of the reaction and the type of drug; for a mild allergic reaction, it was lowest for the oral sulfonamides and clindamycin (1 in 688 and 1 in 856 dispensed prescriptions, respectively); for a moderate to severe allergic reaction, the NNH was lowest for quinolones (1 in 2525), followed by sulfonamides, clindamycin, and, only thereafter, penicillins (1 in 8658) and cephalosporins.

Natural History of Benign Maculopapular Exanthema in Children

Scarce data exist on whether children carry a drug hypersensitivity (DH) into adulthood. Several facts and reasonings have been acknowledged so far: (1) Proven DHR is less common in children than in adults; (2) the immunoglobulin E (IgE) response (to β-lactams) is known to decrease with time (in adults)[36]; and (3) T cell–mediated response is long lasting.[18,37] The validity of a negative drug allergy workup performed in adults who have had a reaction suggesting DH in childhood can be questioned because of the time that has elapsed since the occurrence of the reaction. In a study involving 3275 patients, Rubio and colleagues[38] reported that when the first reaction occurred during childhood, the prevalence rate of positive tests was similar whether the test was carried out during childhood (10.6%) or adulthood (10.6%). Therefore, it could be extrapolated that DH in childhood does not resolve with time, although prescription habits have dramatically changed over the last decades, with increasing use of antibiotics in particular. The most poignant recent data come from the group of Caubet and associates,[39] who performed a follow-up drug provocation test (DPT) after 3.5 years in 18 children with a positive DPT to a β-lactam for an initial clinical history of benign nonimmediate DHR to β-lactams (occurring in all but two cases at age younger than 10 years). Of 18 patients, 16 (89%) had a negative result for follow-up DPT, and, among these patients, 11 tolerated a subsequent treatment with the incriminated β-lactams. The underlying immunologic explanations for this are lacking. Although the generalizability and strength of the conclusions are hampered by the small sample size, these data support the fact that the majority of children with confirmed β-lactam allergy during childhood become tolerant after 3 years.

In children, the drugs most frequently involved in suspected DHRs are similar to those in the adult population: β-lactam antibiotics, NSAIDs, other antibiotics, acetaminophen/paracetamol, and local anesthetics.[38]

Particular Aspects of Drug Allergy Workup in Children

Evaluation of the Clinical History

The suspicion for DHR arises from several factors elicited from the clinical history. The following details should be addressed: (1) the timing of the reaction (with respect to drug administration), (2) the nature of the drugs involved, (3) the history of a previous exposure to the same drug or cross-reactive drugs, (4) the medical and genetic background, (5) the circumstances of the occurrence of the reaction, and (6) the differential diagnosis.[28] If possible, these details should be compiled in a standardized manner.[11] Documentation of the presence and severity of signs and symptoms (Table 42.2) is mandatory because they will tailor the drug allergy workup and establish contraindications to reexposure.

In adults the drug allergy workup may occur decades after the reaction,[40] and information on the initial alleged DHR is lacking in 30% of cases; however, in children the alleged DHR is often better characterized (although most of the time not severe),[41] and the culprit drug is typically known and can be specifically targeted during tests for a precise diagnosis.

Skin Tests

Benign Nonimmediate Reactions to β-Lactams. The pain of intradermal tests may limit their use in young children, and, in the absence of therapeutic necessity, a waiting approach could be adopted until the patient is older. On the other hand, viral infections are thought to be the most common cause of maculopapular or urticarial eruptions in children,[32] and this hypothesis is strongly favored after a negative drug allergy workup. With these two considerations in mind and a growing body of evidence showing suboptimal sensitivity of skin tests, a shorter algorithm of testing, that is, bypassing skin tests, in highly selected pediatric patients with a proven benign nonimmediate reaction after β-lactam treatment has been recommended by the pediatric task force of the EAACI Drug Allergy Interest Group[23]; the appropriateness of this recommendation has been since enhanced by further experience.[41–43]

Another approach could be reducing the number of skin tests. By testing the suspected drug before considering DPT, Diaferio and associates[44] avoided unnecessary DPT in 50% of children.

Immediate Reactions. The evidence to support DPT without skin testing in benign immediate reactions remains limited,

TABLE 42.2	Severity and Danger Signs and Symptoms in Drug Hypersensitivity Reactions	
	Visible Severity Signs and Symptoms	Invisible Severity Parameters
Immediate reactions	Sudden onset of multisystem symptoms (respiratory, skin, and mucosal)	High levels of serum tryptase[a]
	Reduced blood pressure	
	Dyspnea	
	Dysphonia	
	Sialorrhea	
Nonimmediate reactions	General	Changes in blood count[b]
	Lymphadenopathy	Cytopenia
	Fever >38.5°C	Eosinophilia
	Organ specific	Alteration of liver function tests[b]
	Painful skin	
	Skin extension >50%	Alteration of kidney function[b]
	Atypical target lesions	
	Erosions of mucosa	
	Skin blisters, bullae	
	Centrofacial edema	
	Purpuric infiltrated papules, cutaneous necrosis	

[a]No clinical utility in the acute setting.

[b]If a severe delayed drug hypersensitivity reaction is suspected, all patients should have complete blood count and liver and kidney function tests.

With permission from Chiriac AM, Demoly P. Drug allergy diagnosis. Immunol Allergy Clin North Am 2014;34:461–71.

and larger studies are still needed to confirm the safety of this approach. Mill and co-workers[45] performed graded DPTs to amoxicillin without skin tests in 818 children with a suspected amoxicillin allergy, of whom 100 had a history of mild immediate reactions. All the reactions elicited by the DPT in this specific subgroup were mild cutaneous eruptions.

Immediate reactions with danger signs are considered[7,28] clear indications of skin testing before considering DPT. Although not studied in a pediatric population, the positive predictive value of skin testing for β-lactam antibiotics is 100% in the case of a clinical history of anaphylaxis.[46]

Reagents. Classically, a certain number of reagents are considered essential for the diagnosis of β-lactam allergy in adults.[7,18] In children, however, if skin tests are appropriate, testing with the culprit drug may be sufficient as a first-step procedure.[44] In the case of a positive result, other reagents could be added to better characterize the profile (e.g., β-lactam ring, side chains) and find alternatives thereafter.

Of note, a few reports point out the role of selective clavulanic acid hypersensitivity in reactions attributed to the combination of amoxicillin and clavulanic acid. Some authors[47,48] performed skin tests with purified clavulanic acid alone (the drug is unstable in solution, requiring the use of excipients and limiting its availability) and obtained positive results at concentrations that proved negative in exposed controls. In the largest retrospective study to date on β-lactam allergy in children (1431 patients evaluated over a 20-year period), Ponvert and colleagues[49] observed that up to 37 of the 87 (42.5%) children diagnosed as hypersensitive (by positive DPT result) to combined amoxicillin–clavulanic acid were actually selective responders to the latter and tolerated amoxicillin. However, in another large pediatric European study, tackling immediate DHRs to penicillins and cephalosporins in 1170 children,[50] no such case was mentioned.

β-Lactam skin tests have been used for decades, and systemic reactions (ranging from generalized cutaneous reactions to anaphylactic shock, including a few cases of fatalities)[46] have been described, especially in relation to IgE-mediated allergy. The safety of skin tests to β-lactams in children appears to be better than in adults,[51,52] with an overall prevalence of reactions ranging between 0 and 1.2%[50,53] of the tested patients and 2.6% and 3.8% of the allergic children.[49,53]

Drug Provocation Tests

The DPT is performed at the end of a stepwise approach in the drug allergy workup. Most patients (or parents of children undergoing the procedure) accept DPT for diagnostic purposes, irrespective of the final test results, think that it is useful, and state that they would recommend it to others.[54]

General considerations in DPTs, with regard to indications, contraindications, methods, limitations, and interpretation, have been thoroughly addressed[13] and protocols published.[4,14,15,18,55] Nevertheless, the precise DPT procedure may vary considerably from one team to the next. Most protocols are based on empirical protocols. Data-driven protocols also have been published[56–58] for β-lactams and other drugs.

Methodology of DPTs

In a child with negative skin test results (where appropriate) and in the absence of contraindications, DHR should be ruled out or confirmed by administering an age- and weight-appropriate cumulative dose of the drug to which the patient initially reacted.

An observation period should then follow, before discharging the child, to ensure no life-threatening reaction occurs. Informed consent should be obtained (ideally from both parents).

A maximum single dose of the specific drug must be achieved, and the administration of the defined daily dose is desirable.

Duration of the DPT

Depending on the type of the drug, the severity of the DHR under investigation, and the expected time latency between application and reaction, the DPT may take hours, days, or, occasionally, weeks before it is complete.[13]

There is a controversy among different groups as to whether one full therapeutic dose (of the tested drug) is sufficient to elicit reactions in nonimmediate responders, particularly in children. Therefore, prolonged[32,49] courses have been suggested to increase the sensitivity of DPTs. Of note, most of the reactions reported by the patients were mild and nonimmediate. Considering that the NNH (i.e., number of patients who need to be exposed to a prolonged DPT to capture one nonimmediate nonsevere reaction) varies from 9 to 50,[59] the decision to perform a prolonged DPT should be carefully weighted according to a risk (i.e., cost and medical implications) to benefit (i.e., diagnostic improvement) balance. Moreover, a single head-to-head comparison[60] between 1-day and prolonged DPT (i.e., nonimmediate nonsevere reactions, the methodology obeyed a wash-out period after the 1-day DPT) in an adult cohort was published in 2016. The results do not prove the superiority of prolonged DPT over 1-day DPT in terms of sensitivity. Ratzon and colleagues[61] noticed a 100% rate of repeat administration of β-lactams with negative test results in prolonged DPT in a pediatric population versus 75% in 1-day DPT ($P = 0.02$). In this study, the calculated NNH was 9.

Another matter for discussion concerning nonimmediate reactions in children is the duration of the DPT and also, for some authors, the location. Theoretically, DPT should be performed in the hospital, under medical supervision, but in this specific subgroup of children DPT has been safely performed in ambulatory practice[41] and even at home.[49]

Step Dosing

There is substantial evidence that in children with benign nonimmediate cutaneous reactions to β-lactams,[32,41] performing a single-dose DPT can be considered safe. This procedure requires careful primary evaluation and should not be performed in patients suspected of having a more severe reaction. Such a level of certainty about the initial reaction history is possible only if the clinician has observed the reaction first hand or if there is clear documentation of the reaction in the medical record. Otherwise, in case of doubt, a complete drug allergy workup should be performed, including skin testing, before a more progressive DPT and under hospital surveillance.

DPT Contraindications

DPT should never be performed on patients who have experienced severe, life-threatening immunocytotoxic reactions, vasculitic syndromes, exfoliative dermatitis, erythema multiforme major/Stevens-Johnson syndrome, drug-induced hypersensitivity reactions (with eosinophilia)/drug-related eosinophilia with systemic symptoms (DRESS) syndrome, toxic epidermal necrolysis, or organ involvement. In a large retrospective study regarding β-lactam allergy in children, Ponvert and colleagues[49] suggested that serum sick–like reaction (SSLR), erythema multiforme, and Stevens-Johnson syndrome in children are mainly due to viral infections and that in such patients with a negative allergy workup based on late-reading intradermal and patch tests, DPT might be considered for essential (future necessity) β-lactams. However, this course of action must be regarded with the utmost caution, given that supporting evidence is lacking and because of the high risk of recurrence of such reactions.[62]

Follow-Up in Real-Life Settings

The negative predictive value (NPV) of DPTs is important for both the patient and the physician. One of the main limitations of DPT is that a negative test does not prove beyond any doubt tolerance for the drug in the future, but rather that there is no DHR at the time of the test. Studies regarding the NPV of DPTs are, however, encouraging and display virtually the same results in both adult and pediatric populations. Moreover, the NPV in prolonged DPTs is very similar to the one found in adult 1-day protocols (97% for Ponvert and colleagues,[5] 93.3% for Misirioglu and associates,[63] and 96.4% for Tonson La Tour and co-workers[39]). This information should reassure the patients and their doctors about prescription of drugs after negative DPT.

Desensitization

To confirm or rule out DHR, elective testing (i.e., performing a drug allergy workup in children labeled allergic to important drugs [β-lactams, NSAIDs, local anesthetics, antineoplastic drugs, and biologic agents]) is always preferred to testing during situations of acute need. However, in cases in which testing could not be performed before the situation that required therapeutic administration, and in the absence of contraindication, desensitization is an option. Referral to successfully applied existing protocols is recommended because there are no generally accepted protocols for drug desensitization in immediate DHRs.[19,28,64] For nonimmediate DHRs the literature is more controversial, and desensitization should be restricted to uncomplicated exanthems or fixed drug eruption because of the unpredictability and limited therapeutic options in severe DHRs.[25]

Non–β-Lactam Antibiotics

Children suspected of having DHRs for antibiotics other than β-lactams are not generally subjected to elective testing. The attitude most frequently adopted by physicians is definitive avoidance, mainly because these drugs are rarely used as a first-line treatment. Apart from β-lactams, the two antibiotic classes most commonly involved in pediatric DHRs are sulfonamides and macrolides.[33,65] Because they are not systematically studied, the bulk of the data derives from case reports, case series, or studies in specific populations (i.e., human immunodeficiency virus [HIV]-infected subjects for sulfonamides). Moreover, the true prevalence of DHRs to these antibiotics is difficult to determine because of the following issues interfering with the drug allergy workup:

1. The lack of standardized, nonirritating concentrations for skin tests, with most of the diagnosis relying therefore on DPTs.
2. The relative use of DPT as a diagnostic procedure, because of alternative approaches:
   - For macrolides, the use of an alternative drug, as a matter of principle in most cases, without prior confirmation of DHRs to the culprit macrolide
   - For sulfonamides, the use of desensitization for therapeutic purposes

Sulfonamides

Antibacterial sulfonamides (e.g., sulfamethoxazole, sulfadoxine, and sulfapyridine), which are derivates of sulfanilamides, are of allergenic importance. Patients with an allergy to a sulfanilamide might experience a cross-reaction with other sulfanilamides with a different side chain but not with sulfonamides in general.[66] Although they can induce a broad spectrum of DHRs (including type 1 and type 2 allergies, i.e., hemolytic anemia), they are known and feared elicitors of severe cutaneous adverse reactions (SCARs) such as DRESS, Stevens-Johnson syndrome, and toxic epidermal necrolysis. The drug allergy workup obeys the general rules but with the following peculiarities:

1. Positive skin tests have been described,[66] but their sensitivity is low and certain groups support the use of in vitro tests (the lymphocyte transformation test) to increase sensitivity (with the advantage of using compounds that are not available for in vivo testing).
2. In a clinical situation requiring treatment and in the absence of contraindications, desensitization has been an option for many years (it is extensively used in the HIV-infected population), and protocols have been published.[25,67]

Macrolides

Macrolide antibiotics are considered one of the safest antibiotic treatments available, with a DHR prevalence of 0.4% to 3% of all treatments.[55,68] The NNH for a mild reaction to macrolides was estimated at 3874 in an epidemiologic study in the United States.[35] Their chemical structure is characterized by a large lactone ring, which can vary from 12 to 16 atoms, with one or more sugar chains attached. Cross-reactivity among different macrolides has not been extensively studied, but when it was tested, a majority of patients with a demonstrated DHR to a certain macrolide could tolerate another macrolide with a different number of atoms in the lactone ring. Moreover, macrolide antibiotics are unlikely to cross-react with macrolide immunosuppressants such as 23-C tacrolimus and 29-C sirolimus. Published series reveal that, after performing DPT, DHRs to macrolides are confirmed in only 2.7% to 17% of cases.[55,68]

Nonsteroidal Antiinflammatory Drugs

Together with β-lactams, NSAIDs are the most common elicitors of DHRs in children and in adults. Some considerations are worth mentioning with regard to the pediatric population:

1. The infrequent use of acetylsalicylic acid (ASA) because of concerns about the exceptional Reye's syndrome in children.
2. The use of NSAIDs that are known to be generally well-tolerated alternatives in adults is regulated by prescription restrictions. Nimesulide was removed from the market in several countries because of concerns about hepatic ADRs, and oxicams and coxibs are approved only for children older than 15 years and adults, respectively.

Five major clinical entities are recognized in the new nomenclature proposed by the EAACI,[24,69] although overlaps may exist: (1) NSAID-exacerbated respiratory disease (NERD); (2) NSAID-exacerbated cutaneous disease (NECD), (3) NSAID-induced urticaria/angioedema (NIUA); (4) single NSAID–induced urticaria/angioedema or anaphylaxis (SNIUAA); and (5) NSAID-induced delayed hypersensitivity reactions (NIDHRs). These entities underpin two reactive patterns: the cross-reactive types (1, 2, and

3), or cross-intolerant, involving nonallergic mechanisms, and the single-drug–induced types (4 and 5), presumably allergic in nature, involving putative IgE and T cell–mediated mechanisms.

Several studies have confirmed that isolated angioedema is the most common manifestation of confirmed NSAID DHRs in children, with ibuprofen being the most frequently involved drug in the clinical history[24,70] and in proven NSAID DHRs.

As with adults, the diagnosis is mainly based on clinical history and DPT.[24,57,58] For nonallergic type 1 to 3 DHRs, neither skin nor laboratory tests are of value. However, for patients experiencing type 4 and 5 allergic reactions, skin tests and some in vitro tests can be of value, although with limitations.

Some authors perform ASA challenge to confirm or discard cross-reactive status in patients whose clinical history is not reliable, that is, patients who developed a reaction with one or two NSAIDs. However, when challenged with ASA, ibuprofen-sensitive children reacted faster, at a lower total cumulative dose, and occasionally with more severe reactions (including respiratory symptoms such as rhinoconjunctivitis and asthma) than their index reactions.[71]

Corzo and colleagues[72] studied paracetamol and etoricoxib tolerance in 41 children with DHR (proven by means of DPT) to ASA and ibuprofen and found that all of them tolerated these alternative drugs. All but two patients had clinical histories of NIUA (83.3% with angioedema). When challenged with meloxicam, only two patients (4.9%) reacted. The authors concluded that there was better tolerance to these drugs than in the adult NSAID hypersensitive population.[73] However, it cannot be ruled out that, in the natural evolution of NSAID DHR, reactions to these drugs may appear in initially tolerant children. Moreover, although their results indicate that paracetamol can be a safe alternative in these children, the authors underline that this needs to be verified by a DPT, because the estimated reaction to paracetamol varies in other studies and may be as high as 40%.[70,74,75] This high cross-reactive rate was found in a pediatric study (carrying the pitfall of a smaller sample size with only a few DPTs to find safe alternatives), in which the tolerability rate for nimesulide was 88.8%.[70]

The clinical phenotype of NERD is less common in children. Reactions to cyclooxygenase 1 (COX-1) inhibitors can be life threatening as well in children, and simple avoidance is often preferred, followed by a coxib DPT and NASID desensitization.[76]

Vaccines

Vaccines are complex preparations and hold a special place in preventive medicine by generating a protective immune response against various infectious diseases. Withholding vaccination from patients with histories of possible or even confirmed DHRs to any component of the culprit vaccine may result in significant individual and social consequences because of the need for vaccination coverage of the population. Generally, the risks of vaccination are outweighed by the risks of not vaccinating.[8,77] Given these considerations and the growing body of evidence about the rarity of true DHRs to vaccines, recommendations regarding the readministration of vaccines to a patient with a clinical history are somewhat different and more critical than in other areas of DHR, as underlined in the International Consensus on allergic reactions to vaccines.[17]

Allergic-like reactions elicited by vaccines can be attributed to the microbial components, the residual components of the culture medium or the preservatives, stabilizers, and adjuvants added to the vaccines.[77] Both food (e.g., gelatin, egg) and drug (i.e., neomycin,

gentamicin, polymyxin B, streptomycin) hypersensitivities must be considered when evaluating vaccine DHRs. Local reactions are by far the most frequent adverse event after immunization, whereas systemic reactions (either immediate or nonimmediate) occur with an estimated incidence ranging between 1 and 3 reactions per million vaccine doses. Systemic reactions carry the risk of life-threatening anaphylaxis if the patient is reexposed. Drug allergy workup is therefore mandatory before the patient is reexposed.

Vaccination is subject to immunization schedules but "catch-up" booster doses can be administered to children whose vaccination has been delayed because of a suspicion of DHR. If skin testing, especially intradermal testing, to the vaccine itself is unreliable (because it may cause false and clinically irrelevant positive reactions), measuring levels of IgG antibodies to the immunizing agents in a vaccine suspected of causing a serious DHR can be considered as a first step in the drug allergy workup in these patients.[8,77] Determining whether they are at protective levels can help determine whether subsequent doses of the vaccine are required. If patients reach the established level associated with protection from disease, consideration can be given to withholding additional doses, although the induced immunity might be lower than if all doses were injected. Follow-up of levels of protection is then recommended.

Diagnosis and Management of a Patient With a Clinical History of Local Reaction After Vaccine Administration

Patients developing local reactions after vaccine administration do not have a higher rate of systemic reactions on re-exposure, so tests are not needed except in patients with an extremely large local inflammatory reaction. If there is a suspicion of Arthus reaction, measurement of serum vaccine-specific antibodies (IgM/IgG) is indicated to detect a hyperimmunized status.

Patch tests can be useful in patients developing eczema or persistent nodules after vaccine administration. They can demonstrate a delayed DHR to preservatives or adjuvants and guide the physician to avoid vaccines and other products containing these incriminated components. However, a positive patch test is not accurate for the purpose of assessing a patient's ability to tolerate a vaccine and is not a contraindication to administering the vaccine after a risk-to-benefit analysis.[8] There are no contraindications for booster injections in patients who are seronegative for the relevant infectious agent, even if they are positive for aluminum or thimerosal patch test.[8,77]

General Management of Patients With a History of Systemic Reaction to Vaccines

In children with systemic reactions, skin testing (and/or specific IgE) to the vaccine itself but also to the potential single components that may have caused the reaction (when commercially available) is required. Although the sensitivity and specificity of skin tests with the vaccine itself have not been studied and false positive reactions occur, the result can guide the approach. Patients with negative skin test results can receive the full dose of vaccine, whereas in patients with positive skin test results to the vaccine itself (or with confirmed allergy to one of its components) the ratio between risk and therapeutic benefit should be assessed (including measurement of protective antibody levels) and the physician should determine whether subsequent doses of the suspected vaccine or other vaccines with similar components are required. If needed, the vaccine can still be administered after the protocol proposed by the American Academy of Pediatrics.[8]

Multiple Drug Hypersensitivity Syndrome

About one-third of the patients seen in a drug allergy consultation report multiple drug allergies.[50,78] True multidrug hypersensitivity (MDH) syndrome, as opposed to self-reported MDH, is rare and has been estimated in the range of 0.3% to 0.6% in large series of patients presenting with a suspicion of DHR.[79,80] However, its incidence is definitely higher in delayed-type reactions, including SCARs.[37] Interestingly, although the prevalence of proven DHR in children is lower than in adults, Atanaskovic-Markovich et al[50] reported MDH in 7 of 279 children (2.5%) evaluated for suspected DHR over a 5-year period. In this series, one patient had a history of SCAR, that is, Stevens-Johnson syndrome.

Economic Impact of Penicillin Allergy in Children and Antibiotic Stewardship

Although true DHR is relatively uncommon, many children are labeled as being "allergic" to various medications, particularly antibiotics such as penicillins (or more widely, β-lactams). They carry this label into adulthood. These patients are more likely to be treated with alternative antibiotics, which may be less effective, more toxic, more expensive, and lead to the development and spread of certain types of drug-resistant bacteria.

Although subject to limitations related to assigning of insufficient or incorrect ICD-9-CM codes; underreporting; overdiagnosis by lack of allergologic proof of the alleged DHR; and studies approaching DHR through large national or regional databases, in which individual chart review is time-consuming and therefore may not be performed, contribute to our understanding of DHR and its impact from a different angle.

As for adults, hospitalizations in children labeled as allergic to penicillin are associated with a significant increase in comorbidities, longer hospital stays, and a tendency toward higher hospitalization costs,[81] indicating a greater use of hospital resources in this group. To date, studies using allergy management as an antimicrobial stewardship tool have focused on adults.[82] Risk-stratification strategies are essential to encourage care providers other than allergists to endorse such programs. Delabeling children with suspicions of allergies to antibiotics should be encouraged all the more by the rarity of severe reactions (e.g., anaphylaxis[10]) in the pediatric population and therefore by a simpler risk stratification.

Conclusions

Drug allergy workup in children faces similar issues, challenges, and unmet needs as in adults. Just like bypassing skin testing or performing single-dose DPT, which have been accepted as standard practice in selected pediatric patients based on careful risk stratification, specific approaches (e.g., retesting after a few years) seem increasingly attractive to the groups working in pediatric settings. However, a growing body of evidence should be provided before its possible acceptance and adoption as a standard practice in the diagnosis of β-lactam allergy in children. The place of prolonged DPT is debatable.[83,84] Programs in which researchers prioritize pediatric populations in antibiotic stewardship programs are warranted.

The reference list can be found on the companion Expert Consult website at http://www.expertconsult.inkling.com.

43

Insect Sting Allergy

HANNEKE (JOANNE) N.G. OUDE ELBERINK,
LISA ARZT-GRADWOHL, GUNTER J. STURM

KEY POINTS

- The majority of insect sting reactions in children are mild and frequently only dermal (i.e., hives, angioedema).
- A clinically important number of children with moderate to severe sting reactions do not outgrow insect sting allergy.
- Venom immunotherapy (VIT) is highly effective and prevents future systemic sting reactions in 95% of patients.
- VIT is associated with an improvement in quality of life in contrast to use of an epinephrine auto-injector (EAI).

- For most individuals, 3 to 5 years of therapy appears adequate despite the persistence of specific immunoglobulin E.
- In children, the prescription of an EAI should carefully take into account the risks of the disease versus the risks of having an EAI (i.e., diminished quality of life) versus the benefits (i.e., preparedness for treating a potentially life-threatening event).

Introduction

Hymenoptera stings are the major cause of anaphylaxis in adults in Europe and North America[1–4] and the second leading cause of anaphylactic reactions in childhood after food allergy.[3] An allergic reaction can occur at any age, often after a number of uneventful stings. The rate of self-reported systemic sting reactions in epidemiologic studies is up to 3.4%,[5,6] and large local reactions occur in 0.9% to 20.5%[7,8] of children stung by a Hymenoptera spp. Children tend to suffer from less serious reactions, a large local reaction being the most common manifestation in this age group. Stinging insect allergy is responsible for considerable anxiety that is detrimental to lifestyle.

This chapter reviews the general concepts relating to insect sting allergy and, in particular, addresses those aspects that are more relevant to children

The Insects

Biting insects are different from stinging insects. The former primarily cause reactions because of the saliva they inject when feeding, whereas stinging insects inject venom with the stinging apparatus at the back of their abdomen. Salivary gland secretions have no relation to venom allergens. Whereas the venom of a sting typically causes an intense, burning pain, the saliva of a biting insect is a chemical cocktail of substances designed to make blood flow quickly and painlessly to avoid being squished. Unlike insect stings, insect bites rarely cause anaphylaxis.

Biting Insects

The most common biting insects are mosquitoes, flies, midges, gnats, fleas, ticks, and bedbugs.

Itching and a wheal may develop immediately and mostly disappear after about 2 hours, but they are often followed by a small itchy lump (papule) that develops up to 24 hours later and may last for several days before fading away. Large local reactions from mosquito bites are more common in young children.[9] Over time and with repeated exposure the reactions become less intense and are less frequent problems in adolescents and adults. Anaphylaxis has been described after the bites of mosquitoes,[10,11] horse flies,[12] bed bugs, and black flies.

Mosquito bites may be associated with immunoglobulin E (IgE) and perhaps IgG antibodies. Elevated titers correlate with the intensity of the local reactions and appear to be the immunologic mediators responsible for the reactions.[9]

Skeeter syndrome describes a localized (allergic) reaction to mosquito bites masquerading as cellulitis and accompanied by lethargy, fever, and general malaise.[9] Skeeter syndrome usually progresses over the course of hours, whereas cellulitis typically will evolve over the course of several days. Therefore, diagnosis can be made clinically by the course of the symptoms and can be confirmed by measuring IgE and IgG antibodies to mosquito saliva antigens.

A mild reaction to an insect bite will probably resolve itself within a day or two without any need for treatment. In some cases, the use of a topical corticosteroid may assist in reducing inflammation, and an antipruritic may relieve itchiness. There is a scarcity of quantitative scientific studies into the various treatments for insect bite reactions.

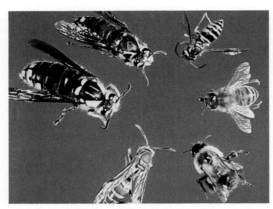

Stinging Insects

Insects that sting are members of the order Hymenoptera. The Hymenoptera represent an insect order comprising over 100,000 species worldwide. It is almost exclusively the social Aculeata of the families Apidae, Vespidae, and Formicidae that cause significant allergic reactions in human beings. The four major subfamilies are Vespinae, which include the yellow jacket, hornet, and wasp; Apinae, which include the honeybee and bumblebee; Myrmicinae, including fire ants; and the Myrmeciinae, including jack jumper ants (Fig. 43.1). An overview of the Hymenoptera is given in Fig. 43.2.

The Aculeata share in common a stinging apparatus that originates in the abdomen of the female insect and actually is a modified ovipositor; therefore, only female insects can sting. The sting consists of a sac containing venom attached to a barbed stinger. The honeybee's stinger has multiple barbs, which usually cause the stinging apparatus to detach from the insect, leading to its death. In contrast, the stingers of vespids have few and finer barbs than honeybees and usually do not autotomize, so vespids can inflict multiple stings (Fig. 43.3).

Vespidae

The Vespidae are divided into the subfamilies Vespinae (yellow jackets and hornets) and Polistinae (wasps). The Vespinae are split into three genera: *Vespula* (yellow jackets), *Dolichovespula,* and *Vespa* (hornets). The common names in general usage can be misleading: in Europe the term "wasps" refers generally to any of the social wasps rather than just to *Polistes* species (Table 43.1).

In most parts of the United States and Europe, yellow jackets are the principal cause of allergic reactions, whereas *Polistes* spp. are more commonly implicated in the Gulf Coast areas of the United States and along the Mediterranean coast of Europe.

Vespula spp. (yellow jackets) preferably build their nests underground, but also can be found under the roof and in window shutters. They live mostly in proximity to humans. Their nests are often encountered by children playing in the garden or are disturbed by lawn mowing, gardening, or other outdoor activities. Yellow jackets are scavengers and are often seen at outdoor events when food and drinks abound. Most stings occur in summer.[13,14]

Vespa spp. include the European hornet *(V. crabro),* which also exists in significant numbers in eastern North America, and the Asian hornet *(V. orientalis).* Hornets nest in shrubs, trees, and birds' nest-boxes. Near their nests, hornets are very aggressive. However, they are attracted much less to meat and sweet foodstuffs than *Vespula* spp. Therefore, hornet stings are rare.

The common paper wasps (*Polistes* spp.) build honeycomb nests in shrubs or under the eaves of houses. Their nests are generally limited to a single layer of open cells (or comb) with minimal outer covering. They are important predators, preying on agricultural and horticultural pests. Important *Polistes* spp. in Europe are *P. dominula* and *P. gallicus,* whereas in North America other species such as *P. annularis, P. apachus, P. exclamans, P. fuscatus,* and *P. metricus* are dominant. *P. dominula* has increasingly spread across the North American continent and central and northern parts of Europe. The coloring of wasps varies greatly: they can be brown, black, red, or striped. The European species, the Mediterranean wasp *(P. dominula),* is difficult to distinguish from a yellow jacket because it has the same bright yellow and black stripes. Outwardly, they are distinguishable by differences at the junction of thorax and abdomen: the waist becomes thicker more rapidly in the Vespinae compared with the Polistinae, and they have characteristic dangling legs when in flight (Fig. 43.4). *Polistes* are more prevalent early in the summer season. In some areas of the United States, such as Texas, they are the most frequent cause of sting reactions.

Apidae

The Apidae are divided into the genera *Apis* (honeybees) and *Bombus* (bumblebees). Honeybees and bumblebees are docile and sting only when provoked. The most significant species in causing allergic reactions is the domesticated *A. mellifera,* cultured all over the world for honey production and to pollinate fruit trees.

American "killer bees" (Africanized honey bees) are hybrid varieties of European and African subspecies showing much greater defensiveness, but their venom does not differ with regard to allergenicity and toxicity. They were introduced into Brazil from Africa in 1956 for the purpose of more productive pollination and have gradually spread north into the United States. The venom components of the Africanized honeybees and the domesticated European honeybees are similar. African honeybees are much more aggressive. Massive stinging incidents have occurred, leading to death from venom toxicity.

Members of the genus *Bombus,* the bumblebees, also live in colonies. The nests are usually in the earth. Most bumblebee species are bigger than honeybees, more heavily built, and more hairy. Bumblebees are not aggressive; children can incur stings when walking on grass. Systemic sting reactions occur in particular in workers of greenhouses where bumblebees are kept for pollination of plants.[15]

Formicids

One subfamily of the family Formicidae is Myrmicinae with the genus *Solenopsis* (imported fire ants). The main two members of the *Solenopsis* genus are the red fire ant *(S. invicta)* and the black fire ant *(S. richteri).* Fire ants build characteristic nests, which can grow to 40 cm in height, and often migrate in trails.

Red fire ants are found in the southeastern and south central United States, especially along the Gulf Coast. They have now spread to California. In Australia they are found only in the Brisbane region.

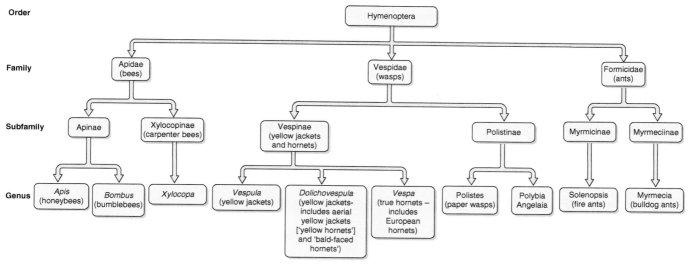

• **Fig. 43.2** Overview of taxonomy of common Hymenoptera (stinging insects).

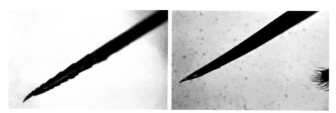

• **Fig. 43.3** The honeybee stinger on the left has multiple barbs. The yellow jacket stinger on the right is smooth.

TABLE 43.1   Popular Names for Vespids in Europe and the United States

Genus	Europe	United States
Vespula	Wasp	Yellow jacket
Dolichovespula	Wasp	Hornet, white-faced hornet, aerial yellow jacket
Vespa	Hornet	European hornet
Polistes	Paper wasp	Wasp

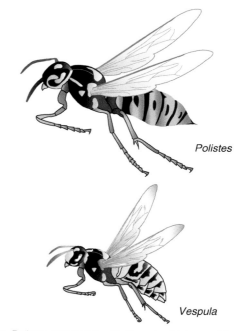

• **Fig. 43.4** *Polistes* compared with *Vespula*: thicker waist and dangling legs when in flight. (From http://crawford.tardigrade.net/bugs/Bugof-Month16.html.)

Stings occur most frequently in summer, most commonly in children, and typically on the lower extremities. The fire ant attaches itself to a person by biting with its powerful mandibles to hold onto the skin. It then pivots around its head and stings at multiple sites in a circular pattern with the stinger located at the tip of its abdomen. Within 24 hours a sterile pustule develops, which is diagnostic of the fire ant sting. Allergic reactions to fire ant stings are becoming increasingly common in the southern United States.[16,17]

Another subfamily is Myrmeciinae with the genus *Myrmecia* (jack jumper ants). Jack jumper ants are native to Australia. Workers and males are large and about the same size ranging between 12 to 14 mm. Furthermore, they are accomplished jumpers, with leaps ranging from 51 to 76 mm. They are known for their aggression toward humans, attraction to movement, and well-developed vision, being able to observe and follow intruders from 1 m away.

Insect Venoms. Venoms contain vasoactive amines (e.g., histamine, dopamine, norepinephrine), acetylcholine, and kinins, which account for the burning, pain, and itching normally experienced from a sting. They increase permeability, allowing the spread of the venom through the body of the victim. The different venom components known to date can be found in the Allergen Nomenclature database (http://www.allergen.org) and are listed in Table 43.2.[18]

The major allergenic components of Hymenoptera venoms are phospholipase A2 in honeybee venom and antigen 5 in vespids. The venom of fire ants differs markedly from the other venoms by consisting approximately of 95% water-insoluble alkaloids. The alkaloids produce a sterile pustule. The protein content is only 5%, with a higher content in summer.[19]

Commercial Hymenoptera venom products are available in many countries as lyophilized protein extracts of honeybee, yellow jacket, and *Polistes* wasp venoms.

Cross-Reactivity

A common problem of in vivo and in vitro diagnosis of insect venom allergy using venom extracts is that patients may have double positive test results for honeybee venom (HBV) and yellow jacket venom (YJV).[18] Three main reasons for double positivity are currently known: (1) true double sensitization to different bee and vespid venom allergens, (2) double positivity caused by cross-reactive specific IgE (sIgE) antibodies that recognize similar

TABLE 43.2 Overview of the Presently Known Hymenoptera Venom Allergens, Including the Percentage Dry Weight and Glycosylation Sites[18]

Allergen	Name/Function	MW (kD)	% DW	Potential N-Glycosylation	Eukaryotic Expression
Bees *(Apis mellifera, A. cerana, A. dorsata)*					
Api m 1, Api c 1, Api d 1	Phospholipase A2	17	12	1	+
Api m 2	Hyaluronidase	45	2	3	+
Api m 3	Acid phosphatase	49	1–2	2	+
Api m 4	Melittin	3	50	0	–
Api m 5	DPP IV	100	<1	6	+
Api m 6	Protease inhibitor	8	1–2	0	+
Api m 7	CUB serine protease	39	?	3	+
Api m 8	Carboxylesterase	70	?	4	+
Api m 9	Serine carboxypeptidase	60	?	4	+
Api m 10	Icarapin variant 2	55	<1	2	+
Api m 11.0101	Major royal jelly protein 8	65	?	6	+
Api m 11.0201	Major royal jelly protein 9	60	?	3	+
Api m 12	Vitellogenin	200	?	1	+
Bumblebee *(Bombus pensylvanicus, B. terrestris)*					
Bom p 1, Bom t 1	Phospholipase A2	16		1	–
Bom p 4, Bom t 4	Protease	27		0, 1	–
Yellow Jackets *(Vespula vulgaris, V. flavopilosa, V. germanica, V. maculifrons, V. pensylvanica, V. squamosa, V. vidua)*					
Ves v 1, Ves m 1, Ves s 1	Phospholipase A1	35	6–14	0, 0,2	+
Ves v 2.0101, Ves m 2	Hyaluronidase	45	1–3	4	+
Ves v 2.0201	Hyaluronidase[a]	45	?	2	+
Ves v 3	DPP IV	100	?	6	+
Ves v 5, Ves f 5, Ves g 5, Ves m 5, Ves p 5, Ves s 5, Ves vi 5	Antigen 5	25	5–10	0	+
Ves v 6	Vitellogenin	200	?	4	+
White-Faced Hornet, Yellow Hornet *(Dolichovespula maculata, D. arenaria)*					
Dol m 1	Phospholipase A1	34		2	–
Dol m 2	Hyaluronidase	42		2	–
Dol m 5, Dol a 5	Antigen 5	23		0	+

TABLE 43.2	Overview of the Presently Known Hymenoptera Venom Allergens, Including the Percentage Dry Weight and Glycosylation Sites[18]—cont'd				
Allergen	Name/Function	MW (kD)	% DW	Potential N-Glycosylation	Eukaryotic Expression
HORNETS (Vespa crabro, V. magnifica, V. mandarinia)					
Vesp c 1, Vesp m 1	Phospholipase A1	34		0	–
Vesp ma 2	Hyaluronidase	35		4	
Vesp c 5, Vesp ma 5, Vesp m 5	Antigen 5	23		0	–
European Paper Wasps (Polistes dominula, P. gallicus)					
Pol d 1, Pol g 1	Phospholipase A1	34		1	–
Pol d 2	Hyaluronidase	50			
Pol d 3	DPP IV	100			
Pol d 4	Protease	33		6	–
Pol d 5, Pol g 5	Antigen 5	23		0	–
American Paper Wasps (Polistes annularis, P. exclamans, P. fuscatus, P. metricus)					
Pol a 1, Pol e 1	Phospholipase A1	34		0	–
Pol a 2	Hyaluronidase	38		2	–
Pol e 4	Protease	?			
Pol a 5, Pol e 5, Pol f 5, Pol m 5	Antigen 5	23		0	+
Fire Ants (Solenopsis invicta, S. geminata, S. richteri, S. saevissima)					
Sol i 1	Phospholipase A1	35	<1	3	–
Sol i 2, Sol g 2, Sol r 2, Sol s 2		14		0	+
Sol i 3, Sol g 3, Sol r 3, Sol s 3	Antigen 5	26		2	+
Sol i v4, Sol g 4		12		0	–

CUB, Domain found in complement component C1r/C1s, Uegf, Bmp1; *CRR*, carbohydrate-rich protein; *DPP IV*, dipeptidyl peptidase IV; *DW*, dry weight; *MRJP*, major royal jelly protein.
[a]Inactive isoform.

protein epitopes of the hyaluronidase (Api m 2—Ves v 2), dipeptidyl peptidase (Api m 5—Ves v 3), or vitellogenin (Api m 12—Ves v 6) of both venoms[20]; (3) the presence of sIgE to cross-reactive carbohydrate determinants (CCDs) in bee and vespid venom allergens.[21]

Causative for the latter are IgE antibodies that are directed against an alpha 1,3-linked fucose residue of the *N*-glycan core established by insects and plants. Most HBV and YJV allergens are glycoproteins with one or more such carbohydrate structures (see Table 43.2). CCD sIgE antibodies have been reported to be responsible for more than 50% of double sensitizations to HBV and YJV.[22] The clinical relevance of CCD-reactive IgE antibodies in the case of insect venom allergy appears to be low or nonexistent.[18,23,24] *Polistes* spp. seem to lack the alpha 1,3-linked fucose residue that is responsible for IgE reactivity to CCDs.[25]

Recombinant allergens lack CCDs, allowing for a more precise distinction between true double sensitization and cross-reactivity

between different venoms.[26] By using CCD-free, correctly folded Ves v 2.0101 and Ves v 2.0201, it also could be demonstrated that hyaluronidases, contrary to previous assumptions, do not play a significant role as major allergens of YJV.[22]

Vespid venoms have been extensively analyzed. Venom allergens of diverse *Vespidae* spp. such as the white-faced hornet (*Dolichovespula maculata*) or the European hornet (*V. crabro*) are fairly similar to those of the yellow jacket,[27] allowing patients allergic to *V. crabro* to be treated with yellow jacket venom.[28]

The IgE cross-reactivity between European and American *Polistes* spp. is described as low because they belong to different subgenera. In contrast, cross-reactivity between Polistinae and Vespinae (*Vespula, Dolichovespula,* and *Vespa*) venoms and purified venom proteins[29] is frequently observed, especially for *Vespula* and both American and European *Polistes* venoms.[30] The converse is also true: half of the people who have had *Polistes* sting reactions have positive skin tests to yellow jacket or hornet venom and require treatment with *Polistes* venom only.

Within the *Apidae* there is cross-reactivity in that people initially sensitized to honeybee venom then react to bumblebee venom because of cross-reactive allergens. In this case, honeybee venom should be sufficient for immunotherapy. However, bumblebees have particular importance for pollination industry workers. Workers who were frequently stung by bumblebees and therefore primarily sensitized to bumblebee venom need to be treated with bumblebee venom.[15,31]

There is only limited cross-reactivity between the phospholipases of fire ant and vespid venom with no more than 40% sequence identity (http://www.allergome.org). Therefore, it is unlikely that this cross-reactivity is clinically relevant.

Epidemiology and Etiology

The rate of self-reported systemic sting reactions in epidemiologic studies is up to 3.4%.[5,6] The majority of reactions that do occur are in younger individuals, although the fatality rate is greater in adults.[15,17,32] Data on fatal reactions are scarce. It is estimated that 40 to 50 deaths per year occur in the United States and 16 to 38 in France as the result of insect sting anaphylaxis.[33,34] Most of these individuals have had no warning or indication of their allergies and had tolerated earlier stings with no difficulty. Fatal reactions can be associated with mastocytosis, particularly in adults.[35]

Development of Insect Sting Allergy

Studies indicate that 56.6% to 94.5% of the general population has been stung at least once in their lifetime by a Hymenoptera spp.[36] The younger the child, the more often they are re-stung; in contrast, prevalence of systemic reactions to field stings was significantly lower in preschool (3.4%) and school-age children (4.3%) compared with adolescents (15.6%).[26]

No immunologic criterion, such as skin test reactivity or titers of serum venom sIgE or sIgG, distinguishes or identifies sting reactors from nonreactors.[37]

The chance of developing insect sting allergy increases with sting frequency.[38] In general, no time relationship exists between the last uneventful sting and the subsequent sting that leads to an allergic reaction,[39] although multiple stings or repeated stings in close temporal proximity (within 2 months) have been associated with a greater risk of developing an allergic reaction.[40]

Classification of Reactions

Normal Reaction

The usual reaction to an insect sting consists of localized pain, slight swelling, and erythema at the site of the sting. This reaction usually subsides within several hours. Little treatment is needed other than analgesics and cold compresses.

Large Local Reactions

A large local reaction has been defined as a swelling exceeding a diameter of 10 cm that lasts for more than 24 hours,[41] and the prevalence ranges from 0.9% to 20.5% in children.[7,8] Swellings often peak at 24 to 48 hours and take 5 to 10 days to resolve. For example, the swelling from a sting on the finger may extend to the wrist or elbow. Fatigue and nausea may develop in addition. For a general clinician it might be difficult to distinguish large local reactions from cellulitis, resulting in misdiagnosis and unnecessary antibiotic treatment. The cause of these large local reactions has not been established, but it is thought to be an IgE-mediated late-phase reaction.[42]

Toxic Reactions

Large numbers of simultaneous stings (50–100) may result in a toxic reaction because of the vasoactive properties of the venom. Symptoms can have the same clinical characteristics as anaphylaxis, including nausea, vomiting, diarrhea, headache, vertigo, syncope, convulsions, and fever. Hemolysis, cardiac complications, renal failure, and rhabdomyolysis also have been described.[43]

Because insect venom is highly sensitizing, most patients will develop sIgE, making the differentiation from an allergic reaction difficult.

Unusual Reactions

There have been rare reports of acute encephalopathy, neurologic reactions, myasthenia gravis, peripheral neuritis, and Guillain-Barré syndrome related to insect stings. Rhabdomyolysis and prior reports of thrombocytopenic purpura and vasculitis, nephrosis, neuritis, encephalitis, and serum sickness occurred in a temporal relationship to insect stings as well.[44,45]

Some patients develop cold-induced urticaria days to weeks after Hymenoptera stings, not necessarily accompanied by an allergic reaction to the sting.[46]

Systemic Sting Reactions

A systemic sting reaction consists of signs and symptoms distant from the site of the sting and may range from mild to life threatening in one or more anatomic systems. Severe sting reactions usually have a rapid onset after the sting. A time interval of less than 5 minutes from sting to the reaction is a risk factor for severe symptoms.[47] Although the mean time span between the sting and the appearance of mild systemic reactions is 15 minutes, severe systemic reactions have occurred already after 6.5 minutes.[48]

The clinical features of systemic sting reactions are the same as those of anaphylaxis from any other cause. Diagnosis of the acute reaction can be quite difficult if hypotension or cardiac manifestations occur with no other signs or symptoms.

Studies from children with venom allergy usually report a milder clinical presentation (predominantly isolated cutaneous symptoms) than in adults.[49–51] In one study including more than 500 children, more than 60% suffered only from mild cutaneous reactions.[52] In a more recent study, however, half of the children suffered from respiratory or cardiovascular symptoms.[53]

Natural History

To assess appropriate intervention, it is necessary to understand the natural history of any disease process. This is particularly true of insect sting allergy. Observations of individuals who have been stung without suffering a reaction and reports from individuals who had allergic reactions from insect stings and who did not receive VIT have provided insight into the natural history of this allergy and suggest that insect sting allergy is a self-limiting process for many people, especially children.[52]

Immunoglobulin E Sensitization

Insect venom is a strong IgE inducer. In the general population, 27.1% to 40.7% have detectable sIgE to Hymenoptera venoms.[54,55] In 30% to 50% of these individuals these tests become negative after 2 to 5 years.[56] In a study of asymptomatically sensitized patients who were sting challenged, only 5% experienced a systemic reaction, whereas 44% had a large local reaction. The risk of systemic sting reaction was not increased compared with that of the general population, whereas there was a 10-fold higher risk for large local reactions.[37]

Taken together, sIgE for venom, either measured by skin test or serologically, without a history of an allergic reaction, does not indicate a risk of systemic sting reactions.

Natural History of Large Local Reactions

In the past, there was a common misconception that large local reactions after insect stings, particularly those that increased in size with each sting, might precede an anaphylactic reaction. Clinical observations in more recent years indicate that these large local reactions tend to be repetitive.[57]

In children with large local reactions, the risk of anaphylaxis is between 2% and 7%.[52,58]

People who have had large local reactions do not require venom skin tests and generally are not candidates for VIT, although VIT might be helpful in reducing size and duration of the large local reaction as demonstrated in a placebo-controlled study.[59]

Natural History of Insect Sting Allergy

A clinically important number of children do not outgrow allergic reactions to insect stings. Systemic sting reactions occurred less frequently in patients who had received venom immunotherapy (VIT) than in untreated patients.[52]

Two factors increase the risk for a repeated systemic sting reaction. The first is age, with the risk for recurrence higher in adults than in children.[51,52,60] In adults the risk varies between 23.5% and 73%.[39,61-65] The second is the culprit insect; those who are allergic to honeybee venom have a higher risk compared with those with a vespid allergy.[61,65] In a sting challenge study in which no reactions occurred at the first sting, a repeated sting caused a systemic reaction in 20% of the patients.[62] It is hypothesized that this variability may be due to variation of the allergen during the season,[19] variation in the insect species,[66] or variations in the patient's physiology or immune status.

The Severity of the Initial Sting Reaction Is of Particular Prognostic Value

Children who have dermal reactions (i.e., urticaria, angioedema) only, without other allergic symptoms, are a specific subgroup. These children have a particularly low reaction rate to re-stings, varying from 13%[52] to 18%,[51,60] and when a reaction occurs, it tends to be of similar intensity. In adults with dermal reactions not treated with VIT, the risk varies from 14% in patients who are allergic to wasp venom and up to 40% in patients with bee venom allergy.[65] In children with more severe reactions (moderate to severe), the risk is about 32%,[52] again with generally milder symptoms or symptoms that had occurred previously. Overall, these data suggest that children who only have dermal reactions have a very benign prognosis and generally do not retain their allergic sensitivity.

In contrast to winged Hymenoptera venom allergy, the natural history of imported fire ant venom allergy is not well known. The prevalence of allergic sensitization to imported fire ant has been studied in 183 children living in an area endemic for imported fire ants.[67] Serum fire ant sIgE was detected in 7.1% of children younger than 1 year, 57.1% of those aged 2 to 5 years, and 64.4% of those aged 6 to 10 years. Despite this high sensitization rate, the number of anaphylactic reactions to imported fire ant stings was low. These limited data suggest a benign prognosis for children who have had large local or generalized cutaneous reactions only from fire ant stings, analogous to experience with winged Hymenoptera.[68]

In an observational study[47] of 657 patients, of which 73% suffered from yellow jacket allergy, four significant indicators and risk factors were identified: elevation of basal serum tryptase (BST), absence of urticaria or angioedema during anaphylaxis, a time interval of less than 5 minutes from sting to onset of symptoms, and senior age. The absence of urticaria or angioedema was significantly related to BST elevation, suggestive for mastocytosis. In children with preexisting insect venom hypersensitivity, minor increases in BST levels (>5 μg/L) within the normal range are associated with a higher risk of severe systemic reactions.[53]

Diagnosis and Detection of Venom Specific Immunoglobulin E

The diagnosis of potential allergy to Hymenoptera venom requires both a history of a sting event that resulted in a systemic sting reaction and the presence of venom sIgE sensitization, assessed by skin testing or in vitro testing (e.g., IgE immunoassay). Both of these components are necessary to document the diagnosis of insect sting allergy and the possibility of administering VIT.

History

Insect stings always cause pain; therefore, the history in this regard seems reliable. A comprehensive history should review the patient's past stings and risk for future stings and determine whether the patient's reaction was local or systemic. Relevant questions are listed in Box 43.1.

Venom Skin Tests

For diagnostic and therapeutic purposes, generally venom preparations are used because whole body extracts contain little or no

---

• **BOX 43.1 Relevant Questions in Eliciting a History of Insect Venom Reactions**

- When did the sting event occur?
- How many stings occurred?
- Where was the patient when stung? (For example, on the terrace, in a wood, on vacation in the south, etc.)
- Could the patient identify the insect? (Notoriously unreliable part of the history.)
- Where on the body did the sting occur? (As an example, a sting on the face could cause extensive facial angioedema as part of a local reaction, but the same symptoms from a sting on the leg would indicate a systemic response.)
  - Did the stinger remain in the skin?
- Which symptoms occurred? (Ask about all symptoms, not only the major symptoms.)
- Was the patient taking any daily medication?
- Were there any previous or subsequent stings? If so, what symptoms developed?
- Is there regular exposure to Hymenoptera insects? (For example, beekeeper or occupational activities)

venom.[63,69] The exception is fire ant, for which skin tests with extracts prepared from whole bodies appear to be reliable.[17,26,32,34]

Skin tests can be performed either as prick or intradermal tests. Sensitivity of the skin prick test is comparable in vespid venom allergy[70] but may be lower in bee venom allergy.

Intradermal skin tests are performed starting with venom doses usually around 0.001 mcg/mL and testing up to a concentration of 1 mcg/mL.[71] Greater venom concentrations may cause irritant and local toxic reactions that are not immunologically specific. Simultaneous testing of all concentrations of two venoms (bee and wasp) is safe.[72,73] The skin test should be performed with a fixed amount of allergen (0.02 or 0.03 mL) and also include a negative diluent (human albumin-saline) control and a positive histamine control. Prick tests and intradermal tests are considered to be positive in the presence of a wheal 3 mm or greater and 5mm or greater in diameter with concomitant erythema, respectively.[70]

Skin tests are clearly positive in the majority of patients with a convincing history, but might be falsely negative if patients are tested too soon after a systemic reaction (attributable to a refractory period of "anergy"),[74] in patients with mastocytosis[75] or because of a lack of particular allergens that are lost or degraded during processing.[76] Generally, guidelines recommend sIgE determination and skin testing not earlier than 2 weeks after the sting because sIgE levels could be decreased or even undetectable.[77] However, there is only weak evidence in the literature for this recommendation. Considerations on IgE consumption rely on older studies showing that sIgE levels turned positive or increased markedly 4 weeks after the sting. Actually, it is not a matter of consumption that is only at decimal level but rather a booster effect caused by the sting.[37]

In Vitro Measurement of Venom Specific Immunoglobulin E

Venom sIgE can be measured in the serum by in vitro tests, performed by many commercial laboratories with variable assays and variable outcomes. Therefore, especially in the United States, skin tests remain the preferred test for the diagnosis of venom allergy and are considered to be more sensitive than the in vitro test.[50,78] ImmunoCAP (Thermo Fisher Scientific) is recognized as a reliable commercial assay and is used worldwide.

False negative results might be partly the result the same problems as in a skin test with loss or degradation of particular allergens during the processing.[76] Of patients with a well-documented history of yellow jacket sting anaphylaxis but negative IgE test results to YJV extract, 84% were subsequently diagnosed using recombinant Ves v 5 as allergen. This discrepancy could be resolved by spiking the diagnostic venom preparation with rVes v 5.[79]

Tryptase Diagnostic Test

Baseline serum tryptase should be measured to screen for an underlying mast cell disorder, particularly if urticaria or angioedema was absent.[75] Reports about the relevance of mast cell disorders in children allergic to insect venom are lacking. BST levels are found to be significantly higher in younger infants compared with older ones, with a gradual decrease to levels similar to those in adults.[80]

Tryptase also can be measured in connection with signs and symptoms of anaphylaxis: an increase from baseline serum tryptase is highly suggestive of IgE-mediated mast cell activation. Concentrations of serum tryptase peak at 60 to 90 minutes after anaphylaxis and decrease to baseline levels over subsequent hours. Total tryptase levels greater than 11.4 µg/L in serum are consistent with systemic anaphylaxis.[81] The tryptase measured immediately after the anaphylactic reaction preferably should be compared with a baseline tryptase sample collected several days after all signs and symptoms have been resolved. Other mast cell metabolites that can be used either to screen for mastocytosis or to determine anaphylaxis are urinary histamine metabolites.[82,83]

Sting Challenge Tests

A live sting challenge has been assumed to be the gold standard, especially to evaluate the efficacy of VIT. Live sting challenges are mainly performed in research settings. Routine use of a live sting challenge as a diagnostic procedure for selection of patients for immunotherapy has drawbacks, partly ethical[84] but also as a result of its limited significance because of the lack of reproducibility of one sting.[62,85]

Therapy

Large Local Reaction

The treatment of large local reactions is symptomatic. There are no studies comparing different treatments. Cold compresses can be used to soothe, antihistamines may reduce pruritus, oral corticosteroids can reduce swelling, and nonsteroidal antiinflammatory drugs can relieve pain and additional flulike symptoms of nausea and fever. A combination of oral antihistamines and corticosteroids is usually prescribed to prevent large local reactions in individuals with previous large local reactions.

Acute Systemic Sting Reaction

The medical treatment for acute systemic sting reactions is the same as that for anaphylaxis from any cause and is detailed in Chapter 44.

Because venom is injected very quickly after the sting, prompt removal of the stinger is not able to prevent an allergic reaction. It has been shown that the method of sting removal does not affect the quantity of venom received.[86] The sting continues to inject venom, but it is a valve system, not contraction or external compression of the venom sac that pumps the venom. Therefore, the method of removal is irrelevant, but even slight delays in removal caused by concerns about the correct procedure are likely to increase the dose of venom received, because 90% of the venom is injected in 20 seconds.[87]

Before discharge from the acute care setting, patients should receive a prescription for an epinephrine auto-injector (EAI), with instructions about how and when to use it and a referral to an allergist to determine whether the patient is really at risk and needs to carry an EAI and if the patient is a candidate for VIT.

Prevention of Acute Systemic Sting Reaction

The optimal approach in the prevention of any IgE-mediated disease is avoidance of the antigen. Although patients allergic to insect venom are able to reduce the frequency of their stings,[88–90] this is difficult in practice (e.g., yellow jackets live in close proximity to humans and have unpredictable and pugnacious behavior). Avoidance advice is not evidence based (Box 43.2).

- Wear slacks, long-sleeved shirts, and shoes when outside, especially when involved in activities that might increase insect exposure such as gardening.
- Cosmetics, perfumes, and hair sprays might attract insects.
- Light-colored clothing is less likely to attract insects.
- Take care outside around food and garbage, which especially attracts yellow jackets.

Epinephrine Auto-injector

Individuals at risk for systemic sting reactions are advised to carry epinephrine, available in preloaded syringes for self-administration.

Current practice regarding prescribing of EAIs varies widely before, during, and/or after stopping VIT,[77,91,92] with some practitioners prescribing them lifelong and also during and/or after stopping VIT. Findings from studies evaluating effects on quality of life suggest the adoption of a more selective approach to prescribing an EAI.

In a randomized study evaluating VIT versus EAI in adults, patients randomized to treatment solely carrying an EAI deteriorated in health-related quality of life (HRQL)[85] and carrying an EAI was associated with a significant burden.[93] After 1 year of carrying an EAI, almost 80% of the patients preferred to start VIT. The same results were found in dermal reactors,[94] a subgroup of patients who are often prescribed an EAI without being given the option of starting VIT.[77,91] It is not known if the reduced quality of life relates to the prescription of an EAI or actually having to carry one.

The effects of the different treatment options on HRQL have not been studied so far in children with an insect venom allergy. In children with a food allergy it has been shown that carrying an EAI can have a detrimental effect on quality of life, independent of other factors that can also affect quality of life such as whether they have previously experienced anaphylaxis.[95] These studies emphasize that physicians prescribing an EAI should carefully take into account the risks of the disease versus the risks of having an EAI (i.e., diminished quality of life) versus benefits (i.e., preparedness for treating a potentially life-threatening event).

Venom Immunotherapy

Therapy with venom is remarkably effective, preventing subsequent allergic reactions in the great majority of treated patients and, in many instances, providing a permanent "cure." Venom preparations should be used because whole body extracts contain little or no venom.[63,69] However, immunotherapy with whole body fire ant extract appears to be quite effective.[96–98] In jack jumper ant allergy, venom is used and is as effective as honeybee therapy.[99]

Major remaining issues relate to the refining of the selection process for people requiring VIT, choosing the right venom, and refining criteria for duration of treatment.

Indications

According to the guidelines on allergen immunotherapy of the European Academy of Allergy and Clinical Immunology (EAACI), VIT is indicated in children after a systemic allergic reaction exceeding generalized skin symptoms with a documented

sensitization to the venom of the culprit insect.[100] The risk of future systemic sting reactions and recommendations for treatment can be found in Table 43.3. As noted, studies of the natural history of insect sting allergy have shown that only approximately 60% or less of these individuals will have a subsequent reaction when re-stung[39,63]; in children the rate is even lower.

Children with only dermal (hives, angioedema) reactions have a very benign prognosis, and they do not necessarily require immunotherapy.[52,60] The risk to both adults and children, including very young children who have had severe allergic reactions is increased.

Anaphylactic reactions after insect stings can have a great impact on the quality of life in both adults and children allergic to insect sting.[90,101] HRQL is an important therapeutic target in the treatment of patients with allergy, because re-sting rates are generally low,[28,52] and mortality is surprisingly low, especially in children. In a 2012 review evaluating the cost-effectiveness of VIT, Hockenhull and colleagues[102] concluded that VIT is only cost-effective if it is able to improve HRQL or in the case of a high re-sting rate.

VIT has been shown to improve HRQL in contrast to EAI prescription only.[90] In a randomized study evaluating VIT versus EAI in adults, VIT—with information about the risks and benefits of the treatment—was preferred by most patients and shown to improve HRQL[93] in patients with moderate to severe reactions and those with only dermal reactions,[94] even if patients are not re-stung. The effect of VIT on HRQL has not been studied so far in children. It is not known what the burden of this treatment (e.g., receiving injections in addition to frequent visits to the doctor) will be for children.

Venom Selection

There is general agreement that a positive skin test cannot be used as the sole criterion to start VIT, because at least 25% of the population has sIgE to one or more venoms without a history of anaphylaxis.[77,91,92] Unnecessary use of additional venoms should be prevented. The administration of a single venom is much better tolerated than the administration of three or four venoms, especially in children, and VIT is a costly treatment.

Knowledge of cross-reactions is necessary to select the correct venom (see discussion of cross-reactivity).

Dosing Schedule

Treatment was usually initiated with very small doses such as 0.02 mcg. Recently it has been shown that initiating immunotherapy with 1 mcg is safe as well.[103,104] Incremental doses are given until the maintenance dose is reached, traditionally 100 mcg. In the United States mixed vespid venom preparations are available for therapy containing the two hornet venoms and yellow jacket venom, with a top dose of 300 mcg.

There is agreement about the efficacy of 100 mcg, originally selected based on the estimated venom protein content of two to four stings. However, the amount of venom of the different species is different. The amount of honeybee venom is in the range of 50 mcg; the amount of vespids is less consistent, ranging from 2 to 20 mcg.[105] Patients who are not adequately protected might be protected with higher doses.[106]

VIT consists of an up-dosing phase and a maintenance phase, which is necessary to ensure a persistent effect of VIT. Several up-dosing protocols are available: the conventional protocol, in which venom preparations are administered weekly, with increasing venom doses until the maintenance dose of 100 mcg is

TABLE 43.3	Indications for Venom Immunotherapy in Patients With Positive Venom Skin Tests or Serologically Positive Specific Immunoglobulin E			
Previous Reaction		**Skin Test or Serum sIgE**	**Risk of a Systemic Reaction**	**Advice**
No reaction	Children and adults	Unknown	1%–3%[38]	None
		Positive	5%[37]	None
Large local	Children	Not relevant (negative or positive)	2%–7%[52,58]	None
	Adults	Not relevant (negative or positive)	4%[42,57]	None
Systemic reaction—dermal	Children	Positive	13%[52]	No VIT, no EAI[a]
	Adults	Positive	14% (YJ)[65] 40% (bee)[65]	EAI[a] and VIT[b,94]
Systemic reaction—grade 2–4	Children <5 yr	Positive	?	EAI[a] and VIT—decisions should be made on an individual basis
	Children >5 yr	Positive	32%[52]	EAI[a] and VIT
	Adults (>15 yr)	Positive	34%–81%[39,61,65]	EAI[a] and VIT
		Negative	?	Further considerations: • Check values 0.1–0.35 kU/L if tIgE is low • Combine tests • Consider basophil activation test • If all tests are negative: consider nonallergic reaction (e.g., panic reaction)

[a]The decision to provide an EAI will depend on the practice patterns in each country.

[b]Quality of life is an important target.

EAI, Epinephrine auto-injector; *sIgE*, specific immunoglobulin E; *tIgE*, total IgE; *YJ*, yellow jacket.

usually reached in 11 to 15 weeks, can be administered in outpatient clinics.[107] With rush[107–111] and ultrarush[112–115] protocols, maintenance dose is reached much faster. Using rush protocols, patients receive several injections with increasing venom doses on consecutive days until the maintenance dose is reached after 5 days. With the ultrarush protocol, patients reach the maintenance dose within a few hours, after receiving several injections. Both rush and ultrarush protocols are performed only in hospitals during an inpatient stay. That these protocols are also safe for children has been demonstrated in several studies.[116–120] Cluster protocols (several injections per day, usually 1–2 weeks apart) are another alternative to conventional protocols.[121,122] In general, conventional protocols appear to be best tolerated, whereas rush and ultrarush protocols are more frequently associated with side effects.[123]

The recommended starting dose for up-dosing protocols ranges from 0.001 to 0.1 mcg. However, it has been shown that a starting dose of 1 mcg is safe in adults and children.[103] The recommended interval for the maintenance dose is 4 to 6 weeks for aqueous preparations and 6 to 8 weeks for depot preparations.[124] Two studies demonstrated an efficacy of 50-mcg maintenance doses in children and therefore favor the use of reduced doses to improve safety and decrease treatment costs.[125,126] However, given the clear dose-dependency of VIT[106] and the fact that children tolerate 100-mcg

doses well lead to the recommendation to use a maintenance dose of 100 mcg in pediatric patients as well.[117–119,127] Table 43.4 presents examples of schedules.

It has been shown that pretreatment with histamine 1 antihistamines improves the tolerability of VIT.[128–131] In detail, it was reported that levocetirizine decreased the rate of systemic sting reactions[131] and fexofenadine decreased the rate of large local and cutaneous systemic sting reaction.[130]

Side Effects

Local swelling may occur, as may generalized fatigue. Systemic side effects are usually mild and respond well to antiallergic treatment.[132,133] VIT-related side effects in children are similar to those in adults.[117] The most important risk factor is treatment with honeybee venom: it has been reported that there is a 3.1- to 6-fold higher risk for systemic side effects as a result of treatment with honeybee venom compared with vespid venom.[103,111,123] Rapid dose increase during the up-dosing phase is an established risk factor as well.[123,134] Whether mastocytosis and/or elevated tryptase levels is a risk factor is still a debated issue.[123,135–137] Several approaches are available to minimize these reactions (Box 43.3).

Effectiveness. VIT induced long-term protection in most children: 84.4% of patients treated with honeybee venom and 94.1% of patients treated with vespid venom were fully protected

TABLE 43.4   Representative Examples of Venom Immunotherapy Dosing Schedules[a]

	Conventional	Cluster	Modified Rush	Rush	Modified Conventional[104]
Day					
1	0.1	0.01	0.1	0.1[b]	1.0
		0.1	0.3	0.3	
		1	0.6	0.6	
				1.0	
				3.0	
				6.0	
				15.0	
2				30.0	
				50.0[c]	
				75.0	
3				100.0	
Week					
1	0.3		1.0		5
			3.0		
			6.0		
2	0.6	2.0	10.0	100	10
		4.0			
			15.0	Repeat every 4 wk	
3	1.0	6.0	30.0		20
		10.0			
4	3.0	10.0	40.0		40
		20.0			
5	6.0	30.0	50.0[‡]		60
		30.0			
6	15.0	50.0	65.0		80
		50.0			
7	30.0	100.0	80.0		100
8	50.0[c]		100.0		
9	65.0				
10	80.0		100.0		
11	100.0	Repeat every 4–6 wk	Repeat every 4 wk		
12					
13	100.0				
	Repeat every 4 wk				

[a]Doses expressed in micrograms.
[b]Sequential venom doses administered on the same day at 20- to 30-minute intervals.
[c]50 mcg may be used as the top dose.

• BOX 43.3 Approaches in the Case of Side Effects

Large Local Reaction

- The venom dose can be split into two injections, limiting the amount delivered at one site.
- Administration of an antihistamine is given 30 to 60 minutes before the venom injection.
- In the case of extensive delayed-onset swelling, topical corticosteroids can be used.

Systemic Reaction

- A temporary reduction of the venom dose (e.g., going one to two steps back in the protocol) may be recommended to avoid further adverse events.
- Pretreatment with antihistamine is provided 30 to 60 minutes before the venom injection.
- If individuals are receiving multiple venoms, it might be advisable to administer single venoms on separate days.
- Check (again) for mastocytosis.

at accidental re-stings: 32 of 54 of patients treated with bee venom and 17 of 34 patients treated with vespid venom were re-stung by the respective venom.[88] VIT is highly effective in preventing subsequent anaphylaxis in children at risk, with efficacy comparable to that in adults. In a study by Golden and associates[52] in 512 patients the efficacy was 95% in patients with moderate to severe symptoms, and 100% in dermal reactors; the culprit insects were not mentioned.

Graft and colleagues[138] reported that during a 3- to 6-year period, 200 re-stings in 49 children treated with VIT resulted in only four mild systemic reactions (98% efficacy).

A study by Rüeff and co-workers included more than 1500 adults receiving a sting challenge 1 year after start of VIT, with a protection rate of 84% for bee VIT and 96% for yellow jacket VIT.[139] These findings confirm previous studies that patients treated with honeybee venom are at higher risk for treatment failure and relapse compared with those who were treated with vespid venom.[140–142] Recent studies demonstrated that more than 50% of patients with allergy to HBV display IgE reactivity to low-abundance proteins such as Api m 3, Api m 5, and Api m 10.[18,20] Two of these allergens, Api m 3 and Api m 10, are present in the crude venom abstract but absent or underrepresented in therapeutic venom preparations.[76] Based on these findings, it is tempting to speculate that the relative lack of these two allergens in therapeutic venom preparations may account for the reduced efficacy of VIT in patients allergic to bee venom, a hypothesis that is currently under investigation.

Treatment Duration

Termination after about 1 or 2 years leads to a relapse in 22% to 27% of cases in both adults and children,[143,144] and several studies conclude that a minimum of a 5-year treatment is superior for long-term effectiveness.[34,141,145,146] Fiedler and associates[147] reported that among 40 children treated with mean 3-year VIT, 50% developed another systemic sting reaction at a median follow-up of 13 years.[147] Therefore, it is suggested that even in pediatric patients, VIT duration should be at least 5 years.[148]

The reference list can be found on the companion Expert Consult website at http://www.expertconsult.inkling.com.

44

Anaphylaxis: Assessment and Management

JULIE WANG

KEY POINTS

- Most episodes of anaphylaxis occur in the community, not in healthcare settings. Food is by far the most common trigger. Concomitant asthma increases the risk of severe or fatal anaphylaxis.
- Diagnosis of anaphylaxis is based on recognition of symptoms and signs that occur suddenly (minutes to a few hours) after exposure to a known or likely trigger.
- Prompt treatment of anaphylaxis is essential. Inject epinephrine intramuscularly in the mid-outer thigh, call for assistance, and place the patient supine or in a position of comfort. Provide

oxygen, intravenous fluids, and other interventions as needed.
- Patients at risk of anaphylaxis should carry one or more epinephrine auto-injectors and a written, personalized anaphylaxis emergency action plan and have medical identification.
- Anaphylaxis triggers should be confirmed and vigilantly avoided. Immunotherapy effectively prevents venom anaphylaxis. Regular follow-up and anaphylaxis education are important aspects of long-term management.

Introduction

Anaphylaxis is defined as a serious generalized allergic or hypersensitivity reaction that is rapid in onset and might cause death.[1] It typically occurs within minutes to a few hours after exposure to the trigger (Box 44.1). The presence of hypotension or shock is not required to make the diagnosis.

The areas covered in this chapter on anaphylaxis in infants, children, and teenagers include epidemiology, risk factors, mechanisms, triggers, diagnosis, treatment of the acute anaphylactic episode, and long-term management.

Epidemiology

Based on a systematic review, prevalence of anaphylaxis in children varies widely worldwide, ranging from 1 to 761 per 100,000 person years.[2] In the general population the incidence of anaphylaxis significantly increased between 2001 and 2010, with an average increase of 4.3% per year (P <.001).[3] Among children, significantly more boys than girls are affected.[3] Rates of emergency department (ED) visits for anaphylaxis increased from 2005 to 2014, with a higher increase for those 5 to 17 years (196% increase, P <.001).[4] Similarly, increases in hospitalization rates for anaphylaxis also have been observed, with the most prominent increases in children 14 years and under, which has been primarily driven by food allergen triggers.[5–8] Despite these increases, the fatality rate remains low.[5,9]

Patients at Increased Risk of Severe Anaphylaxis

Presence of concomitant atopic diseases is a predictor of life-threatening anaphylactic episodes. Persistent asthma, especially if not optimally controlled, is an important risk factor for fatal anaphylaxis. Urticaria pigmentosa with extensive (>90%) involvement of the skin increases the risk of anaphylaxis in infants and children. Studies report that concurrent use of antihypertensive medications such as β-adrenergic blockers and angiotensin-converting enzyme inhibitors is associated with increased risk and severity of anaphylaxis; this may be confounded by underlying cardiovascular disease or other factors such as older age, which would lead to patients requiring such treatment.[10,11] Additionally, infants, teenagers, and pregnant teens can be uniquely vulnerable in anaphylactic episodes because of issues with underrecognition and undertreatment.[12–14]

Co-factors that can amplify anaphylaxis include exercise, ethanol, nonsteroidal antiinflammatory drugs (NSAIDs), febrile illness, perimenstrual status, and emotional stress. Some amplification mechanisms are better understood than others; for example, exercise, ethanol, and NSAIDs increase food allergen bioavailability from the gastrointestinal (GI) tract, and acute viral infections decrease the mast cell activation threshold.[15–17]

Anaphylaxis is highly likely when any *one* of the following three criteria is fulfilled:

1. Acute onset of an illness (minutes to several hours) with involvement of the skin, mucosal tissue, or both (e.g., *generalized* hives, pruritus or flushing, swollen lips/tongue/uvula)
   AND AT LEAST ONE OF THE FOLLOWING:
   • Respiratory compromise (e.g., dyspnea, wheeze/bronchospasm, stridor, hypoxemia)[a]
   • Reduced BP[b] or associated symptoms of end organ dysfunction (e.g., hypotonia [collapse], syncope, incontinence)
2. Two or more of the following that occur rapidly after exposure to a *likely allergen for that patient* (minutes to several hours):
   • Involvement of the skin/mucosal tissue (e.g., generalized hives, itch/flush, swollen lips/tongue/uvula)
   • Respiratory compromise (e.g., dyspnea, wheeze/bronchospasm, stridor, hypoxemia)[a]
   • Reduced BP[b] or associated symptoms (e.g., hypotonia [collapse], syncope, incontinence)
   • Gastrointestinal symptoms (e.g., crampy abdominal pain, *persistent vomiting*)
3. Reduced BP[b] after exposure to a *known allergen for that patient* (minutes to several hours):
   • *Infants and children*: Low systolic BP[b] (age-specific) or >30% decrease in systolic BP[b]
   • *Adults*: Systolic BP[b] or <90 mm Hg or <30% decrease from that person's baseline

[a]*Another example is reduced peak expiratory flow.*

[b]*Low systolic BP for children is defined as <70 mm Hg from 1 month to 1 year, less than (70 mm Hg + [2 × age]) from 1–10 years, and <90 mm Hg from 11–17 years.*

BP, Blood pressure.

From Sampson HA, Muñoz-Furlong A, Campbell RL, et al. Second symposium on the definition and management of anaphylaxis: summary report–Second National Institute of Allergy and Infectious Disease/Food Allergy and Anaphylaxis Network symposium. J Allergy Clin Immunol 2006;117(2):391–7.

Pathologic Mechanisms in Anaphylaxis

In the pediatric population, anaphylaxis typically involves IgE specific to food, venom, or other allergen, high-affinity immunoglobulin E (IgE) receptors (FcεR1 receptors) on mast cells and basophils, and release of mediators of inflammation (including histamine, tryptase, platelet-activating factor, leukotrienes, prostaglandins, cytokines, and chemokines)[18] (Fig. 44.1).

Recruitment of other inflammatory pathways has been reported. These include activation of the complement cascade leading to formation of C3a, activation of the coagulation pathway, and activation of the kallikrein-kinin system pathway with kinin formation. Direct activation of mast cells by physical factors such as exercise, exposure to cold water or cold air, or ingestion of medications such as opioids can also trigger anaphylaxis.[19]

Triggers

Food allergens are responsible for approximately 50% of pediatric anaphylaxis cases seen in the ED where a trigger is identifiable.[4] Milk, egg, peanut, tree nuts such as cashew, crustacean shellfish such as shrimp, and finned fish are the predominant food triggers in many geographic areas, and sesame, wheat, and soy

predominate in others. The relative importance of food triggers also differs with age; for example, in infants, milk, egg, and peanut are the common concerns[8,20] (Box 44.2).

Potential food triggers include hidden, substituted, cross-reacting, or cross-contacting foods, red meats containing the carbohydrate allergen galactose-α-1,3,-galactose, contaminants such as storage mites in flour, and food parasites such as the live nematode *Anisakis simplex* in fish.[17,21,22] Food-induced anaphylaxis is primarily triggered by allergen ingestion. Rarely, anaphylaxis is triggered by skin contact from food or inhalation of actively aerosolized food allergens, such as boiling milk or steaming fish.[23]

Other anaphylaxis triggers include venom from stinging insects such as bees, yellow jackets, wasps, hornets, fire ants, and, less commonly, saliva from biting insects such as mosquitoes and ticks.[24–26]

Medication triggers include penicillins, cephalosporins, and other antibiotics; NSAIDs such as ibuprofen; and antineoplastic agents. Contaminants in medications, including traces of food, can also trigger anaphylaxis. Perioperative anaphylaxis can be triggered by antibiotics or by neuromuscular blockers/muscle relaxants such as suxamethonium, but any inhaled, injected, or topically applied agent can be implicated, including antiseptics such as chlorhexidine.[27–30] Other medication triggers include biologic agents such as the monoclonal antibodies infliximab and omalizumab, allergen skin tests (especially intradermal tests), allergen challenge tests, and allergen immunotherapy by any route.[31]

Vaccines that protect against infectious diseases seldom trigger anaphylaxis. If they do, the culprit is usually an excipient (e.g., gelatin, yeast, dextran, polysorbate-80), other vaccine ingredient (e.g., egg in yellow fever vaccine), or latex from the vaccine vial, *not* the microbial content.[32]

In exercise-induced anaphylaxis, common co-triggers and cofactors include foods (e.g., wheat, shrimp, celery), NSAIDs, ethanol, and concurrent exposure to cold water or cold air, which can also trigger anaphylaxis independently of exercise.[33]

Idiopathic anaphylaxis is uncommon in infants, children, and teenagers[31,34–36] (see also "Idiopathic Anaphylaxis" section, page 398, and Box 44.7).

Diagnosis

In the pediatric population, diagnosis of anaphylaxis depends almost entirely on the history and physical findings.

Clinical Diagnosis

Diagnosis of anaphylaxis is based on recognition of the sudden onset of characteristic symptoms and signs within minutes to hours after exposure to a known or likely trigger or activity (Fig. 44.2). Clinical criteria have been developed and validated as an instrument for rapid assessment of patients who present with a possible diagnosis of anaphylaxis in EDs and other medical settings, for those who present to their physician after the acute event, and for use in epidemiologic studies (see Box 44.1).[1] These criteria have high sensitivity for identification of anaphylaxis, good specificity, and a high negative predictive value.[37]

Anaphylaxis is underreported in the pediatric population.[38] First episodes might not be recognized as such, especially if symptoms are mild and/or transient. Skin involvement (i.e., itching, flushing, generalized urticaria, and/or angioedema) is helpful in making the diagnosis; however, it is absent in 10% to 20% of anaphylactic episodes and can be unrecognized if itching is absent, if a partial skin examination is performed, or if a histamine 1 (H1)

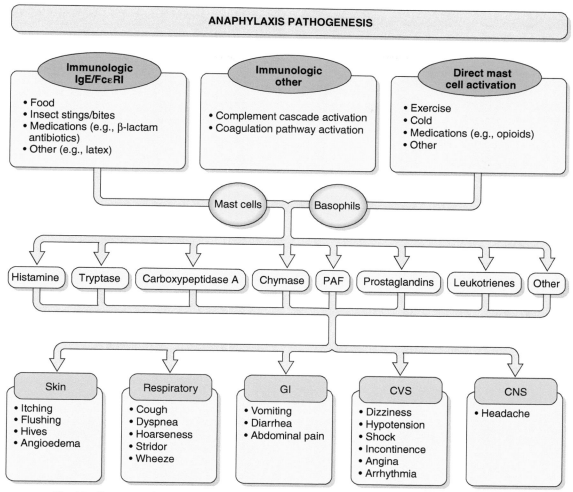

• **Fig. 44.1** Summary of the pathogenesis of anaphylaxis. Details about mechanisms, triggers, key cells, and mediators are found in the text. Two or more target organ systems are typically involved in anaphylaxis. *CNS,* Central nervous system; *CVS,* cardiovascular system; *FcεRI,* high-affinity immunoglobulin E receptor; *GI,* gastrointestinal; *IgE,* immunoglobulin E; *PAF,* platelet activating factor. (Modified from Lieberman P, Nicklas RA, Randolph C, et al. Anaphylaxis: a practice parameter update—2015. Ann Allergy Asthma Immunol 2015;115(5):341–84; Simons FE, Ardusso LR, Dimov V, et al. World Allergy Organization anaphylaxis guidelines: 2013 update of the evidence base. Int Arch Allergy Immunol 2013;162(3):193–204; and Simons FE, Ebisawa M, Sanchez-Borges M, et al. 2015 update of the evidence base: World Allergy Organization anaphylaxis guidelines. World Allergy Organ J 2015;8(1):32.)

antihistamine has been given. Patients with dysphonia, dyspnea, or shock might not be able to describe their symptoms. Anaphylaxis might not be recognized as such in a patient with asthma with acute respiratory symptoms if concomitant cutaneous or GI symptoms are not reported. Lack of recognition or delayed recognition of anaphylaxis may also occur because of patient or caregiver impairment (e.g., depression or substance abuse).[39]

In infants, a high index of suspicion is needed to diagnose anaphylaxis.[12,40] They cannot describe their symptoms, and some of their signs can be difficult to interpret because they also occur in healthy babies (Table 44.1). Hypotension is often undocumented, for example, in settings where infant-size blood pressure cuffs are unavailable.

Differential Diagnosis

The differential diagnosis of anaphylaxis in children includes age-unique entities (Box 44.3).[12,41] Acute generalized hives associated with viral infection, acute asthma, syncope, anxiety or panic attack, and aspiration of a foreign body are common entities to consider. Less common disorders include excess histamine syndromes (e.g., mast cell activation syndromes, ruptured or leaking hydatid cyst); restaurant syndromes (e.g., food poisoning, scombroid poisoning); and nonorganic diseases (e.g., vocal cord dysfunction, Munchausen syndrome, or Munchausen syndrome by proxy). Flush syndromes are rare in the pediatric population except for nonallergic red man syndrome triggered by vancomycin. Seizures and stroke and other forms of shock (i.e., septic, hypovolemic, or cardiogenic) also should be considered in the differential diagnosis.

Laboratory Tests to Support the Clinical Diagnosis

Anaphylaxis is a clinical diagnosis.[1,42] In the pediatric population, laboratory tests (see Fig. 44.2) are seldom helpful in confirming

• BOX 44.2 Anaphylaxis Triggers

Allergen Triggers (IgE-Dependent Immunologic Mechanisms)
- Foods, such as milk, egg, peanut, tree nut, finned fish, crustacean shellfish, soy, and wheat
- Food additives, such as spices, colorants, vegetable gums, and contaminants
- Stinging insects: *Hymenoptera* spp., such as bees, yellow jackets, wasps, hornets, and fire ants
- Medications, such as penicillin, cephalosporins, and other antibiotics; ibuprofen and other NSAIDs; and chemotherapeutic agents
- Biologic agents, such as monoclonal antibodies and allergens (challenge tests, allergen-specific immunotherapy)
- Natural rubber latex
- Inhalants (rare), such as horse dander and grass pollen
- Uncommon triggers[a]
- Novel allergens

Direct Mast Cell Activators
- Physical factors
  - Exercise[b]
  - Cold water or cold air
  - Heat
  - Sunlight/ultraviolet radiation
- Medications (e.g., opioids)

Idiopathic Anaphylaxis[c]

[a]*In the pediatric population, uncommon triggers include vaccines to prevent infectious disease (excipients are the most likely allergen in these cases).*
[b]*With or without co-triggers and co-factors such as foods, ethanol, NSAIDs, cold water, or cold air.*
[c]*Idiopathic anaphylaxis is uncommon in children. The possibility of a novel trigger or a mast cell activation syndrome should be ruled out.*
IgE, Immunoglobulin E; NSAIDs, nonsteroidal antiinflammatory drugs.
Modified from Lieberman P, Nicklas RA, Randolph C, et al. Anaphylaxis: a practice parameter update 2015. Ann Allergy Asthma Immunol 2015;115(5):341–84.

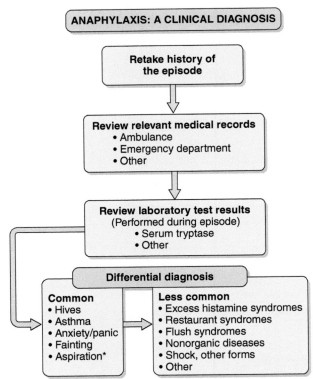

• **Fig. 44.2** Algorithm for confirming the clinical diagnosis of anaphylaxis. Details about the importance of the history, the role of serum tryptase levels and other laboratory tests, and the differential diagnosis are found in the text and in Box 44.3. *Of a foreign body. (Modified from Simons FE, Sampson HA. Anaphylaxis: unique aspects of clinical diagnosis and management in infants (birth to age 2 years). J Allergy Clin Immunol 2015;135(5):1125–31; Lieberman P, Nicklas RA, Randolph C, et al. Anaphylaxis: a practice parameter update—2015. Ann Allergy Asthma Immunol 2015;115(5):341–84; Simons FE, Ardusso LR, Dimov V, et al. World Allergy Organization Anaphylaxis Guidelines: 2013 update of the evidence base. Int Arch Allergy Immunol 2013;162(3):193–204; and Simons FE, Ebisawa M, Sanchez-Borges M, et al. 2015 update of the evidence base: World Allergy Organization anaphylaxis guidelines. World Allergy Organ J 2015;8(1):32.)

anaphylaxis. Tryptase levels can be elevated in anaphylaxis (between 15 minutes and 3 hours after symptom onset),[43] but testing is not available on an emergency basis and levels are seldom elevated in children and in food-induced anaphylaxis.[44,45] Therefore, initial treatment of anaphylaxis should *never* be delayed waiting for a tryptase measurement nor should the diagnosis of anaphylaxis be refuted based on a level within the normal range.

In young infants, interpretation of tryptase levels presents additional complexities, because *baseline* tryptase levels are elevated because of an increased mast cell burden in the developing immune system. In infants younger than 3 months, median *baseline* tryptase levels are reported as 14.2 ± 10.2 µg/L in infants with atopy and 6.1 ± 3.47 µg/L in healthy infants.[46] Levels gradually decline, and by the age of 9 to 12 months, they reach those found in older infants and young children.

Plasma histamine levels and 24-hour urine levels of histamine and its metabolite, *N*-methylhistamine, can be measured by some clinical laboratories. Other mast cell mediators such as platelet-activating factor are measured only in research laboratories.[47,48]

Treatment of the Acute Anaphylactic Episode

The essentials of prompt initial anaphylaxis treatment are outlined in Box 44.4.[19,49,50] It is important to have a printed protocol in the office that is posted and rehearsed regularly; to have emergency medications, supplies, and equipment readily available; and to predesignate staff responsibilities (Box 44.5). Initial steps include removing

any suspected relevant trigger; rapidly assessing the patient's airway, breathing, circulation, skin, and body weight; and injecting epinephrine. Simultaneously, personnel should call to request help from a resuscitation team or from emergency medical services (EMS) and place the patient supine or semireclining in a position of comfort.

Epinephrine (Adrenaline)

Epinephrine has life-saving α_1-adrenergic vasoconstrictor effects that prevent and relieve airway obstruction, hypotension, and shock, and life-saving β_2-adrenergic effects, including bronchodilation and suppression of mediator release from mast cells and basophils (see Box 44.4 and Table 44.2).[39,49,50]

Epinephrine should be promptly injected intramuscularly (IM) in the mid-outer thigh (vastus lateralis muscle) to achieve peak plasma and tissue concentrations rapidly.[51] The epinephrine dose is 0.01 mg/kg IM for first aid treatment (maximum 0.15 mg in an infant; maximum 0.3 mg in a child; maximum 0.5 mg in a teenager).[39] If indicated, it can be repeated several times at 5- to 15-minute intervals. Failure to inject it promptly increases

TABLE 44.1   **Symptoms and Signs of Anaphylaxis in Infants**

Anaphylaxis Symptoms That Infants Cannot Describe	Anaphylaxis Signs That May Be Difficult to Interpret/Unhelpful in Infants, and Why	Anaphylaxis Signs in Infants
General		
Feeling of warmth, weakness, anxiety, apprehension, impending doom	Behavioral changes such as persistent crying, fussing, clinging, irritability, fright	
Skin/Mucous Membranes		
Itching of lips, tongue, palate, uvula, ears, throat, nose, eyes, etc.; mouth tingling or metallic taste	Flushing (may also occur with fever, hyperthermia, or crying spells)	Sudden onset of generalized hives (potentially difficult to discern in infants with acute atopic dermatitis; scratching and excoriations will be absent in young infants); also, angioedema (face, tongue, oropharynx)
Respiratory		
Throat tightness; chest tightness; shortness of breath	Hoarseness, dysphonia (common after a crying spell); drooling/increased secretions (common in teething infants)	Sudden onset of coughing, stridor, wheezing, dyspnea, apnea, cyanosis
Gastrointestinal		
Dysphagia, nausea, abdominal pain/cramping	Drooling, spitting up/regurgitation (common after feeds), loose stools (normal in infants, especially if breastfed); colicky abdominal pain	Sudden onset of persistent vomiting
Cardiovascular		
Feeling faint or dizzy (presyncope), confusion, blurred vision, difficulty in hearing	Hypotension (need appropriate-size blood pressure cuff; low systolic blood pressure for infants is defined as <70 mm Hg from 1 month to 1 year, and <(70 mm Hg + [2 × age in years]) in the first and second years of life; tachycardia, defined as >120–130 beats/min from 3 months to 2 years, inclusive; loss of bowel and bladder control (ubiquitous in infants)	Weak pulse, arrhythmia, diaphoresis/sweating, collapse/unconsciousness
Central Nervous System		
Headache	Behavioral changes (see earlier), drowsiness, somnolence (common in infants after feeding)	Sudden onset of lethargy, hypotonia, unresponsiveness, or seizures

Modified from Simons FE, Sampson HA. Anaphylaxis: unique aspects of clinical diagnosis and management in infants (birth to age 2 years). J Allergy Clin Immunol 2015;135(5):1125–31.

the risk of hypoxic-ischemic encephalopathy and death. There is no absolute contraindication to epinephrine treatment (see Box 44.4).

More than one dose of epinephrine is needed in up to 20% of cases.[52,53] This can be due to rapidly progressing anaphylaxis, failure to respond to the initial dose or suboptimal dose, or route of administration.[39] In addition, biphasic reactions can occur in up to 20% of cases.[54–57] Prior anaphylaxis, hypotension, delayed epinephrine administration, and unknown trigger have been identified as risk factors of biphasic reactions.[58,59]

The presentation and severity of an anaphylactic episode can differ from episode to episode in the same patient, and from one patient to another. At the onset, it is impossible to predict whether the patient will respond promptly to treatment, die within minutes, or recover spontaneously as a result of endogenous secretion of epinephrine, angiotensin II, and endothelin I.[60]

Epinephrine seldom causes serious adverse events in the pediatric population. In patients of all ages, intramuscular epinephrine is much safer than an intravenous bolus dose of epinephrine. Intravenous injection can be associated with delayed epinephrine administration because of difficult venous access and with overdose resulting from, for example, overly rapid infusion or use of a 1:1000 epinephrine solution that has not been appropriately diluted (1:10,000 for intravenous use).[61] Intravenous epinephrine should be given by physicians skilled in vasopressor administration through an infusion pump with dose titration based on the clinical information obtained by continuous electronic monitoring of blood pressure and cardiac rate and function. Reasons for failure to inject epinephrine promptly and reasons for occasional apparent failure of response to intramuscular epinephrine injections are listed in Box 44.6.[39,51]

Other Life-Saving Measures

Supplemental oxygen should be administered by facemask at a flow rate of 8 to 10 L/min to patients receiving repeated doses of epinephrine and those with moderate or severe respiratory symptoms or concomitant asthma.[49,50]

Isotonic (0.9%) saline is preferred for intravenous fluid resuscitation in anaphylaxis[49] (see Box 44.4).

For patients with cardiopulmonary arrest, in addition to rescue breathing at a rate of 1 breath every 3 to 5 seconds (12–20 breaths/min), cardiopulmonary resuscitation (CPR) guidelines emphasize chest compressions at a rate of 100 to 120/min and a depth of 4 cm in infants, 5 cm in children, and 5 to 6 cm in adolescents and adults.[62] Interruptions should be minimized (see Box 44.4).

Second-Line Medications

H1 and H2 antihistamines, glucocorticoids, and β2-adrenergic agonists are second-line medications in anaphylaxis and should not be substituted for epinephrine in initial treatment or given as the only treatment because they do not prevent or relieve life-threatening laryngeal edema, hypotension, or shock (see Box 44.4 and Table 44.2).[49,50]

In a Cochrane systematic review, no high-quality evidence from randomized controlled trials (RCTs) was found to support the use of H1 antihistamines in the treatment of anaphylaxis.[63] Histamine is one of many mediators of anaphylaxis, and H1 antihistamines relieve skin symptoms (e.g., itching, urticaria, flushing, and angioedema), but do not relieve life-threatening respiratory or cardiovascular symptoms. Onset of action of an oral liquid formulation of cetirizine takes 30 minutes for relief of itch and 40 minutes for relief of hives. Use of sedating H1 antihistamines can interfere with recognition of anaphylaxis symptoms (see Box 44.4 and Table 44.2).[64,65]

In another systematic review, no high-quality evidence from RCTs was found to support H2 antihistamine use in anaphylaxis.[66] If given in addition to H1 antihistamines, they provide slightly increased relief of hives and flushing, but they do not relieve itching or life-threatening respiratory or cardiovascular symptoms.

In other Cochrane systematic reviews, no high-quality evidence from RCTs has been found to support glucocorticoid use in anaphylaxis treatment.[67] Because their onset of action through transcription of genes encoding proinflammatory proteins is relatively slow (i.e., hours, not minutes), these medications do not relieve acute symptoms and signs. Based on limited evidence, they

---

• BOX 44.3   Differential Diagnosis of Anaphylaxis in Infants

Skin
- Acute episode of urticaria, urticaria pigmentosa/mast cell activation syndrome, hereditary angioedema

Respiratory (Upper or Lower Respiratory Tract)
- Acute onset of symptoms as a result of obstruction, which can be congenital (e.g., laryngeal web, vascular ring, malacias) or acquired (e.g., aspiration of foreign body,[a] croup, bronchiolitis, asthma); asphyxiation/suffocation, breath-holding

Gastrointestinal Tract
- Acute onset of symptoms as a result of obstruction, which can be congenital (e.g., pyloric stenosis, malrotation) or acquired (e.g., intussusception), food protein–induced enterocolitis syndrome with an acute presentation

Cardiovascular System
- Brief resolved unexplained events; different forms of shock: septic, hypovolemic, cardiogenic, distributive (other than anaphylaxis)

Central Nervous System
- Seizure, postictal state, stroke, trauma, child abuse, increased intracranial pressure

Other
- Metabolic disorders
- Infectious diseases: Pertussis, gastroenteritis, meningitis
- Ingestion: Drug overdose, poison, or toxin (e.g., food, chemical, plant)
- Munchausen syndrome by proxy (Meadow's syndrome)

[a]Peanuts and tree nuts are commonly associated with both foreign body aspiration and anaphylaxis.

Modified from Simons FE, Sampson HA. Anaphylaxis: unique aspects of clinical diagnosis and management in infants (birth to age 2 years). J Allergy Clin Immunol 2015;135(5):1125–31.

• BOX 44.4   Treatment of an Acute Anaphylactic Episode

Have a printed, posted emergency protocol for recognition and treatment of anaphylaxis and rehearse it regularly.
- Rapidly assess airway, breathing, circulation, skin, and weight.
- Inject epinephrine (adrenaline) intramuscularly in the mid-outer thigh in a dose of 0.01 mg/kg (up to a maximum dose of 0.15 mg in an infant, 0.3 mg in a child, or 0.5 mg in a teenager); if there is minimal or no response, it can be repeated several times at 5- to 15-minute intervals.[a–c]
- Call for help: Emergency medical services (e.g., 9-1-1) in community settings or resuscitation team in healthcare settings.[a]
- Place the patient supine (or in a position of comfort if dyspneic or vomiting); the patient should not suddenly sit up or stand and should not walk or run.

When indicated:
- Administer high-flow oxygen (8–10 L/min) by facemask.
- Give nebulized albuterol (salbutamol), 1.25 to 2.5 mg every 20 minutes or continuously to relieve bronchospasm that persists despite epinephrine injection.
- Give intravenous fluids (child: 0.9% [isotonic] saline, up to 10–20 mL/kg in the first 5–10 minutes[d]; teen: 0.9% [isotonic] saline, 1–2 L rapidly (5–10 mL/kg in the first 5 minutes).[d]
- Start cardiopulmonary resuscitation.
- Start continuous electronic monitoring of cardiac rate and function, blood pressure, respiratory rate, and monitor oxygen saturation (by pulse oximetry).[e]
- Consider second-line medications[f]:
  - H1 antihistamines such as cetirizine 0.25 mg/kg PO (to a maximum of 10 mg), or diphenhydramine 1 mg/kg IV (to a maximum of 50 mg) to relieve itch/hives
  - Methylprednisolone 1 to 2 mg/kg/day IV (single dose)

[a]Simultaneous steps: Inject epinephrine, call for help, and position the patient.
[b]The epinephrine solution for intramuscular injection is 1 mg/mL (1:1000).
[c]Patients with anaphylaxis refractory to intramuscular injection of epinephrine and fluid resuscitation preferably should be transferred to the care of an emergency medicine team with the training, experience, and equipment to provide skilled management of the airway and ventilation and provide optimal shock management by administering vasopressors safely through an infusion pump, with frequent dose titrations based on continuous electronic monitoring of cardiac rate and function and blood pressure and monitoring of oxygenation using pulse oximetry.
[d]Titrate the rate of volume expansion to the cardiac rate and blood pressure and monitor for volume overload; in many pediatric emergency departments, hand-held ultrasound units are now used to monitor for and prevent volume overload.
[e]If continuous monitoring is not available, monitor vital signs every 1–5 minutes.
[f]These second-line medications do not precede or replace epinephrine.
Modified from Lieberman P, Nicklas RA, Randolph C, et al. Anaphylaxis-a practice parameter update 2015. Ann Allergy Asthma Immunol 2015;115(5):341–84; Sicherer SH, Simons FE; Section on Allergy and Immunology. Epinephrine for first-aid management of anaphylaxis. Pediatrics 2017;139:e2016400. Simons FE, Ardusso LR, Dimov V, et al. World Allergy Organization Anaphylaxis Guidelines: 2013 update of the evidence base. Int Arch Allergy Immunol 2013;162(3):193–204; and Simons FE, Ebisawa M, Sanchez-Borges M, et al. 2015 update of the evidence base: World Allergy Organization anaphylaxis guidelines. World Allergy Organ J 2015;8(1):32.

are given to prevent biphasic anaphylaxis symptoms, but efficacy is unproven[58,68] (see Box 44.4 and Table 44.2).

An inhaled β_2-adrenergic agonist such as albuterol can be given in addition to epinephrine for patients with wheezing (see Box 44.4 and Table 44.2).[19,49,50]

Refractory Anaphylaxis

Patients with anaphylaxis refractory to epinephrine, supplemental oxygen, and intravenous fluids should be transferred to the care of a specialist team for ventilatory and inotropic support and continuous electronic monitoring of blood pressure, cardiac rate and function, and respiratory rate and oxygenation. If continuous

• BOX 44.5 Practical Tips for the Office Setting

- Anaphylaxis in the office setting is not usually a random event. Prevention of anaphylaxis in an office or clinic involves awareness of procedure-related risk factors and patient-related risk factors.
- Diagnostic and therapeutic interventions that have the potential to trigger anaphylaxis should be conducted in well-equipped healthcare facilities staffed by professionals trained and experienced in recognizing and treating anaphylaxis.
- Allergic comorbidities (e.g., asthma) and co-factors that can amplify anaphylaxis should be assessed before interventions to minimize the risk.
- Emergency medication should be readily accessible because anaphylaxis onset and progression can occur rapidly.

monitoring is not available, vital signs should be measured at frequent, regular intervals (every 1–5 minutes).[19,49,50] Based on case reports in adults, methylene blue infusion is life-saving in anaphylaxis refractory to conventional treatment[69]; however, there are no pediatric studies.

Observation and Monitoring

Duration of observation and monitoring in healthcare settings should be individualized; for example, patients with moderate or severe respiratory or cardiovascular symptoms require monitoring for at least 6 to 8 hours.[70] Recommendations for safe observation periods are supported by the finding that mediators measured at intervals during anaphylaxis peak at different times, and some mediators such as histamine, tryptase, interleukin 6 (IL-6), and IL-10 correlate with delayed deterioration[71] (see Box 44.4).

Emergency Preparedness to Treat Anaphylaxis in Community Settings

Anaphylactic episodes can occur despite vigilant efforts to avoid known confirmed triggers.[38,72,73]

Self-Injectable Epinephrine

Those at risk for anaphylaxis in the community and/or their caregivers should be taught how to recognize anaphylaxis and inject epinephrine correctly and safely using an epinephrine auto-injector (EAI) (see Table 44.2 and Box 44.6). Several EAIs containing fixed doses of epinephrine (0.15 mg and 0.3 mg) are available in

TABLE 44.2	Medications for Anaphylaxis Treatment: Epinephrine Is the Initial Medication of Choice			
Medications	**Epinephrine[a]**	**β_2-Adrenergic Agonist**	**H1 Antihistamine[b]**	**Glucocorticoid**
Pharmacologic effects	At α_1-receptor: ↑ Vasoconstriction ↑ Peripheral vascular resistance ↑ Blood pressure ↓ Mucosal edema (e.g., in larynx) At β_1 receptor: ↑ Heart rate ↑ Force of cardiac contraction At β_2 receptor: ↓ Release of mediators ↑ Bronchodilation	At β_2 receptor: ↑ Bronchodilation	At H1 receptor: ↓ Itch (skin, mucous membranes) ↓ Hives and flushing	At glucocorticoid receptor: Given to prevent or diminish the late-phase response and biphasic, multiphasic or protracted symptoms associated with ongoing mediator release
Potential adverse effects when given in standard doses	Transient anxiety, pallor, restlessness, tremor, palpitations, headache, dizziness	Tremor, tachycardia, dizziness, jitteriness	First-generation H1 antihistamines sedate, impair cognitive function, and cause other adverse effects	Adverse effects are unlikely after one or two doses
Current recommendations	Treatment of first choice	*In addition to epinephrine*, an inhaled bronchodilator (e.g., albuterol [salbutamol]) can be given for bronchospasm	Not life-saving; *in addition to epinephrine* can be given for relief of itching and hives, if needed; not for initial or sole treatment	Not life-saving; *in addition to epinephrine*, can be given for the reasons stated previously; not for initial or sole treatment

[a]Epinephrine by intramuscular injection in the mid-outer thigh is the initial treatment of choice for anaphylaxis.

[b]Cetirizine 0.25 mg/kg to a maximum of 10 mg by mouth; for intravenous use, diphenhydramine 1 mg/kg, maximum 50 mg.

Modified from references Sicherer SH, Simons FE, Section on Allergy and Immunology. Epinephrine for first-aid management of anaphylaxis. Pediatrics 2017;139:e2016400; Simons KJ, Simons FE. Epinephrine and its use in anaphylaxis: current issues. Curr Opin Allergy Clin Immunol 2010;10(4):354–61; and Kemp SF, Lockey RF, Simons FE; World Allergy Organization ad hoc Committee on Epinephrine in Anaphylaxis. Epinephrine: the drug of choice for anaphylaxis: a statement of the world allergy organization. World Allergy Organ J 2008;1(7 Suppl):S18–26.

• BOX 44.6 Epinephrine in Anaphylaxis: Barriers to Use

Why Healthcare Professionals Fail to Inject Epinephrine Promptly

- Lack of recognition of anaphylaxis symptoms/failure to diagnose anaphylaxis.
- Episode appears mild, or there is a history of previous mild episode(s).[a]
- Inappropriate concern about transient mild pharmacologic effects of epinephrine (e.g., tremor).
- Lack of awareness that serious adverse effects are nearly always attributable to intravenous administration, especially intravenous bolus, rapid intravenous infusion, or intravenous infusion of a 1:1000 epinephrine solution instead of an appropriately diluted solution (1:10,000 concentration).

Why Patients and Caregivers Fail to Inject Epinephrine Promptly

- Lack of recognition of anaphylaxis symptoms/failure to diagnose anaphylaxis.
- Episode appears mild, or there is a history of previous mild episode(s).[a]
- H1 antihistamine or asthma inhaler is used initially instead, relieving early warning signs such as itch and cough, respectively.
- Prescription for epinephrine auto-injectors (EAIs) not provided by physician.
- Prescription for EAIs provided but not filled at pharmacy (e.g., if not affordable).
- Patients do not carry EAIs consistently (because of size and bulk, or "don't think they'll need it").

- Patients and caregivers are afraid to use EAIs (fear of making an error when giving the injection, or a bad outcome).
- Patients and caregivers are concerned about injury from EAIs.
- Patients and caregivers are unfamiliar with how to use the EAI. Fifteen percent of mothers with no EAI experience could not fire an EAI immediately after a one-on-one demonstration. Competence in using EAIs is associated with regular allergy clinic visits; it decreases as time elapses from first EAI instruction; therefore, regular retraining is needed.
- Errors in EAI use can occur despite education, possibly related to the design of some EAIs.

Why Patients Occasionally Fail to Respond to Epinephrine Injection

- Delayed recognition of anaphylaxis symptoms; delayed diagnosis.
- Error in diagnosis: Problem being treated (e.g., foreign body inhalation) is not anaphylaxis.
- Rapid progression of anaphylaxis.[b]
- Epinephrine[b]:
  - Injected too late, dose too low on milligram-per-kilogram basis, dose too low because epinephrine solution has degraded (e.g., past the expiration date, stored in a hot place).
  - Injection route or site not optimal; dose took too long to be absorbed.
  - Patient suddenly sits up or walks or runs, leading to the empty ventricle syndrome.
  - Concurrent use of certain medications (e.g., β-adrenergic blockers).

[a]Subsequent anaphylaxis episodes can be more severe, less severe. or similar in severity.
[b]Median times to respiratory or cardiac arrest are 5 minutes in iatrogenic anaphylaxis, 15 minutes in stinging insect venom anaphylaxis, and 30 minutes in food anaphylaxis; however, regardless of the trigger, respiratory or cardiac arrest can occur within 1 minute in anaphylaxis.
Modified from references Sampson HA, Berin MC, Plaut M, et al. The Consortium for Food Allergy Research (CoFAR): the first generation. J Allergy Clin Immunol 2019;143(2):486–93; Sicherer SH, Simons FE; Section on Allergy and Immunology. Epinephrine for first-aid management of anaphylaxis. Pediatrics 2017;139:e2016400; Simons KJ, Simons FE. Epinephrine and its use in anaphylaxis: current issues. Curr Opin Allergy Clin Immunol 2010;10(4):354–61; Kemp SF, Lockey RF, Simons FE; World Allergy Organization ad hoc Committee on Epinephrine in Allergy. Epinephrine: the drug of choice for anaphylaxis: a statement of the world allergy organization. World Allergy Organ J 2008;1(7 Suppl):S18–26; Chad L, Ben-Shoshan M, Asai Y, et al. A majority of parents of children with peanut allergy fear using the epinephrine auto-injector. Allergy 2013;68(12):1605–9.

---

the United States, Canada, and several other countries. A 0.1-mg EAI is available in the United States and Canada, and in Europe an EAI containing 0.5 mg is available. Another option available in the United States is a prefilled syringe and needle (0.15 mg and 0.3 mg). The 0.15-mg dose is labeled for patients weighing 15 to 30 kg, but international guidelines suggest that the 0.15-mg dose should be given for children under 25 kg.[39] If the 0.1-mg device is not available (labeled for 7.5–15 kg), the 0.15-mg device should be used for children under 15 kg. Based on expert consensus, it is appropriate to switch children to the 0.3-mg dose when they are 25 to 30 kg to avoid underdosing those approaching 30 kg.[39] Demonstration with trainer devices should be provided because steps for use differ among the various EAIs. Written instructions and/or website links demonstrating correct EAI technique also should be provided so that families may teach other caregivers. EAIs are not available in many countries; therefore, patients at risk of anaphylaxis who travel abroad should carry more than two EAIs.

Though deaths from anaphylaxis are infrequent, when it does occur, it is often in community settings.[74–76] Yet, some physicians fail to prescribe EAIs for their patients at risk of anaphylaxis. Moreover, many patients do not consistently carry their EAIs or use them when anaphylaxis occurs, even for severe symptoms, including throat tightness, difficulty breathing, wheezing, and loss of consciousness.[38,51] Barriers to EAI use include lack of knowledge on indications for use, unrecognized need for epinephrine, unfamiliarity with EAI technique, concern about medication side

effects, and fear of injuring the child with the EAI.[38,51,77] For all these reasons, anaphylaxis education and EAI technique should be reviewed with families at frequent regular intervals (see Box 44.6).

For young children, adult caregivers have the primary responsibility for anaphylaxis recognition and EAI use. As children mature, they should gradually assume these responsibilities of self-care. In a survey of pediatric allergists, most typically expected their patients to begin sharing these responsibilities by age 12 to 14 years.[78] They started to train patients early and individualized the time of transfer based on patient factors such as presence of asthma and absence of cognitive dysfunction. However, caregivers of at-risk children and teenagers expected to begin transfer of responsibilities considerably earlier, when children are age 6 to 11 years.[79]

Anaphylaxis Emergency Action Plan

EAIs should be prescribed in the context of a written, personalized, anaphylaxis emergency action plan[80] (e.g., see http://www.aap.org/anaphylaxis or http://www.foodallergycanada.ca). Such plans typically list common symptoms and signs of anaphylaxis and the steps for initial anaphylaxis treatment: inject epinephrine promptly using an EAI, call 9-1-1 or EMS, and avoid sitting up, standing, walking, or running. Plans should include reminders that H1 antihistamines and asthma inhalers should not be used as initial treatment or as the only treatment.

Medical Identification

Patients at risk for anaphylaxis recurrences should wear or carry medical identification listing their confirmed trigger(s) and their relevant comorbidities such as asthma.[39] These need to be updated regularly.

Investigations to Confirm the Trigger(s)

Patients with a history of an anaphylactic episode benefit from assessment by an allergy/immunology specialist. A detailed history of the event serves the basis for selecting appropriate skin tests, measuring serum specific IgE (sIgE) levels, and interpretation of test results (Fig. 44.3).[19]

Skin prick tests are performed to assess sensitization to foods, stinging insect venoms, medications, natural rubber latex, and other allergens. Fresh foods such as fresh fruits and vegetables can be tested using the prick-prick technique. Intradermal tests are contraindicated in the workup for food-induced anaphylaxis[81]; however, they can be useful in the workup for venom-induced anaphylaxis[24] and drug-induced anaphylaxis.[27]

Interpretation of allergen sIgE levels will vary depending on factors such as history, age, and geography. Cut-off values published for several major food allergens (e.g., milk, egg, and peanut) are based on ImmunoCAP assay (Thermo Fisher Scientific) results, but studies have shown that results from one assay are not necessarily interchangeable with those based on other immunoassays.[81,82]

Positive allergen skin tests and/or increased allergen sIgE levels confirm sensitization to the allergens tested. However, they are not diagnostic of allergy because sensitization can exist without clinical reactivity, and this is common in the general population. Increasing test positivity correlates with increasing probability of clinical reactivity to the allergens tested, but the level of positivity of these tests does not reliably predict the severity of future anaphylactic episodes.[81,83]

Physician-monitored oral challenge tests are sometimes needed to determine the clinical relevance of borderline positive allergen skin tests or low-positive allergen sIgE levels in patients who have an equivocal history of anaphylaxis. Challenge tests should be conducted in well-equipped healthcare facilities staffed by professionals trained and experienced in patient selection, performing and interpreting these tests, and recognizing and treating anaphylaxis. A positive challenge confirms allergy and provides a sound basis for continued allergen avoidance. A negative challenge allows introduction or reintroduction of the food into the diet or allows the medication to be used as a treatment option. Oral challenge tests are generally not needed for patients with a recent, convincing history of a severe reaction with evidence of sensitization to that allergen.[27,81,83]

For food allergies, the need for potentially risky challenge tests can be reduced by use of allergen component tests that differentiate clinical reactivity associated with IgE binding to potent stable allergens such as casein in milk, ovomucoid (Gal d 1) in egg, or Ara h 2 in peanut from less clinically relevant sensitization (allergens binding to heat-labile proteins).[84]

Physician-supervised challenge tests are contraindicated in patients with venom-induced anaphylaxis, unless performed in the context of an RCT.[24] Challenges are indicated in selected patients with a history of drug-induced anaphylaxis.[27]

Before making the diagnosis of idiopathic anaphylaxis, physicians should rule out a hidden or novel anaphylaxis trigger, perform a meticulous examination of the skin, and obtain a baseline serum tryptase level to rule out a mast cell activation syndrome.[19,35]

Avoidance of Trigger(s)

Printed educational materials about avoidance of specific trigger(s) should be provided and reviewed at regular intervals (Box 44.7).

Foods

Complete avoidance of exposure to some foods such as milk, egg, or peanut is easier said than done. Labeling laws have been enacted in several countries mandating clear identification of allergens in packaged food products. Precautionary labeling (i.e., "may contain" or "manufactured on shared equipment") is increasingly used but is not regulated. Given the ubiquity of many major food allergens, unintentional exposures are common.[85,86] The constant vigilance required every day to avoid hidden or cross-contacting food triggers can negatively affect quality of life of patients, caregivers, and family members.[87] Bullying of children and teens with food allergies occurs, but often parents are unaware.[88,89]

Reliable resources for accurate, practical information are maintained and updated by Food Allergy Research & Education (FARE; http://www.foodallergy.org) and by Food Allergy Canada (http://www.foodallergycanada.ca). For patients with multiple dietary restrictions, a licensed dietician can provide helpful information about safe alternatives and ensure optimal growth on an allergen-restricted diet.[90]

Stinging Insects

Avoidance of exposure involves professional extermination of yellow jacket or wasp nests or fire ant mounds around the patient's home and having the patient avoid uncovered sources of food and beverages at barbecues, picnics, and campgrounds and wear protective clothing, including shoes and socks when outdoors. Insect repellents such as DEET are not effective in preventing *Hymenoptera* stings, although they prevent insect bites.[24] Children younger than 6 years are more likely to be stung than older children, but systemic allergic reactions increase with age.[91]

Drugs and Biologic Agents

Culprit drugs or agents should be avoided. An alternative, non–cross-reacting agent should be substituted, preferably from a different therapeutic class, but sometimes an agent from the same class may be used (e.g., a third-generation cephalosporin for a patient with allergy to a first-generation cephalosporin).[27]

Exercise

Patients with exercise-induced anaphylaxis should not entirely avoid exertion; however, they should avoid their relevant co-triggers and co-factors (e.g., foods, ethanol, NSAIDs, cold water or cold air, and high pollen counts). If none can be identified, they should have a trial of fasting for 4 to 6 hours before exertion. In addition, they should never exercise alone, and if any symptom develops, they should stop exercise immediately and avoid running for help. They should carry one or more EAIs and carry a cell phone for dialing 9-1-1 or EMS.[33]

Immune Modulation

Immune modulation is currently recommended for prevention of anaphylaxis triggered by insect venoms and some drugs.

ANAPHYLAXIS: CONFIRM THE TRIGGER

Retake the history of the episode
Get more details regarding:
- Exposures
- Events
- Chronology of symptoms

Retake complete medical history
- Concomitant diagnoses
  - Asthma
  - Mast cell activation disorder
  - Cardiovascular disease
  - Other
- Concurrent medications
  - β-Blockers
  - ACE inhibitors
  - Other

Skin tests
- Prick/puncture
  - Foods
  - Other
- Intradermal
  - Insect venoms
  - β-Lactam antibiotics

Allergen-specific IgE measurements, quantitative

Challenge tests
- May/may not be indicated
- Allergen specific
  - Food ⎱ (proceed with
  - Medication ⎰ caution)
- Allergen nonspecific
  - Exercise
  - Cold
  - Other

Other assessments, as indicated
- Idiopathic anaphylaxis
  - Serum tryptase

• **Fig. 44.3** Algorithm for confirming anaphylaxis triggers. The importance of the history and information about skin tests and specific immunoglobulin E (*IgE*) measurements to determine allergen sensitization are described in detail in the text. In selected patients, physician-monitored challenge tests are needed to determine the clinical relevance of sensitization. *ACE,* Angiotensin-converting enzyme; (Modified from Golden DB, Demain J, Freeman T, et al. Stinging insect hypersensitivity: a practice parameter update 2016. Ann Allergy Asthma Immunol 2017;118(1):28–54; Joint Task Force on Practice Parameters; American Academy of Allergy, Asthma, and Immunology; American College of Allergy, Asthma and Immunology; Joint Council of Allergy, Asthma and Immunology. Drug allergy: an updated practice parameter. Ann Allergy Asthma Immunol 2010;105(4):259–73; Greenberger PA, Lieberman P. Idiopathic anaphylaxis. J Allergy Clin Immunol Pract 2014;2(3):243–50; quiz 51; Simons FE, Ardusso LR, Dimov V, et al. World Allergy organization anaphylaxis guidelines: 2013 update of the evidence base. Int Arch Allergy Immunol 2013;162(3):193–204; Simons FE, Ebisawa M, Sanchez-Borges M, et al. 2015 update of the evidence base: World Allergy Organization anaphylaxis guidelines. World Allergy Organ J 2015;8(1):32; and Sampson HA, Aceves S, Bock SA, et al. Food allergy: a practice parameter update—2014. J Allergy Clin Immunol 2014;134(5):1016–25.e43.)

• BOX 44.7 Strategies to Prevent Anaphylaxis in Community Settings

Avoid Specific Allergen Trigger[a]
- Foods, including hidden or cross-reacting foods and food additives (e.g., spices, colorants, vegetable gums, contaminants)
- Insect stings
- Drugs
- Biologic agents
- Natural rubber latex
- Novel allergens[b]

Avoid Direct Mast Cell Triggers, If Relevant
- Exercise: Do not avoid exertion, but avoid co-triggers and co-factors[c]
- Cold air, cold water
- Heat
- Sunlight/ultraviolet radiation
- Medications (e.g., opioids)

Immune Modulation, if Relevant
- Foods: Immunotherapy (oral, sublingual, and epicutaneous immunotherapy) currently being investigated, additional approaches include vaccines and biologic agents (see text for details)
- Insect venoms: Subcutaneous allergen immunotherapy
- Medications (e.g., penicillins and other antibiotics and chemotherapies: desensitization)

Pharmacologic Prophylaxis, If Relevant
- Idiopathic anaphylaxis: Favorable natural history. Prophylaxis with a glucocorticoid (e.g., prednisone, a H1 antihistamine (e.g., cetirizine and, if indicated, omalizumab can be given

[a]Suggested by the history and confirmed by skin tests and allergen specific immunoglobulin E (sIgE) levels.
[b]Save the allergen (e.g., food or insect for identification, and save the patient's serum for allergen sIgE measurements.
[c]Avoid relevant co-triggers such as foods, cold air, and cold water, and avoid relevant co-factors such as nonsteroidal antiinflammatory drugs.
Modified from Lieberman P, Nicklas RA, Randolph C, et al. Anaphylaxis-a practice parameter update 2015. Ann Allergy Asthma Immunol 2015;115(5):341–84. Golden DB, Demain J, Freeman T, et al. Stinging insect hypersensitivity: a practice parameter update 2016. Ann Allergy Asthma Immunol 2017;118(1):28–54; Greenberger PA, Lieberman P. Idiopathic anaphylaxis. J Allergy Clin Immunol Pract 2014;2(3):243–50; quiz 51; Sampson HA, Berin MC, Plaut M, et al. The Consortium for Food Allergy Research (CoFAR): the first generation. J Allergy Clin Immunol 2019;143(2):486–93. Sampson HA, Aceves S, Bock SA, et al. Food allergy: a practice parameter update—2014. J Allergy Clin Immunol 2014;134(5):1016–25.e43. Virkud YV, Vickery BP. Advances in immunotherapy for food allergy. Discov Med 2012;14(76):159–65.

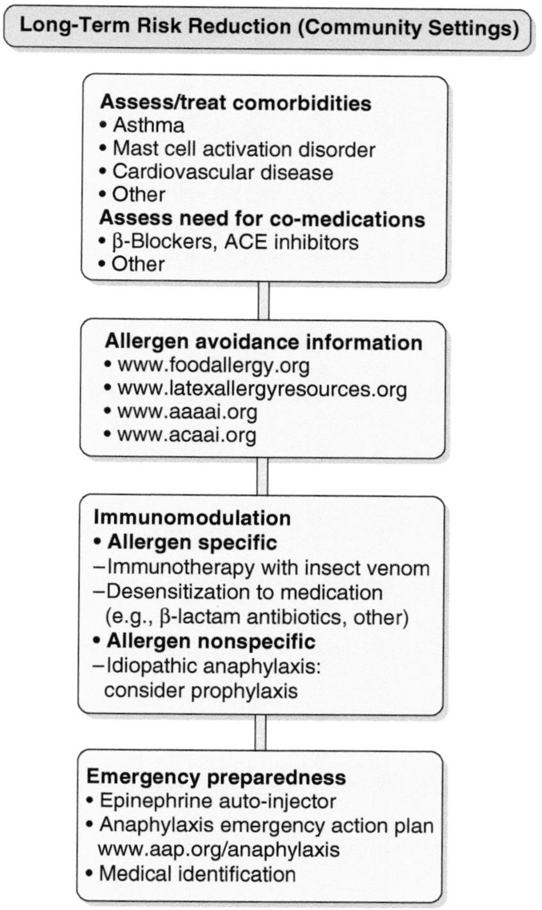

• Fig. 44.4 Summary of the approach to long-term management. Optimal management of comorbidities such as asthma decreases the risk of severe or fatal anaphylaxis. Avoidance measures are allergen specific. Immune modulation is currently used to prevent anaphylaxis recurrences from insect stings and from some medications. Emergency preparedness measures, including epinephrine auto-injectors; written, personalized anaphylaxis emergency action plans; and medical identification (e.g., bracelet, wallet card) are critically important. (Modified from Lieberman P, Nicklas RA, Randolph C, et al. Anaphylaxis: a practice parameter update, 2015. Ann Allergy Asthma Immunol 2015;115(5):341–84; Golden DB, Demain J, Freeman T, et al. Stinging insect hypersensitivity: a practice parameter update 2016. Ann Allergy Asthma Immunol 2017;118(1):28–54. Joint Task Force on Practice Parameters; American Academy of Allergy, Asthma, and Immunology; American College of Allergy, Asthma and Immunology; Joint Council of Allergy, Asthma and Immunology. Drug allergy: an updated practice parameter. Ann Allergy Asthma Immunol 2010;105(4):259–73; Greenberger PA, Lieberman P. Idiopathic anaphylaxis. J Allergy Clin Immunol Pract 2014;2(3):243–50; quiz 51. Sicherer SH, Simons FE, Section on Allergy and Immunology. Epinephrine for first-aid management of anaphylaxis. Pediatrics 2017;139:e2016400; and Wang J, Sicherer SH; Section on Allergy and Immunology. Guidance on completing a written allergy and anaphylaxis emergency plan. Pediatrics 2017;139(3):e20164005.)

Treatments to prevent food-induced anaphylaxis are actively being explored (see Box 44.7 and Fig. 44.4).[92–94]

Food-Induced Anaphylaxis

For many infants and children, milk or egg is outgrown naturally, especially in those with relatively low allergen sIgE levels, small prick test wheal sizes, and history of mild initial reactions. Other food allergies are more likely to be life-long, including peanut, tree nuts, fish, and shellfish.[81]

Mounting evidence supports the potential for oral immunotherapy (OIT) to induce desensitization in many patients.[38,93] Adverse effects are common; therefore, OIT should be undertaken only in well-equipped centers by physicians who are specifically trained and experienced in administering OIT and diagnosing and treating anaphylaxis. Use of adjunctive omalizumab can reduce adverse effects of OIT.[94] Sublingual and epicutaneous immunotherapy are also showing promise for inducing food allergen desensitization.[38,92] Other approaches to treatment include recombinant vaccines and biologic agents targeted at T helper type 2 (T_H2) cytokines.[94]

Insect Sting–Induced Anaphylaxis

Anaphylaxis from bee, yellow jacket, wasp, and hornet venom can be prevented in 97% to 98% of children and teenagers with a history of systemic reactions treated with a 3- to 5-year course of subcutaneous injections of the relevant standardized stinging insect venom.[24] The protective effect can last 10 to 20 years after venom immunotherapy is completed. For prevention of anaphylaxis from fire ant stings, subcutaneous injections with whole body fire ant extract are indicated.

Drug-Induced Anaphylaxis

For prevention of anaphylaxis recurrence from a drug such as an antibiotic, NSAID, chemotherapeutic agent, or monoclonal antibody, when no safe substitute is available, desensitization can be conducted by an experienced allergy/immunology specialist. This technique is safe and effective for one uninterrupted course of treatment; however, long-lasting immunologic tolerance is not achieved and symptoms typically recur when the drug or biologic agent is restarted after being discontinued.[27]

Idiopathic Anaphylaxis

The natural history of idiopathic anaphylaxis is favorable.[35] In the absence of RCTs of pharmacologic prophylaxis, management recommendations are based on expert opinion. If episodes are frequent (≥6 per year, or ≥2 per 2 months), prophylaxis with an oral glucocorticoid such as prednisone and a nonsedating H1 antihistamine such as cetirizine should be considered. Omalizumab can be helpful in patients with symptoms refractory to conventional treatment.[35]

Long-Term Management of Anaphylaxis

Anaphylaxis can lead to impaired quality of life, psychosocial burdens, disrupted activities, and anxiety, as assessed by validated instruments. The impact is highly variable, ranging from minimal psychosocial effects to significant disability. Multiple complexities in anaphylaxis, including differing allergen thresholds for triggering reactions, variable effects of co-factors (such as exercise, febrile illness),[15,19,95] and unpredictability of reaction severity contribute to anxiety. In addition, patients and caregivers often report anxiety about carrying and using EAIs.[77]

Personalized long-term anaphylaxis management aims to achieve a state of minimal impact, in which patients and caregivers are aware of the risk of recurrences but confident that if preventive measures fail, they are prepared to recognize and manage an anaphylactic episode.[19]

Long-term risk reduction measures include identification of allergen triggers and avoidance education, emergency preparedness to treat anaphylaxis in community settings, optimizing management of comorbidities (e.g., asthma), and regular follow-up with a physician, preferably an allergy/immunology specialist.[13,19,50,80] Some patients and families may benefit from support groups (see Box 44.7 and Fig. 44.4).

Prevention of Anaphylaxis in Specific Settings

Unique aspects of anaphylaxis prevention in the physician's office or clinic setting and in school settings will be reviewed briefly.

Physician's Office or Clinic

Anaphylaxis in this setting is not usually a random event. It can be triggered by a food or drug challenge test, infusion of a biologic agent, subcutaneous allergen-specific immunotherapy, and, rarely, allergen skin tests or vaccinations to prevent infectious diseases.[9,24,27,32,83,96] In this setting, the allergen and time of exposure are known and the healthcare professionals involved are likely aware of the patient's comorbidities, concurrent medications, and weight.

Prevention of anaphylaxis in an office or clinic setting involves awareness of procedure-related risk factors and patient-related risk factors, careful selection of patients for diagnostic and therapeutic interventions, reassessment of patients before each intervention, and deferral of interventions when clinically indicated, for example, in a patient with an asthma exacerbation or a forced expiratory volume in 1 second 70% or less of predicted.[24,27,83,96]

Specific wait times after diagnostic and therapeutic interventions are suggested to ensure patient safety; for example, 30 minutes after allergen immunotherapy, at least 1 to 2 hours after completion of a food challenge, and 30 minutes to 2 hours after omalizumab injections for asthma or chronic urticaria.[27,96,97] An EAI should be prescribed, and patients should be trained to recognize anaphylaxis symptoms and use the EAI promptly if symptoms occur after they leave the office or clinic.[19,83,96]

Anaphylaxis in Schools and Other Community Settings

Twenty-five percent of children experience their first anaphylaxis episode at school. Increased availability of stock (unassigned) EAIs that are not prescribed for a specific child but are available for use in any child with anaphylaxis is anticipated to reduce morbidity and mortality in this setting. Prevention of anaphylaxis recurrences in schools and preparedness to recognize and treat it involves the collaborative efforts of the student, family, student's physician, and school (Box 44.8).[98] Anaphylaxis education for teachers and other school staff should emphasize the sudden onset and potentially rapid progression to multisystem involvement and life-threatening symptoms during an anaphylactic episode and the need to be prepared, to recognize the condition and treat it promptly, and to understand the critical role of allergen avoidance in prevention of anaphylaxis recurrences.

In community settings, broader anaphylaxis training for coaches, camp directors, restaurant and food industry workers, airline personnel, and the public would be beneficial.[99–102] The goal of training is to increase awareness that anaphylaxis is a potentially life-threatening reaction that needs to be recognized and treated promptly. Increased availability of stock EAIs in public places such as shopping malls and sports facilities will contribute to decreased morbidity and mortality from anaphylaxis in community settings.

Conclusions

The rate of occurrence of anaphylaxis is increasing in the pediatric population. Food is the most common trigger; however, any allergen can trigger anaphylaxis. Some patients, for example, those with severe or uncontrolled asthma, are at increased risk for severe and fatal anaphylaxis. Diagnosis is based on recognizing the sudden onset of characteristic symptoms and signs that occur within minutes to a few hours after exposure to a known or likely trigger or activity. Validated clinical criteria for diagnosis are available for use (Box 44.9).

Prompt recognition of an acute anaphylactic episode and treatment with epinephrine 0.01 mg/kg IM are essential. Emergency help (call 9-1-1 or EMS) should be activated, and supplemental oxygen, intravenous fluids, and CPR should be provided, if needed. Mild anaphylaxis symptoms can progress quickly, and deterioration (including fatality) can occur within minutes.

• BOX 44.8 Anaphylaxis in Schools

Student's Responsibilities[a]

Food-allergic students at risk of anaphylaxis:

- Avoid ingesting known food allergen(s), trading food with others, or eating snacks or treats containing unknown ingredients.
- All students at risk of anaphylaxis:
  - Notify an adult immediately if inadvertently exposed to trigger or if symptoms develop.
  - Wear medical identification jewelry/carry an anaphylaxis identification card in backpack or wallet.
  - Carry an epinephrine auto-injector if age-appropriate and if permitted by local regulations.

Family's Responsibilities[a]

- Notify the school in writing of the student's risk for anaphylaxis and his/her confirmed trigger(s).
- Educate student about trigger avoidance.
- Provide medical documentation from the student's physician, including a written, personalized, anaphylaxis emergency action plan.
- Discuss the student's personalized anaphylaxis emergency action plan with school personnel.
- Provide a properly labeled epinephrine auto-injector (EAI).
- Replace EAI after use, or if past expiry date.
- Provide emergency contact information for parents/caregivers.

Physician's Responsibilities[a]

- Provide appropriate medical information to student and parents/caregivers.

- Recommend relevant risk reduction strategies (e.g., allergen avoidance, venom immunotherapy).
- Prescribe EAIs.
- Train student and parents to recognize anaphylaxis and use EAI.
- Recommend medical identification.
- Develop a written, personalized anaphylaxis emergency action plan with the family, and/or if age-appropriate, the student, listing allergen trigger(s), relevant concurrent comorbidities such as asthma, and medications.
- If the student has asthma, maintain optimal control of symptoms.[b]

School's Responsibilities[a]

- Develop a comprehensive school policy for prevention, recognition, and treatment of anaphylaxis that includes after-hours events and school-sponsored excursions.
- Identify students at risk of anaphylaxis and review their health records.[b]
- Identify a team: Principal, teachers, school nurses, food service workers, and food suppliers to help prevent anaphylaxis in the school.
- Designate school personnel who are trained to recognize anaphylaxis and administer epinephrine injections using EAIs.
- Rehearse the response to an anaphylactic episode: (1) inject epinephrine promptly; (2) call 9-1-1 or emergency medical services (EMS); (3) do not let the student sit up suddenly, walk, or run; and (4) contact parents/caregivers

[a]All information should be reviewed annually before the start of the school year and at additional intervals as needed, for example, if an episode of anaphylaxis occurs or if a student's allergen triggers change.
[b]Of the many students at risk for anaphylaxis in schools, those with concomitant asthma are at highest risk for severe or fatal anaphylaxis.
Modified from Wang J, Bingemann T, Russell AF, Young MC, Sicherer SH. The allergist's role in anaphylaxis and food allergy management in the school and childcare setting. J Allergy Clin Immunol Pract 2018;6(2):427–35.

• BOX 44.9 Clinical Pearls

- Anaphylaxis is a clinical diagnosis. Laboratory tests are seldom helpful in confirming anaphylaxis, so initiation of treatment should never be delayed by waiting for test results.
- Although skin involvement (i.e., itching, flushing, generalized urticaria, and/or angioedema) is a common finding, it is absent in 10% to 20% of anaphylactic episodes.
- Epinephrine is the treatment of choice and rarely causes serious adverse events in the pediatric population. There is no absolute contraindication to epinephrine treatment for anaphylaxis.
- Children at risk for anaphylaxis should be prescribed epinephrine auto-injectors and provided with written, personalized anaphylaxis emergency action plans.
- Skin tests and serum immunoglobulin E levels do not reliably predict the severity of future anaphylactic episodes.

Patients and caregivers should be prepared for recurrences of anaphylaxis in community settings. Written, personalized anaphylaxis emergency action plans that describe how to recognize symptoms and inject epinephrine promptly using an EAI should be provided. Medical identification should be worn.

Long-term management focuses on prevention of anaphylaxis recurrences. This includes confirmation of anaphylaxis triggers, vigilant avoidance of relevant triggers, and immune modulation, for example, *Hymenoptera* venom immunotherapy, where relevant. Anaphylaxis education aims to increase awareness of the importance of prompt recognition and treatment of acute episodes and the need for prevention of future anaphylactic episodes.

The reference list can be found on the companion Expert Consult website at http://www.expertconsult.inkling.com.

45

Mast Cell Disease and Hypereosinophilic Diseases

MALIKA GUPTA, CEM AKIN, ANNA KOVALSZKI

KEY POINTS

- The majority of mastocytosis cases in children are limited to the skin, termed cutaneous mastocytosis.
- Most cutaneous mastocytosis begins by age 2 and can present with bullous lesions in infants presumably because of edema which causes instability at the dermal-epidermal junction.
- Cutaneous mastocytosis is classified into maculopapular cutaneous mastocytosis, diffuse cutaneous mastocytosis and cutaneous mastocytoma.
- Systemic mastocytosis is seen in less than 10% of children with mastocytosis. Therefore, invasive diagnostic procedures to rule out systemic mastocytosis are not indicated in the majority of children.

- Most early onset mastocytosis resolves by puberty.
- Hypereosinophilia is seen in children as in adults, with a similar broad category of differential diagnostic causes.
- Peak eosinophil counts are higher in children than adults.
- Children are less likely to have idiopathic hypereosinophilic syndrome and more often have secondary associations for their hypereosinophilia including overlap hypereosinophilia (such as in EGIDs), parasitic infections, and underlying immunodeficiencies.
- Hypereosinophilic syndrome in children is treated similarly to that seen adults.
- Natural disease progression is linked to the underlying cause of eosinophilia in children.

Introduction

Mast cells and eosinophils are implicated in almost all allergic disorders, but they are also at play in some primary disorders that affect both adults and children. Although most studies have been done in adults for both mastocytosis and hypereosinophilic diseases, clinical experience and some published data suggest similarities but also differences in the types of entities in which they manifest and their eventual progression and prognosis. We will review mast cell disorders and eosinophilic disorders found in children and the relevant literature, with a focus on disease manifestations and prognosis in this group of patients.

Mastocytosis

Mast cells are important components of the innate immune system found in skin, mucosa, and connective tissues. When activated, they release vasoactive mediators (i.e., histamine, leukotrienes, prostaglandins, heparin, proteases, cytokines, and platelet-activating factor), which produce an inflammatory response needed to protect from microbes, allergens, and toxins. Mastocytosis is characterized by clonal mast cell expansion and abnormal mast cell activation. Mastocytosis is a primary mast cell disorder involving an intrinsic defect in either the progenitors of mast cells or mast cells themselves leading to their clonal expansion. Mastocytosis is a heterogeneous group of diseases associated with the excessive accumulation of mast cells in tissues.[1] Mast cell accumulation can be limited to a single

tissue or multiple tissues. Childhood-onset mastocytosis is most commonly limited to the skin (cutaneous mastocytosis [CM]) compared with adult-onset mastocytosis, which typically involves the bone marrow (systemic mastocytosis [SM]).

In this chapter, we will review the epidemiology, pathogenesis, clinical manifestations, diagnosis, management, natural course, and prognosis of pediatric mastocytosis. We will also highlight some major differences between childhood-onset and adult-onset mastocytosis.

Epidemiology

Mastocytosis is a rare disease, and its exact incidence is unknown. In children, the male-to-female prevalence ratio is reported to be 1.4 to 1:1.[2] There is higher reported prevalence in whites compared with other racial groups.[3] The majority (90%) of mast cell disease in children is initially diagnosed before 2 years of age.[2] Most childhood-onset mast cell disease is limited to the skin, and most resolves or improves by puberty, whereas adults have a more chronic course. Familial mastocytosis limited to first-degree relatives has been reported in approximately 2% to 4% of cases.[2,4]

Pathogenesis

In mastocytosis, mast cells accumulate in excessive numbers in tissues and cause inappropriate mediator release, which often may be exaggerated. Mast cell accumulation in the majority of pediatric mastocytosis is limited to the skin (CM).

Mast cells originate from the yolk sac in embryonic life and in the bone marrow from pluripotent hematopoietic stem cells after birth. They mature and proliferate with the help of stem cell factor (SCF). SCF interacts with its receptor Kit (CD117) with intrinsic tyrosine kinase activity on mast cells. SCF is also known as Kit ligand. *KIT* is the gene encoding the SCF receptor Kit on mast cells. Most cases of mastocytosis are associated with somatic gain-of-function–activating mutations in *KIT*. Mutations in *KIT* affect all aspects of the life cycle of mast cells, including growth, activation, and apoptosis.

The majority of mutations in *KIT* are found in the exon 17, which encodes part of the tyrosine kinase domain. Exon 17 mutations cause a constitutive ligand-independent activation of Kit. Exon 17 mutations most commonly involve codon 816 and cause substitution of valine for aspartate (D816V). In adult-onset SM, *KIT* D816V is the predominant mutation occurring in more than 90% of patients. In their cohort of 50 children with mastocytosis, Bodemer and colleagues[5] reported mutations in *KIT* in most children (86%). Exon 17 mutations in children have been reported in 34% to 42% cases, but a significant percentage (44%) of *KIT* mutations affected exons outside exon 17.[2,5] These involve mutations in exons 8, 9, and 11. However, no clear phenotype-genotype association has been reported.[5]

SCF exists as a membrane-bound form or in a soluble form. The soluble form is generated from the membrane-bound form by proteolytic cleavage at a protease-sensitive site. Increased proteolytic processing and increased levels of soluble SCF in the dermis (but not in the peripheral blood) have been variably reported in patients with CM.[6] This is thought to contribute to an accumulation of mast cells locally in the skin. SCF is also involved in the production of melanin from melanocytes and can potentially explain the increased pigmentation in the lesions of urticaria pigmentosa (discussed later).[6]

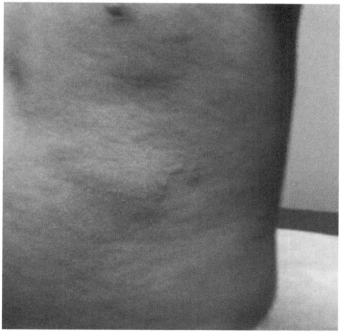

• **Fig. 45.1** Darier's sign. Development of a wheal-flare reaction on stroking a cutaneous lesion with mast cells. (With permission from Gupta M, Akin C, Sanders GM, Chan MP, Ross CW, Castells MC. Blisters, vaccines, and mast cells: a difficult case of diffuse cutaneous mastocytosis. J Allergy and Clin Immunol Pract 2019;7(4):1370–2.)

Infants with CM may have bullous lesions because tissue edema causes the skin to separate at the dermal-epidermal junction, which is relatively poorly developed in early life.[6]

Clinical Manifestations

Cutaneous Mastocytosis

Over 80% of childhood mastocytosis has been reported to be CM.[7] Lesions of CM may be seen at birth but most (80%–90%) appear within the first 2 years of life.[8] Darier's sign (Fig. 45.1) is an important diagnostic finding of mastocytosis and is typically positive in pediatric patients. It is the elicitation of a wheal-and-flare reaction by stroking a CM lesion. Systemic symptoms may be seen from the release of histamine and other mast cell mediators into the circulation and by themselves are not indicative of SM. These symptoms include flushing, pruritus, hives, abdominal pain, diarrhea, vomiting, and, rarely, bronchospasm, hypotension, or anaphylaxis.

Certain triggers are known to provoke mast cell degranulation. These include physical triggers (e.g., changes in temperatures, exercise, skin irritation), spicy foods, certain medications (e.g., antibiotics, opioids, nonsteroidal antiinflammatory drugs [NSAIDs], aspirin, radiocontrast agents, some muscle relaxants), vaccines (especially live viral vaccines),[9] infections, fever, emotional stress, teething, alcohol, surgery,[10] and venom. However, not all triggers will cause symptoms in all patients and avoidance recommendations should be based on individual history and the risk-to-benefit ratio of the intervention. One study found no serious adverse events with anesthesia in 22 pediatric patients with mastocytosis in 29 procedures with or without antihistamine premedication.[11]

CM has been classified into three major types[12]: maculopapular cutaneous mastocytosis (MPCM), diffuse cutaneous mastocytosis (DCM), and cutaneous mastocytoma (Table 45.1 and Fig. 45.2).

Maculopapular Cutaneous Mastocytosis

MPCM (formerly known as urticaria pigmentosa) is the most common form of CM (75%).[2] The lesions typically are oval and red or brown. They vary in size (polymorphic) and can have sharp or indistinct borders. Lesions can be elevated (papular) or flat (macular). Occasionally, lesions may be nodular or plaque-like. At some point all lesions are homogeneous, but these can change character over time.[12] The number of lesions can vary from a few (some may be barely visible) to many hundred. Adults usually have small monomorphic lesions. Monomorphic lesions in children raise suspicion of systemic disease.[13] Lesions in children are typically asymmetric and involve the head, neck, and extremities. Brown lesions on the lateral aspect of the forehead are considered characteristic of the polymorphic version.[12]

Mastocytoma of the Skin

CM manifests as raised brown or yellow plaques with a nodular center. The number of lesions can vary from one to three. If four or more lesions are present, this is classified as MPCM.[12] Mastocytomas can be present at birth (40%) or appear during infancy.[14] Early in their course, mastocytomas may blister, but this tendency decreases over time.[14] Mastocytomas that appear in early childhood (i.e., younger than 2 years of age) have a favorable prognosis and do not have elevated tryptase, systemic involvement, or persistence beyond adolescence. Darier's sign should not be attempted in mastocytomas because systemic symptoms such as hypotension can be caused by excessive mast cell degranulation.

TABLE 45.1 Typical Characteristics of Childhood Mastocytosis

Cutaneous Mastocytosis	
Maculo-papular cutaneous mastocytosis[a] Polymorphic Monomorphic	Most common type. Lesions are typically polymorphic, and involve head, neck, trunk, and extremities. Tryptase level usually is normal or mildly elevated. Typically there is no systemic involvement. Typically resolves by adolescence. Monomorphic form uncommon but when present may be indicative of systemic involvement.
Diffuse cutaneous mastocytosis	Rare. Diffuse skin erythema and thickening, bullous eruptions may be seen. Tryptase level can be significantly elevated, even in the absence of systemic involvement.[b] Premedication before vaccines, procedures, radiography with contrast medium.
Mastocytoma of the skin	Single lesion to a maximum of three lesions. Typically seen in infants and young children. Typical resolution by adolescence. Stroking the lesions can cause systemic symptoms (Darier's sign elicitation *not* recommended).
Systemic mastocytosis	Less than 10% cases of childhood-onset mastocytosis.

[a]Formerly known as urticaria pigmentosa.
[b]See Box 45.1 for reasons to suspect systemic involvement.

From Hartmann K, Escribano L, Grattan C, et al. Cutaneous manifestations in patients with mastocytosis: consensus report of the European Competence Network on Mastocytosis; the American Academy of Allergy, Asthma & Immunology; and the European Academy of Allergology and Clinical Immunology. J Allergy Clin Immunol 2016;137(1):35–45; and Heide R, Zuidema E, Beishuizen A, et al. Clinical aspects of diffuse cutaneous mastocytosis in children: two variants. Dermatology 2009;219(4):309–15.

Diffuse Cutaneous Mastocytosis

DCM is a rare variant of CM (5% of CM)[2] that manifests in early infancy (typically before 6 months of age).[15] The disease may start with erythematous skin and extensive blistering (bullous type) or may start as yellow-orange infiltrates and more limited vesicular blistering (infiltrative small vesicular variant).[15,16] Individual lesions may not be seen, but the skin is usually diffusely erythematous and thickened (pachyderma). Heide and associates[15] reported a broad band of infiltration of mast cells under the epidermis of all patients in their cohort of eight patients with DCM. The infiltration was more prominent in the clinically involved skin compared to the uninvolved skin. Blisters are most prominent during infancy and typically disappear before 4 years of age.[12,15] The involved skin exhibits pronounced dermographism. Blisters and skin wounds are prone to hemorrhages as a result of the release of heparin. Tryptase level can be significantly elevated even in the absence of systemic involvement. This is due to the abundant cutaneous mast cells. Tryptase level declines as the cutaneous lesions resolve.[15] Extensive blistering can ensue after viral illnesses and vaccines.[9] Premedication with corticosteroids and antihistamines before procedures is recommended to prevent extensive mast cell degranulation. Systemic involvement has been rarely reported.

Systemic Mastocytosis of Childhood

SM in which organs other than the skin are affected is rare in childhood and is seen in less than 10% of children affected with the disease. The most common form of SM in children is indolent SM.[17] Patients with MPCM with lesions persisting beyond adolescence may have well-differentiated SM. These patients usually lack the D816V mutation in the *KIT* gene.[18]

SM is classified according to the World Health Organization (WHO) criteria[19] (discussed later) and follows the diagnostic and management guidelines of adulthood-onset systemic disease (discussed in "Management" section).

Diagnosis and Evaluation

The diagnosis of CM is made on clinical grounds and can be confirmed by a skin biopsy. Appearance of typical lesions within the first 2 years of life should raise suspicion of mastocytosis. Darier's sign (a wheal-flare response on stroking a lesion) is considered pathognomic of mastocytosis in skin, but caution should be exercised in eliciting this sign in patients with mastocytomas because it may be associated with systemic mast cell release symptoms such as hives and flushing. Caregivers also usually report symptoms consistent with histamine release.

At the time of initial diagnosis, all children suspected of having CM should have laboratory evaluation consisting of a complete blood count with differential, liver function test, and a baseline serum tryptase (BST) level. A skin biopsy can be used to confirm the diagnosis of CM with special stainings for Kit (CD117) and tryptase. CD117 has a high sensitivity for mast cells because it stains even degranulated mast cells.[20] Analysis of the *KIT* gene for mutations in exon 17 (also exons 8, 9, and 11 in patients with diffuse cutaneous involvement) should be considered.

Based on the European and U.S. consensus report, cutaneous involvement of mastocytosis can be confirmed if the following criteria are met: a skin lesion that is typical of mastocytosis with a positive Darier's sign (major criterion), histologic confirmation of mast cell infiltration into the dermis (minor criterion), and an activating *KIT* mutation in the affected skin (minor criterion).[12,21] We usually use either the major criterion alone or two minor criteria if there is doubt about the typical morphology of the lesions.

Most children can be followed clinically without a bone marrow biopsy and with periodic (e.g., once yearly) measurements of serum tryptase and complete blood count with differential. However, certain features of the physical examination (e.g., monomorphic MPCM lesions, unexplained organomegaly, lymphadenopathy) and laboratory evaluation (e.g., persistent cytopenia, liver function abnormalities, significantly elevated or increasing tryptase level) should prompt an evaluation for systemic involvement (Box 45.1). Bone marrow biopsy is indicated if systemic involvement is suspected. It is important to note that the analysis of the peripheral blood for *KIT* mutation has low sensitivity and can give false negative results even in the presence of the mutation in the lesional skin and/or in the bone marrow.[22]

According to the WHO criteria[19] the diagnosis of SM requires the presence of one major and one minor criterion or the presence of three minor criteria. The presence of multifocal dense aggregates of more than 15 mast cells in the bone marrow or other extracutaneous organs constitutes the major criterion. Minor criteria include (1) the presence of spindle-shaped mast cells or other morphologic abnormalities in more than 25% of mast cells in the bone marrow, (2) the presence of codon 816 mutation (most commonly D816V)

Subforms	Variants	Typical manifestations
Maculopapular cutaneous mastocytosis (formerly known as urticaria pigmentosa)	Monomorphic	
	Polymorphic	
Diffuse cutaneous mastocytosis		
Cutaneous mastocytoma		

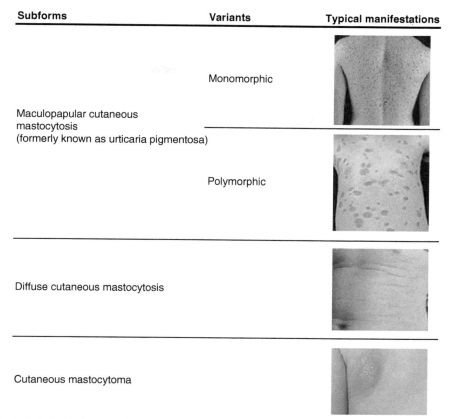

• **Fig. 45.2** Typical lesions of cutaneous mastocytosis: Note that monomorphic lesions are typically associated with systemic disease and adult-onset forms. (With permission from Hartmann K, Escribano L, Grattan C, et al. Cutaneous manifestations in patients with mastocytosis: consensus report of the European Competence Network on Mastocytosis; the American Academy of Allergy, Asthma & Immunology; and the European Academy of Allergology and Clinical Immunology. J Allergy Clin Immunol 2016;137(1):35–45.)

in peripheral blood or other extracutaneous tissue, (3) the expression of surface markers CD2 and/or CD25 on extracutaneous mast cells, and (4) BST level greater than 20 ng/mL (this is not applicable to patients with another clonal non–mast cell hematologic disease). One important consideration is that childhood-onset SM may lack

---

• **BOX 45.1** **Signs That Warrant an Evaluation for Systemic Mastocytosis**

- Persistent cytopenias
- Abnormalities of the liver function test
- Serum tryptase >20 ng/mL[a]
- Persistently elevated or increasing serum tryptase
- Hepatosplenomegaly
- Lymphadenopathy
- Monomorphic cutaneous lesions (in the case of MPCM [formerly known as urticaria pigmentosum])
- Onset of cutaneous lesions beyond 2 years of age
- Cutaneous lesions persist beyond adolescence

---

[a]In diffuse cutaneous mastocytosis, an elevated tryptase level alone does not warrant an evaluation for systemic mastocytosis.
MPCM, Maculopapular cutaneous mastocytosis.
Hartmann K, Escribano L, Grattan C, et al. Cutaneous manifestations in patients with mastocytosis: consensus report of the European Competence Network on Mastocytosis; the American Academy of Allergy, Asthma & Immunology; and the European Academy of Allergology and Clinical Immunology. J Allergy Clin Immunol 2016;137(1):35–45; and Schwartz LB, Irani AM. Serum tryptase and the laboratory diagnosis of systemic mastocytosis. Hematol Oncol Clin North Am 2000;14(3):641–57.

the mast cell aggregates of more than 15 cells that is considered a major criterion to diagnose SM according to the WHO criteria, and thus the diagnosis may require presence of three minor criteria.[17]

Well-differentiated SM is a rare morphologic variant usually observed in children with systemic disease that persists into adulthood. These patients have morphologically normal (i.e., round and fully granulated) mast cell clusters in their bone marrow that do not have CD25 on their mast cells and may lack D816V *KIT* mutation, but are positive for CD30, which is not expressed on normal mast cells.[18]

Management

Most pediatric-onset mastocytosis is cutaneous and self-limited. The management is generally conservative and symptomatic. The highlights of the management are as follows:
1. Avoidance of potential triggers (described previously) that cause flare of lesions and symptoms from mast cell degranulation.
2. Pharmacotherapy for symptoms from inadvertent mast cell degranulation:
   - Oral antihistamines are used to treat symptoms. Some patients (specifically those with elevated BST) may require these prophylactically. Histamine 1 (H1) and H2 antihistamines have both been used. Antileukotriene agents are used in patients with uncontrolled symptoms. Acute flares may require the use of oral corticosteroids and occasionally hospitalization. Patients with DCM who have hemorrhages may require protamine because of the release of heparin from mast cells. Oral cromolyn sodium can be used for patients

with CM with gastrointestinal (GI) symptoms and has been approved for use in children older than 2 years of age. Topical corticosteroids may be used on skin lesions during flares. For children older than 2 years of age, if lesions are confined to less than 10% of the body surface area, topical corticosteroids can be used under an occlusive dressing. Topical cromolyn (0.21%–4%) also has been used to treat pruritus, although the use of this has not been well studied.[10]

3. Preparation before anticipated triggers. Patients should be premedicated with antihistamines and oral corticosteroids before general anesthesia, radiocontrast media administration, and vaccines if they have a history of anaphylaxis or systemic mast cell degranulation symptoms with prior exposure to these triggers. Patients with DCM are particularly susceptible for these events. In the absence of a prior history of a systemic mast cell activation, premedication with an H1 antihistamine alone may suffice, in addition to continuation of their scheduled antimediator regimen.

4. *Preparedness to treat anaphylaxis.* The incidence of anaphylaxis (IgE or non–IgE mediated) is higher in mastocytosis, although it occurs much less frequently in children than in adults.[23] Caregivers should always carry two doses of epinephrine autoinjectors (EAIs) with them. They should be educated about the signs and symptoms of anaphylaxis, and written instructions should be provided. They should be trained on the technique of administration of the EAI. Parents should be educated to lay the child supine during anaphylaxis because this is an effective step in combating hypotension associated with anaphylaxis.

5. *Other measures.* Resection may be indicated rarely for mastocytomas in which symptoms from mast cell degranulation are particularly troublesome. Phototherapy may be useful in selected cases of DCM with extensive symptomatic skin involvement.[24] However, risk for recurrence after stopping therapy and risk for skin cancer make this a less desirable option. Mast cell cytoreductive therapy or tyrosine kinase inhibitors are not recommended in CM because progression to systemic disease is rare.[25]

6. *Monitoring for systemic involvement.* In patients with otherwise stable disease, an annual complete blood count with differential and BST level should be obtained to look for cytopenias or rising tryptase levels. Organomegaly or lymphadenopathy on follow-up physical examinations should also alert the physician to the possibility of systemic disease. Peripheral blood detection of D816V *KIT* mutation by allele-specific polymerase chain reaction (PCR) is also associated with systemic disease and can be used to risk stratify to select patients for bone marrow biopsy if they have other risk factors, as described earlier.

Systemic involvement in pediatric patients is rare. Cytoreductive therapy is rarely indicated for patients who have progressive disease with multisystem involvement. Treatment for SM in children follows the same principles as in adults and is tailored based on the molecular defect, drug side-effect profile, and long-term prognosis. Imatinib, a tyrosine kinase inhibitor, is used in patients without the D816V mutation and has been used in patients with well-differentiated SM (described previously).[26] Treatment of an infant with SM has been described.[27]

Natural Course and Prognosis

In their review of 1747 patients with pediatric mastocytosis, Méni and colleagues[2] reported clinical regression of the disease in 67% of cases and stabilization in 27%. The disease was fatal in 2.9% of cases.[2] The prognosis of early childhood–onset CM (i.e., onset of lesions within first 2 years of life) is generally good, with

spontaneous resolution seen by puberty in most cases. In their cohort of 180 pediatric patients with CM, Ben-Amitai and coworkers[14] reported marked improvement or complete resolution in 92% of their patients with mastocytomas. They reported improvement in 80% of their patients with urticaria pigmentosa (complete resolution in 56%).[14] Given the rarity of the disease, information on the prognosis of DCM is limited to case series. Overall it is considered favorable, although somewhat guarded compared to other forms of early-childhood CM.[15,16] One study showed that the appearance of allergic disease correlates with the resolution of mastocytosis in children.[22]

Risk factors that should prompt evaluation for systemic disease are summarized in Box 45.1. In general, later onset of skin lesions or persistence of lesions beyond adolescence are considered ominous signs.[12] Presence of persistent cytopenias or unexplained hepatomegaly, splenomegaly, or lymphadenopathy are also indicative of systemic involvement. Persistently rising serum tryptase levels have been linked with systemic disease and correlate with skin lesion density and bone marrow pathologic conditions.[28] The extent of skin involvement has not been shown to predict systemic disease.[28] However, characteristics of skin lesions may have some prognostic potential. Although the most common type of childhood-onset MPCM (polymorphic) is benign, MPCM lesions that resemble the small homogeneous lesions of adult-onset disease (monomorphic) are indicative of systemic involvement.[12] Although a *KIT* mutation in the lesional skin does not have prognostic significance,[29] there is some evidence that a *KIT* mutation in the codon D816V of exon 17 in blood may be associated with a risk of progression to systemic disease.[5,18]

Conclusion

Pediatric mastocytosis is usually self-limited, with most patients experiencing regression by adolescence. Treatment is conservative and symptomatic. Avoidance of triggers and preparedness for anaphylaxis are important educational steps. Monitoring for systemic involvement is recommended as the disease can rarely persist and show systemic involvement. Better understanding of the pathogenesis of the disease and prognostic markers to predict systemic involvement are required.

Mast Cell Activation Syndrome

Mast cell activation syndrome (MCAS) is a recently described disorder, generally diagnosed in adults, manifesting with episodic symptoms of mast cell activation meeting the criteria of or resembling anaphylaxis in two or more organ systems, associated with an increase in tryptase levels and a positive response to anti–mast cell mediator targeting therapies.[30,31] It can be caused by a primary mast cell disease (mastocytosis), secondary to IgE- or non–IgE-mediated mast cell activation, or idiopathic. MCAS in children is generally secondary to IgE-mediated disease and, in rare cases, may occur in CM or idiopathically. Investigation for SM by a bone marrow biopsy is usually not necessary in a child presenting with anaphylaxis or mast cell activation symptoms without the skin lesions described earlier in this chapter. Likewise, multiple food intolerances or failure to thrive in a child without objective evidence of CM is unlikely to be associated with a primary mast cell disease.

Hypereosinophilic Diseases

Eosinophils are myeloid cells intimately involved in clearance of parasitic infections and in pathogenesis of allergic disorders. They are found peripherally in the blood and also in the tissues. They exist in certain tissues naturally but can get elevated in certain disease states, and their presence is also abnormal in some parts of the body (e.g., in the lungs). They have a role in antigen presentation and also some role in the clearance of microbes, including bacteria and viruses. They are the targets of newly developed biologic agents for the treatment of asthma and disorders in which they are prevalent and drivers of pathologic processes (e.g., eosinophilic granulomatosis, polyangiitis, and hypereosinophilic syndromes). This section will discuss specific entities not otherwise discussed in other chapters on pediatric presentations of hypereosinophilic states, including hypereosinophilic syndromes, some malignancies, and immunodeficiencies, that are often found in a pediatric population.

Epidemiology

The upper limit of normal for blood eosinophil count is slightly higher in children than in adults. An absolute eosinophil count greater than 700 cells/µL is considered abnormally elevated in children older than 2 years of age.[32] There exists an arbitrary classification of eosinophilia in the blood as mild, moderate, and severe. This definition considers 500 to 1500 cells/µL as mild, 1500 to 5000 cells/µL as moderate, and more than 5000 cells/µL as severe. To be considered persistent, eosinophilia needs to be evaluated on two separate occasions at least 1 month apart and for it to be considered in the hypereosinophilic syndrome range, end-organ damage, cell count above 1500 cells/µL, or evidence of significant tissue eosinophilia with associated blood eosinophilia also must be present.[33]

In tissues, definition of normal varies. In bone marrow, more than 20% eosinophils of all nucleated cells is considered increased, in other tissues the normal numbers are less well defined, and often if the pathologist deems eosinophil presence extensive and mentions it, it is considered abnormal. Occasionally, eosinophils are not present, but if suspicion for their role in pathogenesis of disease exists, laboratory staining for major basic protein, eosinophil peroxidase, or eosinophil-derived neurotoxin can be a surrogate marker of tissue eosinophilia.[34] In the GI tract, eosinophil numbers increase closer to the distal GI tract. In the lungs, they are not present in typical healthy persons, so tissue eosinophilia or bronchoalveolar lavage with more than 5% eosinophils is abnormal.

Hypereosinophilia is defined as having more than 1500 cells/µL on at least two occasions 1 month apart. The differential diagnosis for this level of eosinophilia is large. Some allergic diseases, rheumatologic diseases, parasitic infections, hypereosinophilic syndromes, and underlying malignancy can cause hypereosinophilia.[35] See Box 45.2 for a comprehensive list of entities in which eosinophilia is present. Because of the myriad underlying mechanisms and often waxing and waning cell counts, the prevalence of hypereosinophilia is not known. A 2013 study found 0.3% of 350,000 individuals who underwent routine screening in a primary care setting as having more than 1000 cells/µL at a given time point.[36] Although hypereosinophilia is rare overall, it is even seemingly rarer in the pediatric population. A retrospective analysis of patients with hypereosinophilia evaluated at the National Institutes of Health found that children present with higher peak eosinophil counts, although the differential diagnosis is similar in adults and children.[37] Of the 261 patients without a secondary cause of hypereosinophilia who were included in the study, 12% were children and 88% were adults (diagnosed with hypereosinophilia syndrome

[HES]). The myriad reasons for pediatric eosinophilia are covered in other chapters, including those discussing drug allergy, atopic disorders, asthma, and eosinophilic GI disease (see Box 45.2 for a broad differential diagnosis of eosinophilia). We will subsequently focus our attention on HESs, briefly on malignancy-associated hypereosinophilia, and on eosinophilia related to underlying immunodeficiencies (which are more commonly found in hypereosinophilia manifesting in children).[37,38]

Hypereosinophilic Syndromes

The Hypereosinophilic Diseases Working Group of the International Eosinophil Society published refined criteria for hypereosinophilic syndromes in 2010.[33] Under this definition, there are six subcategories of hypereosinophilia. Pediatric hypereosinophilias can exist in all of the subcategories: idiopathic, myeloproliferative, lymphocytic, overlap, associated, and familial. See Fig. 45.3 for a brief overview of these entities. The incidence of HES in adults and children is not known. It is rare and more infrequent in children. A 2019 review of a single referral center (Cincinnati Children's Hospital Medical Center) found hypereosinophilia mostly to be secondary (i.e., HES overlap and associated mainly with atopic dermatitis, graft-versus-host disease, sickle cell disease, and parasitic infections, which account for the most common conditions seen).[39] Those with higher peak eosinophil counts were more likely to have underlying malignancy or immunodeficiency.

Idiopathic Hypereosinophilic Syndrome

HESs are defined as persistent hypereosinophilia in the setting of end-organ damage. If no specific subtype is identified, they are deemed "idiopathic."

HES in children can manifest with the typical symptoms and end-organ damage found in adults, including most commonly GI, dermatologic, allergic, hematologic, constitutional, and pulmonary manifestations. Treatment of HES depends on subtype, but for most HES initial therapies, glucocorticoids are used followed by corticosteroid-sparing agents in conjunction or after wean, if prolonged therapy is required. These therapies may include hydroxyurea, imatinib mesylate, interferon alpha (IFN-α), methotrexate, cyclosporine, and anti–interleukin 5 (IL-5) therapies. None of these treatments are currently approved by the U.S. Food and Drug Administration (FDA) for treatment of HES, except for imatinib mesylate, and this specific agent is used in myeloid variant HES because of its specific tyrosine kinase inhibitor activity associated with this subvariant. Anti–IL-5 therapies are very promising for nonmyeloid variant HES (both lymphoid and idiopathic), and recent publications provide insight to their role in corticosteroid-sparing therapy of HES. In the two seminal *New England Journal of Medicine* articles published on mepolizumab and benralizumab efficacies in HES (without *FIP1L1-PDGFRA* fusion), the overall percent of patients controlled was 84% (on ≤10 mg of corticosteroid) and 90% of patients had an absolute eosinophil count reduction of 50% or greater, respectively, in the two trials.[40,41]

Myeloid Hypereosinophilic Syndrome

Myeloid HES is a clonal disorder associated with *FIP1L1-PDGFRA, FIP1L1-PDGFRB, FGFR1,* or *JAK2* fusions/activations.[42] Clinical manifestations of myeloid HES include cardiac involvement, typically a male predisposition, and splenomegaly. Other

• BOX 45.2   Eosinophil Associated Diseases and Disorders

Allergic and Atopic Diseases
- Asthma
- Allergic rhinitis
- Eosinophilic esophagitis
- Atopic dermatitis
- Allergic urticaria
- Nasal polyps

Myeloproliferative and Neoplastic Disorders
- Hypereosinophilic syndromes
- Leukemia
- Lymphoma
- Tumor associated
- Mastocytosis

Pulmonary Syndromes
- Parasite induced eosinophilic lung disease:
  - Loeffler syndrome: Patchy migratory infiltrates, resolving over weeks, seen with transpulmonary migration of helminth parasites, especially *Ascaris* spp.
  - Tropical pulmonary eosinophilia: Miliary lesions and fibrosis; heightened immune response causing one form of lymphatic filariasis; increased immunoglobulin E and antifilarial antibodies
  - Pulmonary parenchymal invasion: Paragonimiasis
  - Heavy hematogenous seeding with helminths: Trichinellosis, schistosomiasis, larva migrans
  - Allergic bronchopulmonary aspergillosis
  - Chronic eosinophilic pneumonia: Dense peripheral infiltrates, fever, progressive blood eosinophilia may be absent; corticosteroid responsive
  - Acute eosinophilic pneumonia: Acute presentation diagnosed by bronchoalveolar lavage or biopsy
  - Eosinophilic granulomatosis with polyangiitis vasculitis: Small and medium-sized arteries; granulomas, necrosis; asthma often antecedent; extrapulmonary (neurologic, cutaneous, cardiac, or gastrointestinal) involvement likely
  - Drug and toxin induced eosinophilic lung disease

- Other: Hypereosinophilic syndromes, neoplasia, bronchocentric granulomatosis

Skin and Subcutaneous Diseases
- Skin diseases: Atopic dermatitis; blistering diseases, including bullous pemphigoid, urticarias, drug reactions
- Disease of pregnancy: Pruritic urticarial papules and plaques syndrome (PUPPS), herpes gestationis
- Eosinophilic pustular folliculitis
- Eosinophilic cellulitis (Wells syndrome)
- Angiolymphoid hyperplasia with eosinophilia (AHLE): Idiopathic vasoproliferative papules/plaques or nodules of the skin of the head and neck; and Kimura disease: Chronic inflammatory disease of painless adenopathy and subcutaneous masses of the head and neck
- Eosinophilic fasciitis (Shulman syndrome)

Gastrointestinal Disorders
- Eosinophilic gastroenteritides
- Inflammatory bowel disease: Eosinophils in lesions; occasionally blood eosinophilia with ulcerative colitis

Rheumatologic Diseases
- Vasculitis: Eosinophilic granulomatosis with polyangiitis and cutaneous necrotizing eosinophilic vasculitis

Immunologic Reactions
- Medication-related eosinophilias
- Immunodeficiency diseases: Job syndrome and Omenn syndrome
- Transplant rejections

Endocrine
- Hypoadrenalism

Other Causes of Eosinophilia
- Atheromatous cholesterol embolization
- Hereditary
- Serosal surface irritation, including peritoneal dialysis and pleural eosinophilia

---

myeloid cell lines can be affected, often with elevated B12, tryptase level, and lactate dehydrogenase. These patients may meet the WHO diagnostic criteria for chronic eosinophilic leukemia.

These patients, after induction with corticosteroid therapy (which is usually alone ineffective), are treated with imatinib mesylate, which often causes the disorder to go into remission; efficacy is usually 100% (possibly curative). Patients with myeloid HES are at risk of developing associated myeloid neoplasms. Imatinib mesylate is the only FDA-approved treatment for HES. Myeloid HES typically occurs in adults but has been reported in the pediatric population.[43] There are few reports, but they suggest a male predominance also in children, reported as early as 2 to 16 years and usually treatable with imatinib, as in adults (often to molecular remission). Characteristic bone marrow biopsy samples of myeloid HES have a predominance of abnormal-appearing eosinophils with extensive eosinophilic infiltration (Fig. 45.4).[44]

Lymphocytic Hypereosinophilic Syndrome

Clinical manifestations of lymphocytic variant HES (L-HES) include skin abnormalities with initially difficult to control eczematous-appearing skin lesions that are corticosteroid respondent.

Unfortunately, the continued response depends on remaining on corticosteroid therapy. Patients also can have generalized erythroderma, and skin biopsy samples can have an abnormal T cell population on immunohistochemistry examination. This is thought to be driven by an aberrant T cell clone overproducing IL-5. L-HES is therefore considered a secondary hypereosinophilia. T cells in L-HES are either phenotypically abnormal (most commonly CD3$^-$CD4$^+$, CD3$^+$CD4$^+$CD7$^-$, and CD3$^+$CD4$^-$CD8$^-$ T cell receptor alpha/beta [TCRαβ]$^+$) or associated with clonal TCR gene rearrangements, or both. These patients often remain dependent on low-dose corticosteroid therapy, although anti–IL-5 therapy can decrease their corticosteroid requirements; other corticosteroid-sparing agents such as IFN-α, cyclosporine, and methotrexate also have been used with success.[40,41,45,46] In a French national registry cohort of 21 patients (reported ages 5–75) of lymphocytic variant HES with abnormal T cell surface marker CD3$^-$CD4$^+$ persistently, characteristics included skin manifestations in 81%, followed by peripheral adenopathy in 62% as the most commonly associated symptoms; 76% also had clonal TCRγδ gene rearrangements. There appears to be a mildly increased risk of T cell lymphoma in these patients (1/21 developed this during follow-up). About half of the patient population

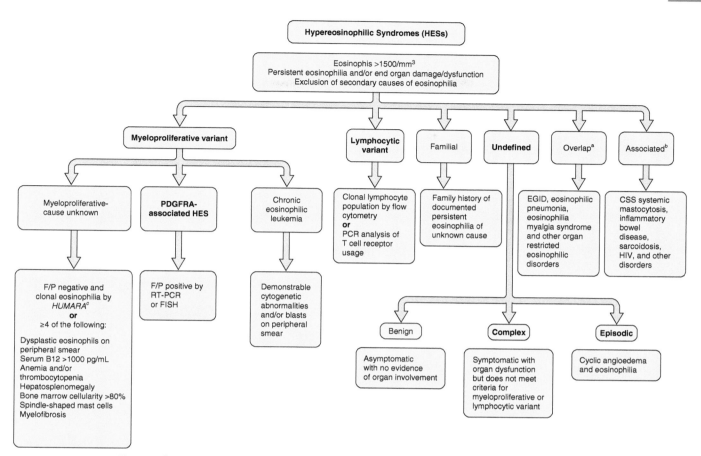

• **Fig. 45.3** Classification of hypereosinophilic syndromes (HESs) based on a workshop summary report. Specific syndromes discussed at the workshop are indicated in bold. [a]Incomplete criteria, apparent restriction to specific tissues/organs. [b]Peripheral eosinophilia, >1500/mm[3] in association with a defined diagnosis. [c]Clonality analysis based on the digestion of the genomic DNA with methylation-sensitive restriction enzymes followed by polymerase chain reaction *(PCR)* amplification of the CAG repeat the human androgen receptor gene *(HUMARA)* locus at the X chromosome. *CSS,* Churg-Strauss syndrome (now referred to as eosinophilic granulomatosis with polyangiitis); *EGID,* eosinophilic gastrointestinal diseases; *FISH,* fluorescence in situ hybridization; *F/P, FLPL1/PDGFRA* mutation; *HIV,* human immunodeficiency virus; *RT-PCR,* reverse-transcriptase PCR. (Originally from Klion AD, Bochner BS, Gleich GJ, et al. Approaches to the treatment of hypereosinophilic syndromes: a workshop summary report. J Allergy Clin Immunol 2006;117:1294, with permission from the American Academy of Allergy, Asthma and Immunology; and Schwartz JT, Fulkerson PC. An approach to the evaluation of persistent hypereosinophilia in pediatric patients. Front Immunol 2018;9:1944.)

had a history of atopy.[47] In the original *New England Journal of Medicine* trial on mepolizumab, 2 of 17 patients evaluated for L-HES response had T cell lymphoma (i.e., cutaneous T cell lymphoma, angioimmunoblastic T cell lymphoma) as final diagnosis in a paper on efficacy of mepolizumab in L-HES (sub-analysis).[45] Clonal and aberrant T cell populations have been reported in children with frequency similar to that with myeloid variant HES.

Episodic angioedema with eosinophilia with elevated immunoglobulin M (IgM) during flares and cyclic monthly flares that spontaneously resolve (historically, Gleich syndrome) has been characterized as a clinical subtype of lymphocytic variant HES, with a cyclical presentation. These patients tend to have abnormal T cell variants similar to those found in lymphocytic HES.[48,49] High-dose corticosteroids during flares are the mainstay of therapy. A 2018 case study published the utility of anti–IL-5 therapy (high-dose mepolizumab 750 mg

intravenously [IV] monthly) in improving the rate of exacerbation phases per year (10 ± 3 versus 2 ± 1; *P* <.005) and decreasing absolute eosinophil counts and serum eosinophil cationic protein levels.[50]

Overlap, Associated, and Familial Hypereosinophilic Syndromes

The overlap disorders with hypereosinophilia have a specific organ-predominant manifestation (e.g., this would include eosinophilic GI diseases in children with hypereosinophilia). Associated hypereosinophilia is found in entities such as rheumatoid arthritis, sarcoidosis, eosinophilic granulomatosis with polyangiitis, ulcerative colitis, and eosinophilic sinus disease and is often associated with aberrant IL-5 production by T cells, hence a secondary phenomenon. Both associated and

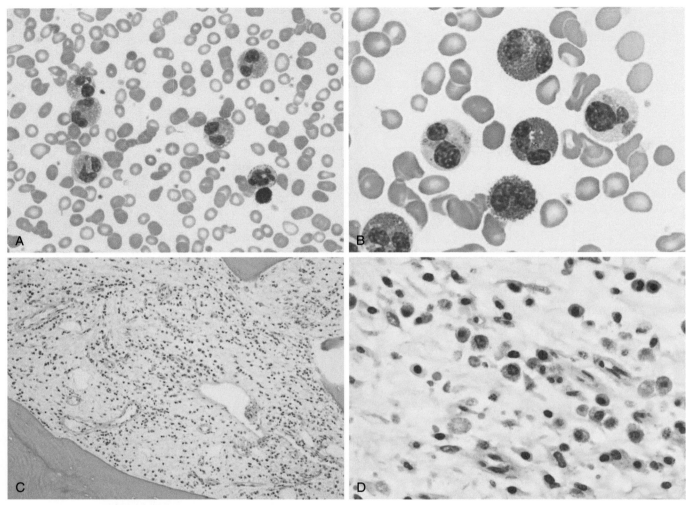

• **Fig. 45.4** Bone marrow biopsy and aspirate in a patient with chronic eosinophilic leukemia carrying the *FIP1L1-PDGFRA* rearrangement. Increased numbers of hypogranulated neoplastic eosinophils observed in the aspirate (A, B) Wright-Giemsa, original magnification, ×100). The infiltrate consists of eosinophils in a background of fibrosis in the biopsy (C, D) Hematoxylin and eosin, original magnification ×400). (With permission from Koval-szki A, Weller PF. Eosinophilia in mast cell disease. Immunol Allergy Clin North Am. 2014;34(2):357–364.)

overlap hypereosinophilias are likely the most common subtypes found in children, as reported at Cincinnati Children's recently.[39]

Familial eosinophilia is rare and is defined by family members and generations in the same family with eosinophilia, often asymptomatic, found in an autosomal dominant fashion. They seem to have less eosinophil activation than typical HES patients. The underlying cause is not known.[51]

Malignancy Associated Hypereosinophilia

Certain solid malignancies elicit abnormal and varied cytokine production (including IL-2, IL-3, IL-5, and granulocyte-macrophage colony-stimulating factor [GM-CSF]) contributing to eosinophil activation and survival (e.g., including lymphomas, breast, colon, lung, renal cell carcinoma, bladder, hepatobiliary, and pancreatic).[52,53] They can present initially with signs and symptoms associated with hypereosinophilia, including pain, fatigue, and

thromboembolic disease. Acute eosinophilic leukemias are very rare; chronic eosinophilic leukemia is somewhat more common. The myeloid variant HES associated with tyrosine kinase–activating mutations, although often categorized as chronic eosinophilic leukemia interchangeably in the past, is currently separated as myeloid/lymphoid neoplasms associated with eosinophilia and rearrangement of PDGFRA, PDGFRB, or FGFR1, or with PCM1-JAK2, whereas chronic eosinophilic leukemia not otherwise specified forms the new category for chronic eosinophilic leukemia currently under classification in the revised WHO criteria from 2016.[54]

In children, malignancies associated with eosinophilia include acute lymphoblastic leukemia. There are case reports of severe eosinophilia up to over 100 thousand eosinophils/mL, with IL3/IGH translocations in acute lymphoblastic leukemia and driven by noneosinophil clones (so actually secondary eosinophilia, not primary).[55–57] This also can manifest initially as part of pediatric hypereosinophilia with clonal B cell population that does not always progress to malignancy. The new WHO criteria have a subcategory of acute lymphoblastic leukemia defined as B cell lymphoblastic leukemia/lymphoma with t(5;14)(q31.1;q32.3) IL3-IGH.[54] Other myeloid neoplasms (such as mastocytosis) also may be associated with peripheral eosinophilia (such as mastocytosis).

Eosinophilia in Underlying Immunodeficiencies

Children are more likely to have a primary immunodeficiency discovered on the basis of hypereosinophilia than adults.[37,39] Immunodeficiencies associated with eosinophilia in the moderate range include hyper-IgE syndrome (HIGES) associated with signal transducer and activator of transcription 3 *(STAT3)* mutations (autosomal dominant HIGES), and DOCK-8 deficiency (formerly thought of as a variant of HIGES but with an autosomal recessive phenotype without significant bone issues). Wiskott-Aldrich syndrome, which affects platelet size, function, and number along with a variety of other cell types as a result of cell cytoskeletal abnormalities and immunologic synapse dysfunction (WAS protein mutation on chromosome X), also has significant eczema associated with elevated eosinophils. Severe combined immunodeficiencies such as Omenn syndrome and adenosine deaminase deficiency also cause significant dermatitis and likely associated eosinophilia. X-linked immunodeficiency with polyendocrinopathy and enteropathy (IPEX) also can manifest with significant eosinophilia and dermatitis. *FOXP3* mutations and dysregulated nonfunctional regulatory T cells cause uncontrolled autoimmunity and atopy. This is an incomplete list of immunodeficiencies more commonly seen with associated hypereosinophilia,[38] and immunodeficiency disorders are discussed in detail in other chapters of this book.

Conclusions

Although the medical literature includes more studies of hypereosinophilias in adults than in children, some case series and reports highlight the similarities and perhaps differences between adults and children diagnosed with hypereosinophilia. Children could potentially have different commonly associated parasitic drivers than adults (*Toxocara* versus myriad others, including *Strongyloides* in adults), have more predominant disease manifestation in different organs (GI manifestations of HES were most common in children and pulmonary manifestations in adults in one review),[37] and have potentially higher mean peak concentrations of eosinophils than adults.[37,39] Yet their overall disease progression, remission, and prognosis were similar to those of adults presenting with hypereosinophilic disease, keeping in mind the variability seen because of the underlying cause.

The reference list can be found on the companion Expert Consult website at http://www.expertconsult.inkling.com

Index

Note: Page numbers followed by '*f*' indicate figures and '*t*' indicate tables and '*b*' indicate boxes.

Structural database of allergenic proteins
(SDAP), 100
Subacute sinusitis
antibiotics for, 154t
antimicrobial therapy for, 153–155
microbiology of, 149, 149t
Subcutaneous immunoglobulin (SCIG), 84
administration of, 87–88
versus IVIG, 87
reactions to, 89
Sublingual immunotherapy (SLIT), 126–128,
312–313
Subtotal C6 deficiency (C6SD), 58
Sulfonamides, allergy to, 372
Sunscreens, 351
Surgery, for sinusitis, 156
Sustained unresponsiveness, definition of, 307
Swimmers, 351–352
Systemic antihistamines, for atopic dermatitis,
324
Systemic contact dermatitis, 346, 347t
Systemic corticosteroids, for asthma, 207
in older children, 225–227
Systemic lupus erythematosus (SLE),
complement deficiency and, 56
Systemic mastocytosis of childhood, 402–404
diagnosis and evaluation of, 402–403, 403b
management of, 403–404
natural course and prognosis of, 404
Systems immunology, to identify mechanisms
of exacerbations, 189

T

T- B- SCID, 47
T cell epitopes, immunotherapy and, 133
T cell immunodeficiencies, 44–54.e4
adenosine deaminase, 44
ataxia-telangiectasia, 52
intravenous immunoglobulins, 51
SCID. *See* Severe combined
immunodeficiency
Wiskott-Aldrich syndrome, 53–54
T cells
autoimmune lymphoproliferative syndrome
and, 79–80
depletion of, in HSCT, 94b
effector, in contact dermatitis, 341
food allergy and, 302
celiac disease, 276–277
eosinophilic esophagitis, 285
food allergy and, mucosal immunology,
257, 258f
immunotherapy effects on, 127–128
tolerance, 259
T helper (Th) cells, in immunotherapy, 127–128
T helper 2 (T$_H$2) cells
allergic rhinitis and, 136–137
cytokines, as targets in asthma, 170–171
paradigm of, 171–172
responses, development of, 170
T helper 3 (T$_H$3) cells, 259–260
T helper 9 (T$_H$9) cells, asthma and, 172

T helper 17 (T$_H$17) cells
asthma and, 172
role of, in allergic rhinitis, 136–137
T helper 22 (T$_H$22) cells, asthma and, 172
T regulatory cells (T$_{REG}$ cells), from
APECED, 75–76
Tacrolimus ointment, 322
Tar preparations, for atopic dermatitis, 324
TCR deficiencies, 47
TCR signaling, defects of, 48
TCRα constant chain *(TRAC)* gene defect, 48
Tear film, 355
Technology-based interventions, for inner city
asthma, 214
Tennis players, 352
Terbutaline, subcutaneous infusions, for
severe, therapy-resistant asthma, 244
Test for Respiratory and Asthma Control in
Kids (TRACK), 198–199
TGF-β, mucosal immunology and, 259
T$_H$2-mediated eosinophilic inflammation, 151
Theophylline, low-dose, for severe, therapy-
resistant asthma, 244
Therapy-resistant asthma, severe, 242–243,
242b
annual assessment of, 246
characteristics of, 239
'difficult asthma' and, 243–244
invasive investigation for, 242–243
monitoring of, 245–246
benefit, 245–246
growth trajectories, 245–246
side-effects, 245
treatment for, 243–244
Thiamin, need for, 298t
Thimerosal, as allergen, 349
Thin-layer rapid use epicutaneous test
(T.R.U.E test), 347, 348t
Thioureas, 350
Thommen's postulates, 110, 110b
Thrombosis, IVIG-related, 89
Thymic medullary epithelial cells (mTECs),
75–76
Thymus, DiGeorge syndrome and, 52
Thyroid, function of, urticaria/angioedema
and, 330
Tic cough, chronic cough and, 161, 161b
Tissue response genes, 28f
Tolerance
definition of, 307
mucosal immunology and, 261
Toll-like receptors (TLRs), mucosal
immunology and, 262–263
Topical calcineurin inhibitors, 322
for allergic contact dermatitis, 352–353
Topical corticosteroids
for contact dermatitis, 352
for eye diseases, 366–367
intranasal, 142–143
Topical medications, dermatitis from, 350
Total serum hemolytic complement assay
(CH$_{50}$), 36

Toxic reactions, to food, 266
Toxicodendron group, allergic plant dermatitis
and, 350
Tracheomalacia, chronic cough and, 163
Transferrin receptor (TFRC) deficiency, 48
Transient hypogammaglobulinemia of infancy
(THI), 41
Transient wheezing, 193–194
Trantas' dots, 358t, 360
Treatment plan, collaboration on, 249–250
Tree nut allergy, food labeling, 292
Tree pollen, 100–101, 111
Triamcinolone, intramuscular, for severe,
therapy-resistant asthma, 244
Trichiasis, 358t
Trimethoprim-sulfamethoxazole (TMP-SMX)
for chronic granulomatous disease, 68
for SCID, 51
Tropomyosin, 101b
Tryptase
mast cell, 106, 390
for venom-specific IgE, 382
Tucson Children's Respiratory Study (CRS),
9–10
Twin studies, 17, 20
TYK2 deficiency, 74
Type 2 immune response, orchestration of,
169, 170f
Type 2 innate lymphoid cells, asthma and, 175

U

Uncontrolled asthma, 199
United States, allergens in, food labeling by,
292t
Upper airway obstruction, refractory
childhood asthma and, 239
Upper airway pathology, chronic cough and,
164
Urban populations, 3–4
Urticaria, 329–339.e3
acute, 331–333
causes of, 331b
chronic, 333–337, 334f
classification of, 329–331
definition of, 329, 330f
diagnostic procedures for, 332, 334–335,
336b
differential diagnosis for, 331, 331f
epidemiology of, 329
etiology of, 331–334
history of, 332, 334
key concepts in, 330b
major syndromes, 335t
pathophysiology, 329–331
physical examination of, 332, 334
treatment of, 332–333, 332b, 335–337
Urticaria pigmentosa. *See* Maculopapular
cutaneous mastocytosis
Urticarial vasculitis, 334
UVB therapy, for atopic dermatitis, 325
Uveal tract, 355
Uveitis, 361